Financial Management of Health Care Organizations

- *To our families, for their love and patience*
- *To our students and colleagues for their invaluable insights and feedback.*

Financial Management of Health Care Organizations

An Introduction to Fundamental Tools, Concepts, and Applications

Second Edition

WILLIAM N. ZELMAN
University of North Carolina, Chapel Hill

MICHAEL J. MCCUE
Virginia Commonwealth University

ALAN R. MILLIKAN
Duke University Health System

NOAH D. GLICK
Integrated Healthcare Information Services, Inc.

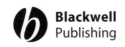
Blackwell
Publishing

BLACKWELL PUBLISHING
350 Main Street, Malden, MA 02148-5020, USA
9600 Garsington Road, Oxford OX4 2DQ, UK
550 Swanston Street, Carlton, Victoria 3053, Australia

First published 2003 by Blackwell Publishing Ltd

11   2009

Library of Congress Cataloging-in-Publication Data has been applied for

ISBN : 978-0-631-23098-4 (hardback)

A catalogue record for this title is available from the British Library.

Set in 10 on 12½ pt Ehrhardt
by Kolam Information Services Pvt. Ltd, Pondicherry, India
Printed and bound in Singapore
by COS Printers Pte Ltd

The publisher's policy is to use permanent paper from mills that operate a sustainable forestry policy, and which has been manufactured from pulp processed using acid-free and elementary chlorine-free practices. Furthermore, the publisher ensures that the text paper and cover board used have met acceptable environmental accreditation standards.

For further information on
Blackwell Publishing, visit our website:
www.blackwellpublishing.com

Brief Contents

Contents

Preface

This book offers an introduction to the most used tools and techniques of health care financial management. It contains numerous examples from a variety of providers, including health maintenance organizations, hospitals, physician practices, home health agencies, nursing units, surgical centers, and integrated health care systems. The book avoids complicated formulas and uses numerous spreadsheet examples so that they can be adapted to problems in the workplace. For those desiring to go beyond the fundamentals, many chapters have additional information included in appendices. Each chapter begins with a detailed outline and concludes with a detailed summary, followed by a set of questions and problems. Finally, a number of perspectives are included in every chapter. Perspectives are intended to provide additional insight into the topic – examples from the real world. In some cases these are abstracted from professional journals and in other cases they are statements from practitioners – in their own words.

The book begins with an overview of some of the key factors affecting the financial management of health care organizations in today's environment. Chapters 2, 3, and 4 focus on the financial statements of the organization. Chapter 2 presents an introduction to the financial statements of health care organizations. The financial statements are (perhaps along with the budget) the most important financial documents of a health care organization, and the bulk of the chapter is designed to help understand these statements, how they are created, and how they link together.

Chapter 3 provides an introduction to health care financial accounting. This chapter focuses on the relationship between the actions of health care providers and administrators and the financial condition of the organization, how the numbers on the financial statements are derived, the distinction between cash and accrual bases of accounting – and the importance of actually defining what is meant by "cost." By the time students complete Chapters 2 and 3, they will have been introduced to a large portion of the terms used in health care financial management.

Building on Chapters 2 and 3, Chapter 4 focuses on interpreting the financial statements of health care organizations. Three approaches to analyzing statements are presented: horizontal, vertical, and ratio analysis. Great care has been taken to show how the ratios are computed and how to summarize the results.

Chapter 5 focuses upon the management of working capital: current assets and current liabilities. This chapter emphasizes the importance of cash management and provides many practical techniques for managing the inflows and outflows of funds through an organization, including managing the billing and collections cycle, and paying off short-term liabilities.

Chapter 6 introduces one of the most important concepts in long-term decision-making – the time value of money. Chapter 7 builds on this concept, incorporating it into the investment decision by presenting several techniques to analyze investment decisions: the payback method, net present value, and internal rate of return. Examples are given for both not-for-profit and for-profit organizations.

Once an investment has been decided upon, it is important to determine how the assets will be financed, which is the focus of Chapter 8, Capital Financing. Whereas Chapter 5 deals with issues of short-term financing, Chapter 8 focuses on long-term investments, with a particular emphasis on issuing bonds.

Chapters 9 through 12 introduce topics typically covered in a managerial accounting course. Chapter 9 focuses on the concept of cost and using cost information for short-term decision-making – including fixed cost, variable cost, and breakeven analysis. In addition to covering the key concepts, it offers a set of rules to guide decision makers in making financial decisions. Chapter 10 explores budget models and the budgeting process. Several different budget models are introduced, including program, performance, and zero-based budgeting. The chapter ends with an example of how to prepare each of the five main budgets: statistics budget, revenue budget, expense budget, cash budget, and capital budget. It also includes examples for various types of payors, including flat fee and capitation.

Chapter 11 deals with responsibility accounting. It discusses the different types of responsibility centers and focuses on the performance measurement in general and budget variance analysis in particular. Chapter 12 discusses methods used by health care providers to determine their costs, primarily focusing on the step-down method and Activity Based Costing. The book concludes with a new chapter, Chapter 13, Provider Payment Systems. This chapter, parts of which were combined with Chapter 12 in the first edition, describes the evolution of the payment system in the United States as well as the specifics of various approaches to managing care and paying providers.

◀MAJOR CHANGES IN THE SECOND EDITION▶

In addition to the specific changes listed for each chapter, the following enhancements were made throughout the text:

- A listing of key terms and key equations at the end of each chapter; each set of key terms now becomes the first question for each chapter.
- An expansion of the use of marginal definitions and key points; all marginal definitions are key terms, and vice versa.
- More questions and problems for almost every chapter; where possible, problems are provided in pairs so that the first can be used as an example, and the second can become part of an assignment.
- Updated perspectives throughout the text.

◀CHAPTER 1: THE CONTEXT OF HEALTH CARE FINANCIAL MANAGEMENT▶

To acknowledge the numerous changes that have occurred in the health care arena since the previous edition, several enhancements were made to Chapter 1. Specifically, the concepts of Ambulatory Payment Classifications (APCs) and the Health Insurance Portability and Accountability Act (HIPAA) are introduced. Rising health care costs includes a discussion of prescription drugs, litigation was expanded to include compliance, and AIDS was expanded to chronic diseases in general. Numerous new tables have been added to illustrate the trends being discussed (e.g. cost increases), and the end of the chapter now includes a set of questions that might lead to classroom or online discussions.

◀CHAPTER 2: HEALTH CARE FINANCIAL STATEMENTS▶

The chapter has been expanded to include an abbreviated financial statement from an investor-owned organization. In addition, an abbreviated set of notes to financial statements has been added so that the student may see their importance to the overall understanding of the balance sheet and income statement. Four new perspectives have replaced the perspectives in the first edition. The questions at the end of the chapter have been updated and three new questions have been added. In addition, 12 new problems at the end of the chapter have been added.

◀CHAPTER 3: PRINCIPLES AND PRACTICES OF HEALTH CARE ACCOUNTING▶

The main example that the chapter is centered on has been updated, and less emphasis has been placed on the intricacies of accounting for donations. Four new perspectives have replaced the perspectives in the first edition. The number of questions has been expanded from four to ten and five new transaction problems have been added.

◀CHAPTER 4: FINANCIAL STATEMENT ANALYSIS▶

Using data from Solucient Incorporated Inc., the benchmark ratios were both updated and expanded to include hospitals of various sizes. The perspectives in the previous edition were replaced with five new ones. In addition, three more questions and seven more ratio analysis problems were added. Four of these are relatively complex, requiring ratio, vertical, and horizontal analyses of the balance sheet and income statement.

◀CHAPTER 5: WORKING CAPITAL MANAGEMENT▶

The chapter has been expanded to include compliance with laws and regulations for health care organizations as set forth by HIPAA. The section on the analysis of working capital strategies has been shortened. Five new perspectives have replaced the perspectives in the previous edition. Six new questions and six new problems have been developed; several relating to the development of a cash budget are quite involved.

◀Chapter 6: The Time Value of Money▶

The chapter places more emphasis on the use of electronic spreadsheets and less emphasis on using tables to make financial calculations. The content has been expanded to include both payment and rate functions. Eighteen additional present and future value problems have been added. The appendices have been modified.

◀Chapter 7: The Investment Decision▶

Changes were made to clarify how to handle depreciation and interest expenses when converting from accrual-based financial statements to cash flows. In addition, a section has been added to help explain the application of IRR. Five new perspectives have replaced the perspectives in the first edition. One question and 13 new problems have been added. Three of the new problems use complex cash flow development for tax-paying entities.

◀Chapter 8: Financing the Organization▶

The discussion of equity financing and pooled financing has been expanded, an exhibit has been expanded, and another exhibit has been developed which provides a listing of key financial ratios for rated hospital bonds in the year 2000. A diagram of the bond rating process has been added, and the discussion on bond amortization has been shifted to an appendix. Five new exhibits replace the exhibits in the first edition. Ten new problems, in the areas of bond valuation, loan amortization, and leasing financing, have been added.

◀Chapter 9: Using Cost Information to Make Special Decisions▶

The material on the breakeven equation has been updated to help the student understand how to apply the basic breakeven equation in cases where direct and indirect costs and/or a desired profit are of concern. The material in the appendix in the first edition which discussed a caution pertaining to the use of unit cost has been integrated into the chapter. Six new perspectives replace the perspectives used in the previous edition. The last three problems are more complex.

◀Chapter 10: Budgeting▶

The budget numbers have been updated, primarily to reflect changes in labor rates. Five new perspectives have been added to replace the perspectives used in the previous edition. The problem section includes new problems.

◀Chapter 11: Responsibility Accounting▶

The discussion on volume and rate variances has been improved and new problems have been added.

◀Chapter 12: Provider Cost Finding Methods▶

The section on activity-based costing has been greatly expanded and now contains an extended example comparing traditional costing to activity-based costing. The step-down method example has been refined. Provider payment systems, which was a section of this chapter in the previous edition, is now a separate chapter. Four new perspectives replace the perspectives used in the first edition. The problems relating to costing have been expanded.

◀Chapter 13: Provider Payment Systems▶

This is a new chapter containing material that was previously contained in Chapter 12 in the first edition. The material has been greatly reorganized to emphasize the history of payment systems in the United States, with an emphasis on the dynamics among payors, providers, and employers. Some of the methods discussed in the first edition have been moved to an appendix. The chapter contains five new perspectives and its own set of questions and problems.

◀Glossary▶

The glossary has been completely updated, and includes each term defined in the text as a marginal definition and key term.

Acknowledgments

We attempted throughout the book to challenge and enlighten. Quantitative as well as qualitative issues are presented in an effort to help the reader better understand the wide range of issues considered under the topic *health care financial management*. We could not have completed this task without our new coauthor, Noah Glick, who has contributed greatly and selflessly to both the first and second editions. We would also like to acknowledge the contributions of: Jason Marks for his review of many of the chapters, exhibits, and problems contained in this text; Matthew Ayotte for his expertise and input into both the format and content of our new chapter on provider payment systems; Lauren Hesler for her excellent secretarial help under pressure; Scott Broome and Angela Nelson for their review and suggestions on the budgeting chapter; Solucient Incorporated for giving us permission to use their data to construct the standards used in Chapter 4; and the many students over the past several years who pointed out errors, offered suggestions and improvements, and provided new ways to solve problems.

Most of all, we would like to thank our families for their encouragement and support, and for their understanding during the countless hours we were not available to them.

The authors and publishers gratefully acknowledge the following for permission to reproduce copyright material:

Perspective 1–1 "Health Care Institutions Need More than Efficiency" (abridged by authors), by James Barba: *Capital District Business Review* (Albany) from the December 11, 2000 print edition. © 2000 American City Business Journals Inc.

Perspective 1–2 Abstract from "Living with Change" (abridged by authors), by Chris Gay: *Wall Street Journal*, October 18, 1999, Eastern Edition.

Perspective 1–3 "Hospital M & A Activity Slow in 2000 as Health Care Industry Begins to Stabilize" (abridged by authors), © 2001 PR Newswire Association, Inc. March 29, 2001.

Perspective 1–4 "A 2020 Vision for American Health Care" (abridged by authors), Commonwealth Fund, www.cmwf.org, December 11, 2000.

Perspective 1–5 "Conflicting Demands" (abridged by authors), by Barbara Kirchheimer. Reprinted with permission from *Modern Healthcare*, August 27, 2001. © 2001 Crain Communications, Inc., 360 N Michigan Avenue, Chicago, IL 60601.

Perspective 2–1 "Buying on Credit" (abridged by authors), by Deanna Bellandi. Reprinted with permission from *Modern Healthcare*, June 18, 2001. © 2001 Crain Communications, Inc., 360 N Michigan Avenue, Chicago, IL 60601.

Perspective 2–2 "HMOs: Some Profits, More Losses" (abridged by authors), by Ashley Gibson: *The Business Journal of Charlotte*, July 12, 2001. © American City Business Journals, Inc.

Perspective 2–3 "Charity Finances Healthcare" (abridged by authors), by Mary Chris Jaklevic. Reprinted with permission from *Modern Healthcare*, July 31, 2000. © 2000 Crain Communications, Inc., 360 N Michigan Avenue, Chicago, IL 60601.

Perspective 2–4 "An Industry Barometer" (abriged by authors), by Cinda Becker, Reprinted with permission from *Modern Healthcare*, June 18, 2001. © 2001 Crain Communications, Inc., 360 N Michigan Avenue, Chicago, IL 60601.

Chapter 2 Appendix "Abbreviated Notes to Financial Statements for Sample Not-For-Profit Hospital, Dec 31, 20X1 and 20X0," permission from the *Audit and Accounting Guide, Health Care Organizations* (new edn), New York: American Institute of Certified Public Accountants, Inc., June 1 1996.

Perspective 3–1 "E-claims Trim Costs, Aid Growth" (abridged by authors), by John Morrissey. Reprinted with permission from *Modern Healthcare*, October 2, 2000, © 2000 Crain Communications, Inc., 360 N Michigan Avenue, Chicago, IL 60601.

Perspective 3–2 "Internal Investigations" (abridged by authors), by Mary Chris Jaklevic. Reprinted with permission from *Modern Healthcare*, September 4, 2000. © 2000 Crain Communications, Inc., 360 N Michigan Avenue, Chicago, IL 60601.

Perspective 3–3 "Revenue Stopper" (abridged by authors), by Mary Chris Jaklevic. Reprinted with permission from *Modern Healthcare*, July 2, 2000, © 2000 Crain Communications, Inc., 360 N Michigan Avenue, Chicago, IL 60601.

Perspective 3–4 "Former HBO Execs Indicted for Fraud" (abridged by authors), by Jeff Tieman. Reprinted with permission from *Modern Healthcare*, October 2, 2000, © 2000 Crain Communications, Inc., 360 N Michigan Avenue, Chicago, IL 60601.

Perspective 3–5 "Debunking Oxford" (abridged by authors), by David Stires. From *Fortune* magazine, March 19 2001. © 2001 Time, Inc.

Perspective 4–1 "100 Top Hospitals: Benchmarks for Success, 1999" (abridged by authors), © 1999 HCIA, L.L.C.

Perspective 4–2 "The Comparative Performance of US Hospitals: The Sourcebook" (abridged by authors), © 2000 HCIA, L.L.C. and Deloitte & Touche LLP.

Perspective 4–4 "The Comparative Performance of US Hospitals: The Sourcebook" (abridged by authors), © 2000 HCIA, L.L.C. and Deloitte & Touche LLP.

Perspective 4–5 "How Health Plans in Phoenix, Arizona Benchmark against Local Market and National Market Ratios" (abridged by authors), *Interstudy Publications Quarterly Newsletter*, Volume 1, Issue 1.

Perspective 5–1 "Stocks are Risky Rx for Hospitals" (abridged by authors), by Dennis Walters. From *Chicago Sun-Times*, October 29, 2000. © Chicago Sun-Times, Inc.

Perspective 5–2 "Funds Management" (abridged by authors), by David Feldheim. From *The Bond Buyer*, September 26, 2000. © 2000 The Bond Buyer, Inc.

Perspective 5–3 "Billing Scam Hits Hospitals" (abridged by authors), by Mark D. Somerson and Mary Beth Lane. From *The Columbus Dispatch*, October 28, 2000. © 2000 Columbus Dispatch.

Perspective 5–4 "Health Plans Create a Rival for WebMD" (abridged by authors), by Ann Carrns. From *The Wall Street Journal*, November 15, 2000. © 2000 Dow Jones & Company, Inc.

Perspective 5–5 "Report Predicts Huge HIPAA Price Tag" (abridged by authors), by Barbara Kirchheimer. Reprinted with permission from *Modern Healthcare*, October 2, 2000. © 2000 Crain Communications, Inc., 360 N Michigan Avenue, Chicago, IL 60601.

Perspective 6–1 "Has the Market Gone Mad?" (abridged by authors), by Shawn Tully. From *Fortune* magazine, January 24, 2000. © 2000 Time, Inc.

Perspective 7–1 "Doctors, St Joseph Get New Tool" (abridged by authors), by Winthrop Quigley. From *Albuquerque Journal*, September 7, 2000. © 2000 Albuquerque Journal.

Perspective 7–2 "McKesson HBOC Announces Next-Generation, Integrated Clinical Solution to Improve Patient Safety and Reduce Cost of Care" (abridged by authors). From *Business Wire*, July 16, 2001. © 2001 Business Wire, Inc.

Perspective 7–3 "New Beckley Clinic to Help Thousands" (abridged by authors). From *The Sunday Gazette Mail*, May 6, 2001. © 2001 Charleston Newspapers.

Perspective 7–4 "Carolina's HealthCare System Gains $326,000 Profit for First Quarter" (abridged by authors), by Mike Stobbe. From *The Charlotte Observer*, June 20, 2001. © 2001 Knight Ridder/Tribune Business News. © 2001 The Charlotte Observer.

Perspective 7–5 "CEO of Nashville, TN-based Healthcare Company Defends Integrity" (abridged by authors), by Bob Gary, Jr. From *Chattanooga Times* and *Free Press*, April 26, 2001. © 2001 Knight Ridder/Tribune Business News. © 2001 Chattanooga Times/Free Press.

Perspective 8–1 "Ailing Stocks Land E-Health Companies in Sick Bay" (abridged by authors), by Robert McCough and Ann Carrns. From *The Wall Street Journal*, April 10, 2000.

Perspective 8–2 "The Fall of the House of AHERF" (abridged by authors), by Lawton R. Burns, John Cacclamani, James Clement, and Welman Aquino. From *Health Affairs*, January/February 2000, Volume 19, Number 1.

Perspective 8–3 "Buying on Credit" (abridged by authors), by Deanna Bellandi. Reprinted with permission from *Modern Healthcare*, June 28, 2001. © 2001 Crain Communications, Inc., 360 N Michigan Avenue, Chicago, IL 60601.

Perspective 8–4 "An Updated Approach to Rating Not-For-Profit Health Care Organizations" (abridged by authors), from *Moody's Rating Methodology Handbook: Public Finance: Nov. 2000*, © 2000 Moody's Investors Service, Inc.

Perspective 8–5 "Ratings firms see fewer downgrades" (abridged by authors), by Mary Chris Jaklevic. Reprinted with permission from *Modern Healthcare*, January 29, 2001. © 2001 Crain Communications, Inc., 360 N Michigan Avenue, Chicago, IL 60601.

Perspective 9–1 "Drkoop.com Lays off Third of Work Force," by Associated Press, August 31, 2000. From *Boston Globe*, © 2000 Globe Newspaper Company.

Perspective 9–2 "Targeting Disease Treatment Could Save States Thousands in Medicaid Costs" (abridged by authors). From *AHA News*, August 28, 2000.

Perspective 9–3 "Length of Stay Has Minimal Impact on the Cost of Hospital Admission" (abridged by authors), by P. A. Taheri, D. A. Butz, and L. J. Greenfield. From *Journal of the American College of Surgeons*, 2000, Aug, 191(2): 123–30. © 2000 American College of Surgeons.

Perspective 9–4 "Speedy Recovery" (abridged by authors), by Laura Johannes. From *The Wall Street Journal*, August 29, 2000. © 2000 Dow Jones & Company, Inc.

Perspective 9–5 "Practices with the Best Practices" (abridged by authors), by Mary Chris Jaklevic. Reprinted with permission from *Modern Healthcare*, February 8, 1999, © 1999 Crain Communications, Inc., 360 N Michigan Avenue, Chicago, IL 60601.

Perspective 9–6 "Mission to Stop Restocking Ambulances" (abridged by authors), by Joel Burgess. From *Times-News Online*, September 14, 2000. © 2000 Times-News.

Perspective 10–2 "Services for Poor Put at Risk" (abridged by authors), by Bonnie Rochman. From *The News & Observer*, July 28, 2000. © 2000 The News & Observer Pub. Co.

Perspective 10–3 "Beth Israel to Cut Back Services" (abridged by authors), by Liz Kowalczyk. From *The Boston Globe*, September 27, 2000. © 2000 Globe Newspaper Company.

Perspective 10–4 "Hospital Makes Work Hour Cuts Voluntary" (abridged by authors), by Jill Doss-Raines. From *The Lexington Dispatch*, July 26, 2000. © 2000 The-Dispatch.

Perspective 10–5 "Shortage of Nurses Looming?" (abridged by authors), by Sara Lindau. From *The Pilot*, August 21, 2000. © 2000 The Pilot LLC.

Perspective 11–1 "Hospital to Shed Its Network of Physician Groups," by Jean P. Fisher. From *Knight-Ridder Tribune Business News: The News & Observer*, August 16, 2001.

Perspective 11–2 "Reviving Ailing Hospitals" (abridged by authors), by Ron Shinkman. Reprinted with permission from *Modern Healthcare*, April 9, 2001. © 2001 Crain Communications, Inc., 360 N Michigan Avenue, Chicago, IL 60601.

Perspective 11–3 "Blue All Over" (abridged by authors), by Barbara Kirchheimer. Reprinted with permission from *Modern Healthcare*, June 25, 2001. © 2001 Crain Communications, Inc., 360 N Michigan Avenue, Chicago, IL 60601.

Perspective 12–1 "House Committee on Public Health Recommendations Relating to Hospital Charity Care & Hospital System Sales, Conversions, Partnerships and Mergers" (abridged by authors), From *Consumers Union*, June 28, 2000. © 2000 Consumers Union.

Perspective 12–2 "Review of Partial Hospitalization Services and Audit of Medicare Cost Report for Community Behavioral Services, a Florida Community Mental Health Center" (abridged by authors), by June Gibbs Brown, Inspector General, January 5, 1998. From the Department of Health and Human Services, Region IV, PO Box 2047, Atlanta, GA 30301.

Perspective 12–3 "Activity Based Costing" (abridged by authors), by Gary Shows. © 2000 Robert Luttman & Associates.

Perspective 12–4 "Cost for Pricing at Blue Cross and Blue Shield of Florida" (abridged by authors), by Kenneth L. Thurston, Dennis M. Deleman and John B. MacArthur. From *Management Accounting Quarterly*, Spring 2000. © 2000 Management Accounting Quarterly.

Perspective 13–1 "The World's Health Care: How Do We Rank?" Susan Landers, AMNews staff. August 28, 2000.

Perspective 13–2 "An Opinion of Managed Care," *Sacramento Business Journal*, December 17, 1999.

Perspective 13–3 "HIPAA Opinion" (abridged by authors), by Jeff Tieman, *Modern Healthcare*, March 26, 2001; exhibit, Jeff Tieman, *Modern Healthcare*, July 16, 2001 (chart source Sheldon Dorenfest and Associates, same article).

Perspective 13–5 "Innovations through Information" (abridged by authors), by Matthew Ayotte, Strategic Planning, Duke University Medical Center, August 2001.

Exhibit 1–2 "The Consumer Price Index vs. Medical Care Inflation," from US Labor Department, Bureau of Labor Statistics (July 2000).

Exhibit 1–3 "Annual Health Care Expenditures in the United States," from Health Care Financing Administration (July 2000).

Exhibit 1–7 "Rising Number of Uninsured," from US Census Bureau (July 2000).

Exhibit 1–8 "Uncompensated Care Costs for the Uninsured," from American Hospital Association (July 2000).

Exhibit 1–9 "Annual Number of Surviving Hospitals," from American Hospital Association (July 2000).

Exhibit 2–3 "Annotated Balance Sheet for Sample Not-For-Profit Hospital." Permission from *Audit and Accounting Guide: Health Care Organizations*, copyright © 1996 by the American Institute of Certified Public Accountants, Inc.

Exhibit 2–4 "Asset Section of the Balance Sheet from Exhibit 2–3 with an Emphasis on Current Assets," reprinted with permission from *Audit and Accounting Guide: Health Care Organizations*, copyright © 1996 by the American Institute of Certified Public Accountants, Inc.

Exhibit 2–6 "Asset Section of the Balance Sheet from Exhibit 2–3 with an Emphasis on Non-current Assets," reprinted with permission from *Audit and Accounting Guide: Health Care Organizations*, copyright © 1996 by the American Institute of Certified Public Accountants, Inc.

Exhibit 2–8 "Liabilities Section of the Balance Sheet from Exhibit 2–3," reprinted with permission from *Audit and Accounting Guide: Health Care Organizations*, copyright © 1996 by the American Institute of Certified Public Accountants, Inc.

Exhibit 2–9 "Net Assets Section of the Balance Sheet from Exhibit 2–3," reprinted with permission from *Audit and Accounting Guide: Health Care Organizations*, copyright © 1996 by the American Institute of Certified Public Accountants, Inc.

Exhibit 2–11 "Illustration of the Owners' Equity Section of the Balance Sheet for an Investor-owned Health Care Organization," adapted from *AICPA Audit and Accounting Guide, Health Care Organizations* (new edn), New York: American Institute of Certified Public Accountants, Inc., June 1, 1996.

Exhibit 2–14 "Annotated Statement of Operations for Sample Not-For-Profit Hospital," reprinted with permission from *Audit and Accounting Guide: Health Care Organizations*, copyright © 1996 by the American Institute of Certified Public Accountants, Inc.

Exhibit 2–15 "Abbreviated Statement of Operations from Exhibit 2–14 Emphasizing Revenues, Gains, and Other Support," reprinted with permission from *Audit and Accounting Guide: Health Care Organizations*, copyright © 1996 by the American Institute of Certified Public Accountants, Inc.

Exhibit 2–17 "Abbreviated Statement of Operations from Exhibit 2–14 Emphasizing Expenses," reprinted with permission from *Audit and Accounting Guide: Health Care Organizations*, copyright © 1996 by the American Institute of Certified Public Accountants, Inc.

Exhibit 2–18 "Statement of Operations from Exhibit 2–14 Emphasizing Items that Do Not Contribute to Excess of Revenues over Expenses," adapted from *AICPA Audit and Accounting Guide, Health Care Organizations* (new edn), New York: American Institute of Certified Public Accountants, Inc., June 1, 1996.

Exhibit 2–19 "Calculation of Increase in Unrestricted Net Assets," reprinted with permission from *Audit and Accounting Guide: Health Care Organizations*, copyright © 1996 by the American Institute of Certified Public Accountants, Inc.

Exhibit 2–20 "Statement of Changes in Net Assets for Sample Not-For-Profit Hospital," reprinted with permission from *Audit and Accounting Guide: Health Care Organizations*, copyright © 1996 by the American Institute of Certified Public Accountants, Inc.

Exhibit 2–21 "Annotated Statement of Cash Flows for Sample Not-For-Profit Hospital," reprinted with permission from *Audit and Accounting Guide: Health Care Organizations*, copyright © 1996 by the American Institute of Certified Public Accountants, Inc.

Exhibit A–1 "Balance Sheet for Sample Not-For-Profit Hospital," reprinted with permission from *Audit and Accounting Guide: Health Care Organizations*, copyright © 1996 by the American Institute of Certified Public Accountants, Inc.

Exhibit A–2 "Statement of Operations for Sample Not-For-Profit Hospital," reprinted with permission from *Audit and Accounting Guide: Health Care Organizations*, copyright © 1996 by the American Institute of Certified Public Accountants, Inc.

Exhibit A–3 "Statement of Changes in Net Assets for Sample Not-For-Profit Hospital," reprinted with permission from *Audit and Accounting Guide: Health Care Organizations*, copyright © 1996 by the American Institute of Certified Public Accountants, Inc.

Exhibit A–4 "Statement of Cash Flows for Sample Not-For-Profit Hospital," reprinted with permission from *Audit and Accounting Guide: Health Care Organizations*, copyright © 1996 by the American Institute of Certified Public Accountants, Inc.

Exhibit A–5 "Consolidated Income Statement for Columbia/HCA Healthcare Corporation," from Columbia/HCA's 10-K report from SEC.

Exhibit A–6 "Consolidated Income Statement for Columbia/HCA Healthcare Corporation," from Columbia/HCA's 10-K report from SEC.

Exhibit A–7 "Consolidated Income Statement for Columbia/HCA Healthcare Corporation," from Columbia/HCA's 10-K report from SEC.

Exhibit 8–5 "Selected Not-for-profit Hospital Industry Bond Ratings and Medians: 2000," from Standard & Poor's Median Health Care Ratios, October 19, 2000.

Exhibit 13–3 "Medicare and Medicaid Entitlement Programs," from http://www.hcfa.gov August 2000.

Exhibit 13–4 "Examples of Diagnostic Related Groups," from http://www.hcfa.gov August 2000.

Exhibit 13–5 "Percent Increase in Medicare Expenditures (IP and OP) 1970–1998," from http://www.hcfa.gov, August 2000.

Exhibit 13–6 "Healthcare Expenditures as a Percent of GNP 1940–2000," from http://www.hcfa.gov, August 2000.

The publishers apologize for any errors or omissions in the above list and would be grateful to be notified of any corrections that should be incorporated in the next edition or reprint of this book.

Chapter One

THE CONTEXT OF HEALTH CARE FINANCIAL MANAGEMENT

LEARNING OBJECTIVES

After completing this chapter, you will be able to:

▶ Identify key factors that have led to rising health care costs.
▶ Identify key approaches to controlling health care costs.
▶ Identify key ethical issues resulting from attempts to control costs.

Chapter Outline

◀INTRODUCTION▶

Never before have health care professionals faced such complex issues and practical difficulties trying to keep their organizations financially viable (see Perspective 1–1). With turbulent changes taking place in payment, delivery, and social systems, health care professionals are faced with trying to meet their organization's health-related mission in an environment of extreme cost pressure. In order to provide a context for the topics covered in this text, this chapter highlights key issues affecting health care providers. It is organized into three sections: rising health care costs, efforts to control costs, and cost control issues with ethical overtones (see Exhibit 1–1).

PERSPECTIVE 1–1

Health Care Institutions Need More than Efficiency

In the past decade, few sectors of the American economy have been as whipsawed as has the health care industry. On one hand, US health consumers continue to demand the highest quality, most accessible care. On the other, current public policy, expressed as dramatically lower payment for care delivered, has caused academic medical centers and community hospitals alike to hemorrhage financially, putting many institutions on the brink of bankruptcy and patient care at serious risk.

Calls for improved economic efficiencies in the American health care system predate early Clinton Administration initiatives. The rise of HMOs was one attempt to use a third party to control costs. But have quality and access been diminished for the sake of controlled economics? The evidence strongly suggests that it has.

In 1997, spurred by the dual ambitions to further constrict health care costs and diminish the federal contribution to national health care, Congress passed the Balanced Budget Act. The BBA was designed to reduce Medicare payments to medical centers and hospitals by $48 billion over five years. But an updated figure by the Congressional Budget Office actually estimated the cuts at $71 billion. While perhaps unintended, the result has been the growing disabling of the American hospital system.

The examples are widespread. In Boston, each of the five academic medical centers is losing tens of millions of dollars annually. The same applies for the eight academic medical centers in the New York metropolitan area. The Association of American Medical Colleges, with 125 member institutions, predicts more than two-thirds of this nation's academic medical centers will run seriously in the red in the year 2000.

Source: James Barba, Chairman of the Board of Directors, President and Chief Executive Officer of Albany Medical Center. *Health Care Quarterly,* December 11, 2000.

Exhibit 1–1   Organization of this Chapter

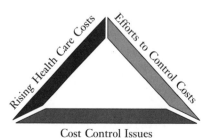

Cost Control Issues
With Ethical Overtones

◄Rising Health Care Costs►

Many factors have led to rising health care costs, which have increased faster than has general inflation over the past decades (see Exhibit 1–2). Though the average life expectancy of the general population has only risen by three years over this time period, the cost to keep people healthy has increased sixfold (Exhibit 1–3). The remainder of this section briefly discusses some of the key factors that have

Exhibit 1–2 The Consumer Price Index versus Medical Care Inflation

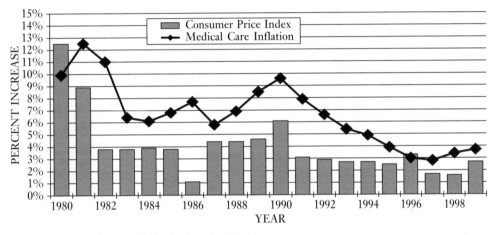

Source: US Labor Department, Bureau of Labor Statistics, July 2000.

Exhibit 1–3 Annual Health Care Expenditures in the United States

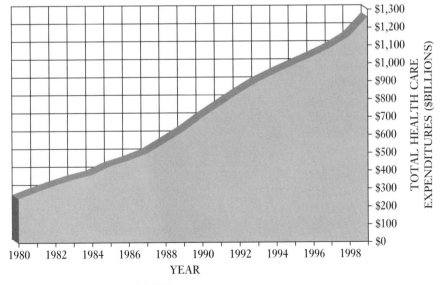

Source: Health Care Financing Administration, July 2001.

contributed to the higher cost of health care: the payment (reimbursement) system, technology, the aging population, chronic diseases, prescription drug costs, litigation, and the uninsured (see Exhibit 1–4).

The Payment System

Ambulatory Payment Classifications (APCs): Enacted by the federal government in 2000, a prospective payment system for outpatient services, similar to DRGs, which reimburses a fixed amount for a bundled set of services.

The introduction of Medicare and Medicaid in 1965 was designed in large part to guarantee health care coverage to the country's most vulnerable populations: the poor and the elderly. Unfortunately, many people at the time failed to recognize that these "Great Society" programs would become the impetus for two interrelated problems that have persisted ever since: rising health care costs far beyond those that were ever predicted, and an increased expectation that access to a high level of affordable health care is a right for all citizens. Since the mid-1960s, the health care payment system in the United States has undergone major changes. The role of the provider has gradually shifted from price-setter to price-taker. The role of the federal government has changed from being a small participant before the mid-1960s to being a major force in both setting amounts of payment and defining payment systems. As the federal government has attempted to control its costs, its inpatient payment systems have evolved from charge-based to cost-based to flat-fee, toward capitation, and now toward mixed systems (see Exhibit 1–5). In 2000, the federal government also introduced a new payment system for outpatient services, called **APCs (Ambulatory Payment Classifications)**, which changed the basis of payment for outpatient services from flat-fee for individual services to fixed reimbursement for bundled services. The federal government, of course, is not the only payor, but its policies greatly influence the practices of other payors, including state governments.

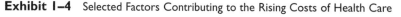

Exhibit 1–4 Selected Factors Contributing to the Rising Costs of Health Care

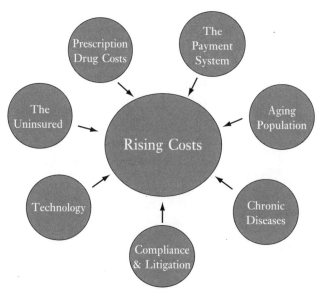

Exhibit 1–5   The Evolution of Payment Systems in the United States Since 1960

Early 1960s	Mid-1960s	Mid-1980s	Late 1990s	2000s
Fee-for-Service	Cost-Based Reimbursement	Prospective Payment (DRGs)	Capitation and Global Payments	APCs and ?

As discussed in depth in Chapter 13, in charge-based and cost-based systems, the provider plays a major role in setting prices. In flat-fee and capitated payment arrangements, the provider assumes an increased financial risk, while the payor potentially has more control over its costs. A major problem caused by payors trying to control their cost has been **cost-shifting**: providers attempting to pass on costs not paid for by one payor onto other payors. This has resulted in a dramatic shift in costs to the private sector, a nearly 500 percent increase over the past two decades: $142.5 billion in 1980 versus $626.4 billion in 1998 (US Health Care Financing Administration, 1999). As a result, employers and insurers are following the government's lead and becoming increasingly more involved in managing care.

> **Cost-shifting**: When providers try to get one payor to pay for costs which have not been covered by another payor. A common example is a provider's trying to compensate for low Medicaid payments by increasing charges to a private insurer.

Technology

No one can deny the benefits of health care technology, but the associated costs have become tremendous. Premature infants, and infants with gross birth defects, who would not have survived just a decade ago, can now survive, but can generate upwards of half a million dollars in the intensive care unit alone, and possibly more afterwards due to developmental disabilities. The total cost in the first year of life for a premature infant can easily surpass $1 million.

Transplants have saved countless lives, and procedure count more than doubled in number in less than 15 years, from 11,163 in 1985 to 25,141 in 1998 (US Department of Health and Human Services, 1999). Many feel that it has not been the individual cost of a transplant, but only the lack of donors that has limited the number of transplants performed. The rise in living-donor transplants (as opposed to cadaverous transplants) has led to more growth in this rapidly evolving field, but these procedures now involve two (or more) living patients who will be operated on, rather than just one. The use of other, more advanced technologies – and their associated costs – have significantly increased as well. For example, the number of MRIs (magnetic resonance imagers) per capita in the United States far exceeds the figure for any other country in the world, as do the figures for CAT (computerized axial tomography) scanners, cardiac catheterization procedures, etc. On the other hand, the United States has become "the place to go" for foreigners who do not have access to these types of advanced technologies in their own countries.

The Aging Population

The average life expectancy of Americans has risen only slightly over the past few decades: from 69.5 to 73.6 for males, and from 77.2 to 79.4 for females (1977–1997, both sets of figures). In the meantime, the overall population has aged significantly, and there are more elderly Americans than ever before. In fact, by the mid-1990s, the age group 85 and older was the fastest growing segment of the population, and the elderly tend to be the heaviest users of health care services. Whereas the leading causes of death in the early part of the last century were sudden illnesses (generally curable today), the current reasons for mortality include more chronic, long-term (and expensive) illnesses, such as heart disease and cancer (see Exhibit 1–6). If a person lives long enough, he or she has a high probability of succumbing to a chronic illness.

The combination of age and technology has increased costs in other ways, too. For example, joint replacements to restore mobility are immensely popular among the elderly, but can become very expensive, especially if complications arise. Though the benefit of such procedures is remarkable in human terms, these technologies have added costs to the system.

The increased need for long-term care for the elderly has also led to increased health care costs. As more working families find that they cannot take care of their aging parents' physical needs, the costs of long-term care become their burden and society's burden. In fact, over half of all Medicaid expenditures in the late 1990s went to elderly patients in nursing homes. A less expensive alternative is home health and live-in nursing aides, but these options are not always covered by insurance and can be unaffordable to the average family: 24-hour nursing coverage, whether home-based or facility-based, now averages well over $100 per day per individual.

Exhibit 1–6   Major Causes of Death and Their Approximate Occurrences in 1999

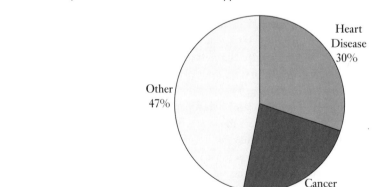

Other 47%

Heart Disease 30%

Cancer 23%

Source: K. D. Kochanek, B. L. Smith, and R. N. Anderson, "Deaths: Preliminary Data for 1999," *National Vital Statistics Reports*, 49(3), 2001, 1–48.

Prescription Drug Costs

A major reason why the population has aged and has survived longer from debilitating chronic diseases has been the advent of increasingly effective – albeit costly – drugs (see Perspective 1–2). A key issue in the 2000 presidential election focused on how to make these prescription medications more affordably to the elderly. Drug manufacturers have received widespread criticism for stifling competition and raising prices, especially as compared to the prices being offered in other countries. However, the manufacturers counter that they can spend hundreds of millions of dollars in research on one drug, and they need to recoup their investments (as well as their investments in numerous other failed drugs that never reached the market). Without the incentive to do research by being granted a patent on new medications (and thus monopoly control), drug manufacturers contend that they would not bring as many promising new drugs to market. While the battle rages on, retail sales of prescription drugs in the United States increased by over 75 percent in just five years from 1995 to 1999, from $68.6 billion to over $121.7 billion (National Association of Chain Drug Stores, 1999).

Chronic Diseases

While chronic diseases are often associated with the elderly, long-term ailments may affect younger segments of the population as well. Sometimes these diseases can be

PERSPECTIVE 1–2

Living with Change – Open Your Wallets

All the technology means we'll be spending less on health care in the years ahead, right? Fat chance. "If the economy continues to grow as it has in this decade, one could see substantial increases in health-care spending with no change in the share of GDP," says Elliott Fisher, a professor of medicine at Dartmouth Medical School in Hanover, NH.

But few doubt we'll be spending more on health in per capita terms. Measured in 1997 dollars, per capita spending on health care rose to $3,925 in 1997 from $765 in 1960, according to the HCFA. Between 1960 and 1990, the health-care component of the consumer price index rose an average of 1.8 percentage of this decade, to as small as 0.4 point, or 22%, in 1997. But it has widened sharply since then.

The ever-expanding array of medical technology – devices and drugs – also drives up health-care costs. While in many industries technology tends to reduce labor costs, in medicine it tends to raise them. "You have more-complex equipment introduced in health care, and you can't have an unskilled person running it," says Paul Starr, a Princeton University sociology professor and author of "The Social Transformation of American Medicine," a history of the profession. Some technological innovations clearly save money; penicillin, for instance, has spared us who-knows-how-many hospital stays. "But relatively little health-care technology has been like that," says Mr Starr. "There's been much more health-care technology that's raised labor costs."

Source: Chris Gay, *Wall Street Journal*, October 18, 1999.
Copyright Dow Jones & Company Inc., New York.

cured, but at other times, only treated. Acquired Immune Deficiency Syndrome, or AIDS, became widespread in the 1980s, and a total of 733,374 cases were reported in the United States between 1981 and 1999 (US Centers for Disease Control and Prevention, 1999). It is a long-term illness that can easily cost $100,000 over the life of a patient, not to render a cure, but only to improve the quality of life and provide palliative support. Other diseases, such as diabetes, liver failure, and cancer, can also affect younger people, who may end up needing expensive treatments for a lifetime. Still other conditions, such as mental illness or debilitating back pain, are expensive to treat and costly in terms of lost productivity. Days of disability have held steady at nearly 4 billion per year: 4.2 billion in 1980 versus 3.8 billion in 1996 (US National Center for Health Statistics, 1996).

Compliance and Litigation

Compliance: The need to abide by governmental regulations, whether they be for the provision of care, billing, privacy, security, etc.

Three interrelated factors have greatly contributed to the rise in healthcare costs: 1) **compliance**, which is the need to comply with governmental regulations, whether they be for provision of care, billing, privacy, security, etc. A noteworthy example of extraordinary compliance costs would be the **Health Insurance Portability and Accountability Act**, or HIPAA (discussed below and described in more detail in Chapter 13); 2) **increased insurance premiums** that providers have to pay insurers to cover the cost of defending against lawsuits and paying large jury awards; and 3) the increased use of **defensive medicine** by practitioners – excessive tests and procedures, oftentimes unnecessary care, simply to ensure that nothing be overlooked should a lawsuit ever arise. And once a patient has undergone a test or procedure, the provider is liable to be aware of and to follow up on all the results, even if the original service were unnecessary.

Health Insurance Portability and Accountability Act (HIPAA): A set of federal compliance regulations enacted in 1996 to ensure standardization of billing, privacy, and reporting as institutions enter a paperless age.

Partially due to concerns over access to health care services as a result of cost-control measures by insurers, the federal government enacted HIPAA in 1996. HIPAA was introduced: to improve the portability and continuity of health insurance coverage; to ensure confidentiality in health care information storage and retrieval; to combat waste, fraud, and abuse in the health insurance and delivery systems; to promote the use of medical savings accounts; to improve access to long-term care; and to simplify the administration of health insurance. Compliance is mandatory by all health care institutions before the year 2005. Though individual state regulations can override HIPAA regulations if they more strictly ensure access to and coverage for health care services, HIPAA imposes minimum standards that must be met by all institutions doing business in any state.

Defensive Medicine: The tendency of health care practitioners to do more testing and to provide more care for patients than might otherwise be necessary, simply to protect themselves against potential litigation.

The cost impact of litigation by patients and their families on health care providers cannot be directly measured, but it is generally believed to be quite significant. On the one hand, patients have a right to expect a reasonable and safe level of care that is dictated by medical necessity, not by profit margins. On the other hand, what is reasonable care seems open to considerable debate, especially on a case-by-case basis. Under tighter reimbursement policies, providers are forced or encouraged to restrict potentially unnecessary tests, while opening themselves up to possible legal battles. The subject of whether or not managed care plan enrollees should be allowed to sue their

HMO or employer has become a heated topic of discussion, as some contend it will ultimately drive costs up even further. Although the legal relationship between provider organizations and their participating providers is beyond the scope of this text, it should be emphasized that litigation and compliance add costs which are not direct (i.e., hands-on) patient care.

The Uninsured

The number of uninsured individuals has risen considerably (see Exhibit 1–7). By the turn of the century, the number of people with no health insurance coverage at some time during the year was approximately 40 million (the number continuously fluctuates as people add or drop coverage). This is due to several factors, including: 1) health insurance premiums have become too costly for many individuals, even if they are working; 2) individuals have been screened out of insurance policies because of "pre-existing conditions"; 3) employers, feeling they cannot afford to continue to provide health insurance as a benefit, have either scaled back their benefits or eliminated them altogether by hiring part-time rather than full-time workers; 4) due to budget restrictions, the federal government and the states have tightened Medicaid eligibility criteria, typically too far below the official federal poverty level for most families to qualify; and 5) individuals have learned that they will be taken care of by providers, especially community hospitals, if they show up at the door (specifically the emergency room), even if they can't pay. Some low-risk people may avoid insurance altogether and assume they will be taken care of if ever need be. Most hospitals are legally

Exhibit 1–7 Number of Uninsured

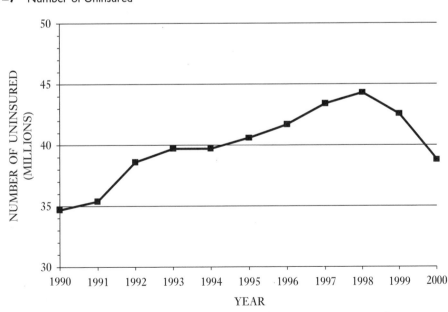

Source: US Census Bureau, July 2001.

Exhibit 1–8   Uncompensated Care Costs for the Uninsured

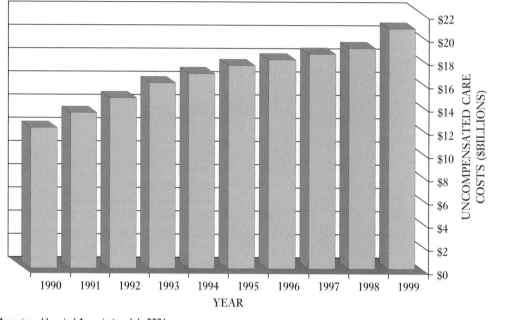

Source: American Hospital Association, July 2001.

obligated to accept these individuals once they have entered the premises. This puts a tremendous burden on health care facilities, especially community hospitals, to continue to provide indigent care, because they can no longer pass on their costs to other payors (see Exhibit 1–8).

◀EFFORTS TO CONTROL COSTS▶

The impact of rising health care costs has had drastic consequences upon the ability of providers to survive financially (see Exhibit 1–9). Hence, keen interest has been fostered by payors and providers to control this rise. The following sections describe measures undertaken to control costs.

Efforts by Payors to Control Health Care Costs

Rising health care costs have forced private and public payors to try a variety of approaches to limit their financial risk. Increasingly, employers and payors have drawn upon their position as the supplier of patients to manage care as well as to manage payments. This has forced hospital administrators to accept payment arrangements that greatly affect the relationships among patients, providers, and payors.

Exhibit 1–9   Annual Number of Surviving Hospitals

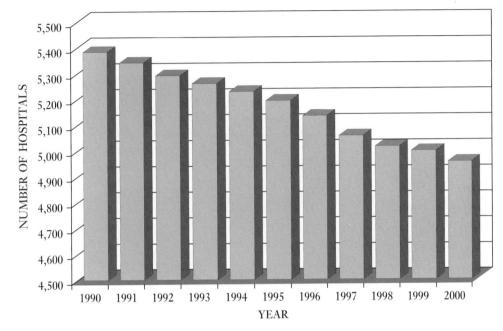

Source: American Hospital Association, July 2001.

The most commonly used methods by payors to control costs are introduced below and illustrated in Exhibit 1–10. These approaches are discussed in more detail in Chapter 13.

- **Retrospective Review:** reviewing services after they have been performed and only reimbursing for those services deemed medically necessary by the payor.
- **Concurrent Review:** monitoring appropriateness and medical necessity of a hospital stay while the patient is in the hospital, and implementing discharge planning.
- **Preadmission Certification and Second Opinions:** requiring prior approval or review of services to determine appropriateness of care.
- **Prospective Payments:** predetermining payments for services in advance based upon common use of resources for that service.
- **Gatekeepers:** requiring a patient to obtain a referral from his or her primary care physician, the "gatekeeper," before going to see a specialist.
- **CON (Certificate of Need):** requiring providers to have their capital expenditures (over a certain dollar amount) preapproved by an independent state agency to avoid unnecessary duplication of services (not implemented in all states).
- **Provider Networks:** requiring a patient to select from a preapproved list of providers.

Prospective Payment System: The payment system used by Medicare to reimburse providers a predetermined amount. Several payment methods fall under the umbrella of PPS, including: DRGs (inpatient admissions); APCs (outpatient visits); RBRVS (professional services); and RUGs (skilled nursing home care). DRGs were the first category to fall under this type of predetermined payment arrangement.

Exhibit 1–10   Selected Methods Implemented by Payors to Control Costs

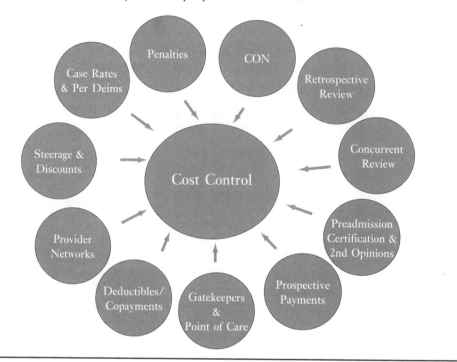

- **Deductibles and Copayments**: requiring patients to pay for part of their own care up to a given amount (*deductible*) or for a portion of each service they receive (*copayment*).
- **Steerage and Discounts**: agreeing to send patients to providers in return for discounted services.
- **Case Rates and Per Diems**: setting reimbursement depending on the type of case (medical, surgical, maternity, etc.) or setting rates per inpatient day based on the type of case (per diems).
- **Penalties**: charging HMO patients a penalty for seeking care outside the HMO network without preapproval. Providers may also be penalized by HMOs for not following managed care rules. Such penalties include reducing or withholding incentive pay.
- **Point of Care**: allowing capitated patients to seek care outside the HMO for an increase in premium.

Because of the enormity of their impact, two payment systems designed to control costs demand special attention: DRGs and capitation. Other payment systems which are emerging, such as global payments and APCs, are also discussed.

DRGs

In an effort to control Medicare inpatient costs, the Reagan administration introduced the **prospective payment** concept in 1984. Under this plan, the government created nearly 500 different categories of illnesses called **Diagnosis Related Groups**, or DRGs, and reimbursed a fixed amount based upon the patient's discharge diagnosis. The goal was to shift the degree of responsibility to the provider to be more efficient, since with few exceptions (called "outliers"), the provider would receive a fixed reimbursement for a patient in a particular category, regardless of the services provided. Several major problems arose from the DRG-based system, which led to searches for alternatives:

- Reimbursement rates did not keep pace with health care inflation, which rose at approximately 11 percent per year through the 1980s and into the early 1990s. Though the health care inflation rate slowed in the late 1990s, it has since picked up again and still exceeds the overall rate of inflation. This trend caused many facilities to lose money on Medicare patients, which encouraged those facilities to steer Medicare patients to other providers.
- Providers began to engage in what became known as "DRG creep," a noticeable (possibly illegal) trend toward patients' being placed into higher-paying DRGs. This led to increased costs.
- Many hospitals find fixed reimbursements to be inconvenient. For example, a patient is admitted for pneumonia, but during the patient's stay, the hospital discovers another problem, poor hearing. If the hospital performs audiology services during the patient's inpatient stay (which would be very convenient), the hospital would not get additional reimbursement for those services because the reimbursement amount is based only upon the patient's discharge diagnosis: pneumonia. To get compensated for audiology services, the hospital must discharge the patient and then bring him back to the hospital later as an outpatient, which has a different and separate payment mechanism. (And even then, to prevent such occurrences, the federal government enacted a "72-hour rule," which in effect states that additional services received within 72 hours of a discharge are considered part of the preceding inpatient visit, and thus are not eligible for separate reimbursement.)

Capitation

One of the newer methods to control costs is *capitation*, whereby the provider receives a set payment to provide health care services to a population for a defined time period. This type of engagement works best with large populations, sometimes referred to as **risk pools**, where risk can be spread out and managed better. Typically, the payment rate is set on a per member per month (PMPM) basis. Under this type of arrangement, the provider receives a fixed amount of money at the beginning of each month (based upon the number of enrollees) and agrees to provide all covered services necessary for

Diagnosis Related Groups (DRGs): A system to classify inpatients based upon their diagnoses. In the most pervasive system, which is used by Medicare, there are approximately 500 different diagnostic categories.

Capitation: A system which pays providers a specific amount in advance to care for the health care needs of a population over a specific time period. Providers are usually paid on per member per month (PMPM) basis. The provider then assumes the risk that the cost of caring for the population will not exceed the aggregate PMPM amount received.

Risk Pools: A generally large population of individuals who are all insured under the same arrangement, regardless of working status. Health care utilization – and therefore cost – is more stable for larger groups than it is for smaller groups, which makes larger groups' cost more predictable for insurers.

Global Payments: A system to pay providers whereby the fees for all providers (i.e. hospitals, physicians, home health care agencies) are included in a single negotiated amount. This is sometimes called "bundling" of services. In non-global payment systems, each provider is paid separately.

those enrollees during that month. Though there are various arrangements to limit financial risk, under a completely capitated arrangement, the burden of cost containment rests entirely on the provider.

Global Payments

Under most of today's payment systems, each provider is paid separately. Under a global payment system, a single price is agreed upon for several providers as a unit (i.e. the hospital, physicians, home health agency, etc.), who have bid a set price for a contract. Payors reduce risk by knowing in advance the amount that they will have to pay. Providers, on the other hand, are able to keep the profit if they can provide all services for less than the negotiated global payment. However, they are at risk for any loss. A particularly interesting problem arises in how the providing parties decide to split any profits or losses on the contract. Global pricing tends to increase: 1) the need for providers to cooperate; and 2) the need to scrutinize practice patterns. Regardless, it can be highly susceptible to unusually complicated and/or high cost patients, called *outliers*.

APCs

APCs, or Ambulatory Payment Classifications, are similar to and based upon the same concept as DRGs, but reimburse fixed amounts for bundled *outpatient* services rather than for *inpatient* services. Implemented in the year 2000 as part of the **Balanced Budget Act** of 1997 (but modified according to the Balanced Budget Refinement Act of 1999), APCs were an effort by the government to control rising outpatient costs. With few exceptions, nearly all outpatient services and supplies were categorized into groupings, each with a fixed reimbursement based upon a hospital's wage index. Because APCs are still relatively new, the impact that APCs have had on providers has not yet been fully researched and realized. Many facilities are believed to be having a difficult time adjusting, both to the provision of outpatient care, and to the fact that they had previously relied on outpatient revenues to help to compensate for financial losses in other areas.

Cutting Delivery Costs

Faced with restrictions on payments, providers have become increasingly concerned with controlling costs. Some of the major trends that have resulted are: the shift to outpatient services; new cost accounting systems; improved information services technology; mergers and acquisitions; and reengineering/redesign.

Shift to Outpatient Services

Many hospitals are offering an increasing number of services on an outpatient basis that have traditionally been performed on an inpatient basis, especially surgical services. In fact, a hospital today commonly performs more than half of all of its surgical cases on an outpatient basis. This has caused problems, however, for many hospitals which were primarily designed to provide inpatient surgical services, including: 1) inadequate preoperative and postoperative holding areas for extended time periods; 2) inefficient processes for preoperative work-up testing, as outpatients must find their own way to various departments throughout the hospital, such as labs and X-ray; and 3) inefficient OR operations, since hospitals must rely on outpatients to arrive at the hospital on time in the early morning, instead of retrieving patients from their inpatient beds when requested. Other less invasive outpatient procedures still have many of the same problems. This shift to outpatient services has forced hospitals to invest in facility enhancements to accommodate their changing needs, and many hospitals find themselves in a bind for funds as well as space.

Cost Accounting Systems

Most hospital accounting systems have a strong billing and collections component, but a very weak cost accounting system. In fact, this is due in large part to the history of reimbursement. Financial incentives were in place to maximize reimbursement, not to control costs. Now that the environment has changed, providers have found it increasingly important to know their precise costs. As a result, there has been a major movement to separate cost accounting systems from financial accounting systems, and to move away from traditional allocation-based cost systems to activity-based cost systems (discussed in depth in Chapter 12). Though an expensive endeavor, declining reimbursement is forcing hospitals to invest in more sophisticated cost accounting systems.

Information Services Technology

With the rapid advances in computer hardware and software applications, many institutions have invested in the latest information technologies in an effort to receive the most accurate information as quickly as possible. Most applications revolve around materials management, budgeting, accounts payable, payroll, and human resource needs. It is essential for institutions to track the flow of materials through their organizations, and to purchase and pay for supplies in the most cost-effective manner. Hospitals can keep funds longer and reduce inventory costs by incorporating "just-in-time" ordering techniques. If they can follow the flow of materials through their organization, they can better track costs and have better reporting and control over their budgets.

Computerization of medical records and information security is also an evolving field requiring significant investments. While institutions are aware of the inefficiencies of trying to manually maintain paper records, eventually many feel they will be forced by competition and by the federal government to resort to a paperless system. And in conjunction with this notion comes investments in telemedicine, the ability to perform services from a distance. Presumably, all these advancements are ultimately designed to save costs and/or lead to better provision of services, but these multi-million dollar investments have to be made now.

Mergers and Acquisitions

Many facilities have invested heavily in mergers and acquisitions under the premise that consolidation of services reduces costs. An acquisition could be as small as acquiring a physician group practice, or as large as merging all the health care institutions in a specific market area. The financial impact of such measures can be tremendous, and health care professionals must have a keen understanding of the local markets and organizational cultures before engaging in such practices. (See Perspective 1–3.) Oftentimes mergers fail or lose money, such as the break-up of Stanford and UCSF medical cen-

PERSPECTIVE 1–3

Hospital M&A Activity Slow in 2000 as Health Care Industry Begins to Stabilize

In 2000, for the third year in a row, the number of US hospital mergers and acquisitions declined, with 22 percent fewer deals announced than in the previous year, according to Irving Levin Associates, Inc., a health care research and publishing firm.

In its seventh edition of "The Health Care Acquisition Report," Levin reports that in 2000, the hospital sector had the greatest number of mergers and acquisitions for the year of any health care services industry segment. Year 2000 hospital M&A activity dropped from 110 deals reported in 1999, 139 deals in 1998, 197 deals in 1997, and 163 deals in 1996. The largest deal of the year was more than 4 times larger than the largest deal of 1999.

While M&A volume decreased, health care stocks and especially hospital stocks improved markedly during the year 2000. "The outlook for 2001 is positive. Reimbursement relief was obtained for certain segments of the industry after two years of suffering from The Balanced Budget Act of 1997. Now the health care industry is beginning to stabilize," stated Kathy Hammell, editor of the report. Hospitals account for the largest share of the more than $1 trillion that Americans spend annually on health care.

For the first time in seven years, for profit hospital acquisitions surpassed non-profit acquisitions in terms of number of hospitals, with 69% of acquisitions involving for profit and only 31% involving non-profit hospitals. Indicative of the rise in corporate acquisitions was the largest deal of the year – the $2.4 billion acquisition of Quorum Health Group by Triad, a spin-off from Columbia/HCA (now HCA-The Healthcare Company), historically a major player in the hospital acquisition market. None of the largest acquirers in 2000 or 1999 were affiliated with Roman Catholic institutions, contrary to the prior year. "While considerably more attention has been focused on the corporate acquisitions of the past five years, this industry will continue to be dominated by nonprofit entities," stated Stephen M. Monroe, a partner at Irving Levin Associates, Inc.

Transaction volume in the managed care sector also dropped in 2000, reflecting the declining financial health of that sector. There were 49 managed care transactions announced, compared to 66 deals in 1999, 62 deals in 1998 and 57 deals in 1997. In the past five years, six managed care deals exceeded a transaction value of $1 billion, but no deals have exceeded this level in the past two years.

Source: Irving Levin Associates, Inc.
Copyright 2001 PR Newswire Association, Inc., March 28, 2001
http://www.prnewswire.com

ters in San Francisco. Other acquisitions, such as those involving Columbia/HCA, were done illegally and resulted in forced break-ups, fines, and jail sentences.

Reengineering/Redesign

As a major measure to cut costs in the last decade, facilities have been learning how to redesign their work processes in order to operate more effectively and efficiently. This involves process analysis, layout redesign, work redesign, total quality management, **care mapping**, and layoff of unnecessary personnel.

Care Mapping: a process which specifies in advance the preferred treatment regimen for patients with particular diagnoses. This is also referred to as a clinical pathway, clinical protocol, or practice guideline.

◀Cost Control Issues with Ethical Overtones▶

Given the myriad efforts to control costs, health care administrators are increasingly faced with ethical dilemmas trying to balance cost with quality and access. Numerous studies have found a direct correlation among income, access, and health status. Administrators must keep in mind that they do not produce widgets, but rather an essential service, often to vulnerable populations. There are literally hundreds of questions with ethical overtones that arise because of pressures to cut costs. Among the most common are:

- How to control costs without cutting quality.
- How to control costs, yet expand access to services, especially in remote or inner-city areas.
- How to control costs and provide services to those who cannot pay.
- How to control costs but offer expensive treatments to special populations, such as the terminally ill or premature infants.
- How to control costs and still offer services that are typically reimbursed below cost, such as certain types of transplants or other special surgical procedures.
- How to control costs and not over-restrict the use of specialty care.
- How to ration health care services based upon medical effectiveness.
- How to weigh societal benefits against individual benefits when there are limited resources.

Perspective 1–4 shows the struggles that health care institutions are facing in regard to several topics discussed in the chapter.

◀Summary▶

The health care administrator today and in the future will be faced with numerous complex issues to consider while making financial decisions. Many factors have led to the rise in increasing health care costs: an aging population, increasingly "high-tech" care,

PERSPECTIVE 1–4

Conflicting Demands: Hospitals' Financial Struggles Pose Legal Obstacle Course for Board Members

Gone are the days when funding a new wing at a hospital was enough to earn someone a seat on its board of directors. To compete with their for-profit competitors, today's not-for-profit hospitals and systems require financially savvy directors who realize that doing good in the community is not enough to keep a hospital afloat.

In an increasingly litigious environment marked by several high-profile hospital bankruptcies, greater state involvement in hospital closures, and increasingly aggressive creditors, hospital board members more frequently are a target of blame for a hospital's financial demise, legal experts say.

If a hospital is approaching insolvency, should a board be focusing on how to continue to provide care for its community? Should it be doing what is best financially for the corporate owner of the hospital? Or should it be concentrating primarily on how to bring in the most cash to pay its creditors? As it turns out, the answers to these fundamental questions are about as clear as mud and vary from state to state, legal experts say.

Take the example of the 30-bed Manhattan Eye, Ear, and Throat Hospital, which tried to exit the acute-care business and sell its real estate assets for $41 million several years ago, only to be challenged in the courts by New York Attorney General Eliot Spitzer. In December 1999, the New York Supreme Court prohibited the hospital's board of trustees from going forward with the deal, despite six months of deliberations, the hiring of a financial adviser, and consideration of alternative bids. The reason, according to Justice Bernard Fried, was that the board breached its fiduciary responsibilities by not considering competing offers that would have allowed the hospital to continue its mission as a specialty facility.

The threat to a not-for-profit hospital's endowment when it approaches insolvency brings board members into the fray. James Schwartz, a partner at Manatt, Phelps & Phillips, Los Angeles, who has represented not-for-profit systems, says board members' shifting duties during insolvency will likely become a major issue in coming years. It could hit California especially hard as hospitals struggle to find the capital to comply with the state's seismic retrofitting mandates, he says. "An awful lot of hospitals are looking at that situation, and to my knowledge, nobody has been giving them much guidance," he says.

Source: Barbara Kirchheimer, *Modern Healthcare*, August 27, 2001.

prescription drug costs, chronic illnesses, compliance, legal concerns, and the ever rising number of uninsured patients. Numerous efforts have been made to counter this rise: changes in reimbursement and the shifting of risk to the providers, a shift towards greater use of outpatient services and shorter inpatient stays, more efficient administrative technologies, mergers and acquisitions, and redesign/reengineering of services in general. But the administrator must constantly maintain a high ethical standard in all decisions, because the health and survival of the population is in the balance.

The remainder of this text focuses on health care financial management topics such as how to analyze financial statements, manage internal funds, make sound business investments, borrow funds, analyze costs, and prepare a budget. It also provides more in-depth analyses of how regulations and restrictions affect how health care institutions must operate. While this knowledge is essential in the financial decision-making process, the health care administrator always needs to carefully weigh non-financial factors as well.

◀Key Terms▶

Ambulatory Payment
   Classifications (APCs)
Capitation
Care Mapping
Compliance

Cost-shifting
Defensive Medicine
Diagnosis Related Groups
   (DRGs)
Global Payments

Health Insurance Portability
   and Accountability Act
   (HIPAA)
Prospective Payment System
Risk Pools

◀Questions and Problems▶

1. **Definitions.** Define the following terms:
   a. Ambulatory Payment Classifications (APCs).
   b. Capitation.
   c. Care Mapping.
   d. Compliance.
   e. Cost-shifting.
   f. Defensive Medicine.
   g. Diagnosis Related Groups (DRGs).
   h. Global Payments.
   i. Health Insurance Portability and Accountability Act (HIPAA).
   j. Prospective Payment System.
   k. Risk Pools.
2. **Increased Costs.** List several factors which have led to the rise in increased costs.
3. **Cost Control.** List several efforts that have been enacted by payors to control costs.
4. **Cost Control.** List several efforts which have been attempted by providers to control costs.
5. **Ethics.** What are some of the ethical issues that must be considered when making any financial decisions?
6. **Capitation.** Explain how and to whom capitation shifts the burden of risk.
7. **Litigation.** Explain the ramifications of allowing/disallowing an individual to be able to sue his or her HMO.
8. **Drugs.** Is the granting of patents good for the development of new drugs? Why or why not?
9. **Ethics.** If an uninsured individual needed expensive medical treatment and did not have the means to pay for it, should the treatment be provided? Would the answer be influenced by the financial status of the institution asked to provide the service? Would the answer be any different if the individual were uninsured voluntarily (e.g. "I'll take my chances and hope nothing happens") or involuntarily (e.g. "It's either health insurance or food for my children")?
10. **Ethics.** Should private for-profit institutions be forced to accept patients who will not reimburse satisfactorily? Why or why not?

Chapter Two

HEALTH CARE FINANCIAL STATEMENTS

LEARNING OBJECTIVES

After completing this chapter, you will be able to:

▶ Identify the four basic financial statements common to all organizations.
▶ Identify and read the four basic financial statements particular to not-for-profit, business-oriented health care organizations: the balance sheet, the statement of operations, the statement of changes in net assets, the statement of cash flows.

Chapter Outline

(Continues)

Chapter Outline (*Contd*)

◀INTRODUCTION▶

Creditors, investors, and governmental and community agencies often require considerable information in order to make judgments about the financial performance of health care organizations. For instance, in order to decide whether to lend money to a home health agency, a lender may want to know how much debt the agency already has, how much cash it has available, and how much profit it is earning. Similarly, in order to make regulatory decisions, a governmental agency may want to know how much charity care is being offered or what the profit margin is for a group of providers. So that standardized financial information needed by outside parties is regularly available, almost all businesses are required to produce four different financial statements at least annually.

- Balance Sheet.
- Income Statement (or Statement of Operations).
- Statement of Changes in Owners' Equity (or Statement of Changes In Net Assets).
- Statement of Cash Flows.

As shown in Perspectives 2–1 and 2–2, the financial statements are not only of interest internally, but may also be of general interest to outside parties. Though the general format of these statements remains the same, they are often modified to reflect the idiosyncrasies of particular industries (e.g. transportation, energy, health care). In health care, four additional subsets of rules apply, depending upon the type of organization: (1) governmental entities; (2) not-for-profit, business-oriented organizations; (3) not-for-profit, non-business-oriented organizations; and (4) investor-owned. The

PERSPECTIVE 2–1

Buying on Credit: Hospital Systems Post Modest Increase in Their Long-term Liabilities

Hospital acquisitions, medical office buildings, transportation systems and equipment purchases all helped to increase the amount of long-term liabilities of the nation's healthcare systems last year. Hospital systems over-all reported a 6% increase in long-term liabilities to $95 billion last year compared with $89.6 billion in 1999, according to Modern Healthcare's 25th annual Hospital Systems Survey (June 4, p. 36). A total of 211 hospital systems provided long-term liability data. Of those, 135 not-for-profit systems reported a 3.3% increase in long-term liabilities to $41 billion last year from $39.7 billion in 1999, while 12 for-profit systems recorded an increase of 7.2% to $12.8 billion last year from $11.9 billion in 1999. Public systems, 21 of them, reported the largest increase in long-term liabilities, 10.2%, to almost $11 billion last year from just under $10 billion in 1999.

Long-term liabilities can include notes, mortgages, capital leases, bonds and obligations under continuing-care contracts. The survey polls systems that own, lease or sponsor at least two acute-care hospitals, and all findings are based on self-reported data. The numbers seem to indicate that healthcare organizations took advantage of a favorable borrowing market in the past year thanks to attractive long-term interest rates, a trend that has con-tinued so far this year....

Unlike for-profit chains, which can raise money without increasing debt thanks to the equities markets, the not-for-profits are limited to borrowing in one way or another because they don't have investors, says Brian McGough, managing director at Banc One Capital Markets in Chicago. He says there were three main reasons systems increased their long-term liabilities last year: not-for-profits borrowing to finance acquisitions of other not-for-profit facilities; not-for-profit systems buying hospitals divested by for-profit companies; and investments in technology, especially costs related to addressing the anticipated Y2K computer problems.

Source: Deanna Bellandi, *Modern Healthcare,* June 18, 2001.
http://www.modernhealthcare.com/archive/article.php3?article=7348

focus of this text is primarily not-for-profit, business-oriented health care organiza-tions, which are referred to hereafter as *not-for-profit health care organizations.* Other types of organizations have a high degree of overlap with the material presented here.

Exhibit 2–1 presents a comparison of the basic financial statements used by investor-owned and not-for-profit health care organizations.

The remainder of this chapter discusses the financial statements and terms used by health care organizations. A complete set of the financial statements discussed

Exhibit 2–1   A Comparison of Generally Used Financial Statements for Investor-Owned and Not-For-Profit Health Care Organizations

Financial Statements Used by Investor-owned Health Care Organizations	Financial Statements Used by Not-for-profit Health Care Organizations
Balance Sheet	Balance Sheet
Income Statement	Statement of Operations
Statement of Changes in Owners' Equity	Statement of Changes in Net Assets
Statement of Cash Flows	Statement of Cash Flows

PERSPECTIVE 2–2

HMOs: Some Profits, More Losses

It was a case of the rich getting richer and the poor getting poorer among HMOs in the Carolinas last year, analysts say. Health maintenance organizations owned by Blue Cross & Blue Shield of N.C. Inc., Cigna Healthcare of N.C. Inc. and United Healthcare of N.C. Inc. registered significant increases in pretax net income from 1999 to 2000. The Wellness Plan of N.C. Inc., now existing under Carolinas HealthCare System to serve only Medicaid patients, saw a tiny dip in membership last year but a $19 million increase in pretax net losses to $27.5 million. . . .

"From an HMO perspective, life is a little tougher than it was a few years ago because physician groups have gotten bigger and stronger," says Will Latham, of Charlotte-based Latham Consulting Group. "At the same time, hospitals have better learned to negotiate and create a challenge for HMOs."

Aetna U.S. Healthcare of the Carolinas Inc. gained more than 8,200 members in 2000 but lost $13.7 million more in pre-tax net income. Its medical and hospital costs shot to $128.5 million in 2000, rising from $84.4 million in 1999, and its administrative costs more than doubled. . . . Last year, Blue Cross & Blue Shield had one of its best financial years, says spokeswoman Michelle Vanstory. . . . She credits much of her company's success to new Chief Executive Robert Greczyn and program offerings such as AltMed Blue, an alternative medicine program, exercise incentives and the strength of the Blue Cross brand. . . .

Source: Ashley M. Gibson, *The Business Journal of Charlotte,* April 23 2001

in this chapter can be found in Appendix A, adapted from the American Institute of Certified Public Accountants' *Audit and Accounting Guide: Health Care Organizations*, 1996.

◀THE BALANCE SHEET▶

The balance sheet of investor-owned organizations presents a summary of the organization's assets, liabilities, and shareholders' equity (see Exhibit 2–2). Similarly, the balance sheet of a not-for-profit health care organization presents a summary of the organization's assets, liabilities, and net assets. (These terms and the relationship among them will be discussed in more detail shortly.) The balance sheet is similar to a snapshot of the organization, for it captures what the organization looks like *at a particular point in time*, usually the last day of the accounting period (i.e. quarter, half-year, fiscal year). Exhibit 2–3 presents an illustration of a balance sheet and serves as an overview of this section of the text.

As with all four financial statements, the balance sheet is organized into three major sections: heading, body, and notes (see Exhibit 2–2). At the top of the balance sheet (and each of the other financial statements) is a three-line **heading** that includes the name of the organization, the name of the statement, and two dates.

The *name of the organization* is important because it provides the reader with the name of the specific entity being summarized. This is not as trivial as it might seem. One health care organization may produce financial statements for more than one entity, depending upon the degree of control and/or economic interest. For example,

Exhibit 2–2 Overview of the Main Balance Sheet Sections of Investor-owned and Not-for-profit Health Care Organizations

Heading	Name of Investor-Owned Organization Balance Sheet Dates	Name of Not-For-Profit Organization Balance Sheet Dates
Body	**Assets** 　Current Assets 　Non-Current Assets *Total Assets* **Liabilities** 　Current Liabilities 　Non-Current Liabilities *Total Liabilities* **Shareholders' Equity**[1] 　Common Stock 　Retained Earnings *Total Shareholders' Equity* *Total Liabilities and Shareholders' Equity*	**Assets** 　Current Assets 　Non-Current Assets *Total Assets* **Liabilities** 　Current Liabilities 　Non-Current Liabilities *Total Liabilities* **Net Assets**[1] 　Unrestricted 　Temporarily Restricted 　Permanently Restricted *Total Net Assets* *Total Liabilities and Net Assets*
Notes	Key pertinent information including: ● Accounting policies ● Payment arrangements with third parties ● Asset restrictions ● Property and equipment ● Long-term debt ● Pension obligations	Key pertinent information including: ● Accounting policies ● Payment arrangements with third parties ● Asset restrictions ● Property and equipment ● Long-term debt ● Pension obligations

[1]A major difference between the balance sheet of an investor-owned and a not-for-profit health care organization is in the owners' equity section. In an investor-owned organization, the section is organized to show the shareholders' ownership stake in the corporation. In a not-for-profit health care organization, the section is termed Net Assets and is organized to show the degree of donor restriction on the assets.

a hospital may produce its own balance sheet or it may be included with other affiliated entities (e.g. managed care, outpatient services, home health). If more than one entity is being summarized, then the report is called a **consolidated** or **combined** balance sheet and the names of the entities being summarized are in the notes.

Below the name of the organization, the term *Balance Sheet* appears in the heading to differentiate it from the other financial statements. Finally, two *dates* are shown. As mentioned earlier, the balance sheet reports what the organization looks like at a particular point in time, usually the last day of the accounting period (i.e. quarter, half-year, fiscal year). Two dates are often shown so that the reader can compare two successive periods. This is called a comparative balance sheet.

Assets are resources that the organization owns, typically recorded at their original costs.

 Key Point The balance sheet reports what the organization's assets, liabilities and equity are at a particular point in time, usually the last day of the accounting period (i.e. quarter, half-year, fiscal year).

Exhibit 2–3 Annotated Balance Sheet for Sample Not-For-Profit Hospital

The balance sheet provides a snapshot of the organization's assets, liabilities and net assets as of a point in time.

1 Title: Gives the name of the organization, the name of the financial statement, and two dates for which the information is being provided.

2 Assets: The resources of the organizations which are eventually used to provide service and generate revenues.

3 Current assets: Assets which will be used or consumed within a year.
- *Cash and cash equivalents:* Coin, currency and checks held within the organization or in financial institutions such as banks.
- *Short-term investments:* Temporary investment accounts which allow the organization to earn interest and have ready access to cash.
- *Assets limited as to use:* The current portion of monies set aside for specific purposes, such as to insure debt repayment.
- *Patient accounts receivable net of estimated uncollectibles:* Money owed to the organization as a result of delivering service to patients, less an estimate of how much will not be collected.
  Uncollectibles: The amount owed to the organization which it expects it will probably not ever receive.
- *Other current assets:* A summary category which may contain smaller accounts.
  Inventory: The supplies used to run the organization and provide services.
  Prepaid expenses: Amounts the organization has paid in advance, such as rent, and insurance.

4 Non-Current Assets: Assets which will benefit the organization for periods longer than a year, such as major equipment and buildings.
- *Assets limited as to use:* Monies set aside for specific purposes such as to ensure debt repayment, less the amount needed this accounting period.
- *Long-term investments:* Investments, such as stocks, bonds and land, which the organization expects to realize a profit from over a period longer than one year.
- *Property and equipment, net:* The buildings and machinery (e.g., x-ray machine) of the organization, less the amount it has been depreciated ("used up") to date, called *accumulated depreciation*.

Total assets: The sum of current and non-current assets.

5 Liabilities: The financial obligations of the organization to pay its creditors.

Current liabilities: The financial obligations which must be paid within one year.
- *Current portion of long-term debt:* That portion of multi-year debt which is due this year.
- *Accounts payable and accrued expenses:* Amounts due this year to suppliers, employees, and others for goods and services which have been received but not yet paid for.
- *Estimated third-party payor settlements:* An estimate of the amount which must be returned to third parties for overpayment of claims.
- *Other:* All other current liabilities not listed above. A major component may be *deferred revenue:* Money that has been received, but not yet earned (e.g., money received in advance from managed care organizations; it will be earned as time passes).

6 Non-Current liabilities: The financial obligations which must be paid-off over a time period longer than one year (e.g. a capital leases). • *Long-term debt, net of current portion:* The amount of multi-year debt due in future years.

7 Net Assets: Assets – Liabilities. This section has traditionally been called *Stockholders' Equity* in investor-owned organizations and *Fund Balance* in not-for-profit organizations.
- *Unrestricted Net Assets:* The amount of the net assets which have no outside restrictions on them.
- *Temporarily restricted net assets:* Assets which have restrictions on their use which will be removed either with the passage of time or the occurrence of some event.
- *Permanently restricted net assets:* Assets which have restrictions on their use which will not be removed.

*An unannotated form of this statement can be found in Appendix A of this chapter.

Source: Reprinted with permission from the Audit and Accounting Guide: Health Care Organizations, copyright ©1996 by the American Institute of Certified Public Accountants, Inc.

Sample Not-For Profit Hospital
Balance Sheet
December 31, 20X1 and 20X0 (in '000)

Assets	20X1	20X0
Current Assets:		
Cash and Cash Equivalents	$4,758	$5,877
Short-Term Investments	15,836	10,740
Assets Limited as to Use	970	1,300
Patient Accounts Receivable, Net Estimated Uncollectibles of $2,500 in 20X1 and $2,400 in 20X0	15,100	14,194
Supplies	2,000	2,000
Prepaid Expenses	670	856
Total Current Assets	39,334	34,967
Non-Current Assets		
Assets Limited as to Use	18,949	19,841
Less Amount Required to Meet Current Obligations	(970)	(1,300)
	17,979	18,541
Long-Term Investments	4,680	4,680
Long-Term Investments Restricted for Capital Acquisition	320	520
Properties and Equipment, Net	51,038	50,492
Other Assets	1,695	1,370
Total Non-Current Assets	75,712	75,603
Total Assets	$115,046	$110,570

Liabilities and Net Assets	20X1	20X0
Current Liabilities		
Current Portion of Long-Term Debt	$1,470	$1,750
Accounts Payable and Accrued Expenses	5,818	5,382
Estimated Third-Party Payor Settlements	2,143	1,942
Deferred Revenues	1,969	2,114
Total Current Liabilities	11,400	11,188
Non-Current Liabilities		
Long-Term Debt, Net of Current Portion	23,144	24,014
Other	3,953	3,166
Total Non-Current Liabilities	27,097	27,180
Total Liabilities	38,497	38,368
Net Assets		
Unrestricted	70,846	66,199
Temporarily Restricted	2,115	2,470
Permanently Restricted	3,588	3,533
Total Net Assets	76,549	72,202
Total Liabilities and Net Assets	$115,046	$110,570

The three major sections comprising the body of the balance sheet are assets, liabilities, and net assets (see Exhibits 2–2 and 2–3). The balance sheet derives its name from the fact that the assets always equal the sum of the liabilities plus the owners' equity (called *shareholders' equity* in investor-owned health care organizations and *net assets* in not-for-profit health care organizations). The relationship among the three major sections of the balance sheet is expressed by the **basic accounting equation**:

$$\text{Assets} = \text{Liabilities} + \text{Owners' Equity}$$

In investor-owned organizations, the equation becomes:

$$\text{Assets} = \text{Liabilities} + \text{Shareholders' Equity}$$

In not-for-profit, business-oriented health care organizations, the equation becomes:

$$\text{Assets} = \text{Liabilities} + \text{Net Assets}$$

In Exhibit 2–3 for the year 20X1, the assets equal $115,046,000 and the liabilities plus the net assets also equal $115,046,000 ($38,497,000 plus $76,549,000). Incidentally, until mid-1996, not-for-profit health care organizations used the term **fund balance** instead of **net assets**, while governmental organizations such as states, cities, and local counties continue to use fund accounting.

Assets

The **assets** of an organization are the resources it owns. Most assets are recorded at their original cost. Assets are divided into two categories, current assets and non-current assets (see Exhibit 2–4).

Current Assets

Current Assets are assets that will be used or consumed within one year (see Exhibit 2–4). They help turn the capacity of the organization (i.e. buildings and equipment) into service. Current assets include:

- Cash and Cash Equivalents.
- Short-term Investments.
- Assets Limited as to Use.
- Patient Accounts Receivable, Net of Estimated Uncollectibles.
- Supplies, Prepaid Expenses and Other Current Assets.

How quickly an asset can be turned into cash is called its **liquidity**, and current assets are always listed in the order noted, which is based upon their relative liquidity in the general business world. Though this order generally reflects the liquidity of many non-health care providers, there are a number of health care providers who find

---

Liabilities are the financial obligations of the organization (i.e. debts).

Net Assets is the difference between an organization's assets and liabilities (assets *minus* liabilities).

Basic Accounting Equation: Assets = Liabilities + Net Assets

Fund Balance: A term used until 1996 for owners' equity by not-for-profit health care organizations. It was replaced with the present term, *net assets,* for non-governmental, not-for-profit organizations.

Liquidity: A measure of how quickly an asset can be converted into cash.

Exhibit 2–4 Asset Section of the Balance Sheet from Exhibit 2–3 with an Emphasis on Current Assets

Assets	20X1	20X0
Current Assets:		
Cash and Cash Equivalents	$4,758	$5,877
Short-Term Investments	15,836	10,740
Assets Limited as to Use	970	1,300
Patient Accounts Receivable, Net of Estimated		
Uncollectibles of $2,500 in 20X1 and $2,400 in 20X0	15,100	14,194
Supplies	2,000	2,000
Prepaid Expenses	670	856
Total Current Assets	39,334	34,967
Non-Current Assets		
Assets Limited as to Use	18,949	19,841
Less Amount Required to Meet Current Obligations	(970)	(1,300)
	17,979	18,541
Long-Term Investments	4,680	4,680
Long-Term Investments Restricted for Capital Acquisition	320	520
Properties and Equipment, Net	51,038	50,492
Other Assets	1,695	1,370
Total Non-Current Assets	75,712	75,603
Total Assets	$115,046	$110,570

Source: Reprinted with permission from the Audit and Accounting Guide: Health Care Organizations, copyright © 1996 by the American Institute of Certified Public Accountants, Inc.

their Patient Accounts Receivable (the money owed to them for services rendered to patients) is their least liquid current asset. Still, by convention, this generally accepted order is followed in the listing of current assets.

Because of their liquidity, current assets require special internal control procedures to ensure that they are handled appropriately and efficiently. For instance, a generally accepted internal control procedure in health care organizations is to have different people send out the bills, open the incoming mail, and record payments – a procedure which, if not followed, lends itself to considerable opportunities for mishandling of funds. Another internal control procedure is to restrict access to supplies and medicines. This leads to a discussion of each of the current asset accounts.

Cash and Cash Equivalents

Cash and cash equivalents are the most liquid current assets (see Exhibit 2–4). This account is composed of actual money on hand as well as money equivalents, such as

Key Point Cash (or cash equivalents) is the most liquid asset on the balance sheet.

savings and checking accounts. It excludes cash that has restrictions regarding withdrawal or for use for other than current operations.

Short-term Investments

Short-term investments include certificates of deposit, commercial paper, and treasury bills. These temporary investment accounts allow a health care facility to earn interest on idle cash and, at the same time, provide almost immediate access to cash for unexpected situations. Short-term investments are discussed in greater detail in Chapter 5.

Assets Limited as to Use

The cash and short-term investments listed above in the current assets section are generally available for management to use to carry out its duties. In addition, a health care organization may have other cash, marketable securities, or other current assets that can be used only under special conditions. For example, in taking out a loan, a health care organization may agree to set aside an amount of funds equal to six months' worth of loan payments. Current assets that fall into this category are classified as Assets Limited as to Use (see Exhibit 2–4). The Assets Limited as to Use accounts for Sample Not-For-Profit Hospital's current assets are $1,300,000 in 20X0 and $970,000 in 20X1.

Patient Accounts Receivable, Net of Estimated Uncollectibles

Charity Care Discounts: Discounts from Gross Patients Accounts Receivable given to those who cannot pay their bills.

Gross Patient Accounts Receivable is the amount owed the health care organization at full charges. However, many payors, such as Medicaid, insurance companies, large employers, and managed care organizations are given discounts, called **contractual allowances**. By subtracting Contractual Allowances and Charity Care Discounts from Gross Patient Accounts Receivable, what remains is Patient Accounts Receivable. Patient Accounts Receivable represents the actual amount the health care organization has the right to collect.

Along with reporting patient accounts receivable (but not *gross* patient accounts receivable) on the balance sheet, health care organizations also present an estimate of how much of their Patient Accounts Receivable they likely will not be able to collect. This estimate is called the Allowance for Uncollectibles.

Assuming Gross Patient Accounts Receivable were $24,800,000, Discounts and Contractual Allowances were $7,200,000, and Allowance for Uncollectibles was $2,500,000, Patient Accounts Receivable, Net of Uncollectibles for 20X1 would be $15,100,000, as shown in Exhibit 2–5.

By convention, the total amount of Patient Accounts Receivable, in this case $17,600,000, is commonly omitted on the balance sheet, since it can be derived by adding the Allowance for Uncollectibles and the Patient Accounts Receivable, Net of Estimated Uncollectibles.

Supplies, Prepaid Expenses, and Other Current Assets

Because of their relatively small size, **supplies and prepaid expenses** are often grouped together under the title Other Current Assets. Two accounts often found in this category are Supplies and Prepaid Assets (see Exhibit 2–4). Supplies include the

Exhibit 2–5   Calculation of Patient Accounts Receivable, Net of Estimated Uncollectibles

Account Title	Amount	Explanation
Gross Patient Accounts Receivable	$24,800	The amount owed to the organization, based on full charges. This amount is not reported on financial statements, because it does not represent how much the health care organization is really owed because of discounts and allowances.
– Discounts and Allowances	7,200	Includes discounts given to third parties (large-scale purchasers of health care services) and discounts for charity care.
Patient Accounts Receivable	17,600	Gross charges less discounts and allowances.
– Allowance for Uncollectibles	2,500	An estimate of how much of Patient Accounts Receivable will likely *not* be collectible.
Patient Accounts Receivable, Net of Estimated Uncollectibles	$15,100	The amount expected to be collected.

Key Point   Supplies are sometimes called inventory.

---

day-to-day supplies used by the organization in the provision of health care services, including food, drugs, office, and medical supplies. Another name for supplies is inventory. A common mistake is to confuse Supplies and Equipment. Supplies refers to small-dollar items that will be "used up" or fully consumed within at least one year, such as pharmaceuticals and office supplies. Equipment refers to relatively expensive items that will be used over a long period of time, such as buildings and radiology equipment. Prepaid Assets, also called Prepaid Expenses, include items the health care organization has paid for in advance, such as rent and insurance. Although they are not tangible, they are still assets – in the form of rights the organization has purchased. For instance, by paying its rent in advance, the organization has a right to use a building for a specified period. To the extent that supplies and prepaid expenses are relatively large, they may be broken out and reported separately rather than grouped together.

Non-current Assets

Whereas current assets will be used or consumed within one year, non-current assets will be used or consumed over periods longer than one year (see Exhibit 2–6). Non-current assets are relatively costly items that allow the organization to deliver service over time. Whereas current assets require special management attention because of their liquidity and transportability, non-current assets require special attention because of their cost and the extensive time horizon it takes to plan, acquire, and manage them. Non-current assets are commonly organized into the following categories:

Non-current Assets: The resources of the organization that will be used or consumed over periods longer than one year.

Exhibit 2–6   Asset Section of the Balance Sheet from Exhibit 2–3 with an Emphasis on Non-current Assets

Assets	20X1	20X0
Current Assets:		
Cash and Cash Equivalents	$4,758	$5,877
Short-term Investments	15,836	10,740
Assets Limited as to Use	970	1,300
Patient Accounts Receivable, Net of Estimated		
Uncollectibles of $2,500 in 20X1 and $2,400 in 20X0	15,100	14,194
Supplies	2,000	2,000
Prepaid Expenses	670	856
Total Current Assets	39,334	34,967
Non-current Assets		
Assets Limited as to Use	18,949	19,841
Less Amount Required to Meet Current Obligations	(970)	(1,300)
	17,979	18,541
Long-term Investments	4,680	4,680
Long-term Investments Restricted for Capital Acquisition	320	520
Properties and Equipment, Net	51,038	50,492
Other Assets	1,695	1,370
Total Non-current Assets	75,712	75,603
Total Assets	$115,046	$110,570

Source: Reprinted with permission from the Audit and Accounting Guide: Health Care Organizations, copyright © 1996 by the American Institute of Certified Public Accountants, Inc.

 Key Point   The terms "non-current" and "long-term" are often used interchangeably.

- Assets Limited as to Use.
- Long-term Investments.
- Property and Equipment, Net.
- Other Assets.

Assets Limited as to Use

With the exception of donor-restricted funds, which are reported elsewhere, this section reports the amount of the assets that have been set aside for long-term purposes and are thus not available for general use. The balance sheet presentation of Assets Limited as to Use must separate internally designated and externally designated amounts either on the statements themselves or in the notes to the financial statements. In the case of Sample Not-For-Profit Hospital in 20X1, this category contains two items: the board has set aside $12,000,000 in order to purchase buildings or equipment, and as part of a loan agreement, the organization has placed

$6,949,000 with a trustee which will be used to pay off the loan (see Exhibit 2–6). Notice that this category begins by presenting all Assets Limited as to Use, and then subtracts the amount required to meet current obligations, which is reported under Current Assets.

Long-term Investments

Long-term Investments are investments with a maturity of more than one year. Securities include various types of stocks and bonds and are discussed in more detail in Chapter 8. Since long-term investments should be classified according to their intended purpose, $4,680,000 is shown in the general account Long-Term Investments and $320,000 is shown in the account Long-Term Investments Restricted for Capital Acquisition.

Properties and Equipment, Net

This category of assets represents the major capital investments in the facility. There are three types of assets included in this category: land, plant, and equipment. Plant refers to buildings (fixed, immovable objects), land refers to property, and equipment includes a wide variety of durable items from beds to CAT scanners. Land, plant, and equipment are recorded on the organization's books at cost, and over time, plant and equipment (but not land!) are depreciated. **Depreciation** is an estimate of how much the plant or equipment has been "used up" during the accounting period.

Depreciation: A measure of how much a tangible asset (such as plant or equipment) has been "used up" or consumed.

The word "net" in "Properties and Equipment, Net" means that the total amount of depreciation taken up to this point in time has been subtracted from the original cost. To derive Properties and Equipment, Net, the total amount of depreciation taken since the asset was put into use (called **Accumulated Depreciation**) is subtracted from the original cost of the asset (called Plant and Equipment). Assuming the original cost is $91,161,000 and accumulated depreciation is $40,123,000, Properties and Equipment, Net would be calculated as shown in Exhibit 2–7.

Accumulated Depreciation is the total amount of depreciation taken on an asset since it was put into use.

By convention, plant and equipment are always kept on the books in their own accounts at their original cost until the assets are modified or sold. Similarly, the total amount of depreciation is kept in a separate account, Accumulated Depreciation. In this way, those looking at the balance sheet are always able to know: (1) the original

Exhibit 2–7   Calculation of Properties and Equipment, Net

Account Title	Amount	Explanation
Properties and Equipment	$91,161	The original cost of the land, plant, and equipment.
Less: Accumulated Depreciation	40,123	An estimate of the amount the assets have been "used up." It is equal to the total amount of depreciation taken since the organization acquired the assets. By convention, plant and equipment depreciate, land does not.
Properties and Equipment, Net	$51,038	The original cost minus the amount the assets have been depreciated (used up).

Exhibit 2–8   Liabilities Section of the Balance Sheet from Exhibit 2–3

Liabilities and Net Assets	20X1	20X0
Current Liabilities		
Current Portion of Long-term Debt	$1,470	$1,750
Accounts Payable and Accrued Expenses	5,818	5,382
Estimated Third-party Payor Settlements	2,143	1,942
Deferred Revenues	1,969	2,114
Total Current Liabilities	11,400	11,188
Non-current Liabilities		
Long-term Debt, Net of Current Portion	23,144	24,014
Other	3,953	3,166
Total Non-current Liabilities	27,097	27,180
Total Liabilities	38,497	38,368

Source: Reprinted with permission from the Audit and Accounting Guide: Health Care Organizations, copyright © 1996 by the American Institute of Certified Public Accountants, Inc.

cost of the assets; (2) how much they have been depreciated; and (3) their current book value (original cost less depreciation).

Other Assets

Other Assets is a catchall account used for those non-current assets not included in the other categories of non-current assets.

Liabilities

Current Liabilities:
Financial obligations
due within one year.

The preceding section focused on how assets are presented on the balance sheet. We now turn to a discussion of the liabilities of a health care organization. **Liabilities** are the obligations of a health care provider to pay its creditors. As with assets, liabilities are divided into two categories: current and non–current (see Exhibit 2–8).

Current Liabilities

Current liabilities are the financial obligations that, due to their contractual terms, will be paid within one year. Common account categories include:

- Current Portion of Long-term Debt.
- Accounts Payable and Accrued Expenses.
- Estimated Third-party Payor Settlements.
- Other Current Liabilities.

Each of these accounts is discussed below.

Current Portion of Long-term Debt

This account contains the amount of the organization's long-term debt that is expected to be paid off within one year. For example, if a home health agency has executed a five-year note payable, the principal amount due this year is reported in this account. The remainder is listed under non-current liabilities. This information is sometimes reported in the account Notes Payable, which reports the amount of short-term (less than one year) obligations for which a formal note has been signed.

Accounts Payable and Accrued Expenses

Accounts Payable are obligations to pay suppliers who have sold the health care organization goods or services on credit. Accrued Expenses are expenses that arise in the normal course of business which have not yet been paid. Included in this category are salaries, wages, and interest. Sometimes accrued expenses are presented in separate accounts, such as:

- Salaries and Wages Payable.
- Interest Payable.

Key Point Accrued expenses are liabilities, and are reflected in the balance sheet and not in the statement of operations.

Estimated Third-party Payor Settlements

This account represents an estimate of funds to be repaid to third-party payors. *Third-party payors* are organizations such as insurance companies and governmental agencies that pay on behalf of patients. This account is necessary because much of the payment process is done using estimates. For example, Medicare (actually, a contractor acting on its behalf) makes periodic payments to a hospital, based on the claims (i.e. bills) it has received and processed. However, the actual rate payable by Medicare to the hospital for some services may not be known until the hospital's fiscal year has been completed and a "cost report" has been submitted to Medicare. As Medicare and Medicaid become more and more fully prospective, settlements should diminish significantly. The amount that appears on the balance sheet under Estimated Third-Party Payor Settlements is an estimate of how much the hospital will need to return to the third parties due to overpayments by the third parties. The estimate is based in large part on the history of such transactions. In addition to amounts based on claims submitted, Estimated Third-party Payor Settlements may also include advances from third parties to support the day-to-day needs of the organization (see Chapter 5). If the provider's experience indicates that third parties need to pay the organization instead, the account Estimated Third-Party Payor Settlements would appear as a current asset similar to accounts receivable, rather than as a current liability.

Third-party Payors: Commonly referred to as third parties, these are organizations that pay on behalf of patients.

Other Current Liabilities

Other Current Liabilities includes all current liabilities not elsewhere presented in the current liabilities section. The accounts summarized in this category may be presented on their own lines or they may be detailed in the notes if they are material in amount. Increasingly, a major item in this account is Deferred Revenues.

Deferred Revenues are fees that have been collected in advance. Although its name implies it is a revenue, it is in fact an obligation. For example, health care organizations receive capitation payments from managed care organizations. Capitated payments are often in the form of a specific amount per member per month (PMPM) and require that the health care organization receiving the capitated payment provide a range of services for the population covered by these payments. When the health care organization receives the capitated payment, it incurs an obligation to provide service. Thus, it records the amount received as an obligation (liability). After the obligation is satisfied (the time the payment covers has passed), the deferred revenue is taken out of the Deferred Revenue account and recorded as revenue.

Non-current Liabilities

Non-current Liabilities: The financial obligations not due within one year.

Non-current Liabilities are obligations that will be paid back over a period longer than one year. Most long-term liabilities fall into two categories: Mortgages Payable and Bonds Payable.

Net Assets

The final category of the balance sheet is Net Assets (see Exhibit 2–9). The term net assets is used to show the community's interest in the assets of the organization. In an investor-owned organization, it equals the stockholders' interest in the organization's assets. It is equal to the organization's assets minus its liabilities. Thus, in not-for-profit health care organizations, the terms in the basic accounting equation are rearranged to derive Net Assets as follows:

Net Assets = Assets – Liabilities

Using the year 20X1 in Exhibit 2–3 as an example, by subtracting the amount of total liabilities ($38,497,000) from the value of the total assets ($115,046,000), Net Assets equals $76,549,000.

Key Point   For not-for-profit health care providers, the net assets section of the balance sheet is analogous to the owner's equity section of a for-profit organization's balance sheet.

Key Point   Although the terms assets and liabilities are used consistently, numerous names have been used for the third section of the balance sheet, including: owners' equity, stockholders' equity, net assets, and fund balance. In any case, the amount reported is equal to the difference between assets and liabilities.

Exhibit 2–9 Net Assets Section of the Balance Sheet from Exhibit 2–3

	20X1	20X0
Net Assets		
Unrestricted	70,846	66,199
Temporarily Restricted	2,115	2,470
Permanently Restricted	3,588	3,533
Total Net Assets	76,549	72,202

Source: Reprinted with permission from the Audit and Accounting Guide: Health Care Organizations, copyright © 1996 by the American Institute of Certified Public Accountants, Inc.

In the presentation of net assets on the balance sheet, not-for-profit health care organizations must categorize net assets into three categories of restrictions:

- Unrestricted Net Assets.
- Temporarily Restricted Net Assets.
- Permanently Restricted Net Assets.

All net assets *not* restricted by donors are considered Unrestricted Net Assets. Net assets that are restricted by donors, on the other hand, must be shown on the balance sheet as temporarily or permanently restricted (see Exhibit 2–10 and Perspective 2–3). An example of a temporary restriction is the donation of land by the county with the provision that the hospital cannot sell it for five years. An example of a permanent restriction is an endowment that allows the health care organization to spend the interest, but never the principal.

Stockholders' Equity

Investor-owned health care organizations use a different form of presentation of the owners' equity section of the balance sheet (see Exhibit 2–11). The terms used in the shareholders' equity section (i.e. *par value of the stock, excess of par value* and *retained earnings*) are quite technical and beyond the scope of this text.

Key Point Stockholders Equity for investor-owned organizations represents the stock and retained earnings.

Exhibit 2–10 Examples of Types of Restrictions on Assets

Temporarily Restricted
Donated land that cannot be sold for five years

Permanently Restricted
An endowment in which only the interest can be spent

PERSPECTIVE 2–3

Charity Finances Healthcare: Donors Are Opening Wallets to Pay for Million-dollar Projects

America's rich tradition of healthcare philanthropy, which waned with the advent of health insurance, is undergoing a revitalization. While philanthropy constitutes a tiny portion of healthcare revenue, some institutions increasingly rely on donations to fund capital projects, research, education, and outreach programs. With operating profits evaporating, philanthropy is becoming a vital funding source and a major concern of hospital chief executives.

"For many years when hospitals were running 5% margins and sometimes 10% margins, philanthropic income was icing on the cake and nobody paid much attention to it," says James DeLauro, vice president of fund development at San Francisco-based Catholic Healthcare West. "But now you've got hospitals struggling to make 1% margins, which is not enough to rebuild and keep up with technology."

A noble cause. Though stingy health plans and soaring costs have tarnished the image of healthcare as a charitable enterprise, some hospital leaders are working to reinforce the image of local healthcare as a noble cause. Max Poll, president and chief executive officer of Scottsdale (Ariz.) Healthcare, spends 20% to 25% of his time on fundraising efforts, such as meeting with potential donors over lunch or giving facility tours. Some weeks, he says, it's as much as half of his time.

The two-hospital system, with revenue of $350 million, typically raises $6 million to $7 million per year. The money has gone to an array of activities, including cancer care and research, a neighborhood outreach bus, capital projects such as a new women's and children's facility, bone density scanners, and nursing scholarships. Still, hospitals generally are struggling to capture their share of the nation's increasing philanthropic wealth. Healthcare fundraising hasn't kept pace with giving in other sectors during the past decade. Giving to all charities has increased nearly 44% to a total of nearly $191 billion since 1990, but the health sector saw an inflation-adjusted increase of 35%, to less than $18 billion.

Healthcare giving suffered in the mid- to late 1990s as a result of for-profit hospital conversions and the creation of regional systems, which alienated contributors, according to the Association for Healthcare Philanthropy, a group that represents fund-raising professionals. Often, the structuring of new foundations was an afterthought in the creation of new systems, says AHP President and CEO William McGinly.

Source: Mary Chris Jaklevic, *Modern Healthcare,* July 31, 2000, p. 26.

Exhibit 2–11   Illustration of the Owners' Equity Section of the Balance Sheet for an Investor-owned Health Care Organization

	20X1	20X0
Shareholders' Equity:		
Common stock, $10 par value; authorized 5,000 shares; issued and outstanding 3,500 shares	$35,000	$35,000
Excess of par value	35,000	35,000
Retained Earnings	6,549	2,202
Total Shareholders' Equity	$76,549	$72,202

Source: Adapted from AICPA Audit and Accounting Guide, Health Care Organizations (new edition). New York NY: American Institute of Certified Public Accountants, Inc., June 1, 1996.

Notes to Financial Statements

The **notes** to the balance sheet are grouped together with the notes of all other financial statements and presented after the financial statements. Although notes might be considered in texts to present somewhat superfluous information, they are an integral part of the financial statements. Since the information in the body of the statement is presented in summary form, additional key information must be presented in the notes. Notes often contain such information as the accounting policies followed by the health care organization, how charity care is determined, the composition of investments, which assets are restricted, the depreciation method used, the market value as well as the initial cost of investments, the maturity and interest rates of the long-term debt, the amount of professional liability insurance for malpractice, and whether there are suits filed against the organization that may adversely affect the financial position of the organization. Exhibit A–8 provides a detailed example of notes in a set of financial statements.

Notes to the financial statements: Notes which follow the four financial statements that provide the reader with key information. The notes for all four financial statements appear together after all four statements have been presented. They are an integral part of the financial statements.

◀THE STATEMENT OF OPERATIONS▶

As opposed to the balance sheet, which summarizes the organization's total assets, liabilities, and net assets at a particular *point in time*, the statement of operations is a summary of the organization's revenues and expenses over a *period of time* (see Exhibit 2–12). The time period is usually the time between statements, such as a quarter, half-year, or fiscal year. The statement of operations is analogous to, but different from, an income statement of a for-profit organization (see Exhibit 2–13). Appendix A contains an example of the financial statements for a for-profit organization. Perspective 2–4 illustrates how the financials of a maker of equipment for the health care industry is used as a barometer of the health care industry as a whole.

Key Point The statement of operations uses the **accrual basis of accounting**, which summarizes how much the organization earned and the resources it used to generate that income during a period of time. It does not use the **cash basis of accounting**, which focuses on the cash that actually came in and went out. This is discussed in detail in the next chapter.

Exhibit 2–12 Comparison of the Time Frame Covered by the Balance Sheet and Statement of Operations

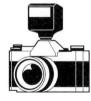

The balance sheet presents a snapshot of the organization as of a point in time.

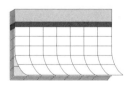

The statement of operations presents a summary of revenues and expenses over a period of time.

Exhibit 2–13   Comparison of the Heading and Major Sections of the Body of the Income Statement for Investor-owned and Not-for-profit Health Care Organizations

	Investor-Owned	**Not-For-Profit**
Title	Income Statement	Statement of Operations
Body	Revenues	Unrestricted Revenues, Gains and Other Support
	– Expenses	– Expenses
	Operating Income	*Operating Income*
	+ Other Income	+ Other Income
	Operating Earnings Before Income Taxes	Excess of Revenues, Gains, and Other Support over Expenses
	– Income Taxes	± Other
	Net Income	*Increase in Unrestricted Net Assets*

Key Point The statement of operations does not represent the cash flow of the organization. Instead, it represents how much the organization earned, its gains and other sources of revenue and the resources it used during the accounting period

The body of the income statement for investor-owned health care organizations is organized into five sections:

- Operating Income.
- Non-operating Income.
- Net Income Before Taxes.
- Provision for Taxes.
- Net Income After Taxes.

The body of the statement of operations for not-for-profit health care organizations includes the following major sections:

- Operating Income.
- Other Income.
- Excess of Revenues, Gains and Other Support over Expenses.
- Other Items.
- Increase in Unrestricted Net Assets.

Exhibit 2–14 is an example of a statement of operations for a not-for-profit health care organization.

This statement does not represent how much cash came into the organization or how much cash went out. Rather, it represents how much the organization earned, its gains and other sources of revenue, and the resources it used during the accounting period. The principle behind focusing on tracking cash and tracking resource use is discussed in detail in Chapter 3.

PERSPECTIVE 2–4

An Industry Barometer

Nestled in the gentle rolling slopes of southern Indiana along a sleepy stretch of the interstate between Indianapolis and Cincinnati, Batesville is to hospital beds and caskets what the Middle East is to oil. Hillenbrand Industries, the deferential company that makes it all happen for this Tudor-style village, found its fortune in the sick and expired.

From its Batesville home, the Fortune 500 company operates two major divisions: Hill-Rom, the hospital bed manufacturer that first "brought the home to the hospital," and Batesville Casket, a company known for no longer calling its products "coffins." ... For years, Hillenbrand has reigned as the undisputed leader in the two major markets. Despite – or because of – these positions, the two units have struggled and thrived along with the industries they supply. ...

People will always get sick and die, but both businesses have their financial downside, especially Hill-Rom. When economics demand that hospitals shed beds and shorten lengths of stay, the town of Batesville suffers from the fallout. As hospitals' capital budgets go, so goes Hill-Rom. "We are kind of like looking at the mercury in the thermometer," says Paul Joyce, Hill-Rom's executive director for North American sales and service administration.

As a result, any clues concerning the long-term survival of the hospital industry might be gleaned from Hill-Rom. Hospital executives may take heart that "after a few rough years," Hill-Rom's outlook is brightening after some internal belt-tightening and external loosening in hospital reimbursements, finds Dhulsini de Zoysa, an analyst with Salomon Smith Barney. ...

The company's financials have remained firmly in the black. Hillenbrand does not break out net income for its operating units, but in 1999, according to its annual report, Hill-Rom earned a gross profit of $402 million on $1.09 billion in revenue from healthcare sales and rentals. Gross profit grew 13% to $454 million on $1.1 billion in 2000. Revenue of $766 million in healthcare sales in 1999 grew to $800 million last year, while revenue from rentals slipped to $312 million in 2000 from $324 million in 1999. Hill-Rom officials say declining revenue in rentals reflects the struggles in the long-term-care and home-care industries. ...

Source: Cinda Becker, *Modern Healthcare,* June 18, 2001.

Unrestricted Revenues, Gains, and Other Support

This section of the statement of operations represents what most people think of as the revenues of the organization (see Exhibit 2–15). Revenues refer to the amounts earned by the organization; Gains come about by selling assets for more than their value on the books (such as selling a building or other investment); and Other Support includes such items as appropriations from governmental organizations and unrestricted donations. Usually Net Patient Service Revenue and Premium Revenue make up the largest portion of Unrestricted Revenues, Gains and Other Support in not-for-profit business organizations.

Key Point — As explained in detail in Chapter 3, revenues represent amounts earned by the organization, not the amount of cash it received during the period.

Net Patient Service Revenues

Gross Patient Service Revenues are the amount the health care organization would have earned if everyone paid full price. However, as discussed under Patient

Exhibit 2–14 Annotated Statement of Operations for Sample Not-For-Profit Hospital

1 The Statement of Operations (also called the *statement of activities*) provides a summary of the organization's revenues and expenses over a period of time.

Title: Gives the name of the organization, the name of the financial statement, and two periods of time for which information is being provided.

2 Unrestricted Revenues, Gains, and Other Support: The income of the organization derived from providing patient service, the sale of assets for more than their book value, contributions, appropriations and assets released from restriction.
- *Net Patient Service Revenues:* Revenues earned from patient care minus the amounts the organization does not expect to collect because of contractual discounts.
- *Premium Revenues:* Revenues earned from capitated contracts.
- *Other Revenues:* Revenues derived from such sources as support services, investments, and certain contributions.
- *Net Assets Released from Restriction:* funds formerly restricted by a donor, now available for general use to run the organization.

3 Expenses: Expenses are a measure of the resources used to generate revenue. (Those expenses listed which are self-evident have not been defined.)
- *Depreciation and Amortization:* Measures of the use of long-lived assets during the accounting period.
- *Provision for Bad Debts:* An estimate of the amount of money owed the organization which it estimates will not be collected.
- *Other:* A catch-all category for miscellaneous expenses and losses including utilities, rent, telephone, travel, etc.

Operating Income: Unrestricted Revenues, Gains, and Other Support minus Expenses and Losses. Traditionally, it is a measure of the income earned from healthcare-related endeavors.

5 Other Income: Income earned from other than healthcare-related endeavors.

6 Excess of Revenues over Expenses: Operating Income plus Other Income. This is analogous to Net Income in for-profit entities.

7 Change in Net Unrealized Gains and Losses on Other than Trading Securities: Changes in the fair value of assets other than trading securities.

8 Net Assets Released from Restrictions Used for Purchase of Property and Equipment: Assets which were previously restricted by a donor, which must now be used to purchase property and equipment. Since they are for the purchase of long-lived assets, they are not considered revenue.

9 Contributions from Sample Hospital Foundation for Property Acquisitions: Self explanatory. Since they are for the purchase of long-lived assets, they are not considered revenue.

10 Transfer to Parent: Transfer of assets from a subsidiary to their parent company.

11 Extraordinary Item: An extremely unusual and infrequent expense.

12 Increase in Unrestricted Net Assets: The increase in unrestricted net assets during the period. It includes operating income, contributions of long-lived assets, transfers to parent and extraordinary items. Restricted revenues are not shown on this financial statement until they become unrestricted.

*An unannotated form of this statement can be found in Appendix A of this chapter.

Sample Not-For Profit Hospital — Statement of Operations — For the Years Ended December 31, 20X1 and 20X0 (in '000)	20X1	20X0
2 Unrestricted Revenues, Gains, and Other Support		
Net Patient Service Revenue	$85,156	$78,942
Premium Revenue	11,150	10,950
Other Revenues	2,601	5,212
Net Assets Released from Restriction Used for Operations	300	0
Total Revenues, Gains and Other Support	99,207	95,104
3 Expenses		
Salaries and Benefits	53,900	49,938
Medical Supplies and Drugs	26,532	22,121
Insurance	8,089	8,526
Depreciation and Amortization	4,782	4,280
Interest	1,752	1,825
4 Provision for Bad Debts	1,000	1,300
Other Expenses	2,000	1,300
Total Expenses	98,055	89,290
5 Operating Income	1,152	5,814
Other Income		
Investment Income	3,900	3,025
6 Excess of Revenues over Expenses	5,052	8,839
7 Change in Net Unrealized Gains and Losses on Other than Trading Securities	300	375
8 Net Assets Released from Restrictions Used for Purchase of Property and Equipment	200	0
9 Contribution from Sample Hospital Foundation for Property Acquisitions	235	485
10 Transfers to Parent	(640)	(3,000)
Increase in Unrestricted Net Assets, Before Extraordinary Item	5,147	6,699
11 Extraordinary Loss (Debt Extinguishment)	(500)	0
12 Increase in Unrestricted Net Assets	$4,647	$6,699

Source: Reprinted with permission from the Audit and Accounting Guide: Health Care Organizations, copyright © 1996 by the American Institute of Certified Public Accountants, Inc.

Exhibit 2–15 Abbreviated Statement of Operations from Exhibit 2–14 Emphasizing Revenues, Gains, and Other Support

	20X1	20X0
Unrestricted Revenues, Gains, and Other Support		
Net Patient Service Revenue	$85,156	$78,942
Premium Revenue	11,150	10,950
Other Revenues	2,601	5,212
Net Assets Released from Restriction Used for Operations	300	
Total Revenues, Gains and Other Support	99,207	95,104
Expenses		
Salaries and Benefits	53,900	49,938
Medical Supplies and Drugs	26,532	22,121
Insurance	8,089	8,526
Depreciation and Amortization	4,782	4,280
Interest	1,752	1,825
Provision for Bad Debts	1,000	1,300
Other Expenses	2,000	1,300
Total Expenses	98,055	89,290
Operating Income	1,152	5,814
Other Income		
Investment Income	3,900	3,025
Excess of Revenues over Expenses	5,052	8,839

Source: Reprinted with permission from the Audit and Accounting Guide: Health Care Organizations, copyright © 1996 by the American Institute of Certified Public Accountants, Inc.

Accounts Receivable, many payors receive discounts, called Contractual Allowances. In addition, most health care organizations also provide some free care to indigent patients, called Charity Care. In reporting Net Patient Service Revenue, a health care organization must subtract amounts both for contractual allowances and for charity care. Thus, the amount reported on the statement of operations is Net Patient Service Revenue, which equals Gross Patient Service Revenues minus Contractual Allowances and Charity Care. For instance, assuming that Gross Patient Service Revenues were $130,284,000, Contractual Allowances $34,898,000, and Charity Care $10,230,000, then the Net Patient Service Revenue for 20X1 would be calculated as shown in Exhibit 2–16.

Premium Revenues

Premium Revenues are revenues earned from capitated contracts. They are not earned solely through the delivery of service, but rather through a combination of the passage of time (during which time the organization is available to provide service when necessary) and actually delivering service as agreed to during the contract period.

Exhibit 2–16   Calculation of Net Patient Service Revenue

Account Title	Amount	Explanation
Gross Patient Service Revenues	$130,284	The amount the health care organization earned at full retail price. This amount cannot be reported on financial statements, since it does not recognize that all payors do not pay full charges.
– Contractual Allowances	34,898	Discounts given to third parties (large-scale purchasers of health care services).
– Charity Care Discounts	10,230	The amount of full charges the organization will not attempt to collect because the patient has been certified as unable to pay. This amount is usually reported only in the footnotes.
Net Patient Service Revenue	$85,156	Full price less contractual allowances and charity care discounts. This amount is reported on the financial statements, for it is felt to be a more realistic estimate of how much revenue the health care organization has actually earned.

Other Revenues

Other Revenues are derived from four major sources: appropriations and grants, support services, income from investments, and revenues from contributions. Appropriations are monies provided by government agencies on an ongoing basis, usually for operating purposes. Grants are funds given to a health care organization for special purposes, usually for a limited time. Support Services include such things as parking fees, cafeteria sales, and revenue from the gift shop. Income from Investments includes unrestricted interest, dividends, and gains from the sale of unrestricted investments. Although some health care organizations report their revenues from support services and investments in this category, it is also possible to report them under Other Income, which is listed after Operating Income (see Exhibit 2–15). This separates revenues earned through health care related activities (termed "Operating Income") and those earned from other than health care related activities (called "Non-Operating Income").

Net Assets Released from Restriction

Net Assets Released from Restriction are funds transferred to unrestricted accounts from temporarily restricted net assets. The income earned from restricted investments and even the investments themselves may be released to unrestricted accounts as certain requirements are met. For example, a donor may stipulate that the release of his or her contribution not occur until after the health care provider raises the required matching funds for a new service line. Net assets released from restrictions that are used to purchase capital items (plant and equipment) are not considered revenues, gains, or other support. They must be reported later in the statement of operations, below Excess of Revenues over Expenses.

Key Point On the statement of operations, expenses are a measure of the amount of resources used or consumed in providing a service, not cash outflows. Using this definition, assets are just expenses waiting to happen!

Expenses

Though most of the expenses listed in Exhibit 2–17 are self-evident, several of them are discussed briefly here.

Depreciation and Amortization

Depreciation and Amortization reflect the amount of a non-current asset used during the accounting period. Depreciation is a measure of how much a tangible asset (such as

Key Point Depreciation and amortization are non-cash expenses.

Exhibit 2–17   Abbreviated Statement of Operations from Exhibit 2–14 Emphasizing Expenses

	20X1	20X0
Unrestricted Revenues, Gains, and Other Support		
Net Patient Service Revenue	$85,156	$78,942
Premium Revenue	11,150	10,950
Other Revenues	2,601	5,212
Net Assets Released from Restriction Used for Operations	300	
Total Revenues, Gains and Other Support	99,207	95,104
Expenses		
Salaries and Benefits	53,900	49,938
Medical Supplies and Drugs	26,532	22,121
Insurance	8,089	8,526
Depreciation and Amortization	4,782	4,280
Interest	1,752	1,825
Provision for Bad Debts	1,000	1,300
Other Expenses	2,000	1,300
Total Expenses	98,055	89,290
Operating Income	1,152	5,814
Other Income		
Investment Income	3,900	3,025
Excess of Revenues over Expenses	5,052	8,839

Source: Reprinted with permission from the Audit and Accounting Guide: Health Care Organizations, copyright © 1996 by the American Institute of Certified Public Accountants, Inc.

Amortization: The allocation of the acquisition cost of debt to the period which it benefits.

a building or equipment) has been "used up" during the accounting period. For example, if a facility buys new examining room equipment for $10,000 and expects it to last 10 years, the accountant might record $1,000 depreciation each year on the assumption that one-tenth of the equipment is "used up" each year. Amortization is a measure of how much of an asset (such as debt issuance cost, capital leases, and goodwill) has been "used up" during the accounting period. Both expenses are non-cash expenses.

Interest

Interest is the cost of borrowing money. If interest is 10 percent per year, then the cost of borrowing $1,000 for one year is $100.

Provision for Bad Debts

Just as a retail business considers bad debts a cost of doing business, so do not-for-profit health care organizations. Provision for Bad Debts, also called Bad Debt Expense or Uncollectibles Expense, is the estimate of Patient Accounts Receivable that will not be collected. It does not include charity care or contractual allowances, for they have already been deducted to derive Patient Accounts Receivable.

Other Expenses

Other Expenses is a catchall category for miscellaneous operating expenses. This category includes all general and administrative expenses, rent, utilities, and contracted services not included in the other categories. Though they are grouped in this example, they may be reported separately.

Operating Income

Operating Income: Income derived from the organization's main line of business.

Operating Income is the income derived from the organization's main line of business: health care. It is calculated by subtracting Expenses from Unrestricted Revenues, Gains and Other Support. In Exhibit 2–14, Operating Income of $1,152,000 in 20X1 is calculated by subtracting Total Expenses of $98,055,000 from Unrestricted Revenues, Gains and Other Support of $99,207,000.

Other Income

Other income includes income earned from activities other than the organization's main line of business. Though there is discretion as to what constitutes operating and non-operating items, interest income, food sales to the public, and parking income are often considered non-operating.

Excess of Revenues over Expenses

Excess of Revenues over Expenses is analogous to Net Income (profit) in a for-profit entity. However, not-for-profit business entities are prohibited from using the more common term, net income. This item, traditionally referred to as *the bottom line* in for-profit entities, is not actually the bottom line in the statement of operations, because accounting rules favor treating not-for-profit, business-oriented health care entities more like traditional not-for-profit organizations than like their for-profit competitors. Thus, there is an emphasis on the change in unrestricted net assets rather than what is traditionally called net income.

Net Income:
Equivalent to Excess of Revenues over Expenses.

Excess of Revenues over Expenses is derived by adding Operating Income and Other Income. In Exhibit 2–17, this is done by adding Operating Income of $1,152,000 and Investment Income of $3,900,000 to get an Excess of Revenues over Expenses of $5,052,000.

Below the Line Items

In addition to the items that contribute to Excess of Revenues over Expenses, several items must appear on the statement of operations below Excess of Revenues over Expenses (see Exhibit 2–18). These are generically referred to as "below the line" items, and include:

- Change in Net Unrealized Gains and Losses on Other than Trading Securities.
- Net Assets Released from Restrictions used for Purchase of Property and Equipment.
- Contributions to Acquire Long-lived Capital Assets.
- Transfer to parent.
- Extraordinary Loss.

Change in Net Unrealized Gains and Losses on Other than Trading Securities

Although the guidelines pertaining to this item are quite complex, for most not-for-profit health care organizations the amount reported here is the change, since the last balance sheet, in the market value of stocks held for investment. It is called *unrealized*, because until the asset is disposed of (i.e. sold), the gain or loss only occurs on the books. Once the investment is disposed of, the gain or loss becomes a *realized* gain or loss.

For example, assume that on the last day of last year an organization purchased $1,000,000 of stock for investment. One year later, the stock is worth $1,300,000. The organization must report a $300,000 *unrealized* gain. On the other hand, if the stocks were sold for $1,300,000 during the last year, the organization would report a $300,000 *realized* gain under either Revenues, Gains, and Other Support or Other

Exhibit 2–18 Statement of Operations from Exhibit 2–14 Emphasizing Items that Do Not Contribute to Excess of Revenues over Expenses

	20X1	20X0
Expenses		
Salaries and Benefits	53,900	49,938
Medical Supplies and Drugs	26,532	22,121
Insurance	8,089	8,526
Depreciation and Amortization	4,782	4,280
Interest	1,752	1,825
Provision for Bad Debts	1,000	1,300
Other Expenses	2,000	1,300
Total Expenses	98,055	89,290
Operating Income	1,152	5,814
Other Income		
Investment Income	3,900	3,025
Excess of Revenues over Expenses	5,052	8,839
Change in Net Unrealized Gains and Losses on Other than Trading Securities	300	375
Net Assets Released from Restrictions Used for Purchase of Property and Equipment	200	
Contribution From Sample Hospital Foundation for Property Acquisitions	235	485
Transfers to Parent	(640)	(3,000)
Increase in Unrestricted Net Assets, before Extraordinary Item	5,147	6,699
Extraordinary Loss (Debt Extinguishment)	(500)	
Increase in Unrestricted Net Assets	$4,647	$6,699

Source: Reprinted with permission from the Audit and Accounting Guide: Health Care Organizations, copyright © 1996 by the American Institute of Certified Public Accountants, Inc.

Income. Note that because of this, *realized* gains affect Excess of Revenues over Expenses, whereas *unrealized* gains do not.

Increases in Long-lived Unrestricted Net Assets

Most increases in unrestricted long-term assets resulting from donations are not considered increases in Revenues, Gains, and Other Support. Rather, they are reported below Excess of Revenues over Expenses in separate accounts. Two examples in the Sample Not-For-Profit Hospital case are:

> **Key Point**
>
> Rather than being reported in Revenues, Gains, and Other Support, increases relating to the donation of unrestricted net assets for capital acquisitions are reported below Excess of Revenues over Expenses.

- Net Assets Released from Restrictions Used for Purchase of Property and Equipment.
- Contributions for the Acquisition of Plant and Equipment.

Transfers to Parent

Another item that affects net assets, but not Excess of Revenues over Expenses, is the transfer of assets to corporate headquarters. In 20X1, Sample Not-For-Profit Hospital transferred $640,000 to its parent corporation.

Extraordinary Items

Extraordinary Items reflect unusual and infrequent gains or losses from such things as paying off loans early, and acts of nature such as hurricanes or earthquakes.

Increase in Unrestricted Net Assets

The final section of the statement of operations is Increase in Unrestricted Net Assets, which is derived by adding or subtracting the remaining items from Net Income, as shown in Exhibit 2–19. There is a subtotal before the extraordinary item so that readers of the financial statements can judge the organization's performance both before and after taking it into account.

◄THE STATEMENT OF CHANGES IN NET ASSETS►

A third financial statement is the statement of changes in net assets. Its purpose is to explain why there was a change from one year to the next in the net asset section of the balance sheet (Exhibit 2–3). There are two major reasons why the net asset section of the balance sheet changes from year to year: increases (decreases) in unrestricted

---

| Key Point | The statement of changes in net assets repeats some of the information found on the statement of operations to explain changes in unrestricted net assets, but adds additional information about changes in restricted net assets. |

Exhibit 2–19 Calculation of Increase in Unrestricted Net Assets

Excess of Revenues over Expenses	5,052
+ Change in Net Unrealized Gains and Losses on Other than Trading Securities	300
+ Net Assets Released from Restrictions Used for Purchase of Property and Equipment	200
+ Contribution from Sample Hospital for Property Acquisitions	235
− Transfers to Parent	(640)
Increase in Unrestricted Net Assets, before Extraordinary Item	5,147
− Extraordinary Loss (Debt Extinguishment)	(500)
Increase in Unrestricted Net Assets	$4,647

net assets (as shown on the statement of operations, Exhibit 2–14), and changes in restricted net assets, which are not included on the statement of operations. Thus, the statement of changes in net assets goes beyond the statement of operations by summarizing all the changes in net assets over the year.

Like the other statements, the statement of changes in net assets has a descriptive heading, a body, and notes. The body of the statement of changes in net assets is organized to represent the changes in each of the three categories of restrictions of net assets: unrestricted, temporarily restricted, and permanently restricted (see Exhibit 2–20). The information in the first section, Unrestricted Net Assets, summarizes the information from the statement of operations. The information in the remainder of the statement of changes in net assets reflects changes in restricted accounts.

To illustrate, the Statement of Changes in Net Assets explains how unrestricted net assets, temporarily restricted net assets, and permanently restricted net assets of Sample-Not-For-Profit-Hospital (see Exhibit 2–3) changed from 20X0 to 20X1.

Changes in Unrestricted Net Assets

Unrestricted Net Assets (see Exhibit 2–20) come directly from the statement of operations. During the year 20X1, Sample Not-For-Profit Hospital made $5,052,000, had an unrealized gain of $300,000 on its investments, received a $235,000 donation of funds to be used for property acquisitions, transferred $640,000 to its parent corporation, released from restriction $200,000 worth of temporarily restricted net assets to be used for the purchase of property and equipment, and lost $500,000 from debt extinguishment, producing an increase in unrestricted net assets of $4,647,000.

Changes in Temporarily Restricted Net Assets

During 20X1, Sample Not-For-Profit Hospital received $140,000 in restricted contributions to pay for charity care, made $5,000 (net) in unrealized and realized gains on temporarily restricted investments, and released $500,000 from temporary restrictions. Since it is to be used for operations, $300,000 of the $500,000 is shown as an increase in Unrestricted Revenues, Gains and Other Support on the statement of operations under the category Net Assets Released from Restriction Used for Operations (see Exhibit 2–14). The $200,000 is also shown below Excess of Revenues over Expenses in the Net Assets Released from Restrictions Used for Purchase of Properties and Equipment account since it is to be used for the acquisition of long-lived assets.

Key Point The "unrestricted" section of the statement of changes in net assets shows how the various items on the statement of operations contributed to the changes in unrestricted net assets.

Exhibit 2–20 Statement of Changes in Net Assets for Sample Not-For-Profit Hospital

Sample Not-For-Profit Hospital
Statement of Changes in Net Assets For the Years Ended December 31, 20X1 and 20X0 (in '000)

	20X1	20X0
Unrestricted Net Assets		
Excess of Revenues over Expenses	$5,052	$8,839
Net Unrealized Gains on Investments Other than Trading Securities	300	375
Contribution from Sample Hospital Foundation for Property Acquisition	235	485
Transfers to Parent	(640)	(3,000)
Net Assets Released from Restrictions Used for Purchase of Properties and Equipment	200	
Increase in Unrestricted Net Assets before Extraordinary Item	5,147	6,699
Extraordinary Loss from Extinguishment of Debt	(500)	
Increase in Unrestricted Net Assets	4,647	6,699
Temporarily Restricted Net Assets		
Contributions for Charity Care	140	996
Net Realized and Unrealized Gains on Investments	5	8
Net Assets Released from Restrictions	(500)	
Increase (Decrease) in Temporarily Restricted Net Assets	(355)	1,004
Permanently Restricted Net Assets		
Contributions for Endowment Funds	50	411
Net Realized and Unrealized Gains on Investments	5	2
Increase in Permanently Restricted Net Assets	55	413
Increase in Net Assets	4,347	8,116
Net Assets, Beginning of Year	72,202	64,086
Net Assets, End of Year	$76,549	$72,202

Source: Reprinted with permission from the Audit and Accounting Guide: Health Care Organizations, copyright © 1996 by the American Institute of Certified Public Accountants, Inc.

Changes in Permanently Restricted Net Assets

For Sample Not-For-Profit Hospital, the only two changes in permanently restricted net assets in 20X1 were an increase of $50,000 for a permanently restricted endowment and $5,000 (net) in unrealized and realized gains on permanently restricted assets (see Exhibit 2–20).

◀THE STATEMENT OF CASH FLOWS▶

The fourth and final major financial statement is the statement of cash flows, which answers the question "Where did cash come from and where did it go?" Though the statement of operations (income statement) may be thought to answer this question, it does not. As noted earlier, it answers the questions "How much was earned?" (not "How much

cash came in?") and "What resources were used?" (not "How much cash went out?").
Hence, the statement of cash flows was developed to report the cash inflows and outflows.

Like the other statements, the statement of cash flows has a descriptive heading, a body, and notes (see Exhibit 2–21). The statement of cash flows covers the same time period as does the statement of operations and the statement of changes in net assets.

The body of the statement is organized into the following sections:

- Cash Flows from Operating Activities.
- Cash Flows from Investing Activities.
- Cash Flows from Financing Activities.
- Net Increase (Decrease) in Cash and Cash Equivalents.

The statement also discloses key non-cash transactions such as the issuance of stock for debt payment or for the acquisition of a company. Though there are two alternative forms of this statement, the most common, called the *indirect method*, has been presented here. The other format is called the *direct method*. The first section of this statement is cash flows from operating activities.

Cash Flows from Operating Activities

This section identifies the cash inflows and outflows resulting from the normal operations of the organization. Since most organizations do not have this information readily available, they derive it by starting with the increase (decrease) in net assets from the statement of changes in net assets, and then make adjustments to convert this accrual-based information into cash flows.

Key Point Cash Flows from Operating Activities identifies cash flow from normal operations of the organization.

Assume for the purposes of illustration that the organization began with no assets or liabilities. During the first week in operation, only two transactions occurred: $150,000 worth of services rendered, and patients paid $50,000 of this amount. Thus, the balance sheet would show Cash of $50,000, Patient Accounts Receivable of $100,000 and Net Assets of $150,000. Hence, the increase in net assets since the last period was $150,000 (see Exhibit 2–22).

However, to estimate cash flows from operations, net assets must be adjusted for changes in accounts that really do not result in cash inflows or outflows. In this case, the $100,000 that is still owed from the $150,000 in Changes in Net Assets is subtracted to determine how much cash actually came in ($150,000 - $100,000 = $50,000). This process occurs in order to convert the Changes in Net Assets account, which was derived using the accrual basis of accounting, into an estimate of actual cash flows: Net Cash Provided from Operating Activities.

Exhibit 2–21 Annotated Statement of Cash Flows for Sample Not-For-Profit Hospital

The Statement of Cash Flows provides a summary of the cash inflows and outflows form one year to the next.

❶ Title: Gives the name of the organization, the name of the financial statement and two periods for which the information is being provided.

❷ Cash Flows from Operating Activities: This section explains the changes in cash resulting from the normal operating activities of the organization. It begins by presenting the change in net assets from the *statement of changes in net assets*. However, since the *statement of changes in net assets* was prepared on the *accrual basis of accounting* to show revenues when earned, not when cash was received, and expenses when resources were used rather than when they were paid, the remainder of this section makes adjustments to convert the changes in current assets and liabilities and other operating accounts to actual cash flows. This is explained in more detail in the next chapter.

❸ Cash Flows from Investing Activities: This section explains cash inflows and outflows of the organization resulting from investing activities such as purchasing and selling investments, or investing in itself such as purchasing or selling plant, property, or equipment.

❹ Cash Flows from Financing Activities: This section explains cash inflows and outflows resulting from financing activities such as obtaining grants and endowments, or from borrowing or paying back long-term debt. It also includes transfers to and from the parent corporation.

❺ Net Increase (Decrease) in Cash and Cash Equivalents: The total of cash flows from operating, investing and financing activities.

❻ Cash and Cash Equivalents at Beginning of Year: The amount of cash and cash equivalents which the organization had at the beginning of the year.

❼ Cash and Cash Equivalents at End of Year: The total of net increases in cash and cash equivalents at the end of the year. It is the same number that appears under this title on the balance sheet.

❽ Supplemental Information: Additional information of use to the reader of the statement.

An unannotated form of this statement can be found in Appendix A of this chapter.

Sample Not-For-Profit Hospital
Statement of Cash Flows (Indirect Method)
For the Years Ended December 31, 20X1 and 20X0 (in '000)

	20X1	20X0
❷ Cash Flows From Operating Activities		
Change in Net Assets	$4,347	$8,116
Adjustments to Reconcile Change in Net Assets to Net Cash Provided by Operating Activities:		
Extraordinary Loss from Debt Extinguishment	500	
Depreciation	4,782	4,280
Net Realized and Unrealized Gains on Investments, Other than Trading	(450)	(575)
Transfers to Parent	640	3,000
Provision for Bad Debt	1,000	1,300
Restricted Contributions and Investment Income Received	(55)	(413)
Increase (Decrease) in:		
Patient Accounts Receivable	(1,906)	(2,036)
Trading Securities	215	
Other Current Assets	186	(2,481)
Other Assets	(325)	(241)
Increase (Decrease) in:		
Accounts Payable and Accrued Expenses	436	679
Estimated Third-Party Payor Settlements	201	305
Other Current Liabilities	(145)	(257)
Other Liabilities	787	(128)
Net Cash Provided by Operating Activities	10,213	11,549
❸ Cash flows from investing activities:		
Purchases of Investment	(3,769)	(2,150)
Capital Expenditures	(4,728)	(5,860)
Net Cash Used in Investing Activities	(8,497)	(8,010)
❹ Cash flows from financing activities:		
Transfer to Parent	(640)	(3,000)
Proceeds from Restricted Contributions and Restricted Investment Income	55	413
Payments on Long-Term Debt	(24,700)	(804)
Payments on Capital Lease Obligations	(150)	(100)
Increase in Long-Term Debt	22,600	500
Net Cash Used in Financing Activities	(2,835)	(2,991)
❺ Net Increase (Decrease) in Cash and Cash Equivalents	(1,119)	548
❻ Cash and Cash Equivalents at Beginning of Year	5,877	5,329
❼ Cash and Cash Equivalents at End of Year	$4,758	$5,877

❽ Supplemental Disclosures and Cash Flow Information:
The Hospital entered into capital lease obligations in the amount of $600,000 for new equipment in 2001.
Cash paid for interest (net of amount capitalized) in 2001 and 2000 was $1,780,000 and $1,856,000 respectively.
See accompanying notes to financial statements.

Source: Reprinted with permission from the Audit and Accounting Guide: Health Care Organizations, copyright © 1996 by the American Institute of Certified Public Accountants, Inc.

Cash Flows from Investing Activities

The second section of the statement of cash flows is Cash Flows from Investing Activities. This section shows cash inflows and outflows from such accounts as:

 Key Point   Investing by an organization includes investing in itself (such as when an organization buys new equipment).

- Purchase of Plant, Property, and Equipment.
- Purchase of Long-term Investments.
- Proceeds from Sale of Plant, Property and Equipment.
- Proceeds from Sale of Long-term Investments.

Information found in this section is derived from changes in the Non-Current Assets section of the balance sheet from one period to the next. It reports both the purchase and/or sale of outside investments and the purchase and/or sale of non-current assets, such as plant and equipment, which will be used to provide services. In the latter case, the organization is investing in itself.

Cash Flows from Financing Activities

In this section of the statement of cash flows, we identify the changes in cash flows resulting from financing activities. These include:

 Key Point   Repayment and Issuance of Long-term Debt are identified in Cash Flow from Financing Activities within the Statement of Cash Flows.

- Transfers to and from Parent.
- Proceeds from Selected Contributions.
- Proceeds from Issuance of Long-term Debt.
- Repayment of Long-term Debt.
- Interest from Restricted Investments if Interest Income Is Also Restricted.

Cash and Cash Equivalents at the End of the Year

This is the "bottom line" of the statement of cash flows and is the same as the Cash and Cash Equivalents amount that appears on the balance sheet. The latter is calculated by adding the net increase (decrease) in cash and cash equivalents for the year to the beginning balance of the cash and cash equivalents. The net increase (decrease) in Cash and Cash Equivalents for the year on the statement of cash flows is computed by adding

Exhibit 2-22 Deriving Net Cash Provided by Operating Activities by Adjusting Change in Net Assets for Items that Do Not Affect Cash Flows

Sample Not-For-Profit Hospital
Balance Sheet
January 7, 20X1 and January 1, 20X1

	1/7/20X1	1/1/20X1		1/7/20X1	1/1/20X1
Cash	$50,000	$0	Liabilities	$0	$0
Patient Accounts Receivable	100,000	0	Net Assets	150,000	0
Total Assets	$150,000	$0	Liabilities and Net Assets	$150,000	$0

Sample Not-For-Profit Hospital
Statement of Cash Flows
For the Period Ended January 7, 20X1

	1/7/20X1	1/1/20X1
Cash Flows from Operating Activities		
Changes in Net Assets	$150,000	$0
Increase in Patient Accounts Receivable	100,000	0
Net Cash Provided by Operating Activities	$50,000	$0

together the cash flows from the operating, investing, and financing activities, respectively. In Exhibit 2–21, the Cash and Cash Equivalents at the end of 20X1 is $4,758,000.

◀SUMMARY▶

This chapter examined the four major statements of not-for-profit, business-oriented health care organizations: the balance sheet, the statement of operations, the statement of changes in net assets, and the statement of cash flows. Each of these statements is organized in the same fashion, with a heading, a body, and notes. The notes are grouped together and presented after all four statements have been provided. They are considered an integral part of the financial statements.

The balance sheet presents a snapshot of the organization at a point in time (usually the last day of the year). The body of the balance sheet has three major sections: assets, liabilities, and net assets. The balance sheet is so named because **assets = liabilities + owners' equity**. This fundamental accounting equation is expressed as **assets = liabilities + shareholders' equity** in investor-owned health care organizations and **assets = liabilities + net assets** in not-for-profit, business-oriented health care organizations.

Assets are the resources of the organization, liabilities are the obligations of the organization to pay its creditors, and net assets are the difference between assets and liabilities. Assets are divided into two main sections: current and non-current. Current assets will be used or consumed within one year. Non-current assets will provide benefit to the organization for periods longer than one year. Assets limited as to use are noted separately from those without such restrictions.

Liabilities are also classified into current and non-current categories. Current liabilities are those that must be paid within one year. Non-current liabilities will be due in more than one year. If part of a liability, such as a mortgage, is due within one year and the rest is due beyond one year, then the part due within one year is classified in the current section, and the remainder is presented under non-current liabilities. Revenues received in advance, such as capitated fees, are liabilities, classified as deferred revenues. They are considered liabilities because the organization has the obligation to deliver service. They are not recognized as revenues until they are earned.

Net assets are the owners' interest in the entity's assets. The owners of not-for-profit entities are generally assumed to be the community. Net assets are presented in three categories: unrestricted, temporarily restricted, and permanently restricted. Unrestricted net assets are not constrained by donors. Restricted net assets are funds that have limitations imposed on them by outside donors.

The statement of operations is analogous to, but not quite the same as, the traditional income statement. Rather than showing how much cash came in or went out, the body of the statement of operations summarizes the changes in unrestricted net assets during a period of time (usually a year). Excess of revenues over expenses is comparable to, but not the same as, the bottom line (net income) in for-profit health care organizations. It is determined by adding operating income and other (non-operating) income. Operating income comprises the organization's unrestricted revenues, gains, and other support less its expenses. Operating income is the income derived from the primary line of business, in this case health care related services, whereas non-operating income is income from all other sources. In addition to the accounts that comprise excess of revenues over expenses, there are a number of "below the line" items that affect the change in unrestricted net assets, but not excess of revenues over expenses. These generally relate to donations of long-lived assets, realized and unrealized gains or losses on other than trading securities, and transfers to parent. Occasionally, there may be an extraordinary item.

The third financial statement is the statement of changes in net assets, which is called the statement of changes in owners' equity in for-profit entities. It summarizes why the net asset account changed during the period covered by the statement of operations, by showing why each of the three main categories of net assets changed: unrestricted net assets, temporarily restricted net assets, and permanently restricted net assets.

The final financial statement of not-for-profit health care organizations is the statement of cash flows. Its purpose is to summarize where the organization's cash came from and how it was spent during the year. It summarizes cash flows in three major categories: cash flows from operating activities, cash flows from investing activities, and cash flows from financing activities. This statement is necessary since the statement of operations is based on the accrual basis of accounting and keeps track of earnings and resources when used, but not actual cash flows.

◄KEY TERMS►

ACCUMULATED DEPRECIATION	DEPRECIATION	NON-CURRENT LIABILITIES
AMORTIZATION	FUND BALANCE	NOTES TO THE FINANCIAL
ASSETS	LIABILITIES	STATEMENTS
BASIC ACCOUNTING EQUATION	LIQUIDITY	OPERATING INCOME
CHARITY CARE DISCOUNTS	NET ASSETS	OWNERS' EQUITY
CURRENT ASSETS	NET INCOME	SHAREHOLDERS' EQUITY
CURRENT LIABILITIES	NON-CURRENT ASSETS	THIRD-PARTY PAYORS

◄KEY EQUATIONS►

General Accounting Equation: Assets = Liabilities + Owners' Equity

Basic Accounting Equation (not-for-profit entities): Assets = Liabilities + Net Assets

Basic Accounting Equation (for-profit entities): Assets = Liabilities + Shareholders' Equity

◀Questions and Problems▶

1. **Definitions.** Define the following terms:
   a. Accumulated Depreciation.
   b. Amortization.
   c. Assets.
   d. Basic Accounting Equation.
   e. Charity Care Discounts.
   f. Current Assets.
   g. Current Liabilities.
   h. Depreciation.
   i. Fund Balance.
   j. Liabilities.
   k. Liquidity.
   l. Net Assets.
   m. Net Income.
   n. Non-current Assets.
   o. Non-current Liabilities.
   p. Notes to the Financial Statements.
   q. Operating Income.
   r. Owners' Equity.
   s. Shareholders' Equity.
   t. Third-party Payors.

2. **Financial Statement Terminology.**
   a. What are each of the major financial statements commonly called in for-profit health care organizations and in not-for-profit health care organizations?
   b. Describe the three major sections common to all financial statements.

3. **Balance Equation.** State the primary accounting equation that describes the balance sheet of a not-for-profit, business-oriented health care organization.

4. **Balance Sheet.** The following questions relate to the balance sheet.
   a. What is the name of this statement in not-for-profit health care organizations?
   b. What are its main sections in investor-owned health care organizations?
   c. What are its main sections in not-for-profit health care organizations?
   d. What are patient accounts receivable?
   e. What is deferred revenue?
   f. What are restricted net assets?

5. **Statement of Operations.** The following questions relate to the statement of operations of not-for-profit health care organizations.
   a. What is the analogous for-profit statement called? What are the main sections of the statement of operations?
   b. What are revenues, gains, and other support?
   c. What are expenses and losses?

    d. Funds released from restricted net assets to unrestricted net assets are presented in what section of the statement of revenue, expenses, and other activities?

6. **Statement of Changes in Net Assets.** The following questions relate to the statement of changes in net assets.
   a. What is the traditional name for this statement?
   b. What is the purpose of this statement?
   c. What are the main sections of this statement?
   d. Discuss the difference between permanently restricted and temporarily restricted net assets.

7. **Statement of Cash Flows.** The following questions relate to the statement of cash flows of a not-for-profit health care organization.
   a. What are its main sections?
   b. What is the purpose of this statement?

8. **Financial Statement Element.** Where in the financial statements would there be important explanatory information?

9. **Financial Statement Element.** In what financial statement would one identify the purchase of long-term investments?

10. **Accounting Methodologies.** How does the accrual basis of accounting differ from the cash basis of accounting?

11. **Balance Sheet.** The following are account balances as of September 30, 20X1 for Zachary Hospital. Prepare a balance sheet at September 30, 20X1 (hint: Net Assets will also need to be calculated).

Gross Plant, Property and Equipment	$6,000,000
Cash	$180,000
Net Accounts Receivable	$650,000
Accrued Expenses	$35,000
Supplies	$100,000
Long-term Debt	$5,000,000
Accounts Payable	$130,000
Accumulated Depreciation	$100,000

12. **Balance Sheet.** The following are account balances as of September 30, 20X1 for Shoemaker Hospital. Prepare a balance sheet at September 30, 20X1 (hint: Net Assets will also need to be calculated).

Gross Plant, Property, and Equipment	$6,000,000
Accrued Expenses	$35,000
Cash	$180,000
Net Accounts Receivable	$650,000
Accounts Payable	$130,000
Long-term Debt	$5,000,000
Supplies	$100,000
Accumulated Depreciation	$100,000

13. **Statement of Operations.** The following are annual account balances as of September 30, 20X1 for Vantage Hospital. Prepare a statement of operations for the 12-month period ending September 30, 20X1.

Net Patient Revenues	$840,000
Transfer to Parent Corporation	$10,000
Net Assets Released from Restriction for Operations	$120,000
Depreciation Expense	$50,000
Labor Expense	$230,000
Interest Expense	$12,000
Supply Expense	$88,000

14. **Statement of Operations.** The following are annual account balances as of September 30, 20X1 for Uptown Hospital. Prepare a statement of operations for the twelve-month period ending September 30, 20X1.

Net Patient Revenues	$960,000
Supply Expense	$65,000
Net Assets Released from Restriction for Operations	$35,000
Depreciation Expense	$45,000
Transfer to Parent Corporation	$12,000
Interest Expense	$16,000
Labor Expense	$400,000

15. **Multiple Statements.** The following are account balances as of September 30, 20X1 for Hightower Outpatient Center. Prepare: (a) balance sheet; (b) statement of operations; and (c) statement of changes in net assets for September 30, 20X1.

Insurance Expense	$25,000
Cash	$100,000
Net Patient Revenues	$600,000
Net Accounts Receivable	$560,000
Ending Balance, Temporarily Restricted Net Assets	$25,000
Wages Payable	$50,000
Prepaid Expenses	$20,000
Long-term Debt	$493,000
Supply Expense	$80,000
Gross Plant, Property, and Equipment	$500,000
Net Assets Released from Temporary Restrictions	$15,000
Depreciation Expense	$5,000
General Expense	$100,000
Transfer to Parent Corporation	$15,000
Beginning Balance, Unrestricted Net Assets	$495,000
Accounts Payable	$100,000
Beginning Balance, Temporarily Restricted Net Assets	$40,000
Interest Expense	$8,000
Labor Expense	$350,000

Accumulated Depreciation	$10,000
Restricted Net Assets	$25,000
Unrestricted Net Assets	$527,000

16. **Multiple Statements.** The following are account balances at September 30, 20X1 for Valley Medical Center. Prepare: (a) balance sheet; (b) statement of operations; and (c) statement of changes in net assets for September 30, 20X1.

Administrative Expense	$350,000
Cash	$20,000
Net Patient Revenues	$960,000
Gross Accounts Receivable	$225,000
Ending Balance, Temporarily Restricted Net Assets	$8,000
Wages Payable	$35,000
Prepaid Expenses	$5,000
Long-term Debt	$650,000
Supply Expense	$200,000
Gross Plant, Property, and Equipment	$800,000
Net Assets Released from Temporary Restriction	$35,000
Less Uncollectibles in Accounts Receivable	$15,000
Inventory	$20,000
Premium Revenues	$150,000
Long-term Investments, Unrestricted	$35,000
Depreciation Expense	$15,000
General Expense	$100,000
Transfer to Parent Corporation	$5,000
Beginning Balance, Unrestricted Net Assets	$474,000
Accounts Payable	$78,000
Beginning Balance, Temporarily Restricted Net Assets	$43,000
Interest Expense	$8,000
Labor Expense	$700,000
Accumulated Depreciation	$45,000
Long-term Investments, Restricted	$8,000
Ending Balance, Unrestricted Net Assets	$247,000
Accrued Expense	$65,000
Temporary Investments	$45,000
Other Revenues	$6,000
Current Portion of Long-term Debt	$15,000

17. **Statement of Cash Flows.** The following are account balances at December 31, 20X1 for Southern Memorial Hospital. Prepare a statement of cash flows for year ended December 31, 20X1. (Hint: the amounts have been stated as positive or negative numbers as they affect cash flow.)

Decrease in Prepaid Expenses	$2,000
Payments on Long-term Debt	($30,000)
Cash and Cash Equivalents at Beginning of the Year	$40,000
Increase in Inventory	($5,000)

Increases in Long-term Debt	$200,000
Decrease in Accrued Expenses	($1,000)
Change in Net Assets	($30,000)
Sale of Long-term Investments	$750,000
Increase in Other Current Liabilities	$4,000
Depreciation	$150,000
Payments on Capital Lease	($25,000)
Purchases of Equipment	($1,000,000)
Increase in Net Account Receivables	($30,000)
Increase in Accounts Payable	$20,000

18. **Statement of Cash Flows.** The following are account balances (in '000) at December 31, 20X1 for Lionville Hospital. Prepare a statement of cash flows for the year ended December 31, 20X1. (Hint: the amounts have been stated as positive or negative numbers as they affect cash flow.)

Increase in Prepaid Expenses	($3,000)
Increase in Accrued Expenses	$8,000
Cash and Cash Equivalents at Beginning of the Year	$65,000
Increase of Capital Lease Obligation	$85,000
Proceeds from Restricted Contribution	$155,000
Change in Net Assets	$50,000
Increase in Net Account Receivables	($90,000)
Sale of Equipment	$40,000
Decrease in Other Current Liabilities	($3,000)
Depreciation	$75,000
Increase in Inventory	($13,000)
Purchase of Long-term Investments	($75,000)
Payments on Long-term Debt	($90,000)
Decrease in Accounts Payable	($15,000)

19. **Multiple Statements.** The following are account balances for Burlington HMO (in '000). Prepare: (a) balance sheet; and (b) income statement for the year ended December 31, 20X0.

Income Tax Benefit of Operating Loss	$7,500
Net Property and Equipment	$22,000
Physician Services Expense	$35,000
Premium Revenue	$90,000
Marketing Expense	$8,000
Compensation Expense	$17,000
Interest Income and Other Revenue	$20,000
Outside Referral Expense	$15,000
Medicare Revenue	$25,000
Occupancy and Depreciation Expense	$4,000
Current Portion of Long-term Debt	$3,200
Accounts Receivable	$6,100
Emergency Room Expense	$7,000

Inpatient Services Expense	$131,000
Interest Expense	$3,000
Medicaid Revenue	$5,000
Owners' equity	$13,300
Cash and Cash Equivalents	$2,800
Long-term Debt	$14,400
Other Administrative Expense	$3,000

20. **Multiple Statements.** The following are account balances (in '000) at September 30, 20X1 for HMO Scotland. Prepare: (a) balance sheet; and (b) income statement.

Income Tax Expense	$2,100
Prepaid Expense	$2,000
Physician Services Expense	$38,000
Long-term Investments	$12,000
Premium Revenues	$118,000
Cash and Cash Equivalents	$68,000
Marketing Expense	$12,500
Compensation Expense	$23,000
Other Non-current Assets	$2,800
Interest Income and Other Revenue	$4,500
Accrued Expense	$3,300
Outside Referral Expense	$7,500
Claims Payable – Medical	$37,000
Medicare Revenues	$13,000
Inventory	$3,500
Occupancy and Depreciation Expense	$5,500
Owners' equity	$66,600
Emergency Room Expense	$3,200
Net Property and Equipment	$13,000
Premium Receivables	$12,000
Inpatient Service Expense	$22,000
Notes Payable	$4,500
Interest Expense	$2,500
Unearned Premium Revenues	$1,500
Medicaid Revenues	$3,000
Long-term Debt	$3,400
Other Administrative Expense	$6,500
Other Receivables	$3,000

21. **Multiple Statements.** The following are account balances at September 30, 20X1 for Appleton Medical Center. Prepare: (a) balance sheet; (b) statement of operations; and (c) statement of changes in net assets for September 30, 20X1.

| Inventory | $12,000 |
| Net Patient Revenues | $898,000 |

Gross Plant, Property, and Equipment	$655,000
Net Accounts Receivable	$235,000
Ending Balance, Temporarily Restricted Net Assets	$20,000
Wages Payable	$45,000
Long-term Debt	$248,100
Supply Expense	$82,000
Net Assets Released from Temporary Restriction	$8,000
Depreciation Expense	$12,000
General Expense	$122,000
Insurance Expense	$26,000
Cash and Cash Equivalents	$85,000
Transfer to Parent Corporation	($8,900)
Beginning Balance, Unrestricted Net Assets	$234,000
Accounts Payable	$76,000
Beginning Balance, Temporarily Restricted Net Assets	$28,000
Interest Expense	$4,200
Labor Expense	$322,000
Accumulated Depreciation	$125,000
Long-term Investments Restricted	$90,000
Ending Balance, Unrestricted Net Assets	$562,900

22. **Multiple Statements.** The following are account balances at September 30, 20X1 for Shively Medical Center. Prepare: (a) balance sheet; (b) statement of operations; and (c) statement of changes in net assets for September 30, 20X1.

Inventory	$10,000
Net Patient Revenues	$1,000,000
Gross Plant, Property, and Equipment	$755,000
Net Accounts Receivable	$225,000
Ending Balance, Temporarily Restricted Net Assets	$6,000
Wages Payable	$25,000
Long-term Debt	$445,000
Supply Expense	$60,000
Net Assets Released from Temporary Restriction	$12,000
Depreciation Expense	$45,000
General Expense	$200,000
Insurance Expense	$35,000
Cash and Cash Equivalents	$50,000
Transfer to Parent Corporation	($13,000)
Beginning Balance, Unrestricted Net Assets	$200,000
Accounts Payable	$66,000
Beginning Balance, Temporarily Restricted Net Assets	$18,000
Interest Expense	$6,000
Labor Expense	$400,000
Accumulated Depreciation	$125,000
Long-term Investments Restricted	$80,000
Ending Balance, Unrestricted Net Assets	$453,000

23. **Multiple Statements.** The following are account balances at September 30, 20X1 for El Paso Outpatient Center. Prepare: (a) balance sheet; (b) statement of operations; and (c) statement of changes in net assets for September 30, 20X1.

Insurance Expense	$35,000
Cash	$75,000
Net Patient Revenues	$980,000
Net Accounts Receivable	$850,000
Ending Balance, Temporarily Restricted Net Assets	$23,000
Wages Payable	$24,000
Prepaid Expense	$25,000
Long-term Debt	$581,000
Supply Expense	$75,000
Gross Plant, Property, and Equipment	$735,000
Net Assets Released from Temporary Restriction	$17,000
Depreciation Expense	$12,000
General Expense	$125,000
Transfer to Parent Corporation	($11,000)
Beginning Balance, Unrestricted Net Assets	$500,000
Accounts Payable	$85,000
Beginning Balance, Temporarily Restricted Net Assets	$40,000
Interest Expense	$3,000
Labor Expense	$344,000
Accumulated Depreciation	$125,000
Long-term Investments Restricted	$45,000
Ending Balance, Unrestricted Net Assets	$892,000

Appendix A

Illustrative Set of Financial Statements for Sample Not-For-Profit Hospital and For-Profit Hospital, and Notes to Financial Statements

Exhibit A–1   Balance Sheet for Sample Not-For-Profit Hospital

Sample Not-For-Profit Hospital
Balance Sheet
December 31, 20X1 and 20X0 (in '000)

Assets	20X1	20X0
Current Assets:		
Cash and Cash Equivalents	$4,758	$5,877
Short-Term Investments	15,836	10,740
Assets Limited as to Use	970	1,300
Patient Accounts Receivable, Net Estimated		
Uncollectibles of $2,500 in 20X1 and $2,400 in 20X0	15,100	14,194
Supplies	2,000	2,000
Prepaid Expenses	670	856
Total Current Assets	39,334	34,967
Non-Current Assets		
Assets Limited as to Use	18,949	19,841
Less Amount Required to Meet Current Obligations	(970)	(1,300)
	17,979	18,541
Long-Term Investments	4,680	4,680
Long-Term Investments Restricted for Capital Acquisition	320	520
Properties and Equipment, Net	51,038	50,492
Other Assets	1,695	1,370
Total Non-Current Assets	75,712	75,603
Total Assets	$115,046	$110,570
Liabilities and Net Assets		
Current Liabilities		
Current Portion of Long-Term Debt	$1,470	$1,750
Accounts Payable and Accrued Expenses	5,818	5,382
Estimated Third-Party Payor Settlements	2,143	1,942
Deferred Revenues	1,969	2,114
Total Current Liabilities	11,400	11,188
Non-Current Liabilities		
Long-Term Debt, Net of Current Portion	23,144	24,014
Other	3,953	3,166
Total Non-Current Liabilities	27,097	27,180
Total Liabilities	38,497	38,368
Net Assets		
Unrestricted	70,846	66,199
Temporarily Restricted	2,115	2,470
Permanently Restricted	3,588	3,533
Total Net Assets	76,549	72,202
Total Liabilities and Net Assets	$115,046	$110,570

Exhibit A–2 Statement of Operations for Sample Not-For-Profit Hospital

Sample Not-For-Profit Hospital
Statement of Operations
For the Years Ended December 31, 20X1 and 20X0 (in '000)

	20X1	20X0
Unrestricted Revenues, Gains, and Other Support		
Net Patient Service Revenue	$85,156	$78,942
Premium Revenue	11,150	10,950
Other Revenues	2,601	5,212
Net Assets Released from Restriction Used for Operations	300	
Total Revenues, Gains and Other Support	99,207	95,104
Expenses		
Salaries and Benefits	53,900	49,938
Medical Supplies and Drugs	26,532	22,121
Insurance	8,089	8,526
Depreciation and Amortization	4,782	4,280
Interest	1,752	1,825
Provision for Bad Debts	1,000	1,300
Other Expenses	2,000	1,300
Total Expenses	98,055	89,290
Operating Income	1,152	5,814
Other Income		
Investment Income	3,900	3,025
Excess of Revenues over Expenses	5,052	8,839
Change in Net Unrealized Gains and Losses on Other than Trading Securities	300	375
Net Assets Released from Restrictions Used for Purchase of Property and Equipment	200	
Contribution From Sample Hospital Foundation for Property Acquisitions	235	485
Transfers to Parent	(640)	(3,000)
Increase in Unrestricted Net Assets, before Extraordinary Item	5,147	6,699
Extraordinary Loss (Debt Extinguishment)	(500)	
Increase in Unrestricted Net Assets	$4,647	$6,699

Source: Reprinted with permission from the Audit and Accounting Guide: Health Care Organizations, copyright © 1996 by the American Institute of Certified Public Accountants, Inc.

Exhibit A–3 Statement of Changes in Net Assets for Sample Not-For-Profit Hospital

Sample Not-For-Profit Hospital
Statement of Changes in Net Assets
For the Years Ended December 31, 20X1 and 20X0 (in '000)

	20X1	20X0
Unrestricted Net Assets		
Excess of Revenues over Expenses	$5,052	$8,839
Net Unrealized Gains on Investments Other than Trading Securities	300	375
Contribution from Sample Hospital Foundation for Property Acquisition	235	485

(Continues)

Exhibit A–3 (Contd)

Transfers to Parent	(640)	(3,000)
Net Assets Released from Restrictions Used for Purchase of Properties and Equipment	200	
Increase in Unrestricted Net Assets before Extraordinary Item	5,147	6,699
Extraordinary Loss from Extinguishment of Debt	(500)	
Increase in Unrestricted Net Assets	4,647	6,699
Temporarily Restricted Net Assets		
Contributions for Charity Care	140	996
Net Realized and Unrealized Gains on Investments	5	8
Net Assets Released from Restrictions	(500)	
Increase (Decrease) in Temporarily Restricted Net Assets	(355)	1,004
Permanently Restricted Net Assets		
Contributions for Endowment Funds	50	411
Net Realized and Unrealized Gains on Investments	5	2
Increase in Permanently Restricted Net Assets	55	413
Increase in Net Assets	4,347	8,116
Net Assets, Beginning of Year	72,202	64,086
Net Assets, End of Year	$76,549	$72,202

Source: Reprinted with permission from the Audit and Accounting Guide: Health Care Organizations, copyright © 1996 by the American Institute of Certified Public Accountants, Inc.

Exhibit A–4   Statement of Cash Flows for Sample Not-For-Profit Hospital

Sample Not-For-Profit Hospital
Statement of Cash Flows (Indirect Method)
December 31, 20X1 and 20X0 (in '000)

	20X1	20X0
Cash Flows From Operating Activities		
Change in Net Assets	$4,347	$8,116
Adjustments to Reconcile Change in Net Assets to		
Net Cash Provided by Operating Activities:		
Extraordinary Loss from Debt Extinguishment	500	
Depreciation	4,782	4,280
Net Realized and Unrealized Gains on Investments, Other than Trading	(450)	(575)
Transfers to Parent	640	3,000
Provision for Bad Debt	1,000	1,300
Restricted Contributions and Investment Income Received	(55)	(413)
(Increase) Decrease in:		
Patient Accounts Receivable	(1,906)	(2,036)
Trading Securities	215	
Other Current Assets	186	(2,481)
Other Assets	(325)	(241)
Increase (Decrease) in:		
Accounts Payable and Accrued Expenses	436	679
Estimated Third-Party Payor Settlements	201	305
Other Current Liabilities	(145)	(257)
Other Liabilities	787	(128)
Net Cash Provided by Operating Activities	10,213	11,549

(Continues)

Exhibit A–4 (Contd)

Cash Flows From Investing Activities		
Purchases of Investment	(3,769)	(2,150)
Capital Expenditures	(4,728)	(5,860)
Net Cash Used in Investing Activities	(8,497)	(8,010)
Cash Flows From Financing Activities		
Transfer to Parent	(640)	(3,000)
Proceeds from Restricted Contributions and Restricted Investment Income	55	413
Payments on Long-Term Debt	(24,700)	(804)
Payments on Capital Lease Obligations	(150)	(100)
Increase in Long-Term Debt	22,600	500
Net Cash Used in Financing Activities	(2,835)	(2,991)
Net Increase (Decrease) in Cash and Cash Equivalents	(1,119)	548
Cash and Cash Equivalents at Beginning of Year	5,877	5,329
Cash and Cash Equivalents at End of Year	$4,758	$5,877

Supplemental Disclosures and Cash Flow Information:
The Hospital entered into capital lease obligations in the amount of $600,000 for new equipment in 2001.
Cash paid for interest (net of amount capitalized) in 2001 and 2000 was $1,780,000 and $1,856,000 respectively.
See accompanying notes to financial statements.

Source: Reprinted with permission from the Audit and Accounting Guide: Health Care Organizations, copyright © 1996 by the American Institute of Certified Public Accountants, Inc.

Exhibit A–5   Consolidated Income Statement for Columbia/HCA Healthcare Corporation

Columbia/HCA Healthcare Corporation
Consolidated Income Statement
For the Years Ended December 31, 1999 and 1998 (in millions)

	1999	1998
Revenues	$16,657	$18,681
Operating expenses:		
Salaries and benefits	6,749	7,811
Supplies	2,645	2,901
Other operating expenses	3,196	3,771
Provision for doubtful accounts	1,269	1,442
Depreciation and amortization	1,094	1,247
Interest expense	471	561
Equity in earnings of affiliates	(90)	(112)
Gains on sales of facilities	(297)	(744)
Impairment of long-lived assets	220	542
Restructuring of operations and investigation related costs	116	111
Total operating expenses	15,373	17,530
Income from continuing operations before minority interests	1,284	1,151
Minority interests in earnings of consolidated entities	57	70
Income from continuing operations before income taxes	1,227	1,081
Provision for income taxes	570	702
Net Income	$657	$379

Source: Columbia/HCA's 10-K report from SEC.

Exhibit A–6   Consolidated Balance Sheet for Columbia/HCA Healthcare Corporation

Columbia/HCA Healthcare Corporation
Consolidated Balance Sheet
December 31, 1999 and 1998 (in millions)

ASSETS	1999	1998
Current assets:		
Cash and cash equivalents	$190	$297
Accounts receivable, less allowances for doubtful accounts of $1,567 and $1,645	1,873	2,096
Inventories	383	434
Income taxes receivable	178	149
Other	973	887
Total current assets	3,597	3,863
Property and equipment, at cost:		
Land	813	925
Buildings	6,108	6,708
Equipment	6,721	7,449
Construction in progress	442	562
	14,084	15,644
Accumulated depreciation	(5,594)	(6,195)
Net Plant and equipment	8,490	9,449
Investments of insurance subsidiary	1,457	1,614
Investments in and advances to affiliates	654	1,275
Intangible assets, net of accumulated amortization of $644 and $596	2,319	2,910
Other	368	318
Total Assets	$16,885	$19,429
LIABILITIES AND STOCKHOLDERS' EQUITY		
Current liabilities:		
Accounts payable	$657	$784
Accrued salaries	403	425
Other accrued expenses	1,112	1,282
Long-term debt due within one year	1,160	1,068
Total current liabilities	3,332	3,559
Long-term debt	5,284	5,685
Professional liability risks, deferred taxes and other liabilities	1,889	1,839
Minority interests in equity of consolidated entities	763	765
Stockholders' equity:		
Common stock $0.01 par; authorized 1,600,000,000 voting shares and 50,000,000 nonvoting shares; outstanding 543,272,900 voting shares and 21,000,000 nonvoting shares (1999) and 621,578,300 voting shares and 21,000,000 nonvoting shares (1998)	6	6
Capital in excess of par value	951	3,498
Other	8	11
Accumulated other comprehensive income	53	80
Retained earnings	4,599	3,986
Total stockholders' equity	5,617	7,581
Total Liabilities & Stockholders' equity	$16,885	$19,429

Source: Columbia/HCA's 10-K report from SEC.

Exhibit A–7 Consolidated Statement of Cash Flows for Columbia/HCA Healthcare Corporation

Columbia/HCA Healthcare Corporation
Consolidated Statement of Cash Flows
For the Years Ended December 31, 1999 and 1998 (in millions)

	1999	1998
Cash flows from continuing operating activities:		
Net income (loss)	$657	$379
Adjustments to reconcile net income (loss) to net cash provided by continuing operating activities:		
Provision for doubtful accounts	1,269	1,442
Depreciation and amortization	1,094	1,247
Income taxes	(66)	351
Gains on sales of facilities	(297)	(744)
Impairment of long-lived assets	220	542
Loss from discontinued operations	0	153
Increase (decrease) in cash from current assets and liabilities:		
Accounts receivable	(1,463)	(1,229)
Inventories and other assets	(119)	(39)
Accounts payable and accrued expenses	(110)	(177)
Other	38	(9)
Net cash provided by continuing operating activities	1,223	1,916
Cash flows from investing activities:		
Purchase of property and equipment	(1,287)	(1,255)
Acquisition of hospitals and health care entities	0	(215)
Spin-off of facilities to stockholders	886	0
Disposal of hospitals and health care entities	805	2,060
Change in investments	565	(294)
Investment in discontinued operations, net	0	677
Other	(44)	(3)
Net cash provided by (used in) investing activities	925	970
Cash flows from financing activities:		
Issuance of long-term debt	1,037	3
Net change in commercial paper and revolving bank credit	200	(2,514)
Repayment of long-term debt	(1,572)	(147)
Issuances (repurchases) of common stock, net	(1,884)	8
Payment of cash dividends and redemption of preferred stock purchase rights	(44)	(52)
Other	8	3
Net cash provided by (used in) financing activities	(2,255)	(2,699)
Change in cash and cash equivalents	(107)	187
Cash and cash equivalents at beginning of period	297	110
Cash and cash equivalents at end of period	$190	$297

Source: Columbia/HCA's 10-K report from SEC.

Exhibit A–8   *Abbreviated Notes to Financial Statements for Sample Not-For-Profit Hospital, December 31, 20X1 and 20X0*

1. Description of Organization and Summary of Significant Accounting Policies

ORGANIZATION

The Sample Not-For-Profit Hospital (the Hospital), located in City, State, is a not-for-profit acute care hospital. The Hospital provides inpatient, outpatient, and emergency care services for residents of northeastern State. Admitting physicians are primarily practitioners in the local area. The Hospital was incorporated in State in 20X0 and is affiliated with the Sample Health System.

USE OF ESTIMATES

The preparation of financial statements in conformity with generally accepted accounting principles requires management to make estimates and assumptions that affect the reported amounts of assets and liabilities, and disclosure of contingent assets and liabilities, at the date of the financial statements, and the reported amounts of revenues and expenses during the reporting period. Actual results could differ from those estimates.

CASH AND CASH EQUIVALENTS

Cash and cash equivalents include certain investments in highly liquid debt instruments with original maturities of three months or less.

The Hospital routinely invests its surplus operating funds in money market mutual funds. These funds generally invest in highly liquid US government and agency obligations.

INVESTMENTS

Investments in equity securities with readily determinable fair values, and all investments in debt securities are measured at fair value in the balance sheet. Investment income or loss (including realized gains and losses on investments, interest, and dividends) is included in the excess of revenues over expenses, unless the income or loss is restricted by donor or law. Unrealized gains and losses on investments are excluded from the excess of revenues over expenses, unless the investments are trading securities.

ASSETS LIMITED AS TO USE

Assets limited as to use primarily include assets held by trustees under indenture agreements, and designated assets set aside by the Board of Trustees for future capital improvements, over which the Board retains control, and which it may at its discretion subsequently use for other purposes. Amounts required to meet current liabilities of the hospital have been reclassified in the balance sheet at December 31, 20X1 and 20X0.

PROPERTY AND EQUIPMENT

Property and equipment acquisitions are recorded at cost. Depreciation is provided over the estimated useful life of each class of depreciable asset and is computed using the straight-line method. Equipment under capital lease obligations is amortized on the straight-line method over the shorter period of the lease term or the estimated useful life of the equipment. Such amortization is included in depreciation and amortization in the financial statements. Interest cost incurred on borrowed funds during the period of construction of capital assets is capitalized as a component of the cost of acquiring those assets.

Gifts of long-lived assets such as land, buildings, or equipment are reported as unrestricted support, and are excluded from the excess of revenues over expenses, unless explicit donor stipulations specify how the donated assets must be used. Gifts of long-lived assets with explicit restrictions that specify how the assets are to be used, and gifts of cash or other assets that must be used to acquire long-lived assets, are reported as restricted support. Absent explicit donor stipulations about how long those long-lived assets must be maintained, expirations of donor restrictions are reported when the donated or acquired long-lived assets are placed in service.

Temporarily and Permanently Restricted Net Assets

Temporarily restricted net assets are those whose use by the Hospital has been limited by donors to a specific time period or purpose. Permanently restricted net assets have been restricted by donors to be maintained by the Hospital in perpetuity.

Excess of Revenues over Expenses

The statement of operations includes excess of revenues over expenses. Changes in unrestricted net assets which are excluded from excess of revenues over expenses, consistent with industry practice, include unrealized gains and losses on investments other than trading securities, permanent transfers of assets to and from affiliates for other than goods and services, and contributions of long-lived assets (including assets acquired using contributions which by donor restriction were to be used for the purposes of acquiring such assets).

Net Patient Service Revenue

The Hospital has agreements with third-party payors that provide for payments to the Hospital at amounts different from its established rates. Payment arrangements include prospectively determined rates per discharge, reimbursed costs, discounted charges, and *per diem* payments. Net patient service revenue is reported at the estimated net realizable amounts from patients, third-party payors, and others for services rendered, including estimated retroactive adjustments under reimbursement agreements with third-party payors. Retroactive adjustments are accrued on an estimated basis in the period the related services are rendered and adjusted in future periods, as final settlements are determined.

Premium Revenue

The Hospital has agreements with various health maintenance organizations (HMOs) to provide medical services to subscribing participants. Under these agreements, the Hospital receives monthly capitation payments based on the number of each HMO's participants, regardless of services actually performed by the Hospital. In addition, the HMOs make fee-for-service payments to the Hospital for certain covered services based upon discounted fee schedules.

Charity Care

The Hospital provides care to patients who meet certain criteria under its charity care policy without charge or at amounts less than its established rates. Because the Hospital does not pursue collection of amounts determined to qualify as charity care, they are not reported as revenue.

Donor-restricted Gifts

Unconditional promises to give cash and other assets to the Hospital are reported at fair value at the date the promise is received. Conditional promises to give and indications of intentions to give are reported at fair value at the date the gift is received. The gifts are reported as either temporarily or permanently restricted support if they are received with donor stipulations that limit the use of the donated assets. When a donor restriction expires – that is, when a stipulated time restriction ends or purpose restriction is accomplished – temporarily restricted net assets are reclassified as unrestricted net assets and reported in the statement of operations as net assets released from restrictions. Donor-restricted contributions whose restrictions are met within the same year as received are reported as unrestricted contributions in the accompanying financial statements.

ESTIMATED MALPRACTICE COSTS

The provision for estimated medical malpractice claims includes estimates of the ultimate costs for both reported claims and claims incurred but not reported.

INCOME TAXES

The Hospital is a not-for-profit corporation and has been recognized as tax-exempt pursuant to Section 501(c)(3) of the Internal Revenue Code.

2. Net Patient Service Revenue

The Hospital has agreements with third-party payors that provide for payments to the Hospital at amounts different from its established rates. A summary of the payment arrangements with major third-party payors follows.

MEDICARE

Inpatient acute care services rendered to Medicare program beneficiaries are paid at prospectively determined rates per discharge. These rates vary according to a patient classification system that is based on clinical, diagnostic, and other factors. Inpatient non-acute services, certain outpatient services, and defined capital and medical education costs related to Medicare beneficiaries are paid based on a cost reimbursement methodology. The Hospital is reimbursed for cost reimbursable items at a tentative rate, with final settlement determined after submission of annual cost reports by the Hospital and audits thereof by the Medicare fiscal intermediary. Beginning in 20X0, the Hospital claimed Medicare payments based on an interpretation of certain "disproportionate share" rules. The intermediary disagreed and declined to pay the excess reimbursement claimed under that interpretation. Through 20X0, the Hospital has not included the claimed excess in net patient revenues pending resolution of the matter. In 20X1, the intermediary accepted the claims and paid the outstanding claims, including $950,000 applicable to 20X0 and $300,000 applicable to 20X1 and prior, which has been included in 20X0 net revenues.

MEDICAID

Inpatient and outpatient services rendered to Medicaid program beneficiaries are reimbursed under a cost reimbursement methodology. The Hospital is reimbursed at a tentative rate with final settlement determined after submission of annual cost reports by the Hospital and audits thereof by the Medicaid fiscal intermediary.

The Hospital also has entered into payment agreements with certain commercial insurance carriers, health maintenance organizations, and preferred provider organizations. The basis for payment to the Hospital under these agreements includes prospectively determined rates per discharge, discounts from established charges, and prospectively determined daily rates.

3. Investments

ASSETS LIMITED AS TO USE

The composition of assets limited as to use at December 31, 20X1 and 20X0 is set forth in the following table. Investments are stated at fair value.

	20X1	20X0
Internally designated for capital acquisition:		
Cash	$545,000	$350,000
US Treasury Obligations	11,435,000	12,115,000
Interest Receivable	20,000	35,000
	12,000,000	12,500,000
Held by trustee under indenture agreement:		
Cash and short-term investments	352,000	260,000
US Treasury obligation	6,505,000	7,007,000
Interest receivable	92,000	74,000
	6,949,000	7,341,000
Total	$18,949,000	$19,841,000

OTHER INVESTMENTS

Other investments, stated at fair value, at December 31, 20X1 and 20X0, include:

	20X1	20X0
Trading:		
US Corporate Bonds	$1,260,000	$1,475,000
Other		
US Treasury Obligations	19,266,000	14,233,000
Interest receivable	310,000	232,000
	20,836,000	15,940,000
Less:		
Long-term investments	4,680,000	4,680,000
Long-term investments restricted for Capital acquisitions	320,000	520,000
Total	$15,836,000	$10,740,000

Investment income and gains for assets limited as to use, cash equivalents, and other investments are comprised of the following for the years ending September 30, 20X1 and 20X0:

	20X1	20X0
Income:		
Interest Income	$3,585,000	$2,725,000
Realized gains on sales of securities	150,000	200,000
Unrealized gains on trading securities	165,000	100,000
	$3,900,000	$3,025,000
Other Changes in Unrestricted Net Assets:		
Unrealized gains on other than trading securities	$300,000	$375,000

4. Property and Equipment

A summary of property and equipment at September 30, 20X1 and 20X0 follows.

	20X1	20X0
Land	$3,000,000	$3,000,000
Land improvements	472,000	472,000
Buildings and improvements	52,047,000	53,975,000
Equipment	29,190,000	26,260,000
Equipment under capital lease obligations	2,851,000	2,752,000
Less accumulated depreciation and amortization	40,123,000	38,000,000
Construction in progress	3,601,000	2,033,000
Property and Equipment (Net)	$51,038,000	$50,492,000

Depreciation expense for the years ended December 31, 20X1 and 20X0 amounted to approximately $4,782,000 and $4,280,000. Accumulated amortization for equipment under capital lease obligations was $689,000 and $453,000 at December 31, 20X1 and 20X0, respectively. Construction contracts of approximately $7,885,000 exist for the remodeling of Hospital facilities. At December 31, 20X1, the remaining commitment on these contracts approximated $4,625,000.

5. Charity Care

The amount of charges forgone for services and supplies furnished under the Hospital's charity policy aggregated approximately $4,5000,000 and $4,100,000, in 20X1 and 20X0, respectively.

Source: Adopted with permission from the *Audit and Accounting Guide: Health Care Organizations*, Copyright © 1996 by the American Institute of Certified Public Accountants, Inc.

Chapter Three

PRINCIPLES AND PRACTICES OF HEALTH CARE ACCOUNTING

LEARNING OBJECTIVES

After completing this chapter, you will be able to:

▶ Record financial transactions.
▶ Understand the basics of accrual accounting.
▶ Summarize transactions into financial statements.

Chapter Outline

◀INTRODUCTION▶

The financial viability of a health care organization results from numerous decisions made by various people, including care givers, administrators, boards, lenders, community members, and politicians.

These decisions eventually result in an organization's acquiring and using resources to provide services, to incur obligations, and to generate revenues. One of the major roles of accounting is to record these transactions and report the results in standardized format to interested parties. This chapter shows how a series of typical transactions at a health center are recorded on the books, and how these records are used to produce the four major financial statements for a not-for-profit, business-oriented health care organization. The recording and reporting process can be quite time consuming, but changes are continually being made to automate it. (See Exhibit 3–1 and Perspective 3–1.)

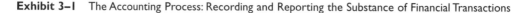

Exhibit 3–1   The Accounting Process: Recording and Reporting the Substance of Financial Transactions

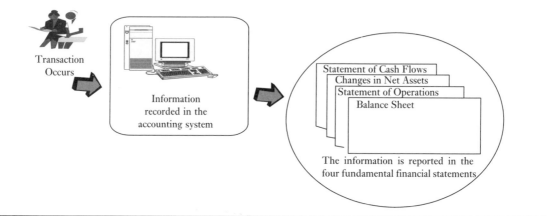

PERSPECTIVE 3–1

E-claims Trim Costs, Aid Growth

Intermountain Health Care's physician-practice division was thriving. You could tell by the number of clerks bent over their computer keyboards, posting claims payments to patient accounts in 72 separate practices across Utah. It took 27 people to handle the postings, reconcile payments with the charges and bill patients for the difference. "That's all they did." For starters, says Wierz, implementing electronic transaction formats in the billing process can play a big part in "eliminating a lot of handwork, a lot of manual transactions." That directly attacks the twin beasts of overhead expense – bulging payroll and rejected claims – by requiring fewer people to do the detail work and cutting down on manual mistakes that result in claims denials. The benefits, as chronicled at Intermountain, can be quantified in fewer full-time-equivalent employees and more productivity per employee.

Source: John Morrissey, *Modern Healthcare*, October 2, 2000.

The Books

As transactions of a health care organization occur (such as the purchase of supplies), they are recorded chronologically in a "book" called a **journal**. Today, this "book" is more likely to be a computer than a journal requiring manual entries. Periodically (simultaneously with most computer programs), these transactions are summarized by account (i.e. Cash, Equipment, Revenues, etc.) into another book called a **ledger**. With these two books, the organization has both a chronological listing of transactions and the current balance in each account (see Exhibit 3–2). The totals for each account in the ledger are used to prepare the four financial statements. Although this procedure is quite simple to conceptualize, ensuring the financial statements are prepared accurately and in a timely manner is quite involved, as Perspective 3–1 shows.

There is a fairly standard set of account categories used by all health care organizations, which is listed in a book entitled **chart of accounts**. The accounts that are used in the financial statements in Chapter 2 comprise an important part of the standard set of account categories (though there may be subcategories in each one).

The Cash and Accrual Bases of Accounting

Before introducing examples of recording and reporting transactions, we discuss the difference between cash and accrual accounting. The **cash basis of accounting** focuses on the flows of cash in and out of the organization, whereas the **accrual basis of accounting** focuses on the flows of resources and the revenues those resources help to generate. This discussion begins with a focus on the cash basis of accounting,

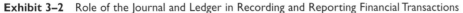

Exhibit 3–2   Role of the Journal and Ledger in Recording and Reporting Financial Transactions

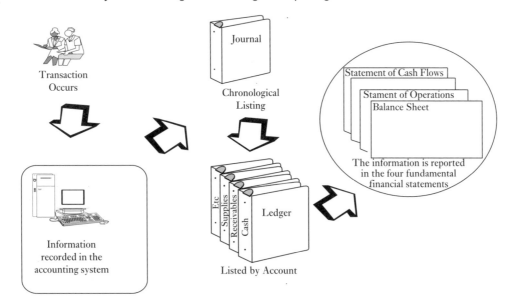

for it is more intuitive. The focus then turns to the accrual basis of accounting, which is the system the accounting profession applies to health care organizations.

The Cash Basis of Accounting

Cash Basis of Accounting: An accounting method which tracks when cash was received and when cash was expended, regardless of when services were provided or resources were used.

The cash basis of accounting records transactions similarly to the way most people keep their personal checkbooks: revenues are recorded when cash is received, and expenses are recorded when cash is paid out (see Exhibit 3–3). For example, if an organization delivers a service to a patient, the revenue from that patient is recorded when received. Expenses are recorded as they are paid (such as when the staff are paid). The advantages of this method of accounting are: 1) cash flows can be tracked; and 2) it is simple. Its main disadvantages are: 1) it does not match revenues with the resources used to generate those revenues; and 2) the financial reports under the cash basis of accounting are susceptible to managerial manipulation. Incidentally, one of the functions of auditors is to give assurance that the statements have been prepared according to generally accepted accounting principles (GAAP) (see Perspective 3–2).

The Accrual Basis of Accounting

Accrual Basis of Accounting: An accounting method which aligns the flow of resources and the revenues those resources helped to generate. It records revenues when earned and resources when used, regardless of the flow of cash in or out of the organization. This is the standard method in use today.

The accrual basis of accounting overcomes the disadvantages of the cash basis of accounting by recognizing revenues when they are earned and expenses when resources are used (see Exhibit 3–3). The advantages of the accrual basis of accounting are that: 1) it keeps track of revenues generated and resources used as well as cash flows; 2) it matches revenues with the resources used to generate those revenues; and 3) the financial statements provide a broader picture of the provider's operation. Its main disadvantages are that: 1) it is more difficult to implement; and 2) it, too, is open to manipulation, often by bending accounting rules. Keeping track of revenues and resource use can be a technologically intensive endeavor (see Perspective 3–3).

An Example of the Effects of Cash Flows on Profit Reporting Under Cash and Accrual Accounting

Exhibit 3–4 illustrates how the cash basis of accounting is vulnerable to management's manipulation of revenues and expenses. Assume a health care organization earned $12,000 in revenues and had $4,000 in expenses. In Scenario 1, management wants to show a high profit, so although it collects full payment of $12,000, it delays paying its bills until after

Exhibit 3–3   Comparison of the Cash and Accrual Bases of Accounting

	Cash Basis of Accounting	Accrual Basis of Accounting
Revenues Are Recognized	When Cash Is Received	When Revenues Are Earned
Expenses Are Recognized	When Cash Is Paid Out	When Resources Are Used

PERSPECTIVE 3–2

Internal Investigations: Healthcare Systems Are Deploying More Internal Auditors to Monitor All Aspects of Operations

A recent survey published by the Healthcare Financial Management Association found that from 1990 to 1998, the duties and responsibilities of healthcare internal auditors shifted from verifying and analyzing data to assessing operations to supporting managerial decision making. The same survey found that more internal audit directors had earned the status of certified public accountant or certified internal auditor, a status granted by the Institute of Internal Auditors.

"Healthcare is probably one of the biggest growth areas for internal auditors," says Michael Fabrizius, Bon Secours' vice president of internal audit. Internal auditors can assess technology, review corporate compliance programs, oversee the transition to new Medicare payment schemes and coordinate coding and billing, Fabrizius says. Bon Secours President and Chief Executive Officer Christopher Carney says an important factor in Bon Secours' financial success is its heavy use of internal auditors to monitor all aspects of financial and operational performance.

The system's team of 20 internal auditors nose through everything from corporate compliance programs to managed-care collections to billing functions at ancillary sites, looking for opportunities to reduce financial risk. Bon Secours officials say the internal audit department, with an annual budget exceeding $1 million in salaries and travel, saves more money for the system than it consumes. "They really become consultants to Management to help us do a better job," Carney says. Some organizations that lack dedicated internal auditors have hired consultants to perform some of the same functions. Last fall, Newtown Square, Pa.-based Catholic Health East hired accounting firm Deloitte & Touche to assess the effectiveness of its corporate compliance programs and provide consistency in financial and accounting reporting by its 32 hospitals.

Source: Adapted from Mary Chris Jaklevic, *Modern Healthcare*, September 4, 2000, p. 64.

Exhibit 3–4 Illustration of Management Manipulation under the Cash Basis of Accounting

---

Situation: During the accounting period, a health care organization has earned $12,000 in revenues, and consumed $4,000 in resources.

Assume 3 scenarios:
1. Management wants to show a high profit, so although it collects full payment of $12,000, it delays paying its bills until after the end of the accounting period.
2. Management wants to show low profit, perhaps to encourage more donations. It pays the bills, $4000, but discourages patients and third parties from paying until after the end of the accounting period.
3. Accrual basis of accounting rules are followed, and the organization records revenues earned of $12,000, and resources used to generate those revenues of $4,000.

	Scenario 1	Scenario 2	Scenario 3
Revenues Reported	$12,000	$0	$12,000
Expenses Reported	$0	$4,000	$4,000
Profit Reported	$12,000	($4,000)	$8,000

Points:
1. Management can manipulate reported profits through its payment and collection policies under the cash basis of accounting.
2. Revenues are not necessarily matched with the resources used to generate those revenues under the cash basis of accounting.

PERSPECTIVE 3–3

Revenue Stopper: Bungled Billing System Conversions Are Plaguing the Hospital Industry

Like many hospitals and healthcare systems, University of Chicago Hospitals rushed to install Y2K-compliant patient accounting software. The goal was to protect the system's cash flow by ensuring that it could continue to bill for services and collect revenue without a hiccup after Jan. 1, 2000. . . .

For about two months after the new system went live in February 1999, the medical center struggled to generate bills. Normally, the academic medical center produced 70,000 claims monthly. The average time it took to collect a payment ballooned from about 45 days to nearly 70. Because the software had not been fully customized and tested, less than 40% of claims that were issued were complete and accurate, according to staff who worked on the project. The result was a cash crunch, with collections 6.3% below budgeted projections for the 1999 fiscal year.

To meet expenses, the hospital took out a bank line of credit, which cost it more than $1 million in interest and delayed some capital projects. . . . Though not widely reported, bungled billing system conversions have clogged cash flows at many hospitals, which often installed new systems to avoid problems associated with the turnover to the year 2000. In the industry, stories abound of patient-accounting departments that were unable to generate bills for months or were forced to write off millions of dollars in revenue because data needed to submit a clean claim could not be converted to new software. . . . Billing glitches can lead to credit downgrades, layoffs and even bankruptcy. . . . Even a small spike in the number of days it takes hospitals to collect money can drain millions of dollars, eroding investment income and impairing access to capital markets.

Source: Adapted from Mary Chris Jaklevic, *Modern Healthcare*, July 2, 2001, p. 36.

the end of the accounting period; therefore, the reported profit is $12,000. In Scenario 2, management wants to show low profit (perhaps so it can encourage more donations). In this case, management pays all of its bills, $4,000, but sends out its own bills late so that payment is not received from patients and third parties until after the end of the accounting period; reported profit under this scenario is −$4,000. Scenario 3 follows the accrual basis of accounting rules and records revenues earned of $12,000 and resources used to generate those revenues of $4,000, which shows a profit of $8,000. Thus, under accrual accounting the organization cannot influence reported profit by accelerating or slowing cash inflows and outflows. Revenues *must* be recorded when they are earned and expenses recorded when resources are used. Perspectives 3–4 and 3–5 exhibit the importance of accurate record keeping, and show how systems can go astray.

Generally accepted accounting principles recommend that health care organizations use the accrual basis of accounting. This does not mean that having information about cash flows is any less important than is having information about revenues and the resources used to generate those revenues.

◀RECORDING TRANSACTIONS▶

Assume Windmill Point Outpatient Center is a not-for-profit, business-oriented, health care organization which had the transactions summarized in Exhibit 3–5 during 20X1, its

PERSPECTIVE 3–4

Former HBO Execs Indicted for Fraud

Two former executives of McKesson HBOC were indicted late last week in what was called one of the largest financial reporting frauds in US history. The government accused the pair of falsely inflating company revenue from 1997 to 1999 by hundreds of millions of dollars.

A 17-count indictment announced late last week by federal prosecutors in San Francisco alleges that Albert Bergonzi, 50, and Jay Gilbertson, 40, former HBO & Co. co-president and cochief operating officer, "systematically defrauded HBO shareholders and the investing public" in a scheme that resulted in shareholder losses of $9 billion. Bergonzi and Gilbertson shared the top post at Atlanta-based HBO before it was acquired by San Francisco-based drug distributor McKesson Corp. in January 1999 for $14 billion and renamed McKesson HBOC.

"This case is the poster child for the devastating effect of financial fraud by corporate management," US Attorney Robert Mueller said in a written statement. "The defendants violated the antifraud, internal controls, and books and records provisions of the federal securities laws," SEC officials said in a written statement. The SEC also alleges that "Gilbertson violated the rule against lying to auditors." A Wall Street darling throughout the 1990s, HBO's shady accounting practices first came to light in April 1999, when an annual review by auditors unveiled the first signs of irregularities. Shares slid almost 50% on the news to $34 per share from $65 per share, socking a $9 billion punch to McKesson HBOC's market value in a single day. According to the indictment, Bergonzi and Gilbertson went to great lengths to help HBO meet or beat Wall Street analysts' expectations of the company's performance.

Source: Adapted from Jeff Tieman, Deanna Bellandi, and Ed Lovern, *Modern Healthcare*, October 2, 2000, p. 2.

PERSPECTIVE 3–5

Debunking Oxford. Oxford Health Has Convinced Wall Street It Has Pulled off a Turnaround that Is Nothing Short of Legendary. This Legend – Like Many – May not Be True

But as the company's financial statements reveal, there may also be a more troubling reason for Oxford's low loss ratio. The insurer has been steadily releasing money from its reserve for future medical claims. Specifically, it has been letting money out of a reserve for what's known as incurred-but-not-reported claims, or IBNR. In HMO accounting, IBNR is an actuarial estimate of medical claims that plan members have incurred (for doctor's visits, diagnostic tests, surgical procedures, etc.) but that have not hit the books because the provider or member has not yet reported the claim to the insurer. Some have expressed concern that Oxford is feeding off its reserve, which is meant to pay for patients' medical care. But on Wall Street, there are few raised eyebrows. Instead, the practice is considered more evidence of Payson's magical touch. "I don't know of any other HMO that has consistently been able to release its reserves," marvels analyst Robert Mains of Advest, a financial advisory firm in Hartford, Conn., who rates Oxford's stock a buy. He says releases from reserves demonstrate how impressive Oxford is as a "medical-cost-containment story" since they indicate that the company's medical expenses have been lower than it had estimated.

But here's the problem: The amount that's released reduces the "health-care expense" component in calculating the medical-loss ratio, making that MLR look better. In translation, Oxford's cost of care looks cheaper than it actually is. It's a fine tactic, but one that works for only a limited time.

Source: David Stires, *Fortune Magazine*, March 19, 2001.

Exhibit 3–5 Sample Transactions for Windmill Point Outpatient Center, January 1, 20X1 to December 31, 20X1

1. The center received $600,000 in unrestricted contributions.
2. The center obtained a $500,000 bank loan at 6% interest; $20,000 in principal is due this year.
3. The center purchased $450,000 of plant and equipment (P&E). It paid cash for the purchase.
4. The center purchased $100,000 of supplies on credit. The vendor expects payment within 30 days.
5. The center provided $500,000 of non-discounted, billable services to non-capitated patients. Payment has not yet been received.
6. On the first day of the year, the center received $250,000 in capitation payment from an HMO. This means an HMO paid the center $250,000 in advance on a per member per year (PMPY) basis to provide for the health care needs of its enrollees over the next year.
7. In the provision of services to all patients, the center incurred $300,000 in labor expenses, which it paid for in cash.
8. In the provision of services to all patients, the center used $80,000 of supplies.
9. The center paid $10,000 in advance for one year's insurance.
10. The center paid for $90,000 of the $100,000 of supplies purchased in Transaction 4.
11. Patients or their third parties paid the center $400,000 of the $500,000 they owed (see Transaction 5).
12. During the year, the center made a $50,000 cash payment toward its bank loan; $20,000 was for principal and $30,000 was to pay the full amount of interest due.
13. The center transferred $25,000 to its parent corporation.

At the end of the year, the center recognized the following:
14. Since the last payday, employees have earned wages of $35,000.
15. Equipment has depreciated $45,000.
16. The $10,000 of insurance premium was for one year. That time has now expired.
17. The Health Center has fulfilled the health care service obligation it took on for the $250,000 in capitated payments for one year (Transaction 6), which has now expired. This revenue is now considered earned.
18. $20,000 of the note payable in Transaction 2 is due within the next year.
19. Bad debt is estimated to be $5,000.
20. $60,000 is set aside for the beginning of the next fiscal year to be used towards purchase of new computer equipment.

first year of operation. Exhibit 3–6 presents the journal and ledger entries to record the transactions listed in Exhibit 3–5. Since the transactions are recorded chronologically by row, the rows serve as the journal. Since each account has its own column summarized at the bottom, the columns serve as a ledger. These transactions are being recorded in part so that the four financial statements can be prepared. These statements allow interested parties to make informed judgments about the financial health of the organization.

Rules for Recording Transactions

Two rules must be followed to record transactions under the accrual basis of accounting:

1. **At least two accounts must be used to record a transaction.**
   a. Increase (decrease) an *asset* account whenever assets are acquired (used).
   b. Increase (decrease) a *liability* account whenever obligations are incurred (paid for).

Exhibit 3-6 Listing of Financial Transactions for Windmill Point Outpatient Center

Windmill Point Outpatient Clinic
Journal and Ledger
For the Period January 1 - December 31, 20X1.

Transaction	Cash	Assets Limited as to Use	Accounts Receivable	Allowance for Doubtful Accounts	Supplies	Prepaid Expenses	Long-term Investments	Plant & Equipment (P&E)	Accumulated Depreciation	Current Liabilities	Deferred Revenues	Non-Current Liabilities	Revenues, Gains and Other Support	Expenses	Transfer to Parent	Unrestricted Net Assets	Restricted Net Assets
					ASSETS						LIABILITIES				NET ASSETS		
Beginning Balance	$0	$0	$0	$0	$0	$0	$0	$0	$0	$0	$0	$0	$0	$0	$0	$0	$0
1 Contribution	600,000												600,000				
2 Long-term bank loan	500,000									20,000		480,000					
3 Purchased P & E with cash	-450,000							450,000									
4 Purchased supplies on credit					100,000					100,000							
5 Patient services on credit			500,000										500,000				
6 Received HMO capitation	250,000										250,000						
7 Paid labor	-300,000													-300,000			
8 Used supplies					-80,000									-80,000			
9 Prepaid insurance	-10,000					10,000											
10 Paid cash for supplies	-90,000									-90,000							
11 Patients paid accounts	400,000		-400,000														
12 Paid bank loan & interest	-50,000									-20,000		-30,000		-30,000			
13 Transferred funds to parent	-25,000														-25,000		
Adjustments																	
14 Wages earned but not paid										35,000				-35,000			
15 Depreciation									-45,000					-45,000			
16 Expired insurance						-10,000								-10,000			
17 Capitation earned											-250,000		250,000				
18 Current portion of Debt										20,000		-20,000					
19 Bad debt				-5,000										-5,000			
20 Board funds set aside	-60,000	60,000															
Balances after adjustments	765,000	60,000	100,000	-5,000	20,000	0	0	450,000	-45,000	65,000	0	460,000	1,350,000	-505,000	-25,000	0	0
Operating income													-505,000				
Closing income from operations to unrestricted net assets													845,000			845,000	
Transfer to parent																-25,000	
Ending Balances	765,000	60,000	100,000	-5,000	20,000	0	0	450,000	-45,000	65,000	0	460,000				820,000	
Balances with Summarized Net Assets	$765,000	$60,000	$100,000	-$5,000	$20,000	$0	$0	$450,000	-$45,000	$65,000	$0	$460,000				$820,000	$0

Summary:
Total Assets = 1,345,000
Liabilities + Net Assets = 1,345,000
Current Assets = 940,000
Non-Current Assets = 405,000

   c. Increase a *revenue, gain, or other support* account when revenues are earned, a gain occurs, or other support is received.

   d. Increase an *expense* account when an asset is used. Net Assets increase when Unrestricted Revenues, Gains, and Other Support increase, and Net Assets decrease when Expenses occur.

There are additional rules which must be followed for donations; however, these rules can become quite complex and are beyond the scope of this text.

2. After each transaction, the fundamental accounting equation must be in balance:

$$\text{Assets} = \text{Liabilities} + \text{Net Assets}$$

The Recording Process (see Exhibit 3–6)

1. The center received $600,000 in unrestricted contributions.

   a. Since cash was received, Cash (an asset) is increased by $600,000.

   b. Since an unrestricted contribution for operating purposes was received, Revenues, Gains, and Other Support is increased by $600,000. If Exhibit 3–6 were not constrained for space, the transaction would be more accurately recorded in a subcategory of Revenues, Gains, and Other Support, called Other Revenue.

 Caution   Under accrual accounting, revenues are recognized when earned. Since the receipt of an unrestricted donation *that can be used for operating purposes* is not earned in the same sense that patient revenues are, such donations are recorded in the related account Other Revenue, under Revenue, Gains, and Other Support.

2. The center obtained a $500,000 bank loan at 6 percent interest; $20,000 in principal is due this year.

   a. Since cash was received, Cash (an asset) is increased by $500,000.

   b. Since the center borrowed $500,000, it must recognize this as a liability. The part due this year ($20,000) is a current liability. The part not due this year ($480,000) is a non–current liability. Thus, Notes Payable under current liabilities is increased by $20,000, and Notes Payable under non-current liabilities is increased by $480,000.

 Caution   Notice that although cash was received, no revenues were recognized. Under accrual accounting, revenues are recognized when they are earned. In this case, the cash received did not represent earnings, just the borrowing of funds. Also note that this transaction involved three accounts, not just two: Cash, Current Liabilities, and Non-Current Liabilities. However, the fundamental accounting equation still remains in balance.

A common error is to record interest expense at this time. Since interest is a "usage" fee, interest is recognized as the borrower keeps the funds, not when the borrowing takes place. (This is shown in Transaction 12.)

3. **The center purchased $450,000 of properties and equipment (P&E). It paid cash for the purchase.**
   a. Since cash was paid, Cash (an asset) is decreased by $450,000.
   b. Since properties and equipment were purchased, Properties and Equipment (an asset) is increased by $450,000.

Caution

Notice that although cash was paid, no expense was recognized. Under accrual accounting, expenses are recognized as assets are used, and the center has not yet used the plant and equipment. (This is shown in Transaction 15.)

4. **The center purchased $100,000 of supplies on credit. The vendor expects payment within 30 days.**
   a. Since supplies increased, Supplies (an asset) is increased by $100,000.
   b. Since the vendor is owed $100,000, and the payment is due within 30 days, the current liability, Accounts Payable, is increased by $100,000.

Caution

Notice that although supplies were purchased, no supplies expense was recognized. Under accrual accounting, expenses are recognized when resources are used or consumed, and the center has not yet used the supplies. (This is shown in Transaction 8.)

5. **The center provided $500,000 of non-discounted, billable services to non-capitated patients. Payment has not yet been received.**
   a. Although the patients received services, they have not paid. Therefore, Accounts Receivable (an asset) is increased by $500,000 to show that the organization has a right to collect the money it is owed.
   b. Since revenue was earned by providing services, Patient Revenues, a net asset sub-account, is increased by $500,000.

Caution

Under accrual accounting, revenues are recognized when earned. Therefore, although no cash was received, revenues are increased because the service was performed.

6. **On the first day of the year, the center received $250,000 in capitation pre-payment from an HMO. This means the HMO paid the center $250,000 in advance on a per member per year (PMPY) basis to take care of the medical needs of all its enrollees over the next year.**
   a. Since cash was received, Cash (an asset) is increased by $250,000.
   b. The center has an obligation to provide services to the capitated patients. Therefore, Deferred Revenues (a liability) is increased by $250,000.

Caution

Under accrual accounting, revenues are recognized when they are earned. Although cash was received, the revenues will only be earned as the "coverage period" expires. (This is shown in Transaction 17.)

7. **In the provision of services to all patients, the center incurred $300,000 in labor expenses, which it paid for in cash.**
   a. Since cash was paid out, Cash (an asset) is decreased by $300,000.
   b. Since labor, a resource, was used, Expenses, a net asset, is increased. Since expenses decrease net assets, it is recorded as a negative number.

Caution

Since cash was paid in recognition of the use of resources, expenses would have been recognized under either the cash or accrual basis of accounting.

8. **In the provision of services to all patients, the center used $80,000 of supplies.**
   a. The organization now has $80,000 less in supplies. Therefore, Supplies (an asset) is decreased by $80,000.
   b. Since $80,000 of supplies has been used, Supplies Expense is increased by $80,000. Since expenses decrease net assets, it is recorded as a negative number.

Caution

Although no cash was paid, the expense is recognized because resources have been used. Recall that no expense was recognized when the resource was purchased in Transaction 4.

9. **The center paid a $10,000 premium in advance for one year's insurance coverage.**
   a. Since cash was paid out, Cash (an asset) is decreased by $10,000.
   b. $10,000 purchased the right to be covered by insurance for the entire year. Therefore, Prepaid Insurance (an asset) is increased by $10,000.

Caution

Under accrual accounting, expenses are recognized when assets are used. Thus, although cash has been paid out, no expense was recognized. The expense will be recognized as the right to be covered by insurance is "used up" (with the passage of time). (This is shown in Transaction 16.)

10. **The center paid for $90,000 of the $100,000 of supplies purchased in Transaction 4.**
    a. Since cash was paid, Cash (an asset) is decreased by $90,000.
    b. Since it no longer owes $90,000 of the $100,000 liability, Accounts Payable (a liability) is decreased by $90,000.

Caution

Although cash has been paid out, no expense was recognized since no resources were used.

11. **Patients or their third parties paid the center $400,000 of the $500,000 they owed (see Transaction 5).**
   a. Since cash was received, Cash (an asset) is increased by $400,000.
   b. Since payment has been received, the organization no longer has the right to collect this $400,000 from patients. Therefore, Accounts Receivable (an asset) is decreased by $400,000.

 Notice that although cash was received, no revenues were recognized. Under accrual accounting, revenues are recognized when they are earned. The revenue was recognized when it was earned in Transaction 5.

12. **During the year, the center made a $50,000 cash payment toward its bank loan; $20,000 was for principal and $30,000 was to pay the full amount of interest due.**
   a. Since cash was paid out, Cash (an asset) is decreased by $50,000.
   b. Since $20,000 of the loan has been paid off, Notes Payable (a liability) is decreased by $20,000.
   c. Since the center paid $30,000 for the use of the $500,000 loan (6 percent interest rate), Interest Expense (a net asset) is increased by $30,000. Since expenses decrease net assets, it is recorded as a negative.

 Remember, interest expense was not recognized when the loan was taken in Transaction 2. Interest, the right to use someone else's money, is recognized over time, as the loan is outstanding.

13. **The center transferred $25,000 to its parent corporation.**
   a. Since cash was paid out, Cash (an asset) is decreased by $25,000.
   b. Since the organization now has $25,000 less assets, Transfer to Parent (a net asset) is decreased by $25,000 dollars. This is recorded as a negative because it has the effect of decreasing Unrestricted Net Assets (like expenses that are also recorded as negatives).

 Although cash has been paid out, no expense is recognized since no resources were used.

14. **Since the last payday, employees have earned wages of $35,000.**
   a. Since the center owes its employees $35,000, it must recognize this obligation by increasing Wages Payable (a liability) by $35,000.
   b. Since the center used $35,000 of labor, it must increase Labor Expense (a liability) by $35,000. Since expenses decrease net assets, the increase in expenses is recorded as a negative number.

 Although no cash was paid, the expense was recognized because labor resources have been used.

Contra-asset: An
asset which, when
increased, decreases
the value of a related
asset on the books.
Two primary examples
are Accumulated
Depreciation, which is
the contra-asset to
Properties and
Equipment, and the
Allowance for
Uncollectibles, which
is the contra-asset to
Accounts Receivable.

15. Equipment has depreciated $45,000.

a. To keep a cumulative record of the amount of depreciation taken on the assets, the center must increase Accumulated Depreciation (a contra-asset account) by $45,000. An increase in a contra-asset account results in a decrease in the value of the assets. Thus, the accumulated depreciation is subtracted from the amount in the equipment account to find the book value of the equipment.

b. Since the organization has "used up" $45,000 of the equipment, it must increase Depreciation Expense (a net asset account) by $45,000. Since expenses decrease net assets, the increase in expenses is recorded as a negative number.

Caution

Although no cash was paid, the depreciation expense is recognized because resources have been used.

16. The $10,000 of insurance coverage was for one year. That time has now expired.

a. Since the organization no longer has the $10,000 of insurance coverage it purchased, it must decrease Prepaid Insurance (an asset) by $10,000.

b. Since the organization "used up" the right it purchased to be covered by insurance for one year, it must increase the Insurance Expense account by $10,000. The expense is recognized as the resource is used, not when the insurance is purchased (see Transaction 9). Since expenses decrease net assets, the increase in expenses is recorded as a negative number.

Caution

Although no cash was paid, the insurance expense is recognized because the right to be covered by insurance has been "used up."

17. The Center has fulfilled its health care service obligations under the $250,000 capitated arrangement in transaction 6. This revenue is now considered earned.

a. The center no longer has the obligation to provide service to these HMO enrollees. Therefore, it must reduce Unearned HMO Revenues (a liability) by $250,000.

b. By covering the health care needs of the HMO enrollees for one year, the center earned $250,000. Therefore, Revenues, Gains, and Other Support are increased by $250,000. The specific account that would be increased under Revenues, Gains, and Other Support is Premium Revenues. Incidentally, note that revenue was not recognized when the cash was received (see Transaction 6).

Caution

Although no cash was received, revenues are recognized when earned.

18. **$20,000 of the note payable is due within the next year.**
   a. Since the organization must pay $20,000 next year, the center must increase Notes Payable (a current liability) by $20,000.
   b. Since it no longer owes $20,000 over the long term, the center decreases Notes Payable (a non-current liability) by $20,000.

19. **Bad debt is estimated to be $5,000.**
   a. The estimate of how much of the accounts receivable will *not* be paid is placed in a contra-asset account called the Allowance for Uncollectibles. Therefore, the Allowance for Uncollectibles is increased by $5,000. By increasing the allowance for uncollectibles, Net Patient Accounts Receivable is decreased.
   b. By estimating uncollectibles, the organization is recognizing that there are certain patient accounts receivable it will not be able to collect. This is part of doing business. Essentially, the organization is "using up" the right to collect the funds without actually collecting anything. It recognizes this use of resources by increasing Bad Debt Expense by $5,000. Since expenses decrease net assets, the increase in expenses is recorded as a negative number.

Caution Although no cash was paid, the bad debt expense (Provision for Bad Debt) is recognized in the same time period as the earning occurred. If the organization did not recognize this expense at this time, it would be matching one year's bad debt with the revenues earned in a future year.

Key Point The terms Allowance for Doubtful Accounts, Allowance for Uncollectible Accounts, and Allowance for Bad Debt are used interchangeably in practice. Similarly, the terms Provision for Bad Debt and Bad Debt Expenses are used interchangeably in practice. In this text, the terms "Allowance for Uncollectibles" and "Bad Debt Expense" are used throughout.

Key Point If nothing else were done, the value of the Allowance for Uncollectibles would grow indefinitely. To avoid this, when deemed uncollectible, specific accounts are written off, and both the Allowance for Uncollectibles and Accounts Receivable are reduced by an equal amount.

20. **$60,000 is set aside by the Board to be used next year to help purchase a new information system.**
   a. Since Cash was set aside, Cash (an asset) is decreased by $60,000.
   b. Since the Board designated these funds for a specific use next year, Assets Limited as to Use (a current asset) is increased by $60,000.

Caution Because no resource has been consumed, there is no expense.

◀DEVELOPING THE FINANCIAL STATEMENTS▶

Once the transactions have been analyzed and recorded, the organization can develop the four financial statements: the balance sheet, the statement of operations, the statement of changes in net assets, and the statement of cash flows.

The Balance Sheet

The balance sheet presents the assets, liabilities, and net assets for a health care provider (see Exhibit 3–7). To construct a balance sheet for Windmill Point Outpatient Clinic, the information from the transaction-recording sheet (see Exhibit 3–6) is used to develop a snapshot of the organization's financial position at year's end.

Assets

For Windmill Point Outpatient Center, Total Current Assets ($940,000) equals the sum of all Cash ($765,000), Assets Limited as to Use ($60,000), Net Accounts Receivable ($95,000: Accounts Receivable of $100,000 less the Allowance for Uncollectibles of $5,000), Supplies ($20,000), and Prepaid Assets ($0). The Properties and Equipment, Net is $405,000. This is computed by taking the original purchase of $450,000 and subtracting the $45,000 of accumulated depreciation. Thus, Total Assets are $1,345,000, which is the sum of current and non-current assets.

Liabilities

Windmill Point Outpatient Center has a balance of $65,000 in current liabilities: $10,000 for supplies ($100,000 purchased minus $90,000 paid for); $35,000 in wages payable; and $20,000, the current portion of the long-term debt. There are no deferred revenues but there is $460,000 of the long-term portion of the loan remaining, which is a non-current liability. The sum of these accounts, $525,000, is the total liabilities.

Net Assets

Net assets equal $820,000. This net asset balance is computed by summing the beginning balance of $0, plus the increase in unrestricted net assets of $820,000 and $0 in temporarily restricted and permanently restricted net assets.

The Statement of Operations

As with the balance sheet, the information in Exhibit 3–6 is used to develop a statement of operations for Windmill Point Outpatient Center (see Exhibit 3–8).

Exhibit 3-7 Balance Sheet for Windmill Point Outpatient Center

Windmill Point Outpatient Center Balance Sheet
For the Periods Ending December 31, 20X1 and 20X0

		12/31/20X1	12/31/20X0			12/31/20X1	12/31/20X0
Current Assets				**Current Liabilities**			
Cash		$765,000	$0	Accounts Payable		$10,000	$0
Gross Accounts Receivable	100,000			Wages Payable		35,000	0
(less Allowance for Uncollectibles)	(5,000)			Notes Payable		20,000	0
Net Accounts Receivable		95,000	0	Total Current Liabilities		65,000	0
Supplies		20,000	0				
Assets Limited as to Use		60,000		Non-Current Liabilities		460,000	0
Prepaid Expenses		0	0				
Total Current Assets		940,000	0	Total Liabilities		525,000	0
Non-Current Assets				**Net Assets**			
Long-Term Investments (Net)		0	0	Unrestricted		820,000	0
Plant, Property & Equipment	450,000			Temporarily Restricted		0	0
(less Accumulated Depreciation)	(45,000)			Permanently Restricted		0	0
Net Plant, Property & Equipment		405,000	0	Total Net Assets		820,000	0
Total Non-Current Assets		405,000	0	Total Liabilities & Net Assets		$1,345,000	$0
Total Assets		$1,345,000	$0				

Exhibit 3–8   Statement of Operations for Windmill Point Outpatient Center

Windmill Point Outpatient Center
Statement of Operations
For the Periods Ending December 31, 20X1 and 20X0

	12/31/20X1	12/31/20X0
Revenues		
Unrestricted Revenues, Gains and Other Support		
Net Patient Revenue	$500,000	$0
Premium Revenue	250,000	0
Other Revenue	600,000	0
Total Revenues	1,350,000	0
Expenses		
Labor Expense	335,000	0
Supplies Expense	80,000	0
Interest Expense	30,000	0
Insurance Expense	10,000	0
Provision for Bad Debt	5,000	0
Depreciation and Amortization	45,000	0
Total Expenses	505,000	0
Operating Income	845,000	0
Excess of Revenues Over Expenses	845,000	0
Contribution of Long-Lived Assets	0	0
Transfers to Parent	(25,000)	0
Increase in Unrestricted Net Assets	$820,000	$0

However, since the transactions that comprise this statement were recorded in an abbreviated form, it is necessary to refer also to the first column of Exhibit 3–6 to identify the specific nature of the transactions classified under Unrestricted Revenues, Gains, and Other Support as well as Expenses.

Unrestricted Revenues, Gains, and Other Support

The revenues of Windmill Point Outpatient Center are classified into three categories: net patient revenues earned from non-capitated patients ($500,000); premium revenue earned from capitated patients ($250,000); and unrestricted contributions, which are presented in the category Other Revenue ($600,000). These revenues total $1,350,000.

Operating Expenses

Operating Expenses are costs that are incurred in the day-to-day operation of the business. Exhibit 3–8 shows that the operating expense of $505,000 is made up of

$335,000 labor expense ($300,000 paid for and $35,000 not yet paid for); $80,000 supplies expense; $30,000 interest expense; $10,000 insurance expense; $5,000 provision for bad debt; and $45,000 depreciation expense.

Operating Income and Excess of Revenues over Expenses

Operating Income is the difference between Unrestricted Revenues, Gains, and Other Support and Expenses. For Windmill Point Outpatient Center, operating income is $845,000. Since there are no "non-operating income" items, this is also equal to Excess of Revenues over Expenses, the net income of the organization.

Increase in Unrestricted Net Assets

As shown in Exhibit 3–8, the increase in unrestricted net assets, $820,000, for Windmill Point Outpatient Center is operating income ($845,000) minus the transfers to parent ($25,000).

The Statement of Changes in Net Assets

The third financial statement is the statement of changes in net assets, or the statement of changes in owners' equity or stockholders' equity for a for-profit business. Its purpose is to explain the changes in net assets from one period to the next (see Exhibit 3–9). This statement reflects increases and decreases in net assets for both restricted and unrestricted net asset accounts. For Windmill Point Outpatient Center, the ending balance of net assets, $820,000, is the sum of the beginning total net asset account for the year, $0, plus the changes in unrestricted net assets for the year, $820,000 (from the statement of operations), plus changes made to restricted net asset accounts, $0.

The Statement of Cash Flows

Since accrual accounting is used, the statement of operations provides information about how much revenue was generated and the amount of resources used to generate those revenues. However, the statement of operations does not tell how much cash came into the organization and how much went out. That is the purpose of the statement of cash flows (see Exhibit 3–10). The construction of the statement of cash flows is beyond this introductory text. Most standard introductory accounting texts can provide more detailed information.

This statement is organized into three major sections: cash flows from operating activities, cash flows from investing activities, and cash flows from financing activities. Whereas the sections on investing and financing activities are relatively straightforward, the section on cash flows from operating activities is not. The latter begins with

Exhibit 3–9   Statement of Changes in Net Assets for Windmill Point Outpatient Center

Windmill Point Outpatient Center
Statement of Changes in Net Assests
For the Periods Ending December 31, 20X1 and 20X0

	12/31/20X1	12/31/20X0
Unrestricted Net Assets		
Excess of Revenues Over Expenses	$845,000	$0
Contribution of Long-Lived Assets	0	0
Transfer to Parent	(25,000)	0
Increase in Unrestricted Net Assets	820,000	0
Temporarily Restricted Net Assets		
Restricted Contribution	0	0
Increase in Temporarily Restricted Net Assets	0	0
Permanently Restricted Net Assets		
Increase in Permanently Restricted Net Assets	0	0
Increase in Net Assets	820,000	0
Net Assets, Beginning of Year	0	0
Net Assets, End of Year	**$820,000**	**$0**

changes in net assets and then makes adjustments required by the accrual basis of accounting.

Cash flows from investing activities include cash transactions involving the purchase or sale of properties and equipment, and the purchase or sale of long-term investments. Cash flows from financing activities include changes in non-current liability accounts, such as an increase or decrease in long-term debt (including the current portion), any increase in temporarily or permanently restricted assets, and the recognition of the transfer of cash funds to the parent corporation.

That Transfer to Parent appears twice in this statement can be confusing. It appears in the cash flows from operating activities section to show that there was $25,000 more cash available from operations than is shown in changes in net assets, which is the beginning point for calculating cash flows from operating activities. Since the inflow is included in the cash flows from operating activities, the cash outflow is then shown as a cash flow from financing activities.

◄SUMMARY►

The financial viability of a health care organization is the result of numerous decisions made by a variety of people, including caregivers, administrators, boards, lenders, community members, and politicians. These decisions eventually result in the organization's acquiring and using resources to provide services, to incur obligations, and to generate revenues. One of the major roles of accounting is to record these transac-

Exhibit 3–10 Statement of Cash Flows for Windmill Point Outpatient Center

Windmill Point Outpatient Center
Statement of Cash Flows
For the Periods Ending December 31, 20X1 and 20X0

	12/31/20X1	12/31/20X0
Cash Flows from Operating Activities		
Change in Net Assets	$820,000	$0
Depreciation Expense	45,000	0
− Increase in Temporarily Restricted Net Assets	0	0
+ Transfers to Parent	25,000	0
− Increase in Net Accounts Receivable	(95,000)	0
− Increase in Inventory	(20,000)	0
+ Increase in Accounts Payable	10,000	0
+ Increase in Wages Payable	35,000	0
Net Cash Provided by Operating Activities	820,000	0
Cash Flows from Investing Activities		
Purchase of assets limited as to use	(60,000)	0
Purchase of Plant, Property, & Equipment	(450,000)	0
Net Cash Flow Used in Investing Activities	(510,000)	0
Cash Flows from Financing Activities		
Transfers to Parent	(25,000)	0
Increase in Long-Term Debt	480,000	0
Net Cash Provided by Financing Activities	455,000	0
Net Increase in Cash & Cash Equivalents	765,000	0
Cash and Cash Equivalents, Beginning of Year	0	0
Cash and Cash Equivalents, End of Year	**$765,000**	**$0**

tions in a standardized format and to report the results to interested parties. This chapter shows how a series of typical transactions of a health center are recorded on the books, and how these records are used to produce the four major financial statements of a not-for-profit, business-oriented health care organization.

Transactions are recorded using either the cash basis of accounting or the accrual basis of accounting. In the *cash basis* of accounting, revenues are recognized when cash is received, and expenses are recognized when cash is paid. In the *accrual basis* of accounting, revenues are recognized when earned, and expenses are recognized when resources are used. The accrual basis of accounting must be used by health care organizations.

Major rules for recording transactions using the accrual basis of accounting include:

1. **At least two accounts must be used to record a transaction.**
   a. Increase (decrease) an *asset* account whenever assets are acquired (used).
   b. Increase (decrease) a *liability* account whenever obligations are incurred (paid for).

      c. Increase a *revenue, gain, or other support* account when revenues are earned, a gain occurs, or other support is received.

      d. Increase an *expense* account when an asset is used. Net Assets increase when Unrestricted Revenues, Gains, and Other Support increase, and Net Assets decrease when Expenses occur.

There are additional rules which must be followed for donations; however, these rules can become quite complex and are beyond the scope of this text.

2. After each transaction, the fundamental accounting equation must be in balance:

$$\text{Assets} = \text{Liabilities} + \text{Net Assets}$$

◀Key Terms▶

Accrual Basis of Accounting	Cash Basis of Accounting	Contra-asset

---

◀Questions and Problems▶

1. **Definitions.** Define the following terms:
   a. Accrual basis of accounting
   b. Cash basis of accounting
   c. Contra-asset
2. **Accrual versus Cash Basis of Accounting.** Explain the difference between the accrual basis of accounting and the cash basis of accounting. What are the major reasons for using accrual accounting?
3. **Accrual Accounting.** How are revenues and expenses defined under accrual accounting?
4. **Journal versus Ledger.** What are the purposes of a journal and a ledger?
5. **Adjustment of Three Accounts.** Give two examples of transactions which involve the adjustment of three accounts, rather than the usual two accounts.
6. **Contra-asset.** Give an example of a contra-asset, and explain how it is recorded on the ledger as a transaction.
7. **Prepaid Expense.** Explain what a "prepaid expense" is and how it is recorded on the ledger as a transaction.
8. **Timing of Transactions.** How would transactions differ if Supplies were completely paid for and consumed in one period, or paid for in one period but not used until the next period?
9. **Timing of Transactions.** Are transactions recorded on a fiscal-year basis or a calendar-year basis? Does it have to be one or the other, and if so, why?
10. **For-profit versus Not-for-profit Transactions.** What are the major differences in recording transactions for a for-profit organization versus a not-for-profit, or are there any?
11. **Transactions + Multiple Statements.** List and record each transaction for S. Zee Outpatient Clinic under the accrual basis of accounting at

December 31, 20X1. Then develop a balance sheet as of December 31, 20X1, and a statement of operations for the year ended December 31, 20X1.

a. The clinic received a $3,000,000 unrestricted cash contribution from the community. (Hint: this transaction increases the unrestricted net assets account.)

b. The clinic purchased $2,000,000 of equipment. The clinic paid cash for the equipment.

c. The clinic borrowed $1,000,000 from the bank on a long-term basis.

d. The clinic purchased $1,500,000 of supplies on credit.

e. The clinic provided $5,500,000 of services on credit.

f. In the provision of these services, the clinic used $1,000,000 of supplies.

g. The clinic received $500,000 in advance to care for capitated patients.

h. The clinic incurred $2,000,000 in labor expenses and paid cash for them.

i. The clinic incurred $1,500,000 in general expenses and paid cash for them.

j. The clinic received $4,500,000 from patients and their third parties in payment of outstanding accounts.

k. The clinic met $300,000 of its obligation to capitated patients in Transaction g.

l. The clinic made a $100,000 cash payment on the long-term loan.

m. The clinic also made a cash interest payment of $50,000.

n. A donor made a temporarily restricted donation of $100,000 to be used for operations.

o. The clinic recognized $200,000 in depreciation for the year.

p. The clinic estimated that $500,000 of patient accounts would not be received.

12. **Transactions + Multiple Statements.** The following are the financial transactions for Family Home Health Care Center, a not-for-profit, business-oriented organization. Beginning balances at January 1, 20X1 for its assets, liabilities, and net asset accounts were:

Cash	$5,000
Accounts Receivable	$55,000
Allowance for Uncollectibles	$5,000
Supplies	$20,000
Long-term Investments	$5,000
Properties and Equipment	$300,000
Accumulated Depreciation	$10,000
Short-term Accounts Payable	$20,000
Wages Payable	$10,000
Long-term Debt	$200,000
Unrestricted Net Assets	$135,000
Permanently Restricted Net Assets	$5,000

List and record each transaction under the accrual basis of accounting. Then develop a balance sheet as of December 31, 20X1 and 20X0, and a statement of operations for the year ended December 31, 20X1.

a. The center purchased $10,000 of supplies on credit.

    b. The center provided $150,000 of home health services on credit.

    c. The center consumed $5,000 of supplies in the provision of its home health services.

    d. The center provided $100,000 of home health services and patients paid for services in cash.

    e. The center paid cash for $15,000 of supplies in the provision of its home health services.

    f. The center paid $15,000 in cash for supplies previously purchased on credit.

    g. A donor established a $10,000 permanent endowment fund (in the form of long-term investments) for the center. (Hint: this transaction increases the permanently restricted net assets account.)

    h. The center collected $100,000 from patients for outstanding receivables.

    i. The center recognized $50,000 in labor expense.

    j. The center paid $50,000 in cash toward its long-term loan.

    k. The center purchased $75,000 in small equipment on credit. Amount is due within one year.

    l. The center incurred $8,000 in general expenses. The center used cash to pay for the general expenses.

    m. The center incurred $2,000 in interest expense for the year. Cash payment of $2,000 was made to the bank.

    n. The center made a $1,000 cash transfer to its parent corporation.

    o. The center owes its staff wages of $3,000.

    p. The center recognized depreciation expenses of $10,000.

    q. The center estimated it would not collect $25,000 of the patient accounts receivable.

13. **Statement of Operations.** The following is a list of account balances for Krakower Healthcare Services, Inc. on December 31, 20X1. Prepare a Statement of Operations as of December 31, 20X1. (Hint: when net assets are released from restriction, the restricted account is decreased, and the unrestricted account is increased. It is recognized under revenues, gains and other support).

Supply Expense	$110,000
Transfer to Parent Corporation	$25,000
Bad Debt Expense	$30,000
Depreciation Expense	$60,000
Labor Expense	$350,000
Interest Expense	$15,000
Administrative Expense	$75,000
Net Patient Service Revenues	$960,000
Net Assets Released from Restriction	$180,000

14. **Statement of Operations.** The following is a list of account balances for Northland Hospital on September 30, 20X1. Prepare a Statement of

Operations as of September 30, 20X1. (Hint: unrestricted donations are recognized under revenues, gains, and other support.)

Labor Expense	$500,000
Provision for Bad Debt	$50,000
Supplies Expense	$200,000
Unrestricted Cash Donation for Operations	$10,000
Net Patient Revenue	$1,800,000
Professional Fees	$300,000
Transfer to Parent Corporation	$25,000
Other Revenues from Cafeteria and Gift Shop	$30,000
Depreciation Expense	$50,000
Income from Investments (Unrestricted Investments)	$15,000
Administrative Expense	$100,000

15. **Statement of Cash Flows.** The following is a list of account balances for Dover Hospital on June 30, 20X1. Prepare a Statement of Cash Flows as of June 30, 20X1.

Transfer to Parent Corporation	$125,000
Proceeds from Sale of Fixed Equipment	$400,000
Principal Payment on Bonds Payable	$700,000
Beginning Cash Balance	$500,000
Cash from Operating Activities	$225,000
Principal Payment on Notes Payable	$20,000

16. **Multiple Statements.** The following is a list of accounts for Bauer Biomedical Supplies on December 31, 20X1. Prepare a Balance Sheet and Statement of Operations as of December 31, 20X1. (Hint: unrestricted contributions increase the unrestricted net assets account, and they are a part of revenues, gains, and other support.)

Interest Expense	$5,000
Cash	$4,000
Gross Accounts Receivable	$55,500
Accrued Expenses	$9,000
Long-term Debt	$145,000
Labor Expenses	$236,000
Supplies	$4,000
Accumulated Depreciation	$147,000
Net Sales Revenues	$484,500
Other Non-current Assets	$5,000
Professional Expenses	$42,000
Short-term Accounts Payable	$35,000
Administrative Expenses	$104,000
Prepaid Expenses	$2,000
Depreciation Expense	$37,000
Non-operating Gains	$5,000

Unrestricted Cash Contributions	$20,000
Short-term Investments	$18,000
Other Current Liabilities	$8,000
Other Revenues	$125,500
Gross Plant and Equipment	$462,000
Deferred Revenue	$3,000
Bad Debt Expense	$12,000
Allowance for Bad Debt	$4,500

17. **Transactions + Multiple Statements.** St. Catherine's Diagnostic Center had the following beginning balances at January 1, 20X0, for its assets, liabilities, and net assets accounts.

Cash	$30,000
Accounts receivable	$250,000
Allowance for Bad Debts	$50,000
Supplies	$6,000
Plant and Equipment	$500,000
Accumulated Depreciation	$50,000
Accounts payable	$8,000
Short-term Notes Payable	$130,000
Bonds Payable	$300,000
Unrestricted Net Assets	$248,000
Restricted Net Assets	$0

List and record each 20X1 transaction under the accrual basis of accounting. Then develop a Balance Sheet for end-of-years 20X0 and 20X1, a Statement of Operations, and a Statement of Changes in Net Assets for the year ended December 31, 20X1.

a. The center collected $200,000 in cash from outstanding accounts receivable.

b. The center purchased $20,000 of supplies on credit.

c. The center provided $500,000 of patient services on credit.

d. The center incurred $200,000 of labor expenses, which it paid in cash.

e. The center consumed $15,000 of supplies in the provision of its diagnostic services.

f. The center paid $15,000 in cash for outstanding short-term notes payable.

g. The center collected $150,000 in cash from outstanding accounts receivable.

h. The center paid $18,000 in cash for outstanding accounts payable.

i. The center issued $2,000,000 in long-term bonds that they must pay back.

j. The center purchased $1,800,000 in equipment on credit.

k. The center recognized $40,000 in interest expense.

l. The center incurred $70,000 in general expenses, which it paid in cash.

m. The center paid in cash $200,000 principal payment toward its outstanding bonds.

n. A local corporation gave an unrestricted $25,000 cash donation. (Hint: this transaction increases the unrestricted net assets account.)

o. The center earned but did not receive $1,000 in interest income from unrestricted short-term investments.

p. The center transferred $7,000 in cash to its parent corporation.

q. The center incurred annual depreciation expense of $50,000.

r. The center estimated the ending balance of the Allowance of Uncollectible Accounts is $60,000.

18. **Transactions + Multiple Statements.** Ambulatory Center Inc. had the following beginning balances for its assets, liabilities, and net accounts as of December 31, 20X0.

Cash	$20,000
Accounts Receivable	$55,000
Allowance for Uncollectibles	$5,000
Supplies	$15,000
Prepaid Insurance	$2,000
Long-term Investments	$50,000
Plant and Equipment	$2,000,000
Accumulated Depreciation	$150,000
Short-term Accounts Payable	$20,000
Accrued Expenses	$5,000
Long-term Debt	$1,000,000
Unrestricted Net Assets	$912,000
Permanently Restricted Net Assets	$50,000

List and record each 20X1 transaction under the accrual basis of accounting. Then develop a Balance Sheet for end-of-years 20X0 and 20X1, a Statement of Operations, and a Statement of Changes in Net Assets for the year ended December 31, 20X1.

a. The center made cash payment of $10,000 to pay off outstanding accounts payable.

b. The center received $25,000 in cash from a donor who temporarily restricted its use. (Hint: this transaction increases the temporarily restricted net assets account.)

c. The center provided $750,000 of services on credit.

d. The center consumed $10,000 of supplies in the provision of its ambulatory services.

e. The center paid off its accrued interest expense of $5,000 in cash.

f. The center collected $125,000 in cash from outstanding accounts receivable.

g. The center incurred $50,000 in general expenses that it paid for in cash.

h. The center made a $25,000 cash principal payment toward its long-term debt.

i. The center collected $600,000 in cash from outstanding accounts receivable.

j. The center received $50,000 in cash from an HMO for future capitated services.

k. The center purchased $12,000 of supplies on credit.
l. The center earned, but did not receive, $5,000 in income from its restricted net assets. The income can be used for general operations. (Hint: this transaction increases interest receivable and is also recorded under revenues, gains and other support.)
m. The center's temporarily restricted asset account released $1,000 from its restricted account to its unrestricted account for operations. (Hint: the transfer gets recorded under revenues, gains, and other support.)
n. The center incurred $5,000 in interest expense. The interest expense was recorded, but not yet paid in cash.
o. The center incurred $500,000 in labor expenses, which it paid for in cash.
p. The center paid $2,000 in advance for insurance expense.
q. The center transferred $10,000 in cash to its parent corporation.
r. The center incurred $150,000 in depreciation expense.
s. The center's prepaid insurance of $2,000 expired for the year.
t. The center recognized $15,000 for bad debt for the year.

Chapter Four

FINANCIAL STATEMENT ANALYSIS

LEARNING OBJECTIVES

After completing this chapter, you will be able to:

▶ Analyze the financial statements of health care organizations using horizontal analysis, vertical (common-size) analysis, and ratio analysis.
▶ Calculate and interpret liquidity ratios, profitability ratios, activity ratios, and capital structure ratios.

Chapter Outline

◀INTRODUCTION▶

The financial performance of health care organizations is of interest to numerous individuals and groups, including administrators, board members, creditors, bondholders, community members, and government agencies (see Perspectives 4–1 and 4–2). Chapters 2 and 3 examined the four main financial statements of health care organizations and the accounting methods underlying the preparation of these statements. This chapter shows how to analyze the financial statements of health care organizations to help answer questions about the organization that produced them:

- Is the organization profitable? Why or why not?
- How effective is the organization in collecting its receivables?
- Is the organization in a good position to pay its bills?
- How efficiently is the organization using its assets?
- Are the organization's plant and equipment in need of replacement?
- Is the organization in a good position to take on additional debt?

PERSPECTIVE 4–1

Using Clinical and Financial Ratios: Performance of the 100 Top Hospitals

In 1993, HCIA (now Solucient) created a model that identifies benchmark hospitals around the country, based solely on empirical, publicly available performance data. The *100 Top Hospitals™ : Benchmarks for Success* study rates hospitals by nine measures of clinical, operational, and financial performance. Generally, *100 Top Hospitals*:

- **have better outcomes.** Their median Medicare case mix indices are 20 percent higher, but their quality of care, as measured by mortality and complications, is as much as 17 percent better than the rest of the country's hospitals.
- **do more with less.** With fewer staff, yet 23 percent higher occupancy rates, they are twice as profitable. Moreover, the *100 Top* hospitals have maintained this level of efficiency over the years, while their peers have steadily increased staffing ratios.
- **manage their debt better.** Debt service ratios are two times higher at *100 Top* hospitals than at their peers. A popular measure of creditworthiness, this ratio measures the amount of funds a hospital has available to cover its debts.
- **have growing occupancy rates.** In 1998, the *100 Top* hospitals' median occupancy rate was 62 percent, compared with the peer hospitals' 50 percent median. Benchmark hospitals grew their occupancy an average of 4.2 percent a year between 1996 and 1998, compared with only 0.3 percent at peer hospitals.
- **invest more in plant modernization and patient services.** Although higher capital costs (per adjusted discharge) are often viewed as unfavorable, benchmark hospitals have been able to maintain these figures without increasing overall operating expenses per discharge.

The *100 Top Hospitals* exhibit high-quality care, operate efficiently, and produce superior financial results. These benchmarks in turn provide the health care industry with some indications and directions for positive change. If all US acute hospitals were to operate like the *100 Top Hospitals*, expenses would decline by an aggregate $31.7 billion yearly, resulting in lower costs and savings across the board.

(Continues)

Perspective 4–1 (*Contd*)

National Performance Comparisons for 1999 Top 100

Performance Measure	Median 1999 Benchmark Hospitals	Median 1998 Benchmark Hospitals	Peer Group of US Hospitals	% Benchmark Exceeds Peer Group
Mortality index[2]	0.86	0.84	1.10	14.9%
Complications[2]	0.89	0.85	1.01	11.9%
Average length of stay	4.3	4.2	4.5	6.0%
Expenses per adjusted discharge	$3,452	$3,509	$4,249	18.8%
Cash flow margin	16.9%	16.3%	10.5%	6.5%[1]
Proportion of outpatient revenue	37.0%	36.6%	41.6%	–4.6%[1]
Occupancy rate	62.0%	60.4%	50.3%	11.7%[1]
Growth in occupancy rate	4.2%	2.0%	27.0%	
Total asset turnover ratio	1.08	1.04	0.92	17.4%

HCIA 100 Top Hospital Performance

Mortality index[2]	# of actual deaths/# of expected deaths
Complications[2]	# of cases with complications/# of expected cases with complications
Average length of stay	average length of stay adjusted for severity of illness
Expenses per adjusted discharge	total operating expenses/discharges adjusted by casemix and wage index
Cash flow margin	(net income + depreciation + interest)/(net patient revenues + other income)
Proportion of outpatient revenue	proportion of outpatient revenue
Occupancy rate	occupancy rate
Growth in occupancy rate	% change in occupancy rate 1996–1998
Total asset turnover ratio	net patient revenue/total assets

[1]Values are percentage point difference between current benchmark and peer group value.
[2]Clinical indexes used in these measures assign a value of one to the expected level of mortality and complications assigned to pre-existing conditions. Less than one means deaths or complications were below expectations.

Source: *100 Top Hospitals* ™ : *Benchmarks for Success*, 1999. © 1999 by HCIA, L.L.C. Reprinted with permission.

PERSPECTIVE 4–2

Use of Financial Ratios to Benchmark Hospital Performance

The performance of the country's hospital industry is not unidimensional. It can be appraised in a number of ways. Performance measures have traditionally relied upon ratios calculated from a hospital's income statement and balance sheet. These chart a hospital's historical financial performance and suggest its future. However, other measures, such as a hospital's occupancy rate and staffing ratios, are equally important because they illuminate the underlying causes of favorable or unfavorable financial performance.

There are seven major categories of hospital performance measures.

- **Capacity and utilization** – A hospital's productive capacity and the utilization of that capacity are key predictors of financial performance. Some of these measures are number of beds, total discharges, occupancy rate, and average length of stay.

(Continues)

Perspective 4–2 (*Contd*)

- **Patient and payer mix** – Hospital financial performance is tied to the illness complexity of the patients treated by the hospital and to the source and nature of third-party reimbursement for patient services. Measures include percentage of Medicare and Medicaid acute care discharges, Medicare case mix index, and percentage of outpatient revenue.
- **Capital structure** – Measures of a hospital's capital structure are key indicators of its ability to incur additional long-term debt and gain access to similar sources of outside funding or financing for growth and expansion. Similarly, these measures often predict a hospital's long-term creditworthiness and solvency. These measures include plant age; debt per bed; capital costs as a percentage of operating expense and per adjusted discharge; long-term debt to total assets, to net fixed assets, and to capitalization; cash flow to total debt; debt service coverage ratio; and capital acquisitions as a percentage of net patient revenue.
- **Liquidity** is a measure of a hospital's ability to meet its short term obligations with the hospital's cash on hand plus its assets that are most easily convertible to cash. These include current ratio, acid test ratio, days in accounts receivable, and average payment period.
- **Revenues, expenses, and profitability** – Profitability refers to a hospital's ability to generate an excess of revenues over expenses. Some measures of profitability are gross patient revenue per adjusted discharge, operating revenue per adjusted discharge, operating profit margin, total profit margin, cash flow margin, return on assets, and cash flow per bed.
- **Productivity and efficiency** – Measures of productivity and efficiency often display the underlying causes of financial performance. These measures include full-time equivalent personnel (FTEs) per adjusted average daily census, salary and benefits per FTE, overhead expense as a percentage of operating expense, and total asset turnover ratio.
- **Pricing strategies** – A hospital's ability to generate profits is a function of its ability to operate efficiently and of its pricing strategies. By examining some of the important markup ratios, such as medical supplies sold, drugs sold, laboratory, diagnostic radiology, and ancillary services, a hospital can examine their pricing strategies to meet the demands of a competitive marketplace.

When analyzing the performance of an individual hospital, it is crucial to evaluate the hospital against a comparison group of similar hospitals. But even after controlling for the effects of structural, locational, and functional differences, there can still be substantial variations in performance. These remaining performance differences should be given special consideration because they are the ones most susceptible to scrutiny and modification by hospital management.

Source: The Comparative Performance of US Hospitals: The Sourcebook. © 2000 by HCIA, L.L.C. and Deloitte & Touche LLP. Reprinted with permission.

Three approaches are commonly used to analyze financial statements: horizontal analysis, vertical analysis, and ratio analysis. Each of these approaches is examined using the financial statements shown in Exhibit 4–1, Newport Hospital's statement of operations and balance sheet. For simplicity, the statement of operations only contains operating items.

Caution

The financial statements presented in this chapter have been simplified from those presented in Chapter 2 in order to facilitate the application of the tools and techniques presented in this chapter.

Exhibit 4–1 Statement of Operations and Balance Sheet for Newport Hospital

Newport Hospital Statement of Operations For Years Ended December 31, 20X1 and 20X0

	12/31/20X1	12/31/20X0
Operating Revenues		
Net Patient Revenues	$10,778,272	$10,566,176
Other Operating Revenues	233,749	253,517
Total Operating Revenues	11,012,021	10,819,693
Operating Expenses		
Salaries and Benefits	5,644,880	5,345,498
Supplies	1,660,000	1,529,680
Insurance	1,536,357	1,551,579
Depreciation	383,493	420,238
Interest	500,000	276,379
Bad debt	456,289	365,678
Other	500,093	276,455
Total Operating Expenses	10,681,112	9,765,507
Operating Income	330,909	1,054,186
Non–Operating Revenue	185,000	165,000
Excess of Revenues Over Expenses	515,909	1,219,186
Increase (Decrease) in Unrestricted Net Assets	**$515,909**	**$1,219,186**

Newport Hospital Balance Sheet For Years Ended December 31, 20X1 and 20X0

	12/31/20X1	12/31/20X0
ASSETS		
Current Assets		
Cash & Marketable Securities	$363,181	$158,458
Patient Accounts Receivables		
Net of Uncollectible Accounts	1,541,244	1,400,013
Inventories	346,176	316,875
Prepaid Expenses	163,734	78,788
Other Current Assets	100,000	0
Total Current Assets	2,514,335	1,954,134
Non–Current Assets		
Gross Plant, Property, & Equipment	7,088,495	6,893,370
(less Accumulated Depreciation)	(2,781,741)	(2,398,248)
Net Plant, Property, and Equipment	4,306,754	4,495,122
Long–term Investments	3,414,732	4,525,476
Other Assets	640,915	340,853
Total Non–Current Assets	8,362,401	9,361,451
Total Assets	**$10,876,736**	**$11,315,585**
LIABILITIES AND NET ASSETS		
Current Liabilities		
Accounts Payable	$387,646	$166,600
Salaries Payable	135,512	529,298
Notes Payable	500,000	2,359,524
Current Portion of Long–term Debt	372,032	338,996
Total Current Liabilities	1,395,190	3,394,418
Long–term Liabilities		
Bonds Payable	6,938,891	6,009,484
Total Long–term Liabilities	6,938,891	6,009,484
Total Liabilities	8,334,081	9,403,902
Net Assets		
Unrestricted	1,901,739	1,570,830
Temporary Restricted	328,000	40,853
Permanently Restricted	312,916	300,000
Total Net Assets	2,542,655	1,911,683
Total Liabilities and Net Assets	**$10,876,736**	**$11,315,585**

◀HORIZONTAL ANALYSIS▶

Horizontal and vertical analyses are two of the most commonly used techniques to analyze financial statements; each is based on percentages. Horizontal analysis looks at the percentage change in a line item from one year to the next. A horizontal analysis of Newport Hospital's statement of operations and balance sheet is presented in Exhibit 4–2 and serves as the basis for the discussion in this section. Horizontal analysis uses the formula:

$$\left(\frac{\text{subsequent year} - \text{previous year}}{\text{previous year}} \right) 100 = \text{percentage change}$$

The goal is to answer the question, "What is the percentage change in a line item from one year to the next year?" For example, from Newport Hospital's statement of operations in Exhibit 4–2, the change in operating income from 20X0 (where 20X0 is the base year) to 20X1 using horizontal analysis would be:

$$\left(\frac{\$330,909 - \$1,054,186}{\$1,054,186} \right) 100 = -68.6\%$$

A problem with horizontal analysis is that percentage changes can hide major dollar effects. For example, there is an 80.9 percent change in interest expense from the statement of operations, which was the result of a $223,621 change from 20X0 to 20X1 ($500,000 – $276,379) (Exhibit 4–1); on the other hand, the 9.4 percent change in total operating expenses was a $915,605 change (Exhibit 4–2).

Key Point   Three approaches to analyze financial statements: horizontal analysis, vertical analysis, and ratio analysis.

Horizontal analysis is also often used to compare changes from one year to the next over several years. The following example analyzes five consecutive years of Newport Hospital's operating income (not shown in the exhibits):

Key Point   When using horizontal analysis: 1) small percentage changes can mask large dollar changes from one year to the next; 2) large percentage changes from year to year may be relatively inconsequential in terms of dollar amounts. This usually occurs when the base year is a small dollar amount.

	20X0	20X1	20X2	20X3	20X4
Operating Income	$1,054,186	$330,909	$500,098	$1,232,565	$1,453,567
Percentage Change from Previous Year		–68.6	51.1	146.5	17.9

The change from 20X1 to 20X2 is calculated as follows:

$$\left(\frac{\$500,098 - \$330,909}{\$330,909}\right)100 = 51.1\%$$

This analysis shows how successful the organization was in increasing operating income from one year to the next. A disadvantage of this approach is that it does not answer the question, "How much overall change has there been since 20X0?" Trend analysis supplies an answer to this question.

Horizontal Analysis: A method of analyzing financial statements which looks at the percentage change in a line item from one year to the next. It is computed by the formula [(subsequent year – previous year)/ previous year] × 100.

◄TREND ANALYSIS►

Instead of looking at single year changes, trend analysis compares changes over a longer period of time by comparing each year to a base year. The formula for a trend analysis is:

Exhibit 4–2 Horizontal Analysis of the Statement of Operations and Balance Sheet for Newport Hospital

Newport Hospital Statement of Operations For the Years Ended December 31, 20X1 and 20X0

	12/31/20X1	12/31/20X0	% Change 20X1–20X0
Operating Revenues			
Net Patient Revenues	$10,778,272	$10,566,176	2.0%
Other Operating Revenues	233,749	253,517	–7.8%
Total Operating Revenues	11,012,021	10,819,693	1.8%
Operating Expenses			
Total Operating Expenses	10,681,112	9,765,507	9.4%
Operating Income	330,909	1,054,186	– 68.6%
Non-Operating Revenue	185,000	165,000	12.1%
Excess of Revenues Over Expenses	515,909	1,219,186	–57.7%
Increase (Decrease) in Unrestricted Net Assets	**$515,909**	**$1,219,186**	–57.7%

Newport Hospital Balance Sheet December 31, 20X1 and 20X0

	20X1	20X0	% Change 20X1–20X0
Assets			
Current Assets	$2,514,335	$1,954,134	28.7%
Non–current Assets	8,362,401	9,361,451	–10.7%
Total Assets	$10,876,736	$11,315,585	–3.9%
Liabilities			
Current Liabilities	$1,395,190	$3,394,418	–58.9%
Long–term Liabilities	6,938,891	6,009,484	15.5%
Total Liabilities	8,334,081	9,403,902	
Net Assets			
Total Net Assets	2,542,655	1,911,683	33.0%
Total Liabilities and Net Assets	**$10,876,736**	**$11,315,585**	–3.9%

$$\left(\frac{\text{subsequent year} - \text{base year}}{\text{base year}} \right) 100$$

Applying this formula to operating income for the same five-year period used to illustrate horizontal analysis yields the following results:

	20X0	20X1	20X2	20X3	20X4
Operating Income	$1,054,186	$330,909	$500,098	$1,232,565	$1,453,567
% Change from 20X0		−68.6%	−52.6%	16.9%	37.9%

Trend Analysis:
A type of horizontal analysis that looks at changes in line items compared to a base year. It is calculated: [(any subsequent year − base year)/ base year] × 100.

For instance, the change from 20X0 to 20X4 is calculated as follows:

$$\left(\frac{\$1,453,567 - \$1,054,186}{\$1,054,186} \right) 100 = 37.9\%$$

Thus, from 20X0 (the base year) to 20X4, operating income rose 37.9 percent. Note that the average annual increase of 9.5 percent (37.9 percent/4 years) is different from that of simply averaging the increases or decreases each year.

◄VERTICAL (COMMON-SIZE) ANALYSIS►

The purpose of vertical analysis is to answer the general question, "What percentage of one line item is another line item?" The formula to use in this case is:

$$\left(\frac{\text{line item of interest}}{\text{base line item}} \right) 100$$

Vertical Analysis: A method to analyze financial statements which answers the general question: What percentage of one line item is another line item? Also called common-size analysis because it converts every line item to a percentage, thus allowing comparisons among the financial statements of different organizations. Since all items are stated as percentages, this methodology can be used to compare several different organizations to determine, for example, "Which organization has the highest percentage of its assets as current assets?"

For instance, Newport Hospital might want to know if Net Patient Revenues has increased as a percent of Total Operating Revenues or, similarly, what percentage of its Operating Revenues are the Operating Expenses. The top of Exhibit 4–3 computes all line items for Newport Hospital's statement of operations as a percentage of Total Operating Revenues. In 20X0, Total Operating Expenses were 90.3 percent of Total Operating Revenues [($9,765,507/ $10,819,693) × 100], but by 20X1, they had increased to 97 percent of total operating revenues [($10,681,112/$11,012,021) × 100]. This information provides some insight as to why Newport Hospital experienced the 68.6 percent decrease in operating income observed in the horizontal analysis.

Though the focus up until now has been on the statement of operations, vertical analysis is very useful for analyzing the balance sheet as well, as shown in the bottom of Exhibit 4–3, which presents all line items as a percentage of total assets. By using total assets as a base, the reader can ask such questions as: "Has the composition of the balance sheet changed appreciably from 20X0 to 20X1?" In this example, total liabilities decreased from 83.1 percent of total assets in 20X0 to 76.6 percent in 20X1.

Exhibit 4–3 Vertical (Common-Size) Analysis for the Statement of Operations and Balance Sheet for Newport Hospital

Newport Hospital
Statement of Operations
For Years Ended December 31, 20X1 and 20X0

	12/3120X1	% of Total Revenues	12/3120X0	% of Total Revenues
Operating Revenues				
Net Patient Revenues	$10,778,272	97.9%	$10,566,176	97.7%
Other Operating Revenues	233,749	2.1%	253,517	2.3%
Total Operating Revenues	11,012,021	100.0%	10,819,693	100.0%
Operating Expenses:				
Total Operating Expenses	10,681,112	97.0%	9,765,507	90.3%
Operating Income	330,909	3.0%	1,054,186	9.7%
Non-Operating revenue	185,000	1.7%	165,000	1.5%
Excess of Revenues over Expenses	515,909	4.7%	1,219,186	11.3%
Increase (Decrease) in Unrestricted Net Assets	$515,909	4.7%	$1,219,186	11.3%

Newport Hospital
Balance Sheet
For Years Ended December 31, 20X1 and 20X0

	20X1	% of Total Assets	20X0	% of Total Assets
Assets				
Current Assets	$2,514,335	23.1%	$1,954,134	17.3%
Non-Current Assets	8,362,401	76.9%	9,361,451	82.7%
Total Assets	$10,876,736	100.0%	$11,315,585	100.0%
Liabilities				
Current Liabilities	$1,395,190	12.8%	$3,394,418	30.0%
Long-Term Liabilities	6,938,891	63.8%	6,009,484	53.1%
Total Liabilities	8,334,081	76.6%	9,403,902	83.1%
Net Assets				
Total Net Assets	2,542,655	23.4%	1,911,683	16.9%
Total Liabilities and Net Assets	$10,876,736	100.0%	$11,315,585	100.0%

Two points can be noted from this information: 1) in 20X1, debt was used to finance 76.6 percent of Newport Hospital's assets, whereas in 20X0 it was used to finance over 83 percent; and 2) the use of long-term debt to finance assets grew from 53.1 percent of total assets in 20X0 to 63.8 percent in 20X1. In other words, Newport is more highly leveraged in 20X1 than it was in 20X0.

Financial Leverage:
The degree to which an organization is financed by debt.

Exhibit 4–4 presents common-size financial statements for a small community hospital and a large community hospital. The larger facility has a smaller percentage of its assets in plant and equipment, 75 percent, compared to 88 percent for the smaller facility. However, the smaller facility has a lower proportion of its capital structure in total debt, 58 percent, compared to 70 percent for the larger facility. The larger facility also has a higher percentage of its revenues from net patient revenues (97 percent) than does the smaller facility (83 percent). While there are no standards to compare these percentages to, they can elicit questions as to why the differences exist.

◀Ratio Analysis▶

Although horizontal and vertical analyses are easy to calculate and commonly used, ratio analysis is the preferred approach to gain an in-depth understanding of financial statements. A ratio expresses the relationship between two numbers as a single number. For instance, the current ratio expresses the relationship between current assets and current liabilities. This provides an indication of the organization's ability to cover current obligations with current assets (the ability to pay short-term debt).

$$\text{Current Ratio} = \frac{\text{Current Assets}}{\text{Current Liabilities}}$$

Categories of Ratios

Ratios are generally grouped into four categories: liquidity, profitability, activity, and capital structure.

Ratio: An expression of the relationship between two numbers as a single number.

- *Liquidity ratios* answer the question: "How well is the organization positioned to meet its short-term obligations?"
- *Profitability ratios* answer the question: "How profitable is the organization?"
- *Activity ratios* answer the question: "How efficiently is the organization using its assets to produce revenues?"
- *Capital structure ratios* answer the questions: "How are the organization's assets financed?" and "How able is the organization to take on new debt?"

Exhibit 4–4 Common-Size Financial Statements for a Small and a Large Hospital

<table>
<tr><th colspan="3">Small Community Hospital
Balance Sheet December 31, 20X0</th><th colspan="3">Small Community Hospital Statement of
Operations December 31, 20X0</th></tr>
<tr><td></td><td></td><td>% Total
Assets</td><td></td><td></td><td>% Total
Revenues</td></tr>
<tr><td>Current Assets</td><td>$1,000</td><td>10%</td><td>Net Patient Revenues</td><td>$10,000</td><td>83%</td></tr>
<tr><td>Net Plant and Equipment</td><td>9,000</td><td>88%</td><td>Investment Income</td><td>2,000</td><td>17%</td></tr>
<tr><td>Other Assets</td><td>200</td><td>2%</td><td>Total Operating Revenues</td><td>12,000</td><td>100%</td></tr>
<tr><td>Total Assets</td><td>$10,200</td><td>100%</td><td>Operating Expenses</td><td>10,000</td><td>83%</td></tr>
<tr><td>Current Liabilities</td><td>$900</td><td>9%</td><td>Income from Operations</td><td>2,000</td><td>17%</td></tr>
<tr><td>Long-Term Debt</td><td>5,000</td><td>49%</td><td></td><td></td><td></td></tr>
<tr><td>Total Liabilities</td><td>5,900</td><td>58%</td><td>Excess of Revenues Over Expenses</td><td>2,000</td><td>17%</td></tr>
<tr><td>Net Assets</td><td>4,300</td><td>42%</td><td>Increase in Net Assets</td><td>$2,000</td><td>17%</td></tr>
<tr><td>Total Liabilities and Net Assets</td><td>$10,200</td><td>100%</td><td></td><td></td><td></td></tr>
</table>

<table>
<tr><th colspan="3">Large Community Hospital
Balance Sheet December 31, 20X0</th><th colspan="3">Large Community Hospital Statement of
Operations December 31, 20X0</th></tr>
<tr><td></td><td></td><td>% Total
Assets</td><td></td><td></td><td>% Total
Revenues</td></tr>
<tr><td>Current Assets</td><td>$15,000</td><td>22%</td><td>Net Patient Revenues</td><td>$68,000</td><td>97%</td></tr>
<tr><td>Net Plant and Equipment</td><td>50,000</td><td>75%</td><td>Investment Income</td><td>2,000</td><td>3%</td></tr>
<tr><td>Other Assets</td><td>2,000</td><td>3%</td><td>Total Operating Revenues</td><td>70,000</td><td>100%</td></tr>
<tr><td>Total Assets</td><td>$67,000</td><td>100%</td><td>Operating Expenses</td><td>65,000</td><td>93%</td></tr>
<tr><td>Current Liabilities</td><td>$12,000</td><td>18%</td><td>Income from Operations</td><td>5,000</td><td>7%</td></tr>
<tr><td>Long-Term Debt</td><td>35,000</td><td>52%</td><td></td><td></td><td></td></tr>
<tr><td>Total Liabilities</td><td>47,000</td><td>70%</td><td>Excess of Revenues Over Expenses</td><td>5,000</td><td>7%</td></tr>
<tr><td></td><td></td><td></td><td>Increase in Net Assets</td><td>$5,000</td><td>7%</td></tr>
<tr><td>Net Assets</td><td>20,000</td><td>30%</td><td></td><td></td><td></td></tr>
<tr><td>Total Liabilities and Net Assets</td><td>$67,000</td><td>100%</td><td></td><td></td><td></td></tr>
</table>

Note: All figures expressed in '000.

Exhibit 4–5 shows what the ratios would be for Newport Hospital and compares them to industry norms. The remaining sections of this chapter will describe how these results were derived.

Key Points to Consider When Using and Interpreting Ratios

1. **No one ratio is necessarily better than any other ratio.** It is often useful to use more than one ratio to help answer a question.
2. **Each ratio's terms offer clues about how to fix a problem.** For example, if the current ratio (current assets/current liabilities) is too low, it can be

Exhibit 4-5   Newport Hospital Ratios for 20X0 and 20X1, and HCIA & HCFA Median Ratio Values

Ratios	Standard Small Hospitals' HCIA & HCFA Median Ratio[1]	Desired Position	Newport Trend Analysis 20X1	Newport Trend Analysis 20X0	Year Position	Current Trend Position	Possible Explanation Current Year Relative to Standards
Liquidity Ratios							
Current Ratio	2.18	Above	1.80	0.58	Below	Increasing	Liquidity improving, but many ratios are still
Quick Ratio[2]	1.76	Above	1.36	0.46	Below	Increasing	considerably below standard. Mixed picture on
Acid Test Ratio	0.35	Above	0.26	0.05	Below	Increasing	cash available:acid test ratio low while days in
Days in Accounts Receivable	67	Below	52	48	Below	Increasing	accounts receivable favorable. Its days cash on
Days Cash on Hand[2]	46	Above	13	6	Below	Increasing	hand is 70% below standard. Average payment
Average Payment Period	54	Below	49	133	Below	Decreasing	period is moving toward standard.
Profitability Ratios							
Operating Margin	0.02	Above	0.03	0.10	Above	Decreasing	At or above the standard for two of the four
Non-Operating Revenue[2]	0.05	Varies	0.02	0.02	Below	Increasing	profitability ratios, but shows a precipitous
Return on Total Assets	0.03	Above	0.05	0.11	Above	Decreasing	drop in three of the four. This raises concerns
Return on Equity Net Assets[2]	0.06	Above	0.20	0.64	Above	Decreasing	about control of revenues and expenses.
Activity Ratios							
Total Asset Turnover Ratio	1.02	Above	1.01	0.96	Below	Increasing	Near standard on its TAT, but ~ 25% below std. on FAT. Though improving, still of
Net Fixed Assets Turnover Ratio	3.59	Above	2.56	2.41	Below	Increasing	concern. Avg. age of plant increase a
Age of Plant Ratio	9.86	Below	7.25	5.71	Below	Increasing	concern.
Capital Structure Ratios							
Long-Term Debt to Net Assets Ratio	0.21	Below	2.73	3.14	Above	Decreasing	Though decreased its debt position, still well
Net Assets to Total Assets Ratio[2]	0.62	Above	0.23	0.17	Below	Increasing	above std. The proportion of debt to net assets
Times Interest Earned Ratio[2]	2.85	Above	2.03	5.41	Below	Decreasing	is still too high, but decreasing. Ability to
Debt Service Coverage Ratio	3.35	Above	2.00	4.02	Below	Decreasing	pay debt is of considerable concern.

[1]Since Newport Hospital was less than 100 beds, HCIA–Sachs Standard ratio values for Beds less than 100 were used
[2]These values were obtained from: the Health Care Financing Administration's (HCFA) Hospital Cost Report Information System Files for financial statements ending in 1998 and HCIA–Sachs Standard's 1998 median values, *The Comparative Performance of US Hospitals: The Sourcebook 2000*, HCIA Publications, Baltimore, MD.

improved by increasing the numerator (current assets), decreasing the denominator (current liabilities), or both. However, changing the conditions to improve one ratio may affect other ratios as well.

3. **Most ratios are interpreted as follows: "There are N dollars in the numerator for every dollar in the denominator."** Thus, a current ratio of 2 indicates that there is $2 in current assets for every $1 in current liabilities.

4. **A ratio can best be interpreted relative to a standard.** The standard may be the organization's past performance, a goal set by the organization, a comparison group (such as similar organizations), or some combination thereof. For example, a current ratio of 2.00 probably would be interpreted favorably if the industry standard were 1.75; however, it probably would be interpreted unfavorably if the industry standard were 2.50.

5. **There are several problems with using standards for comparison in the health care industry.** Two of the most prominent are the availability and reliability of the data:

   - **Finding appropriate data.** Not all segments of the health care industry have data available that can be used for standards. For example, there are no complete, national-level ratio data on health departments or mental health centers. On the other hand, certain segments of the industry have excellent data. The Center for Healthcare Industry Performance Studies (CHIPS) and HCIA-Sachs both provide excellent ratio information on hospitals on both a national and regional basis. In addition, many cooperatives, such as Premier, provide benchmarking standards to their members. Alternatively, individual providers may join together to develop their own standards. Even if data are available, it is important to compare an organization to similar organizations. It might be highly inappropriate for a small rural hospital in North Dakota to use the ratios of large academic medical centers in Boston for comparison. Services such as CHIPS can provide data by size and location. The data are presented by both median and percentile, which means that an organization can set its own standards relative to what it considers an appropriate comparison group.

   - **The reliability of the data.** The same ratio may be calculated differently by different organizations and/or different sources of industry standards. For example, in calculating the days in accounts receivable, one organization may use the ending balance in accounts receivable, whereas another organization may use the average daily balance. *Therefore, when comparing organizations to one another or to standards, it is necessary to make sure the same formula is being used* (see Perspective 4–3). There may be differences in practices and procedures among organizations that may not be immediately apparent to those using the information. For example, hospitals may use different depreciation or inventory valuation methods. This could have a profound effect on certain ratios.

6. **In general, a ratio should be neither too high nor too low relative to the standard.** For example, the acid test ratio [(cash + marketable securities)/current liabilities] looks at an organization's ability to meet its

PERSPECTIVE 4–3

Formulas Hospitals Report Using to Calculate Net Days in Accounts Receivable

Hospital	Formula
Hospital 1	Gross Accounts Receivable – Uncollectibles ÷ [(Gross Charges – Deductions) ÷ Number of Days in Period]
Hospital 2	Net Patient Accounts Receivable ÷ (Net Patient Service Revenue ÷ 365)
Hospital 3	Net Accounts Receivable ÷ Net Charges per Day
Hospital 4	Net Accounts Receivable ÷ [(Gross Patient Service Revenue – Charity – Contractual Allowances – Bad Debt) ÷ 365]
Hospital 5	Accounts Receivable + Reserve for Bad Debt + Contractual Adjustments ÷ (Net Patient Revenue ÷ Number of Days in the Period)
Hospital 6	Accounts Receivable ÷ (Revenue Available ÷ Days in Current Year)
Hospital 7	Net Patient Revenue ÷ Operating Margin
Hospital 8	Net Accounts Receivable ÷ (Net Revenue Past 3 months ÷ Days in Period)

Source: Contributed by Denise R. Smith, FHFMA, CMPA. DSS Data Analyst Columbia Cape Fear Memorial Hospital.

short-term debt. Though an organization would like to have this ratio above the standard, a value too high may indicate too much cash on hand, which likely could be better invested elsewhere.

7. **Not only should a ratio be compared to a standard, but also the trend of the ratio can help to interpret how well an organization is doing.** For example, an organization would feel differently if a ratio were at the standard and declining versus being at the standard and rising over the past five years.

8. **Since ratios are usually relatively small, relatively small differences may indicate large percentage deviations from the standard.** For example, if the organization's current ratio were 1.5 and the industry standard 2.0, while this is only a 0.5 difference, the organization would be 25 percent below standard.

Caution

When comparing organizations to one another or to standards, it is necessary to make sure the same formula is being used.

The remainder of this chapter uses ratio analysis to analyze the statement of operations and balance sheet for Newport Hospital (see Exhibit 4–1) using industry standards for small hospitals.

Liquidity Ratios

Liquidity ratios answer the question, "How well is the organization positioned to meet its current obligations?" Six key ratios fall into this category: the current ratio, quick ratio, acid test ratio, days in accounts receivable, days cash on hand, and average payment period (Exhibit 4–6). Incidentally, by convention, the current ratio, quick ratio and acid test ratio all have the word "ratio" in their title, while the other three do not.

Key Point | Liquidity ratios measure a facility's ability to meet short-term obligations, collect receivables, and maintain a cash position.

Each of these liquidity ratios provides a different insight into Newport Hospital's liquidity. Notice that the first three ratios focus only on the balance sheet, each giving a little more stringent picture of the organization's ability to pay off its current liabilities. The last three ratios use information from both the statement of operations and the balance sheet to look at different aspects of liquidity: the ability of the organization to turn its receivables into cash, the actual amount of cash it has on hand to meet its short-term obligations, and how long it takes the organization to pay its bills, respectively.

Current Ratio

The **current ratio** (current assets/current liabilities) is one of the most commonly used ratios. The current ratio is the proportion of all current assets to all current liabilities. Values above the standard indicate either too many current assets, too few current liabilities, or both. Values below the standard indicate either too few current assets, too many current liabilities, or both. To calculate the current ratio (see Exhibit 4–6a):

Step 1. Identify the dollar amount of current assets on the balance sheet.
Step 2. Identify the dollar amount of current liabilities on the balance sheet.
Step 3. Divide the current assets by the current liabilities.

Newport Hospital's current ratio increased from 0.58 in 20X0 to 1.80 in 20X1. The standard used for comparison is 2.18. Although the 20X1 value is still below the industry median, this dramatic increase in Newport's current ratio reflects a major improvement in liquidity according to this measure.

Quick Ratio

The **quick ratio** [(cash + marketable securities + net accounts receivable)/current liabilities] is commonly used in industries in which net accounts receivable is relatively liquid.

Exhibit 4–6 Selected Liquidity Ratios

Ratio	Formula	Standard[1]	Desired Position
Current Ratio	$\dfrac{\text{Current Assets}}{\text{Current Liabilities}}$	2.18	Above
Quick Ratio	$\dfrac{\text{Cash} + \text{Marketable Securities} + \text{Net Receivables}}{\text{Current Liabilities}}$	1.76	Above
Acid Test Ratio	$\dfrac{\text{Cash} + \text{Marketable Securities}}{\text{Current Liabilities}}$	0.35	Above
Days in Accounts Receivable	$\dfrac{\text{Net Patient Accounts Receivable}}{\text{Net Patient Revenues}/365}$	67	Below
Days Cash on Hand	$\dfrac{\text{Cash} + \text{Marketable Securities}}{(\text{Operating Expenses} - \text{Depreciation Expense})/365}$	46	Above
Average Payment Period (Days)	$\dfrac{\text{Current Liabilities}}{(\text{Operating Expenses} - \text{Depreciation Expense})/365}$	54	Organizationally Dependent

[1] Based upon HCIA-Sachs' 1998 approximate hospital median values in mid-1990s

Exhibit 4–6a   Newport's Current Ratio for 20X0 and 20X1

Year	Current Ratio	=	Current Assets	÷	Current Liabilities
20X1	1.80	=	$2,514,335	÷	$1,395,190
20X0	0.58	=	$1,954,134	÷	$3,394,418

Standard = 2.18

Exhibit 4–6b   Newport's Quick Ratio for 20X0 and 20X1

Year	Quick Ratio	=	(Cash + Marketable Securities	+	Net Accounts Receivable)	÷	Current Liabilities
20X1	1.36	=	$363,181	+	$1,541,244	÷	$1,395,190
20X0	0.46	=	$158,458	+	$1,400,013	÷	$3,394,418

Standard = 1.76

Traditionally, this has not been the case in health care organizations. To compute the quick ratio (see Exhibit 4–6b):

> Step 1. Identify the dollar amount of cash, marketable securities, and net accounts receivable on the balance sheet.
> Step 2. Identify the dollar amount of current liabilities on the balance sheet.
> Step 3. Divide the sum of cash, marketable securities, and net accounts receivable by current liabilities.

As with the current ratio, Newport Hospital's quick ratio improved from 20X0 to 20X1, but it is still approximately 25 percent below the industry standard of 1.76. In order to improve this ratio, Newport Hospital must either increase its current assets or decrease its current liabilities or both.

Acid Test Ratio

The **acid test ratio** [(cash + marketable securities)/current liabilities] provides the most stringent test of liquidity. It looks at how much cash is on hand or readily available from marketable securities to pay off all current liabilities. This ratio is particularly useful if current liabilities contain a high percentage of accounts that must be paid off soon (such as wages payable), and/or if collections of accounts receivable are slow. To compute the acid test ratio (see Exhibit 4–6c):

> Step 1. Identify the dollar amount of cash and marketable securities on the balance sheet.
> Step 2. Identify the dollar amount of current liabilities on the balance sheet.
> Step 3. Divide the sum of cash and temporary investments by current liabilities.

Newport's acid test ratio increased from 0.05 to 0.26 from 20X0 to 20X1. In this case, there is a favorable trend, but a concern might be raised because Newport is still about 25 percent below the industry standard of 0.35. This means that Newport needs to increase its cash and marketable securities or decrease its current liabilities in order to meet the target figure.

Key Point   The current ratio, quick ratio and acid test ratio all measure the relationship of various current assets to current liabilities. The acid test ratio provides the most stringent test of liquidity of the three.

Days in Accounts Receivable

The **days in accounts receivable** ratio [net patient accounts receivable/(net patient revenues/365)] provides an indication of how quickly a hospital is converting its receivables into cash. By dividing net patient accounts receivable by an average day's revenue (net patient revenues/365), this ratio provides an estimate of how many days' revenues have not yet been collected. Values above the standard indicate problems relating to credit and/or collection policies. To calculate the days in accounts receivable ratio (see Exhibit 4–6d):

Key Point   The term **Average Collection Period** can also be used interchangeably with **Days in Accounts Receivable**.

Exhibit 4–6c   Newport's Acid Test Ratio for 20X0 and 20X1

Year	Acid Test Ratio	=	(Cash + Marketable Securities)	÷	Current Liabilities
20X1	0.26	=	$363,181	÷	$1,395,190
20X0	0.05	=	$158,458	÷	$3,394,418

Standard = 0.35

Exhibit 4–6d   Newport's Days in Accounts Receivable Ratio of 20X0 and 20X1

Steps 1,2

Year	Average Net Patient Revenues/Day	=	Net Patient Revenues	÷	365 days
20X1	$29,530 /day	=	$10,778,272	÷	365 days
20X0	$28,948 /day	=	$10,566,176	÷	365 days

Steps 3,4

Year	Days in Accounts Receivable	=	Net Patient Accounts Receivable	÷	Average Net Patient Revenues/Day
20X1	52 days	=	$1,541,244	÷	$29,530 /day
20X0	48 days	=	$1,400,013	÷	$28,948 /days

Standard = 67 days

Step 1. Identify the dollar amount of net patient revenues on the statement of operations.

Step 2. Divide net patient revenues by 365 to compute average net patient revenues per day.

Step 3. Identify the dollar amount of net patient accounts receivable on the balance sheet.

Step 4. Divide net patient accounts receivable by average net patient revenues per day.

Though it took four days longer on average to collect receivables in 20X1 than it did in 20X0, Newport Hospital is well below the standard (67 days) for both 20X0 (48 days) and 20X1 (52 days). This generally indicates excellent performance in this area.

Days Cash on Hand

The **days cash on hand** ratio {(cash + marketable securities)/[(operating expenses − depreciation expense)/365]} provides an indication of the number of days' worth of expenses an organization can cover with its most liquid assets: cash and marketable securities. The denominator [(operating expenses − depreciation expense)/365] measures an average day's cash outflow. Depreciation is subtracted from operating expenses in the denominator since it is an operating expense, but requires no cash outflow. To compute the days cash on hand ratio (see Exhibit 4–6e):

Step 1. Identify the dollar amount of operating expenses and depreciation expense on the statement of operations.

Step 2. Divide operating expenses minus depreciation expense by 365 days to compute average cash operating expense per day.

Step 3. Identify the dollar amount of cash and marketable securities on the balance sheet.

Step 4. Divide cash and marketable securities by the average cash operating expense per day (from Step 2).

Exhibit 4–6e   Newport's Days Cash on Hand Ratio for 20X0 and 20X1

Year	Operating Expense per Day	=	(Operating Expenses	−	Depreciation Expense)	÷	365 days
20X1	$28,213/day	=	$10,681,112	−	$383,493	÷	365 days
20X0	$25,603/day	=	$9,765,507	−	$420,238	÷	365 days

Year	Days Cash On Hand	=	(Cash + Marketable Securities)	÷	Operating Expense per Day
20X1	13 days	=	$363,181	÷	$28,213/day
20X0	6 days	=	$158,458	÷	$25,603/day

Standard = 46 days

Newport Hospital has more than doubled its days cash on hand from six days (20X0) to thirteen days (20X1). However, it is still 33 days below the standard, indicating that it should consider either increasing its cash and marketable securities or decreasing its operating expenses. When examining a hospital's days cash on hand ratio, be aware that system-affiliated hospitals may keep a very low balance of cash on hand, since they may transfer a large portion of cash to their parent each day. If an unusual amount of cash is needed, the parent will transfer back the needed amount. By doing this, the parent organization has larger amounts of cash available for investment purposes, and in many cases is in a better position to invest cash than are the subsidiaries. In such cases, a low days cash on hand ratio of the subsidiary organization is not indicative of a problem.

Average Payment Period

The **average payment period** ratio {current liabilities/[(operating expenses − depreciation expense)/365]} is the counterpart to the days in accounts receivable ratio. It is a measure of how long, on average, it takes an organization to pay its bills. Since the denominator is a measure of an average day's payments for bills, dividing current liabilities by an average day's payment provides a measure of how many days' bills have not been paid. In order to develop a creditworthy relationship and goodwill with vendors and suppliers, health care organizations should attempt to pay their bills on time. To calculate the average payment period ratio (see Exhibit 4–6f):

 Key Point

Days in accounts receivable, cash on hand, and average payment period are all liquidity ratios which give an insight into how quickly cash is flowing in and out of the organization.

Step 1. Identify the dollar amount of total expenses and depreciation expense on the statement of operations.
Step 2. Divide operating expenses minus depreciation expense by 365 days to compute average cash expense per day.

Exhibit 4–6f   Newport's Average Payment Period Ratio for 20X0 and 20X1

Steps 1, 2

Year	Average Cash Expense per Day	=	(Operating Expenses	−	Depreciation Expense)	÷	365 days
20X1	$28,213 /day	=	($10,681,112	−	$383,493)	÷	365 days
20X0	$25,603 /day	=	($9,765,507	−	$420,238)	÷	365 days

Steps 3, 4

Year	Average Payment Period	=	Current Liabilities	÷	Average Cash Expense per Day
20X1	49 days	=	$1,395,190	÷	$28,213/day
20X0	133 days	=	$3,394,418	÷	$25,603/day

Standard = 54 days

Step 3. Identify the dollar amount of current liabilities on the balance sheet.
Step 4. Divide the current liabilities by average cash expense per day.

In the period of one year, Newport Hospital has decreased its average payment period from 133 days to 49 days and is now below the industry standard of 54 days.

Liquidity Summary

From 20X0 to 20X1, Newport Hospital improved its ability to meet current obligations with current assets as indicated by its current, quick, acid test and days cash on hand ratios, though all are still considerably below their standards (Exhibit 4–7). In terms of the relative amount of cash actually available, a mixed picture emerges. On the one hand, the acid test ratio, which indicates the amount of cash and marketable securities available to meet current liabilities, is below its desired position of being at the standard. On the other hand, it is favorably positioned on its days in accounts receivable, which (see Exhibit 4–8) indicates that the organization is performing well in turning its receivables into cash. Its days cash on hand is over 70 per cent below standard.

In regard to collecting the money owed it and paying its bills, Newport's days in accounts receivable is increasing toward the standard (which means revenues will be converted to cash more slowly), while it has greatly decreased its average payment period (which will likely be well received by its suppliers). Unfortunately, days cash on hand is still quite low, which should cause some concern to the organization.

Profitability Ratios

There are several profitability ratios, each providing a different insight into the ability of a health care organization to produce a profit. The most commonly used ratios include operating margin, non-patient service revenue, return on net assets, and return on total assets (see Exhibit 4–9 and Perspective 4–4).

Exhibit 4–7 Newport's Hospital's Current, Quick, and Acid Test Ratios for 20X0 and 20X1 as Compared to the Standard

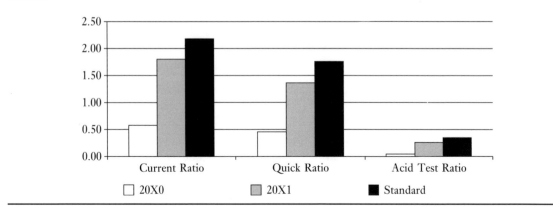

Exhibit 4–8 Newport Hospital's Days in Accounts Receivable, Days Cash on Hand, and Average Payment Period Ratios for 20X0 and 20X1 as Compared to the Standard

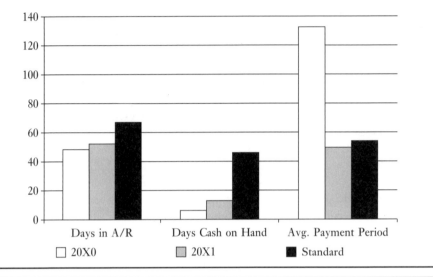

Exhibit 4–9 Selected Profitability Ratios

Ratio	Formula	Standard[1]	Desired Position
Operating Margin	$\dfrac{\text{Operating Income}}{\text{Total Operating Revenues}}$	0.02	Above
Non-Operating Revenue Ratio	$\dfrac{\text{Non-Operating Revenues}}{\text{Total Operating Revenues}}$	0.05	Organizationally Dependent
Return on Total Assets[2]	$\dfrac{\text{Excess of Revenues over Expenses}}{\text{Total Assets}}$	0.03	Above
Return on Net Assets[3]	$\dfrac{\text{Excess of Revenues over Expenses}}{\text{Net Assets}}$	0.06	Above

[1] Based upon HCIA-Sachs's 1998 approximate hospital median values in mid-1990s.

[2] Called *return on assets* and calculated as net income/total assets in for-profit health care organizations.

[3] Called *return on equity* in for-profit health care organizations (net income/owners' equity).

Operating Margin

The **operating margin ratio** (operating income/total operating revenues) measures profits earned from the organization's main line of business. The margin indicates the proportion of profit earned for each dollar of operating revenue; that is, the proportion of profit remaining after subtracting total operating expenses from operating revenues. To compute the operating margin (see Exhibit 4–9a):

Step 1. Identify operating income on the statement of operations.
Step 2. Identify total operating revenues on the statement of operations.
Step 3. Divide operating income by total operating revenues.

PERSPECTIVE 4–4

Key Profitability Performance Measures

HCIA-Sachs considers four profitability measures in its analysis of hospital profitability. Operating profit margin, total profit margin, and cash flow margin are expressed as a percentage of net revenues, while return on assets is expressed as percentage of total assets. Operating profit margin measures a hospital's operating income with respect to the provision of patient care services. Total profit margin measures not only operating income but also non-operating income earned from private philanthropy, interest income, and other income not generated from hospital operations. Cash flow margin measures cash earnings before depreciation and is a critical measure in assessing a hospital's ability to borrow. Return on asset measures the income earned from assets. A downward trend in profitability can impair a hospital's liquidity position.

Source: HCIA, *Comparative Performance of US Hospitals:The Sourcebook 2000.* HCIA Publications, Baltimore, MD.

Exhibit 4–9a   Newport's Operating Margin Ratio for 20X0 and 20X1

Year	Operating Margin	=	Operating Income	÷	Total Operating Revenues
20X1	0.03	=	$330,909	÷	$11,012,021
20X0	0.10	=	$1,054,186	÷	$10,819,693
Standard = 0.02					

In 20X0, Newport Hospital was considerably above the industry standard (0.10 versus 0.02). However, the operating margin ratio has decreased to 0.03 in 20X1, reflecting the fact that total operating expenses have increased faster than have total operating revenues.

Non-Operating Revenue Ratio

The purpose of the **non-operating revenue ratio** (non-operating revenues/total operating revenues) is to find out how dependent the organization is on patient-related net income. The higher the ratio, the less the organization is dependent on direct patient-related income and the more it is dependent on revenues from other sources. This ratio is becoming increasingly difficult to use to compare health care organizations, because under recent accounting rules, there is considerable discretion as to what is classified as operating or non-operating revenues.

This results in two potential problems: 1) to the extent that the ratio for any one organization is not calculated in exactly the same way as the standard, a comparison to the standard may be inappropriate; and 2) when multiple organizations are being compared, to the extent they did not classify various items (such as interest income) in exactly the same way, the comparison may be invalid. Non-operating revenue may include such accounts as interest income, parking lot revenues, sales to the general public of such things as food and gift shop items, gains from investment activities, and assets released from restricted investment accounts (see Exhibit 4–9b):

Exhibit 4–9b Newport's Non-Operating Revenue Ratio for 20X0 and 20X1

Year	Non-Operating Revenue Ratio	=	Non-Operating Revenues	÷	Total Operating Revenues
20X1	0.02	=	$185,000	÷	$11,012,021
20X0	0.02	=	$165,000	÷	$10,819,693
Standard = 0.05					

Step 1. Identify non-operating revenues on the statement of operations.

Step 2. Identify total operating revenues on the statement of operations.

Step 3. Divide non-operating revenues by total operating revenues.

Newport's non-operating revenue ratios in both years are 0.02, slightly below the national standard of 0.05. An increase in contributions and greater investment portfolio performance could raise its ratio value.

Return on Total Assets

In not-for-profit organizations, the **return on total assets ratio** is calculated as (excess of revenues over expenses/total assets). In for-profit organizations it is called return on assets and is calculated as (net income/total assets). It measures how much profit is earned for each dollar invested in assets. To compute the return on total assets ratio (see Exhibit 4–9c):

Step 1. Identify excess of revenues over expenses on the statement of operations.

Step 2. Identify total assets on the balance sheet.

Step 3. Divide excess of revenues over expenses by total assets.

Newport Hospital's return on total assets ratio declined significantly over this time period (0.11 to 0.05), and is currently only slightly above the standard of 0.03 in 20X1. One reason for this decrease could be that Newport's expenses have increased faster than its revenues, thereby reducing the excess of revenues over expenses. To improve this ratio, Newport could increase operating revenues, decrease expenses, and/or decrease total assets.

Return on Net Assets

In not-for-profit organizations this ratio is called **return on net assets** (excess of revenues over expenses/net assets). In for-profit organizations it is called return on equity and is calculated using the formula (net income/owners' equity). In for-profit organizations, it measures the rate of return for each dollar in owners' equity. In not-for-profit health care organizations it measures the rate of return for each dollar in net assets. To calculate the return on net assets ratio (see Exhibit 4–9d):

Exhibit 4–9c Newport's Return on Total Assets Ratio for 20X0 and 20X1

Year	Return on Total Assets	=	Excess of Revenues over Expenses	÷	Total Assets
20X1	0.05	=	$515,909	÷	$10,876,736
20X0	0.11	=	$1,219,186	÷	$11,315,585
Standard = 0.03					

Exhibit 4–9d Newport's Return on Net Assets Ratio for 20X0 and 20X1

Year	Return on Net Assets	=	Excess of Revenues over Expenses	÷	Net Assets
20X1	0.20	=	$515,909	÷	$2,542,655
20X0	0.64	=	$1,219,186	÷	$1,911,683
Standard = 0.06					

Step 1. Identify the excess of revenues over expenses on the statement of operations.

Step 2. Identify the net assets on the balance sheet.

Step 3. Divide excess of revenues over expenses by net assets.

As in the case for the return on total assets ratio, the return on net assets ratio also decreased (from 0.64 in 20X0 to 0.20 in 20X1). Expenses growing faster than revenues contributed to this decrease. However, the return on net assets in 20X1 is still considerably above the industry standard of 0.06.

It is important to note that the return on net assets ratio is magnified by the amount of debt financing. The higher the level of debt relative to net assets, the greater the return on net assets is affected for a given level of profit or loss. Exhibit 4–10 provides an example of this phenomenon.

Key Point Higher debt increases financial risk by magnifying the returns on net assets or equity.

In Case 1, the organization earns a profit (excess of revenues over expenses) of $100,000. Since there is no debt, the return on net assets is 0.1 ($100,000/$1,000,000). However, in Case 2, the assets are financed with 50 percent debt and 50 percent equity. Thus, the return to the owners is doubled (0.2), because they only have half as much invested ($500,000 instead of $1,000,000), the remainder of the assets being financed by debt. Though debt financing results in higher returns when there is a profit (as in both Cases 1 and 2), there is a greater loss in terms of return on net assets when the organization is unprofitable (as illustrated in Cases 3 and 4). As previously noted, financial leverage reflects the proportion of debt used within the organization's capital structure. Thus, these cases show that debt increases the financial risk to the

Exhibit 4–10   Example of How Increased Debt Magnifies Gains and Losses When Computing Return on Net Assets

In Case 1, the organization has no debt. In Case 2, the organization has 50 percent of its assets financed by debt. In both cases, the organization makes a $100,000 profit, but the return on net assets is twice as high in Case 2.

Case 1: $100,000 Excess of Revenues over Expenses; no debt

Balance Sheet				Statement of Operations	
Assets	$1,000,000	Debt	$0	Excess of Revenues over Expenses	$100,000
		Net Assets	$1,000,000		

Return on Net Assets = $100,000/$1,000,000 = **0.10**

Case 2: $100,000 Excess of Revenues over Expenses; 50% debt

Balance Sheet				Statement of Operations	
Assets	$1,000,000	Debt	$500,000	Excess of Revenues over Expenses	$100,000
		Net Assets	$500,000		

Return on Net Assets = $100,000/$500,000 = **0.20**

In Case 3, the organization has no debt. In Case 4, the organization has 50 percent of its assets financed by debt. In both cases, the organization incurs a $100,000 loss, but the negative return on net assets is twice as much in Case 4.

Case 3: ($100,000) Excess of Revenues over Expenses; no debt

Balance Sheet				Statement of Operations	
Assets	$1,000,000	Debt	$0	Excess of Revenues over Expenses	($100,000)
		Net Assets	$1,000,000		

Return on Net Assets = -100,000/$1,000,000 = **–0.10**

Case 4: ($100,000) Excess of Revenues over Expenses; 50% debt

Balance Sheet				Statement of Operations	
Assets	$1,000,000	Debt	$500,000	Excess of Revenues over Expenses	($100,000)
		Net Assets	$500,000		

Return on Net Assets = -$100,000/$500,000 = **–0.20**

Point: Increased debt magnifies both gains and losses when computing Return on Net Assets

owners of a health care organization. It magnifies positive returns when there is a profit, but negative returns when there is a loss. It also carries the added burden of fixed interest payments.

Profitability Summary

Though Newport Hospital is at or above the standard for two of the four profitability ratios in 20X1, it has experienced a precipitous fall from 20X0 to 20X1 in three of the four profitability ratios (see Exhibit 4–11). This raises concerns about control of revenues and expenses.

 Key Point   Because many of the activity ratios ask the general question, "How many dollars in revenue (the numerator) are being generated relative to [specific] assets (the denominator)", activity ratios are also called efficiency ratios. The higher the ratio, the more efficiently the assets are being used.

Exhibit 4–11   Newport Hospital's Profitability Ratios for 20X0 and 20X1 as Compared to the Standard

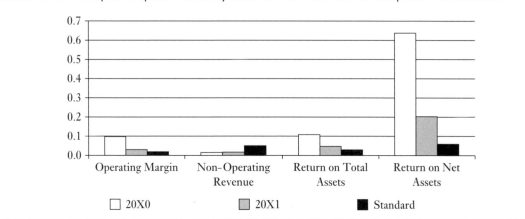

Activity Ratios

In general, activity ratios (see Exhibit 4–12) ask the question, "For every dollar invested in assets, how many dollars of revenue (not excess of revenues over expenses) are being generated?" Most ratios in this category take the general form:

$$\frac{\text{Revenues}}{\text{Assets}}$$

Thus, the more revenue generated, the higher the ratio.

Total Asset Turnover

The **total asset turnover ratio** (total operating revenues/total assets) measures the overall efficiency of the organization's assets to produce revenue. It answers the question, "For every dollar in assets, how many dollars of operating revenue are being generated?" To calculate the total asset turnover ratio:

Exhibit 4–12   Selected Activity Ratios

Ratio	Formula	Standard[1]	Desired Position
Total Asset Turnover Ratio	$\dfrac{\text{Total Operating Revenues}}{\text{Total Assets}}$	1.02	Above
Fixed Asset Turnover Ratio	$\dfrac{\text{Total Operating Revenues}}{\text{Net Plant and Equipment}}$	3.59	Above
Age of Plant Ratio	$\dfrac{\text{Accumulated Depreciation}}{\text{Depreciation Expense}}$	9.86	Below

[1] Based upon HCIA-Sachs's 1998 median values.

Exhibit 4–12a Newport's Total Asset Turnover Ratio for 20X0 and 20X1

Year	Total Asset Turnover	=	Total Operating Revenues	÷	Total Assets
20X1	1.01	=	$11,012,021	÷	$10,876,736
20X0	0.96	=	$10,819,693	÷	$11,315,585

Standard = 1.02

Key Point Asset accounts reflect values at a specific point in time, which, in turn, can fail to account for seasonal changes in asset accounts. To deal with this problem, some analysts use an average of the beginning and ending year values for the fixed asset or current asset accounts. That convention, however, is not used in this text.

Step 1. Identify total operating revenues on the statement of operations.
Step 2. Identify total assets on the balance sheet.
Step 3. Divide total operating revenues by total assets.

For Newport Hospital, the ratio increased slightly from 20X0 to 20X1 and has remained very close to the standard. A value of 1.00 indicates that for every dollar of total assets, one dollar of total revenues is generated, which is approximately the standard (see Exhibit 4–12a).

Fixed Asset Turnover

The **fixed assets turnover ratio** (total operating revenues/net plant and equipment) aids in the evaluation of the most productive assets, plant and equipment. To calculate the fixed assets turnover ratio:

Step 1. Identify total operating revenues on the statement of operations.
Step 2. Identify net plant and equipment assets on the balance sheet.
Step 3. Divide total operating revenues by net plant and equipment (fixed) assets.

Key Point The Fixed Asset Turnover Ratio is a measure of how productive the fixed assets of the organization are in generating operating revenues.

Newport's fixed asset turnover ratio increased from 20X0 to 20X1 (2.41 to 2.56), but is still below the standard of 3.59. The fixed asset turnover value of 2.56 indicates that for every dollar of fixed assets, only $2.56 of operating revenues is being generated (see Exhibit 4–12b).

Caution Note that this text uses Excess of Revenues Over Expenses in the numerator for the Profitability Ratios *Return on Total Assets* and *Return on Net Assets*, and it uses Total Operating Revenues in the numerator for the Activity Ratios *Total Asset Turnover Ratio* and *Net Asset Turnover Ratio*.

Exhibit 4–12b   Newport's Fixed Asset Turnover Ratio for 20X0 and 20X1

Year	Fixed Asset Turnover	=	Total Operating Revenues	÷	Net Plant and Equipment
20X1	2.56	=	$11,012,021	÷	$4,306,754
20X0	2.41	=	$10,819,693	÷	$4,495,122

Standard = 3.59

Age of Plant Ratio

The **age of plant ratio** (accumulated depreciation/depreciation expense) provides an indication of the average age of a hospital's plant and equipment. This ratio complements the fixed asset turnover ratio. High fixed asset turnover ratios may be an indication of a lack of investment in fixed assets. If the average age of plant is high, it may indicate that the organization needs to replace its fixed assets shortly. If so, it would be important to look at other ratios to see how well positioned the organization is to finance the purchase of new assets. To compute the age of plant ratio (see Exhibit 4–12c):

Step 1. Identify accumulated depreciation on the balance sheet.
Step 2. Identify depreciation expense on the statement of operations.
Step 3. Divide accumulated depreciation by depreciation expense.

 Key Point

Asset turnover ratios have an interesting property because of accrual accounting. When revenues (the numerator) stay the same, the ratio will continually increase from year to year because asset values (the denominator) decrease each year due to depreciation. This will occur until the assets are fully depreciated. To check how old the assets are, the age of plant ratio is used.

Newport Hospital's average age of plant ratio has increased by over one and one-half years (5.71 to 7.25), but it is still more than two years under the industry standard of 9.86.

Activity Summary

Though Newport Hospital has been near the standard on its total asset turnover ratio, it is more than 25 percent below the standard on its fixed asset turnover ratios, but

Exhibit 4–12c   Newport's Age of Plant Ratio for 20X0 and 20X1

Year	Age of Plant	=	Accumulated Depreciation	÷	Depreciation Expense
20X1	7.25	=	$2,781,741	÷	$383,493
20X0	5.71	=	$2,398,248	÷	$420,238

Standard = 9.86

Exhibit 4–13   Newport Hospital's Activity Ratios for 20X0 and 20X1 as Compared to the Standard

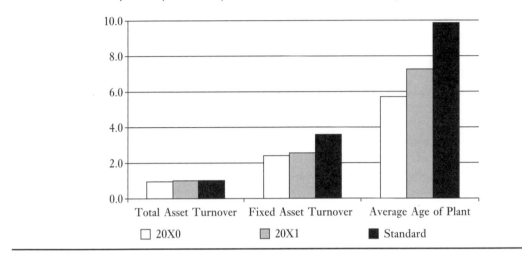

shows improvement from 20X0 to 20X1 (see Exhibit 4–13). Its average age of plant is below the standard of 9.86 years, which indicates that the hospital has newer assets relative to the standard of small hospitals. Thus, because of the fixed asset ratio, a question should be raised regarding how efficiently the fixed assets are being used to generate revenue.

Capital Structure Ratios

Capital structure ratios answer two questions: 1) "How are an organization's assets financed?" and 2) "How able is this organization to take on new debt?" In many cases, a greater understanding of these ratios (and answers to these questions) can be gained by examining the statement of cash flows to see if significant long-term debt has been acquired or paid off, or if there has been a sale or purchase of fixed assets. Capital structure ratios include long-term debt to net

Key Point | Capital structure ratios measure how an organization's assets are financed, and how able the organization is to pay for the new debt.

Key Point | One might also want to measure capital structure ratios by using the unrestricted net asset account rather than the combined restricted and unrestricted net asset values. The unrestricted net asset account represents the claim on assets that the provider could sell in order to meet debt payments.

Exhibit 4–14   Selected Capital Structure Ratios

Ratio	Formula	Standard	Desired Position
Long-Term Debt to Net Assets Ratio	$\dfrac{\text{Long-Term Debt}}{\text{Net Assets}}$	0.21	Below
Net Assets to Total Assets Ratio	$\dfrac{\text{Net Assets}}{\text{Total Assets}}$	0.62	Above
Times Interest Earned Ratio	$\dfrac{\text{(Excess of Revenues over Expenses + Interest Expense)}}{\text{Interest Expense}}$	2.85	Above
Debt Service Coverage Ratio	$\dfrac{\text{(Excess of Revenues over Expenses + Interest Expense + Depreciation Expense)}}{\text{(Interest Expense + Principal Payments)}}$	3.35	Above

assets, net assets to total assets, times interest earned, and debt service coverage (see Exhibit 4–14).

Long-term Debt to Net Assets

The **long-term debt to net assets ratio** (long-term debt/net assets) measures the proportion of debt to net assets. In for-profit organizations, this ratio is called the long-term debt to equity ratio and is calculated by the formula: (long-term debt/owners' equity). Although most organizations certainly want to finance a portion of their assets with debt, at a certain level an organization takes on too much debt and may find itself in a precarious position where it has difficulty both paying back its existing debt and borrowing additional funds. To calculate the long-term debt to net assets ratio (see Exhibit 4–14a):

Key Point 👉 Long-term debt to net assets ratio measures the proportion of assets which are financed by debt relative to those which are not.

Exhibit 4–14a   Newport's Long-Term Debt to Net Assets Ratio for 20X0 and 20X1

Year	Long-Term Debt to Net Assets	=	Long-Term Debt	÷	Net Assets
20X1	2.73	=	$6,938,891	÷	$2,542,655
20X0	3.14	=	$6,009,484	÷	$1,911,683

Standard = 0.21

Step 1. Identify non-current debt on the balance sheet.

Step 2. Identify net assets on the balance sheet.

Step 3. Divide non-current debt by net assets.

For Newport Hospital, despite an increase in non-current debt, the long-term debt to net assets ratio actually decreased from 20X0 to 20X1 due to the increase in net assets. Still, the 20X1 ending value (2.73) is over ten times the industry standard (0.21).

Net Assets to Total Assets

The **net assets to total assets ratio** (net assets/total assets) reflects the proportion of total assets financed by equity. In for-profit organizations, this ratio is called the equity to total assets ratio and is calculated by the formula: (owners' equity/total assets). Creditors desire a strong equity position with sufficient funds to pay off debt obligations. A high net asset or equity position is enhanced either through retention of earnings or through private contributions from the community. In investor-owned facilities, retention of earnings and issuance of stock increase the equity. To calculate the net assets to total assets ratio (see Exhibit 4–14b):

Step 1. Identify net assets on the balance sheet.

Step 2. Identify total assets on the balance sheet.

Step 3. Divide net assets by total assets.

In 20X1, this ratio was less than half of the industry standard (0.62), but it did increase from 0.17 (20X0) to 0.23 (20X1). With this thin equity state, creditors probably would be somewhat cautious about lending funds to this facility in the future.

Times Interest Earned

The **times interest earned ratio** [(excess of revenues over expenses + interest expense)/interest expense] enables creditors and lenders to evaluate a hospital's

Exhibit 4–14b   Newport's Net Assets to Total Assets Ratio for 20X0 and 20X1

Year	Net Assets to Total Assets	=	Net Assets	÷	Total Assets
20X1	0.23	=	$2,542,655	÷	$10,876,736
20X0	0.17	=	$1,911,683	÷	$11,315,585

Standard = 0.62

Exhibit 4–14c   Newport's Times Interest Earned Ratio for 20X0 and 20X1

Year	Times Interest Earned	=	(Excess of Revenues over Expenses	+	Interest Expense)	÷	Interest Expense
20X1	2.03	=	($515,909	+	$500,000)	÷	$500,000
20X0	5.41	=	($1,219,186	+	$276,379)	÷	$276,379

Standard = 2.85

ability to generate earnings necessary to meet interest expense requirements. In for-profit organizations the ratio is calculated by the formula: [(net income + interest expense)/interest expense]. The ratio answers the question: "For every dollar in interest expense, how many dollars are there in profit?" Interest expense is added back into the numerator so that the numerator reflects profit *before* taking interest into account. To calculate the times interest earned ratio (see Exhibit 4–14c):

Step 1. Identify excess of revenues over expenses on the statement of operations.

Step 2. Identify interest expense on the statement of operations.

Step 3. Add together excess of revenues over expenses and interest expense and divide the total by interest expense.

Unfortunately, Newport's times interest earned ratio decreased precipitously from 20X0 (5.41) to 20X1 (2.03), falling to below the standard of 2.85. A continued decline in the times interest earned ratio may affect Newport's ability to borrow in the future.

Debt Service Coverage

A more robust measure of ability to repay a loan is the **debt service coverage ratio** [(excess of revenues over expenses + interest expense + depreciation expense)/(interest expense + principal payments)]. In for-profit organizations it is calculated as: [(net income + interest expense + depreciation expense)/(interest expense + principal payments)]. It answers the question, "For every dollar the organization has to pay on debt service (principal + interest), what is its approximate cash inflow during the year?"

 Key Point | Debt service coverage ratio is a critical ratio used by investment bankers, because it measures what proportion of the cash flow payments is being used to pay off debt.

This ratio is used extensively by investment bankers and bond rating agencies to evaluate a facility's ability to meet its total loan requirements, principal payments plus interest. Principal payments are usually presented in the statement of cash flows. Since it is not provided, assume that Newport's principal payments are $200,000 per year.

Exhibit 4–14d   Newport's Debt Service Coverage Ratio for 20X0 and 20X1

Steps 1–4

Year	Cash Flow Before Interest	=	(Excess of Revenues over Expenses	+	Interest Expense	+	Depreciation Expense)
20X1	$1,399,402	=	($515,909	+	$500,000	+	$383,493)
20X0	$1,915,803	=	($1,219,186	+	$276,379	+	$420,238)

Step 5

Year	Debt Service Coverage	=	Cash Flow Before Interest	÷	(Interest Expense	+	Principal Payments)
20X1	2.00	=	$1,399,402	÷	($500,000	+	$200,000)
20X0	4.02	=	$1,915,803	÷	($276,379	+	$200,000)

Standard = 3.35

Interest expense and depreciation expense are added to the excess of revenues over expenses to develop an indication of cash flow before interest expense. To compute the debt service coverage ratio (see Exhibit 4–14d):

> Step 1. Identify excess of revenues over expenses on the statement of operations.
> Step 2. Identify interest expense on the statement of operations.
> Step 3. Identify principal payments on the statement of cash flows.
> Step 4. Add the excess of revenues over expenses, interest expense, and depreciation expense from the statement of operations.
> Step 5. Divide the sum from Step 4 by the sum of interest expense and principal payments.

Reconfirming the outcome of the times interest earned ratio, Newport also has placed itself in a precarious position in terms of meeting its interest and principal payments. It is considerably below the standard of 3.35 and has dropped in half from 20X0 (4.02) to 20X1 (2.00). It currently has a cash flow before principal and interest payments of only 2.00 times its debt service payments. If this condition were to continue, Newport likely would find itself in technical default on its long-term obligations.

Capital Structure Summary

Newport Hospital decreased its debt position from 20X0 to 20X1; however; this amount of debt is still well above the industry standard. This is reflected in the capital structure ratios, which show that its proportion of debt to net assets is still too high, albeit decreasing. More troublesome for Newport is its ability to pay its debt:

Exhibit 4–15   Newport Hospital's Capital Structure Ratios for 20X0 and 20X1 as Compared to the Standard

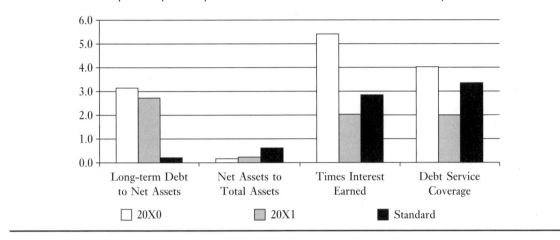

both the times interest earned and debt service coverage ratios are considerably below the standard (see Exhibit 4–15).

Summary of Newport Hospital's Ratios

Newport Hospital's ratios cause some concern. Most problematic are the capital structure ratios, which indicate that Newport Hospital is above the standard in debt and considerably below the standard in ability to pay it off. Though improving in liquidity from 20X0 to 20X1, it is still below the standard in its ability to meet current obligations with current assets, except with its ability to collect on its receivables. The majority of Newport's profitability ratios are above standard, but they are falling precipitously, indicating potential problems in its ability to pay off its short-term obligations. Though Newport Hospital seems to be using its assets more efficiently as indicated by most of the activity ratios, this is likely due to increasing age of plant. Newport's capital structure ratios raise serious concerns about its ability to pay off current debt, or to increase debt financing if needed to replace properties and equipment in the near future.

While this chapter has introduced commonly used financial ratios, there are many others. Perspective 4–5 presents some used by HMOs.

◀Summary▶

The financial performance of health care organizations is of interest to numerous individuals and groups, including administrators, board members, creditors, bond-holders, community members, and government agencies. This chapter presented

PERSPECTIVE 4–5

How Health Plans in Phoenix, Arizona Benchmark against Local Market and National Market Ratios

According to Interstudy Data, the Phoenix-Mesa, AZ market has shown a steady rise in HMO enrollment from 564,000 in 1994 to 1,068,000 in 1999. This market is very competitive with no dominating health plan. The average market has 15 HMOs with one HMO possessing over 30% of the market, while the Phoenix market has only 12 HMOs with no plan sharing more than 20% of the market. Listed below are the key financial ratios for benchmarking of Pacificare of Arizona Health Plan against other local market and national market values for HMOs. Lower medical and administrative expenses for Pacificare contributed to a higher profit margin. Higher premium revenues may also have contributed to this profit position. Given the rising growth in enrollment, one might expect that Pacificare will continue to expand its market share.

HMO 1998 ratios	Pacificare Health Plan	Phoenix Mesa, AZ	Average Large Market
Administrative Expenses	10.0%	14.5%	13.2%
Medical Loss	83.0%	84.7%	88.4%
Operating Margin	0.037	(0.001)	(0.015)
Average PMPM Total Revenue	$268	$171	$159

Source: Interstudy Financial Database 1998. *Interstudy Quarterly Newsletter,* Volume 1, Issue 1, 2000.

three ways to analyze the financial statements of health care organizations: horizontal analysis, vertical analysis, and ratio analysis.

Horizontal analysis examines year-to-year changes in the line items of the financial statements. It answers the question, "What is the percentage change from one year to the next in a particular line item (such as cash, long-term debt, patient accounts receivable)?" The formula for horizontal analysis is [(subsequent year − previous year)/previous year] × 100 = percent increase (decrease) between years.

A variant of horizontal analysis is trend analysis. Instead of comparing one line item with that of the previous year, trend analysis compares a line item from any subsequent year to that of the base year. Trend analysis answers the question, "What is the percentage change from a base year?" For example: "How much have net patient service revenues increased between 20X4 and 20X0?" The formula for trend analysis is [(any subsequent year − base year)/base year]. As the name suggests, trend analysis is most useful when data for multiple periods are available. Generally, there are no recognized national standards for either horizontal or trend analysis.

Vertical analysis compares one line item to another line item for the same period. It answers the question, "What percentage of one line item is another line item?" For example: "What percentage of current assets is cash?" or "What percentage of operating revenues are operating expenses?" Vertical analysis is also called common-size analysis, because it allows comparison of different-sized organizations by converting all items to percentages. As with horizontal analysis, there are no nationally recognized standards.

Exhibit 4–16a Financial Ratios for All US Hospitals by Bed Size

Ratio	HCIA & HCFA Median Ratio[1] Hospital Industry	HCIA & HCFA Median Ratio[1] 1–99 beds	HCIA & HCFA Median Ratio[1] 100–249 beds	HCIA & HCFA Median Ratio[1] 250–399 beds	HCIA & HCFA Median Ratio[1] 400+ beds	Desired Position[2]
Liquidity Ratios						
Current Ratio	2.06	2.18	1.95	1.94	1.84	Above
Quick Ratio	1.69	1.76	1.57	1.54	1.48	Above
Acid Test Ratio	0.26	0.35	0.31	0.31	0.11	Above
Days in Accounts Receivable	66	67	65	64	68	Below
Days Cash on Hand	47	46	43	44	45	Above
Average Payment Period (Days)	58	54	66	69	67	Below
Profitability Ratios						
Operating Margin	0.03	0.02	0.02	0.03	0.04	Above
Non-Operating Revenue	0.05	0.05	0.04	0.06	0.09	Varies
Return on Total Assets	0.04	0.03	0.04	0.05	0.04	Above
Return on Net Assets	0.08	0.06	0.09	0.10	0.10	Above
Activity Ratios						
Total Asset Turnover Ratio	0.93	1.02	0.85	0.79	0.81	Above
Net Fixed Assets Turnover Ratio	3.50	3.59	3.45	3.44	3.62	Above
Age of Plant Ratio	9.53	9.86	10.01	9.93	9.74	Below
Capital Structure Ratios						
Long-Term Debt to Net Assets Ratio	0.38	0.21	0.48	0.56	0.64	Below
Net Assets to Total Assets Ratio	0.60	0.62	0.56	0.55	0.52	Above
Times Interest Earned Ratio	4.29	2.85	4.30	5.39	4.31	Above
Debt Service Coverage Ratio	4.06	3.35	3.73	4.61	5.59	Above

[1] These values were obtained from: The Health Care Financing Administration's (HCFA) Hospital Cost Report Information System Files for financial statements ending in 1998; and HCIA-Sachs Standard's 1998 median values, *The Comparative Performance of US Hospitals: The Sourcebook 2000*, HCIA Publications, Baltimore, MD

[2] These are true to a certain point. For example, for the acid test ratio, in general, the higher the better, but after a certain point, the organization might be better off investing some of the excess cash.

Ratio analysis is the preferred approach for a detailed analysis of the financial statements of health care organizations. Ratio analysis asks the question, "What is the ratio of one line item to another?" For example: "How many dollars are there in current assets compared to current liabilities?" Since ratios are not limited to just one financial statement at a time, they may combine and compare items from several different financial statements. The four categories of ratios are liquidity, profitability, activity, and capital structure.

- *Liquidity ratios* answer the question, "How well is an organization positioned to meet its short-term obligations?"
- *Profitability ratios* answer the question, "How profitable is an organization?"
- *Activity ratios* answer the question, "How efficiently is an organization using its assets to produce revenues?"
- *Capital structure ratios* answer two questions: 1) "How are an organization's assets financed?" and 2) "How able is this organization to take on new debt?"

Once calculated, these ratios are generally compared to some meaningful standard (historical, industry, etc.). Such comparisons yield clues as to how well an entity is functioning and how it might improve its operational performance and financial position. Exhibit 4–16a presents financial ratios for US hospitals overall and by bed size categories. Exhibit 4–16b presents a summary of key financial ratios and their formulas.

◀KEY TERMS▶

FINANCIAL LEVERAGE	RATIO	VERTICAL ANALYSIS
HORIZONTAL ANALYSIS	TREND ANALYSIS	

◀KEY EQUATIONS▶

See Exhibit 4–16b

Exhibit 4–16b   Formulas for Key Financial Ratios

Liquidity Ratios

	Formula
Current Ratio	Current Assets/Current Liabilities
Quick Ratio	(Cash + Marketable Securities + Net Receivables)/Current Liabilities
Acid Test Ratio	(Cash + Marketable Securities)/Current Liabilities
Days in Accounts Receivable	Net Patient Accounts Receivables/(Net Patient Revenues/365)
Days Cash on Hand	(Cash + Marketable Securities)/((Operating Expenses − Depreciation Expense)/365)
Average Payment Period (Days)	Current Liabilities/((Operating Expenses − Depreciation Expense)/365)

Profitability Ratios

	Formula
Operating Margin	Operating Income/Total Operating Revenues
Non-Operating Revenue Ratio	Non-Operating Revenues and Other Income/Total Operating Revenues
Return on Total Assets[1]	Excess of Revenues over Expenses/Total Assets
Return on Net Assets[2]	Excess of Revenues over Expenses/Net Assets

Activity Ratios

	Formula
Total Asset Turnover Ratio	Total Operating Revenues/Total Assets
Net Fixed Assets Turnover Ratio	Total Operating Revenues/Net Plant and Equipment
Age of Plant Ratio	Accumulated Depreciation/Depreciation Expense

Capital Structure Ratios

	Formula
Long-term Debt to Net Assets Ratio[3]	Long-term Debt/Net Assets
Net Assets to Total Assets Ratio[4]	Net Assets/Total Assets
Times Interest Earned Ratio[5]	(Excess of Revenues over Expenses + Interest Expense)/Interest Expense
Debt Service Coverage Ratio[6]	(Excess of Revenues over Expenses + Interest Expense + Depreciation Expense)/(Interest Expense + Principal Payments)

[1] In for-profit health care organizations, calculated as: Net Income/Total Assets.

[2] Called the *Return on Equity* in for-profit health care organizations, and calculated as: Net Income/Owners' Equity.

[3] Called *Long-term Debt to Equity* in for-profit health care organizations, and calculated as: Long-term Debt/Owners' Equity.

[4] Called *Equity to Total Assets* in for-profit health care organizations, and calculated as: Owners' Equity/Total Assets.

[5] In for-profit health care organizations, calculated as: (Net Income + Interest Expense)/Interest Expense.

[6] In for-profit health care organizations, calculated as: (Net Income + Interest Expense + Depreciation Expense)/(Interest Expense + Principal Payments).

◄QUESTIONS AND PROBLEMS►

1. **Definitions.** Define the following terms:
   a. Financial Leverage
   b. Horizontal Analysis
   c. Ratio
   d. Trend Analysis
   e. Vertical Analysis

2. **Horizontal and Vertical Analyses.** Compare horizontal and vertical analyses, including trend analysis. How are they used?

3. **Vertical Analysis.** Explain common-sized analysis.

4. **Ratio Analysis.** What is the purpose of ratio analysis? What are the four standard categories of ratios?

5. **Medians.** Explain why an industry median may not be an appropriate benchmark to which a particular organization wants to compare itself.

6. **Ratio Interpretation.** How do the current, quick, and acid test ratios differ from the average payment period ratio? To what categories do these ratios belong?

7. **Ratio Interpretation.** How do capital structure ratios and liquidity ratios differ in providing insight into an organization's ability to pay debt obligations? Identify two situations where an organization might have increasing activity ratios but declining profitability.

8. **Ratio Interpretation.** What is the difference between the operating margin ratio and a return on total assets ratio? To what categories of ratios do these belong?

9. **Ratio Interpretation.** What capital structure ratio measures the ability to pay debt service payments?

10. **Ratio Interpretation.** Discuss the plant and equipment status of a health care provider with an increasing age of plant ratio.

11. **Profitability Analysis.** Compare the profitability ratios for Glen Hall Hospital with its industry standards. Keep in mind that market conditions reveal that 90 percent of Glen Hall's market is under fixed contract payment with HMOs, Medicare, and Medicaid (see Exhibit 4–17).

12. **Ratio Analysis.** Compare the profitability and capital structure ratios for Buxton Hospital to its industry standards (see Exhibit 4–18).

13. **Ratio Analysis.** The balance sheet and statement of operations for Dogwood Community Hospital for the years ended 20X0 and 20X1 are shown in Exhibits

Exhibit 4–17   Selected Ratios for Glen Hall Hospital and the Industry Standards

Profitibility Ratios	Industry Standard	Glen Hall Hospital
Operating Margin	0.041	(0.031)
Return on Total Assets	0.075	0.024
Non-Operating Ratio	0.040	0.010

Exhibit 4–18 Selected Ratios for Buxton Hospital and the Industry Standards

Ratios	Industry Standard	Buxton Hospital
Return on Total Assets	0.044	0.044
Return on Net Assets	0.065	0.130
Net Assets to Total Assets	0.600	0.300
Long-Term Debt to Net Assets	0.380	0.615

4–19a and 4–19b. Compute the following ratios for both years: current, acid test, days in accounts receivable, average payment period, long-term debt to net assets, net assets to total assets, total asset turnover, fixed asset turnover, return on total assets, and operating margin. After calculating the ratios, comment on Dogwood's liquidity, efficient use of assets or activity ratios, profitability, and capital structure relative to its standards for its respective bed size listed in Exhibit 4–16a. Cite at least two meaningful ratios per category. Assume Dogwood is a 125-bed facility for the analysis. How might the opinion of Dogwood change if it were a 450-bed facility?

14. **Ratio Analysis.** Exhibits 4–20a and 4–20b show the statement of operations and balance sheet for Maryville Community Hospital for the years ended 20X0 and 20X1. Compute the following ratios for both years: current, quick, acid tests, days in accounts receivable, days cash on hand, average payment period, operating margin, non-operating revenue, return on total assets and net assets, total asset turnover, fixed asset turnover, age of plant, long-term debt to net assets, and net assets to total assets. Comment on Maryville's

Exhibit 4–19a Statement of Operations for Dogwood Community Hospital

Dogwood Community Hospital Statement of Operations (in '000)
For the Years Ended December 31, 20X1 and 20X0

	20X1	20X0
Revenues:		
Net Patient Service Revenue	$1,400	$1,200
Other Revenue	200	200
Total Operating Revenues	1,600	1,400
Expenses:		
Nursing Services	1,320	1,150
Administrative Services	110	100
Depreciation	20	15
General Services	50	35
Total Operating Expenses	1,500	1,300
Operating Income	100	100
Excess of Revenues over Expenses	100	100
Increase (Decrease) in Net Assets	$100	$100

Exhibit 4–19b   Balance Sheet for Dogwood Community Hospital

Dogwood Community Hospital Balance Sheet (in '000)
For the Years Ended December 31, 20X1 and 20X0

	20X1	20X0
Current Assets		
Cash and Cash Equivalents	$30	$50
Net Patient Receivables	295	235
Prepaid Expenses	80	80
Total Current Assets	405	365
Non-Current Assets		
Plant, Property, & Equipment		
Gross Plant, Property, & Equipment	350	300
(less Accumulated Depreciation)	(70)	(50)
Net Plant, Property, & Equipment	280	250
Construction in Progress	203	0
Total Assets	$888	$615
Current Liabilities		
Accounts Payable	$220	$190
Salaries Payable	75	50
Total Current Liabilities	295	240
Long-Term Liabilities		
Bonds Payable	100	20
Total Long-Term Liabilities	100	20
Net Assets	493	355
Total Liabilities and Net Assets	$888	$615

liquidity, efficient use of assets, profitability, and capital structure, citing at least one ratio per category. Use the national hospital industry standards listed in Exhibit 4–16a for 250 beds, and then perform an analysis if hospital size were unknown.

15. **Ratio Analysis.** Exhibit 4–21 lists the financial ratios for 227-bed Hollywood Community Hospital. Assess the profitability, liquidity, activity, and capital structure of Hollywood for 20X1. Explain why these financial measures changed between 20X0 and 20X1.

16. **Ratio Analysis.** McGill Healthcare System, an 800-bed institution, is located in a highly competitive, urban market area. Using the financial ratios from Exhibit 4–22 for the current and previous years, evaluate McGill's financial condition, focusing on profitability, liquidity, activity, and capital structure ratios.

17. **Ratio Analysis, Unknown Bed Size.** Compare Hope Community Hospital's liquidity, profitability, activity, and capital structure ratios to its national industry standards using the data from Exhibits 4–16a and 4–23.

Exhibit 4–20a   Statement of Operations for Maryville Community Hospital

Maryville Community Hospital Statement of Operations (in '000)
For the Years Ended December 31, 20X1 and 20X0

	20X1	20X0
Revenues		
Net Patient Service Revenue	$17,500	$18,000
Net Assets Released from Restriction	2,000	100
Other Revenue	500	450
Total Operating Revenues	20,000	18,550
Expenses		
Nursing Services	13,000	15,000
Administrative Services	5,000	3,000
Depreciation	1,000	1,000
General Services	200	100
Total Operating Expenses	19,200	19,100
Operating Income	800	(550)
Excess of Revenues over Expenses	800	(550)
Transfer to Parent	500	0
Increase (Decrease) in Net Assets	$300	($550)

18. **Ratio Analysis, Unknown Bed Size.** In Exhibit 4–24 are the financial ratios for St Jude's Hospital, whose financial condition deteriorated from 20X0 to 20X1. Identify the problem areas relative to the standards, and explain how this downfall came about.

19. **Ratio Analysis.** Swayze Community Hospital, a 265-bed facility, is a sole provider hospital in small, rural New England serving a large area. Assess Swayze's profitability, liquidity, activity and capital structure ratios. Using the financial ratios from Exhibit 4–25 for the current and previous years, evaluate Swayze's financial condition.

20. **Ratio Analysis.** Avon Community Hospital, a small 95-bed hospital, is located in a large metropolitan area and competes with several large teaching facilities as well as other community hospitals. During the past year, one of the large teaching hospitals decided to sponsor a Medicaid and Medicare HMO. As a result Avon has experienced a decline in its government payer mix. Assess Avon's profitability, liquidity, activity, and capital structure ratios. Using the financial ratios from Exhibit 4–26 for the current and previous years, evaluate Avon's financial condition.

21. **Horizontal, Vertical, and Ratio Analyses.** Exhibits 4–27a and 4–27b show the statement of operations and balance sheet for 190-bed Lake Community Hospital for 20X0 and 20X1.
    a. Perform a horizontal analysis on both statements.
    b. Perform a vertical analysis on both statements relative to 20X0.
    c. Compute all the selected ratios listed in Exhibit 4–16a, and compare them to the standard.

Exhibit 4–20b   Balance Sheet for Maryville Community Hospital

Maryville Community Hospital Balance Sheet (in '000)
For the Years Ended December 31, 20X1 and 20X0

	20X1	20X0
Current Assets		
Cash and Cash Equivalents	$750	$650
Net Patient Receivables	2,500	3,800
Inventory	700	800
Total Current Assets	3,950	5,250
Non-current Assets		
Plant, Property, & Equipment		
Gross Plant, Property, & Equipment	20,000	19,000
(less Accumulated Depreciation)	(6,000)	(5,000)
Net Plant, Property, & Equipment	14,000	14,000
Board-designated Funds	7,000	4,500
Total Assets	**24,950**	**23,750**
Current Liabilities		
Accounts Payable	1,500	1,800
Accrued Expenses	500	750
Total Current Liabilities	2,000	2,550
Long-term Liabilities		
Bonds Payable	10,500	11,000
Total Long-term Liabilities	10,500	11,000
Net Assets	12,450	10,200
Total Liabilities and Net Assets	**$24,950**	**$23,750**

Exhibit 4–21   Selected Financial Ratios for Hollywood Community Hospital

Ratio	20X1	20X0
Current Ratio	4.05	2.30
Acid Test Ratio	0.95	0.20
Days in Accounts Receivable	75 days	65 days
Days Cash on Hand	25 days	5 days
Average Payment Period (Days)	55 days	55 days
Fixed Asset Turnover Ratio	3.45	2.60
Total Asset Turnover Ratio	1.15	1.05
Operating Margin	− 0.05	0.02
Return on Net Assets	0.01	0.06
Long-term Debt to Net Assets (Equity)	2.95	1.18
Net Assets to Total Assets	0.34	0.46
Age of Plant	5.05	5.78

Exhibit 4–22   Selected Ratios for McGill Healthcare System

Ratio	12/31/20X1	12/31/20X0
Current Ratio	1.75	2.50
Quick Ratio	1.01	1.85
Acid Test Ratio	0.15	0.35
Days in Accounts Receivable	55 days	65 days
Average Payment Period	40 days	45 days
Days Cash on Hand	12 days	35 days
Fixed Asset Turnover Ratio	0.95	3.20
Total Asset Turnover Ratio	0.65	1.10
Operating Margin	0.03	0.02
Non-Operating Revenue	0.25	0.10
Return on Total Assets	0.06	0.04
Long-term Debt to Equity	0.22	0.25
Equity to Total Assets	0.65	0.35
Debt Service Coverage Ratio	5.55	4.55
Age of Plant	4.50	10.01

Exhibit 4–23   Financial Ratios for Hope Community Hospital

Ratio	20X1	20X0
Liquidity Ratios		
Current Ratio	1.78	1.81
Quick Ratio	1.29	1.39
Acid Test Ratio	0.23	0.18
Average Collection Period	82 days	118 days
Days Cash on Hand	19 days	17 days
Average Payment Period (Days)	81 days	95 days
Profitability Ratios		
Return on Total Assets	0.14	0.14
Return on Net Assets	0.44	0.50
Operating Margin	0.12	0.06
Non-Operating Revenue	0.02	0.11
Activity Ratios		
Total Asset Turnover Ratio	1.07	0.84
Fixed Asset Turnover Ratio	1.96	1.46
Age of Plant	13.00	11.00
Capital Structure Ratios		
Net Assets to Total Assets	0.32	0.27
Long-term Debt to Net Assets	1.47	1.95
Debt Service Coverage Ratio	1.50	1.53
Times Interest Earned	4.00	4.10

Exhibit 4–24   Financial Ratios for St Jude's Hospital

Ratio	20X1	20X0
Current Ratio	2.10	2.20
Acid Test Ratio	0.10	0.25
Days in Accounts Receivable	60 days	45 days
Days Cash on Hand	5 days	15 days
Average Payment Period (Days)	45 days	43 days
Fixed Asset Turnover Ratio	2.54	3.58
Total Asset Turnover Ratio	1.04	1.10
Operating Margin	0.03	0.10
Return on Total Assets	0.12	0.20
Long-term Debt to Equity	2.18	1.10
Equity to Total Assets	0.42	0.55
Debt Service Coverage Ratio	2.10	3.20
Age of Plant	3.50	5.70

Exhibit 4–25   Financial Ratios for Swayze Community Hospital

Ratio	20X1	20X0
Current Ratio	2.25	1.95
Quick Ratio	1.65	1.45
Acid Test Ratio	0.10	0.25
Days in Accounts Receivable	80	50
Average Payment Period	65	75
Days Cash on Hand	15	35
Fixed Asset Turnover Ratio	3.50	3.20
Total Asset Turnover Ratio	1.12	1.10
Operating Margin	0.08	0.06
Return on Total Assets	0.10	0.07
Long-term Debt to Net Assets	0.55	0.68
Net Assets to Total Assets	0.45	0.35
Debt Service Coverage Ratio	3.55	2.25
Age of Plant	7.80	6.80

Exhibit 4–26   Financial Ratios for Avon Hospital

Ratio	20X1	20X0
Current Ratio	0.50	1.60
Acid Test Ratio	0.02	0.35
Days in Accounts Receivable	120 days	80 days
Average Payment Period	95 days	75 days
Days Cash on Hand	5 days	15 days

(Continues)

Exhibit 4–26 (Contd)

Fixed Asset Turnover	0.75	1.00
Total Asset Turnover	0.95	1.20
Operating Margin	−0.08	−0.01
Return on Total Assets	−0.01	0.02
Long-term Debt to Equity	3.11	2.10
Equity to Total Assets	0.10	0.35
Debt Service Coverage Ratio	1.25	2.01
Age of Plant	10.01	7.85

Exhibit 4–27a   Statement of Operations for Lake Community Hospital

Lake Community Hospital
Statement of Operations (in '000)
For the Years Ended 12/31/20X1 and 12/31/20X0

	20X1	20X0
Revenues:		
Net Patient Service Revenue	$20,000	$17,000
Other Operating Revenue	2,500	2,000
Total Operating Revenues	22,500	19,000
Operating Expenses:		
Nursing Services	12,000	10,000
Administrative Services (includes Bad Debt Expense of $100)	4,000	3,500
Depreciation	1,000	1,200
General Services	2,500	2,500
Fiscal Services	400	400
Professional/Ancillary Services	3,500	3,000
Interest	1,000	1,000
Total Operating Expenses	24,400	21,600
Income from Operations	(1,900)	(2,600)
Non-Operating Income:		
Investment Income/Contributions	3,000	3,000
Excess of Revenues over Expenses	1,100	400
Net Income	**$1,100**	**$400**

Exhibit 4–27b   Balance Sheet for Lake Community Hospital

Lake Community Hospital
Balance Sheet (in '000)
For the Years Ended 12/31/20X1 and 12/31/20X0

	20X1	20X0
Current Assets:		
Cash and Cash Equivalents	$1,300	$800
Net Patient Accounts Receivables	3,500	4,000
		(Continues)

Exhibit 4-27b (Contd)

Inventories	2,000	1,800
Other Current Assets	100	80
Total Current Assets	6,900	6,680
Plant, Property, & Equipment		
Gross Plant, Property, & Equipment	21,000	22,000
(less Accumulated Depreciation)	(6,500)	(5,500)
Net Property, Plant and Equipment	14,500	16,500
Funded Depreciation/Board Designated Funds		
Cash and Short-Term Investments	4,000	1,500
Total Assets	**$25,400**	**$24,680**
Current Liabilities:		
Accounts Payable	$3,000	$3,200
Salaries Payable	30	25
Notes Payable	250	300
Total Current Liabilities	3,280	3,525
Long-term Liabilities:		
Bonds Payable	15,000	18,000
Total Long-term Liabilities	15,000	18,000
Net Assets	7,120	3,155
Total Liabilities and Net Assets	**$25,400**	**$24,680**

Using these financial performance measures, evaluate the financial state of Lake Community. The debt principal payments each year are $40,000.

22. **Horizontal, Vertical, and Ratio Analyses.** Exhibits 4–28a and 4–28b show the statement of operations and balance sheet for 375-bed Pine Island Regional Hospital for 20X0 and 20X1.

   a. Perform a horizontal analysis on both statements.

   b. Perform a vertical analysis on both statements relative to 20X0.

   c. Compute all the selected ratios listed in Exhibit 4–16a, and compare them to the standard.

   Using these financial performance measures, evaluate the financial state of Pine Island. The debt principal payments each year are $1,000,000.

23. **Horizontal, Vertical, and Ratio Analyses.** Exhibits 4–29a and 4–29b show the statement of operations and balance sheet for Rocky Mountain Resort Hospital for 20X1 and 20X0. The debt principal payments each year for Rocky Mountain Resort are $500,000 for 20X1 and $1,300,000 for 20X0.

   a. Perform horizontal and vertical analyses using the Statement of Operations.

   b. Perform horizontal and vertical analyses using the Balance Sheet.

   c. Compute all the selected ratios listed in Exhibit 4–16.

Exhibit 4–28a Statement of Operations for Pine Island Regional Hospital

Pine Island Regional Hospital
Statement of Operations (in '000) For the Years Ended 12/31/20X1 and 12/31/20X0

	12/31/20X1	12/31/20X0
Revenues:		
Net Patient Service Revenue	$55,000	$62,000
Net Assets Released from Restriction	5,000	4,000
Other Operating Revenue	3,000	7,000
Total Operating Revenues	63,000	73,000
Expenses:		
Nursing Services	20,000	25,000
Administrative Services	18,000	22,000
Depreciation	5,000	5,000
Interest	4,000	4,000
General Services	8,000	3,000
Total Operating Expenses	55,000	59,000
Operating Income	8,000	14,000
Excess of Revenues over Expenses	8,000	14,000
Increase (Decrease) in Net Assets	**$8,000**	**$14,000**

Exhibit 4–28b Balance Sheet for Pine Island Regional Hospital

Pine Island Regional Hospital
Balance Sheet (in '000) For the Years Ended 12/31/20X1 and 12/31/20X0

	12/31/20X1	12/31/20X0
Current Assets:		
Cash and Cash Equivalents	$4,200	$4,750
Net Patient Receivables	6,000	6,500
Inventory	300	250
Prepaid Expenses	750	800
Total Current Assets	11,250	12,300
Plant, Property, & Equipment		
Gross Plant, Property, & Equipment	55,000	60,000
(less Accumulated Depreciation)	(30,000)	(25,000)
Net Property, Plant and Equipment	25,000	35,000
Long-Term Investments	2,000	1,500
Total Assets	**$38,250**	**$48,800**
Current Liabilities:		
Accounts Payable	$5,500	$4,800
Salaries Payable	1,075	950
Total Current Liabilities	6,575	5,750

(Continues)

Exhibit 4-28b (Contd)

Long-term Liabilities:		
Bonds Payable	20,000	25,000
Total Long-term Liabilities	20,000	25,000
Net Assets	11,675	18,050
Total Liabilities and Net Assets	$38,250	$48,800

Exhibit 4–29a   Statement of Operations for Rocky Mountain Resort Hospital

Rocky Mountain Resort Hospital
Statement of Operations (in '000) For the Years Ended 12/31/20X1 and 12/31/20X0

	12/31/20X1	12/31/20X0
Revenues:		
Net Patient Service Revenue	$45,000	$30,000
Net Assets Released from Restriction	12,000	9,000
Other Operating Revenue	10,000	7,000
Total Operating Revenues	67,000	46,000
Expenses:		
Nursing Services	33,000	31,000
Administrative Services	13,000	12,500
Depreciation Expense	8,000	4,000
Interest Expense	4,000	500
General Services	5,000	4,000
Total Operating Expenses	63,000	52,000
Operating Income	4,000	(6,000)
Excess of Revenues over Expenses	4,000	(6,000)
Increase (Decrease) in Net Assets	**$4,000**	**($6,000)**

Exhibit 4–29b   Balance Sheet for Rocky Mountain Resort Hospital

Rocky Mountain Resort Hospital
Balance Sheet (in '000) For the Years Ended 12/31/20X1 and 12/31/20X0

	12/31/20X1	12/31/20X0
Current Assets:		
Cash and Cash Equivalents	$3,800	$8,750
Net Patient Receivables	15,000	11,500
Inventory	2,300	1,250
Prepaid Expenses	5,500	4,500
Total Current Assets	26,600	26,000

(Continues)

Exhibit 4–29b (Contd)

Plant, Property, & Equipment		
Gross Plant, Property, & Equipment	65,000	40,000
(less Accumulated Depreciation)	(20,000)	(15,000)
Net Property, Plant and Equipment	45,000	25,000
Long-Term Investments	2,000	10,500
Total Assets	**$73,600**	**$61,500**
Current Liabilities:		
Accounts Payable	$8,500	$3,800
Salaries Payable	950	700
Total Current Liabilities	9,450	4,500
Long-term Liabilities:		
Bonds Payable	40,000	5,000
Total Long-term Liabilities	40,000	5,000
Net Assets	24,150	52,000
Total Liabilities and Net Assets	**$73,600**	**$61,500**

Evaluate the financial state of Rocky Mountain Resort, a 60-bed facility, using all of the above measures. Make the basis for the vertical analyses the year 20X0.

24. **Horizontal, Vertical, and Ratio Analyses.** Exhibits 4–30a and 4–30b show the Balance Sheet and Statement of Operations for 660-bed Williamson Academic Medical Center for the years 20X0 and 20X1.
   a. Perform full horizontal and vertical analyses on the Balance Sheet.
   b. Perform full horizontal and vertical analyses on the Statement of Operations.
   c. Calculate every ratio described in the chapter for both years as compared to the standard. (Note: assume that principal payments each year are for $500,000.)

Discuss Williamson's current financial position and future outlook based upon these results. Make the basis for the vertical analyses the year 20X0.

Exhibit 4–30a Balance Sheet for Williamson Academic Medical Center

Williamson Academic Medical Center
Balance Sheet (in '000) For the Years Ended December 31, 20X0 and 20X1

	12/31/20X1	12/31/20X0
Current Assets:		
Cash & Cash Equivalents	$1,000	$800
Patient Accounts Receivables, Net	4,500	5,500
Inventories	2,000	1,800
Other Current Assets	100	80
Total Current Assets	7,600	8,180

(Continues)

Exhibit 4-30a (Contd)

Plant, Property, & Equipment Gross Plant, Property, & Equipment	18,000	18,500
(less Accumulated Depreciation)	(6,500)	(5,500)
Net Property, Plant and Equipment	11,500	13,000
Long-Term Investments	2,000	1,500
Total Assets	$21,100	$22,680
Current Liabilities:		
Accounts Payable	$4,000	$4,200
Salaries Payable	30	25
Notes payable	250	300
Other Current Liabilities	0	0
Total Current Liabilities	4,280	4,525
Non-Current Liabilities:		
Bonds Payable	10,000	12,000
Total Non-Current Liabilities	10,000	12,000
Net Assets	6,820	6,155
Total Liabilities and Net Assets	$21,100	$22,68

Exhibit 4–30b   Statement of Operations for Williamson Academic Medical Center

Williamson Academic Medical Center
Statement of Operations (in '000) For the Years Ended December 31, 20X0 and 20X1

	12/31/20X1	12/31/20X0
Revenues:		
Net Patient Revenues	$20,000	$17,000
Other Operating Revenues	2,500	2,000
Total Operating Revenues	22,500	19,000
Expenses:		
Nursing Services	8,000	7,000
Administrative Services	4,000	3,500
(includes bad debt expense of $100,000)		
Depreciation	500	500
General Services	2,500	2,500
Fiscal Services	400	400
Professional/Ancillary Services	3,500	3,000
Interest	1,000	1,000
Total Operating Expenses	19,900	17,900
Income from Operations	2,600	1,100
Non-Operating Income:		
Investment Income + Contributions	400	2,000
Excess of Revenues over Expenses	3,000	3,100
Increase (Decrease) in Net Assets	$3,000	$3,100

Chapter Five

WORKING CAPITAL MANAGEMENT

LEARNING OBJECTIVES

After completing this chapter you should be able to:

▶ Define working capital.
▶ Understand working capital management strategies.
▶ Construct a cash budget.
▶ Manage receivables and payables.

Chapter Outline

◀INTRODUCTION▶

Working Capital:
Current assets and
current liabilities.

Although non-current assets provide the capability to provide services, it is the combination of current assets and current liabilities that turns that capability into service. For example, an X-ray machine is useless without an adequate supply of film on hand or cash to pay the radiation technologists. This chapter begins with a discussion of working capital and then focuses on the management of two primary components of working capital in the health care industry: cash and accounts receivable.

Net Working Capital:
The difference between
current assets and
current liabilities.

The term "working capital" refers to both current assets *and* current liabilities. A related term, "net working capital," refers to the *difference* between current assets and current liabilities. That is:

$$\text{Net Working Capital} = \text{Current Assets} - \text{Current Liabilities}$$

◀THE WORKING CAPITAL CYCLE▶

In the day-to-day operations of an organization, an ongoing series of cash inflows and outflows pays for day-to-day expenses (such as supplies and salaries). The organization must have sufficient funds available to pay for these items on a timely basis. This is particularly problematic in health care, where it is not unusual for payments to be received more than two months after the patient or third party has been billed for the provided services.

Working Capital Strategy: The amount of working capital that an organization determines it must keep available as a cushion to protect against unforeseen expenditures.

Ideally, a health care organization would earn and receive sufficient funds from providing services to enable it to meet its current obligations with available cash. To do this requires managing the four phases of the working capital cycle (see Exhibit 5–1): 1) obtaining cash; 2) turning cash into resources, such as supplies and labor, and paying bills; 3) using these resources to provide services; and 4) billing patients for the services, and collecting revenues so that the cycle can be continued.

With regard to cash, managing the working capital cycle involves not only ensuring that total cash inflows cover cash outflows, but also managing the timing of these flows. To the extent that payments are due before cash is available, the organization will have to obtain cash from sources other than existing revenues, such as from investments or through short-term borrowing. To illustrate, suppose an organization starts the month of September with no working capital (see Exhibit 5–2). During the month, it delivers $20,000 worth of services, but must pay $9,000 in staff salaries every 15 days and $2,000 for supplies every 30 days. Situation 1 assumes that the full amount owed is collected during the month, but isn't received until the end of the month. Situation 2 assumes that the organization also collects the full amount owed, but in two equal payments of $10,000 each – the first payment arriving after 15 days, and the second payment, after 30 days.

In both cases, cash inflows ($20,000) equal cash outflows ($20,000). However, whereas in Situation 2 there is always sufficient cash on hand to meet the payments

Exhibit 5–1   The Working Capital Cycle: The Importance of Timing in Managing Working Capital

$$\text{Effective Interest Rate} = \frac{(\text{Interest Expense on Amount Borrowed} + \text{Total Fees})}{(\text{Amount Borrowed} - \text{Compensating Balance})}$$

Exhibit 5–2   Illustration of the Effects of Timing on Working Capital Needs

		Situation #1				Situation #2		
	Account	Cash Inflows	Cash Outflows	Balance	Account	Cash Inflows	Cash Outflows	Balance
Day 1				$0				$0
Day 15	Revenues				Revenues	$10,000		
	Salaries		$9,000	($9,000)	Salaries		$9,000	$1,000
Day 30	Revenues	$20,000			Revenues	$10,000		
	Salaries		$9,000		Salaries		$9,000	
	Supplies		$2,000	$0	Supplies		$2,000	$0

when due, in Situation 1 the organization would not be able to meet its first $9,000 payroll on Day 15. To meet this obligation, it either must take cash out of existing reserves or borrow. However, even in Situation 2, there is little margin for error. The amount of working capital that an organization determines it must keep available as a cushion against unforeseen expenses is called its **working capital strategy**.

Working Capital Management Strategies

Working capital management strategy has two components: asset mix and financing mix. **Asset mix** is the amount of working capital an organization keeps on hand relative to its potential working capital obligations. **Financing mix** refers to how an organization chooses to finance its working capital needs.

Asset Mix Strategy

Asset Mix: The amount of working capital an organization keeps on hand relative to its potential working capital obligations.

A health care provider's asset mix strategy falls on a continuum between an aggressive strategy and a conservative strategy (see Exhibit 5–3). Using the aggressive approach, the health care organization attempts to maximize its returns by investing its funds in potentially higher-earning non-liquid assets such as buildings and equipment; yet it does so at the risk of lower liquidity with increased chances of inventory stock-outs, dissatisfied customers from the stringent collections policies to earn revenues more quickly, and lack of cash to pay employees and suppliers.

Liquidity: a measure of how easily an asset can be converted into cash.

Conversely, using a *conservative approach*, a health care organization seeks to minimize its risk of not having sufficient funds readily available by having higher liquidity. However, it does so at the cost of receiving lower returns, since short-term investments typically earn a lower return than do long-term investments (see Perspective 5–1).

 Key Point   A health care organization that utilizes an aggressive asset mix strategy seeks to maximize its returns by investing in non-liquid assets, but faces the risk of lower liquidity.

Financing Mix Strategy

Financing Mix: How an organization chooses to finance its working capital needs.

Financing mix refers to how the organization chooses to finance its working capital needs. Temporary working capital needs result from short-term fluctuations, whereas permanent working capital needs arise from more ongoing factors, such as a permanent increase in patient volume. Borrowing short-term at lower interest costs for short-term needs under normal conditions leads to a higher profit, because working capital is otherwise being invested optimally (everything else being equal), but this places the facility at risk because of possible higher debt payments if the need to borrow arises. If the organization has long-term working capital financing needs, it is better off financing those needs with long-term financing under normal conditions. Facilities borrowing long-term at higher interest costs to support ongoing working capital needs face lower

Exhibit 5–3   Working Capital Management Strategies

	Aggressive Strategy	Conservative Strategy
Goal	Maximize Returns	Minimize Risk
Liquidity	Low	High
Risk	High	Low
Return	High	Low

PERSPECTIVE 5–1

Changing Investment Philosophy of Health Care Providers in the 1990s and 2000

In the 1990s, health care providers started to become more aggressive with their investment strategies. For example, MedAmerica Health Systems Corp. of Dayton Ohio started investing more of its cash in stocks, and that's been good for the nonprofit hospital operator and its bondholders – so far. Currently, 50 percent of its investment portfolio is in stocks, up from 20 percent three years ago. As a result, MedAmerica registered almost a 10 percent compounded annual return. Its investment gains and interest income of $14.9 million in the first half of 2000 exceeded its slimmer operating surplus of $ 4.4 million.

Overall, nonprofit hospitals on average more than tripled their stock holdings from 1995 to 1999, as reported by a recent survey completed by the bond rating agency of Fitch, Inc. However, the rating agency has noted that some hospitals have been utilizing stock investments to shore up for weak operating results, which could turn dangerous with falling stocks prices during the year 2000. Anil Joseph, a Fitch analyst, notes that "they have so little room for error, that it just magnifies the risk they have" if stock losses occur.

As a result, significant investment losses could cause further credit downgrades because they would reduce financial cushions, especially at weaker hospitals with lower cash reserves. Rating analysts note that these returns masked the effect of reduced reimbursement for health care.

Source: Dennis Walters, "Stocks are Risky Rx for Hospitals." *Chicago Sun-Times*, October 29, 2000, Financial Section, p. 48.

| Key Point | Three rules to follow under normal conditions to decide between short-term and long-term borrowing to finance working capital needs: 1) finance short-term working capital needs with short-term debt; 2) finance long-term working capital needs with long-term financing; and 3) when an organization has fluctuating needs for working capital, employ a mixed strategy by financing a certain base amount with long-term financing, and as short-term situations arise, finance those with short-term debt. |

---

earnings, but reduce their risk with lower debt payments. Exhibit 5–4 compares the key characteristics of short–term and long–term borrowing. Overall, an aggressive working capital strategy involves maintaining a relatively low amount of working capital on hand and financing working capital shortfalls with short–term debt. Though this results in a greater return, it also results in lower liquidity and an increased chance of not having the working capital available when needed.

Exhibit 5–4   Comparison of Key Characteristics of Short- and Long-term Borrowing under Normal Conditions

	Short-term	Long-term
Interest Rate[1]	Lower	Higher
Interest Cost	Lower	Higher
Profit	Higher	Lower
Volatility Risks	Variable	Fixed

[1] Short-term rates are typically lower than long-term rates

In reality, most health care organizations follow neither an aggressive nor a conservative approach, but fall somewhere in the middle. A health care provider located in a market with little competition and a high degree of stability for services might consider a more aggressive approach, since it is better able to forecast its working capital needs. On the other hand, a provider in a competitive, unsettled market with fluctuating demand for services should choose a more conservative approach to working capital management.

Key Point	There are three major reasons to hold cash: daily operations, precautionary measures, and speculative needs.

◀Cash Management▶

In general, the term **cash** refers not only to coin and currency, but also to **cash equivalents** such as interest-bearing savings and checking accounts. There are three major reasons for a health care provider to hold cash:

- Daily operations.
- Precautionary purposes.
- Speculative purposes.

Daily operations refers to holding cash so that day-to-day bills may be paid. **Precautionary purposes** refers to holding cash to meet unexpected demands, such as unexpected maintenance of a facility or piece of equipment. **Speculative purposes** refers to holding cash to take advantage of unexpected opportunities, such as a group practice's buying a competing practice that has decided to sell.

Sources of Temporary Cash

Though it would be favorable to always have excess short-term funds available to invest, health care organizations often find that they need to borrow funds for short periods of time to meet their maturing obligations. The three primary sources of short-term funds include:

- Extension of credit from suppliers (i.e. trade payables).
- Bank loans.
- Billings, collections, and disbursement policies that increase the speed with which money is collected.

Bank Loans

There are two major types of *unsecured* (not backed by an asset) short-term loans offered by banks: lines of credit, and transaction notes. The interest expense associated with these alternatives is a function of economic conditions and the credit background of the borrower.

Lines of Credit

There are two types of lines of credit: a normal line of credit, and a revolving line of credit. A **normal line of credit** is an agreement established by the bank and the borrower that establishes the maximum amount of funds that can be borrowed. Thus, the bank is not legally obligated to fulfill the borrower's credit request. On the other hand, **a revolving line of credit** legally requires the bank to fulfill the borrower's credit request up to the pre-negotiated limit.

Commitment Fees

In addition to the interest rate on a line of credit, financial institutions are also compensated through commitment fees and/or compensating balances. A **commitment fee** is a percentage of the *unused* portion of the revolving credit line which is charged to the potential borrower. The annual fee, often between 0.25 and 0.50 percent, is a function of the credit risk of the borrower and the reason for the line of credit. For example, assume a health care organization has a line of credit of $4,000,000 and borrows on average $2,500,000 during the year. If the commitment fee rate were 0.25 percent, then the borrower would pay an annual fee of $3,750 [($4,000,000 − $2,500,000) × 0.0025] to have the right to borrow the full $4,000,000 essentially on demand. Sometimes an organization can negotiate with a bank to reduce or eliminate a commitment fee for a line of credit, especially if it has a favorable long-standing history with the lending institution.

Key Point A revolving line of credit differs from a normal line of credit in that the revolving line of credit legally requires a bank to fulfill the borrower's credit request up to the pre-negotiated limit.

Compensating Balances

Under a **compensating balance**, the borrower is required to maintain a designated dollar amount on deposit with the bank. The balance requirement generally is a percentage (perhaps 10–20 percent) of the total credit line, or a percentage of the unused portion of the credit line. The effect of the compensating balance is to increase the true or effective interest rate that the borrower must pay. The effective interest rate is calculated using the following formula:

$$\text{Effective Interest Rate} = \frac{(\text{Interest Expense on Amount Borrowed} + \text{Total Fees})}{(\text{Amount Borrowed} - \text{Compensating Balance})}$$

Assume Community Healthcare Provider borrowed $600,000 during the year on a credit line of $1,000,000 with an interest rate of 9 percent, with no fees. Using this

---

Normal Line of Credit: an agreement established by a bank and a borrower which establishes the maximum amount of funds that can be borrowed, and the bank may loan the funds at its own discretion.

Revolving Line of Credit: an agreement established by the bank and the borrower that legally requires the bank to loan money to the borrower at any time requested up to the pre-negotiated limit.

Commitment Fee: a percentage of the unused portion of a credit line which is charged to the potential borrower.

Compensating Balance: a designated dollar amount on deposit with a bank which a borrower is required to maintain.

Effective Interest Rate: The true interest rate that a borrower pays.

formula, the interest expense in the numerator is $54,000 (9% × $600,000). The amount borrowed in the denominator is $600,000, and the compensating balance is 10 percent of the unused portion of the line of credit (10% × $400,000), or $40,000. Thus, the effective interest rate is 9.64 percent [($54,000 + $0) / ($600,000 - $40,000)].

$$9.64\% = \frac{(\$54,000+\$0)}{(\$600,000 - \$40,000)}$$

Transaction Notes

Transaction Note: a short-term, unsecured loan made for some specific purpose.

The second type of bank loan commonly used for short-term borrowing by health care providers is a transaction note. A **transaction note** is a short-term, unsecured loan made for some specific purpose, such as the financing of inventory purchases. Transaction notes have compensating balance requirements. The borrower obtains the loan by signing a promissory note or IOU. The terms of transaction (maturity and cost) are similar to that for the line of credit.

Trade Credit/Payables

Trade Credit: Short term credit offered by the supplier of a good or service to the purchaser.

Trade Payables: Short-term debt that results from supplies purchased on credit for a given length time. This allows an organization to use the supplier's money to pay for the purchase up until the time it pays the supplier the amount owed.

Instead of relying solely on the outside to obtain cash, an organization can generate cash by controlling its outflow, but the health care organization must have strict cash disbursement policies and procedures in effect. When a health care organization buys on credit, it is in fact using the supplier's money to pay for the purchase up until the time it pays the supplier the amount owed. These credit obligations are called trade payables (often referred to as accounts payable). Thus, one of the most important areas to address in cash management is that of either accepting or rejecting discounts offered by suppliers for early payment. These discounts are often stated as follows:

2/10 net 30

This example means that the full payment is due within 30 days ("net 30"), but a 2 percent discount is available if the payment is made within 10 days after the sale ("2/10") (see Exhibit 5–5). Although at first glance it may seem optimal to delay

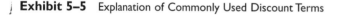

Exhibit 5–5 Explanation of Commonly Used Discount Terms

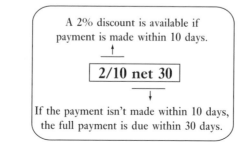

A 2% discount is available if payment is made within 10 days.

↑

2/10 net 30

↓

If the payment isn't made within 10 days, the full payment is due within 30 days.

Exhibit 5–6 Two Approaches to Conceptualize the Cost Associated with Not Taking a Discount

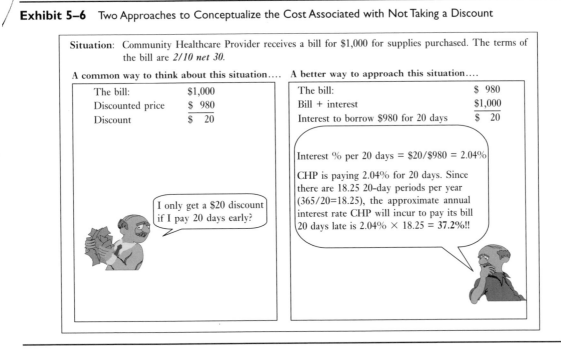

Situation: Community Healthcare Provider receives a bill for $1,000 for supplies purchased. The terms of the bill are *2/10 net 30*.

A common way to think about this situation....   A better way to approach this situation....

The bill:	$1,000
Discounted price	$ 980
Discount	$ 20

The bill:	$ 980
Bill + interest	$1,000
Interest to borrow $980 for 20 days	$ 20

I only get a $20 discount if I pay 20 days early?

Interest % per 20 days = $20/$980 = 2.04%

CHP is paying 2.04% for 20 days. Since there are 18.25 20-day periods per year (365/20=18.25), the approximate annual interest rate CHP will incur to pay its bill 20 days late is 2.04% × 18.25 = 37.2%!!

payment for 30 days to retain cash on hand, in fact, *depending upon the credit terms, it is usually in the best interests of an organization to pay early and take the discount.*

Key Point Depending upon a health care organization's credit terms for its trade payables, it is usually in the best interest of an organization to pay early and take the discount.

To compare the financial implications of taking a discount versus not taking the discount, assume an organization receives an invoice for $1,000 with terms of 2/10 net 30. If the organization pays within 10 days, it receives a 2 percent discount and only has to pay $980 ($1,000 - $20). If the payment isn't made until 30 days, the health care organization has to pay the full $1,000. Although it should be clear that if the organization takes the discount it is paying less as opposed to holding onto its cash longer, the true cost of paying late may not be so apparent. To understand this involves switching perspectives.

A common way to approach this situation would be to think that paying $1,000 after 30 days would be the "normal" management action, and to pay $980 early would be the alternative action. From this perspective, the savings from taking the discount is $20 (see Exhibit 5–6). A better way to approach this decision would be to think of the discounted price ($980) as being the "real" price, and the full price paid after 10 days ($1,000) as being a penalty price with a supplemental interest charge for not paying within the discount period. In other words, the organization would be paying $20 in interest ($1,000 – $980) to keep the $980 for an extra 20 days (the time between day 10 and day 30).

Approximate Interest Rate: The annual interest rate incurred by not taking advantage of a supplier's discount offer to pay bills early. The formula in this chapter gives an approximate annual interest rate. A more precise method of calculation can be found in more advanced texts.

To determine the approximate interest rate the health care organization would pay to keep $980 for an extra 20 days, use the formula in Exhibit 5–7.

The calculation shows that the approximate annual interest rate is 37.2 percent. Thus, by not taking the discount within 10 days and waiting to pay until day 30, the health care organization is paying the equivalent of 37.2 percent on an annual basis to borrow $980. Thus, if the organization has the $980, it should take the discount unless it can earn this much by investing the $980 elsewhere, or it should borrow the $980 on a short-term basis if it can do so at a rate less than 37.2 percent. Incidentally, the higher the discount being offered, the higher the approximate interest rate for not taking (or losing) the discount.

Exhibit 5–8 shows that the approximate interest rate decreases the longer the period of time after the discount date increases until the bill is paid. Therefore, *a prudent approach is to pay as late as possible within the discount period or, if the discount isn't taken, to pay at the end of the "net" period.* Although it is true that the effective interest costs seem to decrease as the number of days the bill is not paid increases, at a certain point after the "net" period, new costs are encountered. These costs include late fees, loss of discounts in the future, loss of priority status with the supplier, etc.

Incidentally, in regard to the above example, organizations which do weekly processing may find it virtually impossible to take advantage of a contract with terms such as "2/10 net 30." In such cases, an organization may try to negotiate terms such as "2/15 net 35" in order to give itself enough time to process the invoice and still meet the early payment deadline.

Exhibit 5–7   Calculating the Approximate Interest Rate Associated with Not Taking a Discount

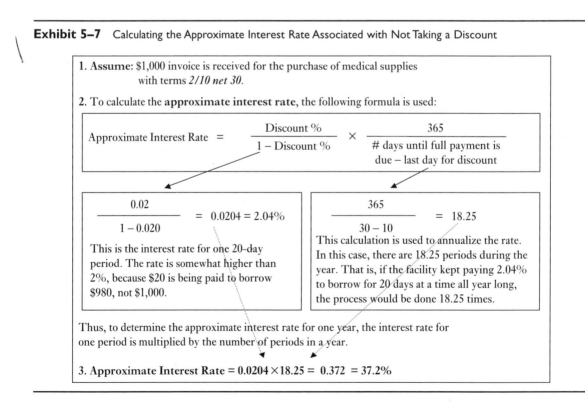

1. **Assume:** $1,000 invoice is received for the purchase of medical supplies with terms *2/10 net 30*.

2. To calculate the **approximate interest rate**, the following formula is used:

$$\text{Approximate Interest Rate} = \frac{\text{Discount \%}}{1 - \text{Discount \%}} \times \frac{365}{\text{\# days until full payment is due} - \text{last day for discount}}$$

$$\frac{0.02}{1 - 0.020} = 0.0204 = 2.04\%$$

This is the interest rate for one 20-day period. The rate is somewhat higher than 2%, because $20 is being paid to borrow $980, not $1,000.

$$\frac{365}{30 - 10} = 18.25$$

This calculation is used to annualize the rate. In this case, there are 18.25 periods during the year. That is, if the facility kept paying 2.04% to borrow for 20 days at a time all year long, the process would be done 18.25 times.

Thus, to determine the approximate interest rate for one year, the interest rate for one period is multiplied by the number of periods in a year.

3. **Approximate Interest Rate** = $0.0204 \times 18.25 = 0.372 = 37.2\%$

Exhibit 5–8 Illustration of How Not Taking a Discount at Various Discount Rates and Extending Payments Affects the Approximate Interest Rate Paid

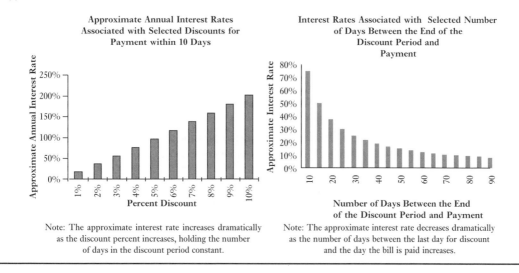

Note: The approximate interest rate increases dramatically as the discount percent increases, holding the number of days in the discount period constant.

Note: The approximate interest rate decreases dramatically as the number of days between the last day for discount and the day the bill is paid increases.

Billing, Collections, and Disbursement Policies, and the Concept of Float

In addition to bank loans and trade credit, billing, collections, and disbursement policies and procedures are also tools used to increase the amount of cash available to the organization. The objective of **billing, credit, and collection policies** is to accelerate cash receipts, while the objective of **cash disbursement policies** is to slow down cash outflows. The concept of float is one of the most useful concepts to implement good collections and disbursement policies. **Float** is the time delay during the process that starts from the assembling of a bill and ends with the deposit of the payment in the bank and subsequent payments to creditors. There are four main categories of float: billing, collection, transit, and disbursement (see Exhibit 5–9).

Float: The time delay of the process of assembling a bill until depositing the payment in the bank and making subsequent payments to creditors.

Billing Float

Billing float is any delay in getting the bill to the patient or third party payor (such as an insurance company). There are two aspects of billing float: assembling the bill

Exhibit 5–9 Types of Float

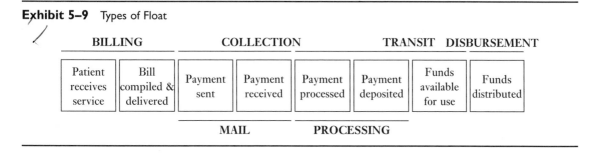

and delivering the bill to the patient or his third-party payor. Ideally, a bill is made up concurrently with service delivery, so that by discharge, or even at any point during the service delivery process, the patient's bill reflects all services received. However, assembling the final bill is a problem for many health care organizations, which for some can take weeks. Although delivering the bill may seem straightforward, a number of problems can delay the billing process:

- Medical records compliance issues and lack of trained coders.
- Patients who use more than one name.
- Name changes.
- Address changes.
- Lack of clarity as to who is responsible to pay the bill.
- Specific requirements demanded by various third-party payors, such as retrospective review.

In recent years, a number of techniques have been developed to help overcome billing-related problems, including:

- **Improved Billing Policies and Procedures.** An essential component of an effective billing process is having up-to-date, well utilized billing policies and procedures. The objective is to ensure that policies and procedures are in place that will result in fair, timely, and accurate bills. Thus, billing policies and procedures define the goals, roles and responsibilities, and appropriate procedures to be used at various stages in the billing process (see Perspectives 5–2 and 5–3).
- **Improved Preadmissions and Admissions Screening.** In preadmission screening, information is gathered and verified before the patient enters the providing organization. Preadmissions and admission screenings are important because they help the health care organization determine a patient's ability to pay, including the verification of name, address, employment status, and insurance coverage. Also in this process, the health care organization can make financial arrangements for patients who are unable to pay. It is important to note that under capitated payment systems, much of the effort in this regard takes place at the time of enrollment and assignment.
- **Management Information Systems.** The health care provider's management information system is a key to gathering, compiling, analyzing, and disseminating information concerning patient accounts. A key problem facing many health care providers is difficulty assembling information about a single patient from throughout the system. Ideally, the information system should allow easy interface among admissions, patient accounts, and medical records in a process that gathers and submits charge data in an accurate and timely manner. The primary objective among these systems is the accurate and timely transfer of data and information.
- **Internal Claims Processing.** The purpose of internal claims processing is to avoid the denial of claims. This involves the proper conduct of utilization

PERSPECTIVE 5–2

Getting One's Due: The Latest Techniques in Collecting Receivables

Receivable collection is the critical element behind the financial viability of any health care organization. Monica Lambert, who owns Netgain Medical Consulting in Fort Myers, Fla., advocates "revenue enhancement." To stop the bleeding in the health care payment process, you have to look where it starts, Lambert says.

And where revenue collection starts is at the registration and scheduling desk. But at most facilities, she notes, this function is treated as the least important. The desk is usually staffed by the most recent hires or by part-time staff, who are often the lowest paid. Yet these are the people who are responsible for collecting insurance information, entering correct information on service dates, and usually collecting any co-pays as well. The cost to fix any problem when the patient is not at the point of service is tremendous, Lambert points out. One of her first projects when called in as a consultant is to convince management of the importance of having skilled and motivated registration staff. This is accomplished by changing the job description, increasing the pay scale, and staffing the positions with competent personnel. This alone cuts errors by 80% to 85% in a matter of months, she contends, and can increase the revenue stream by 10% to 15%.

The accounts receivable department of a health care facility should be able to concentrate on collecting money from patients who do not want to pay their bills, Lambert explains, not to deal with those whose insurance claims were not filed or are being delayed because of errors in the first instance. These days, she says, many medical facilities are writing off 35% to 40% of what they are billing. Much of this is due to faulty claims filing, which needs to be identified and corrected rather than charged as an insurance discount.

Source: David Feldheim, *Bond Buyer 2000*, September 26, 2000.
Copyright © 2000 Thomson Financial Media. All Rights Reserved.

review: preadmission certification and second opinions, verification of patient insurance, appropriate record keeping and patient classification, etc. An important area to address is improper medical records coding, which can result in delays and lost funds. For instance, failure of the medical staff to

PERSPECTIVE 5–3

Billing Scam Hits Hospitals

In their daily operations, hospitals sometime view more than a thousand invoices. However, sometimes these bills are bogus. In the case of Bucyrus Community Hospital, an accounts payable coordinator found a heating repair bill for $3,907. The employee noted, "There was something funny about it." Further investigation on the part of the employee found the invoice to be phony. The employee was able to uncover a scam, whereby a bogus company had sent identical bills to dozens of Ohio hospitals as well as to medical centers in at least nine other states. The hospital notified the Ohio Hospital Association, which alerted the American Hospital Association. They found that this fake invoice was reported by hospitals in several Midwest States. The payables department was also able to find a bogus invoice from a local supply company that indicated that the hospital was past due on a payment of $82.70, but no such company existed.

Source: Mark D. Somerson and Mary Beth Lane, "Billing Scam Hits Hospitals." *The Columbus Dispatch,* October 28, 2000, p. 1B.

assign final diagnosis to the chart as well as to sign the chart can delay the timeliness of the payment. Similarly, miscoding the diagnosis can also impact the funds the organization receives. The health care provider by-laws should state the responsibility of physicians to fulfill these obligations.

- **Electronic Billing.** Electronic billing is a process whereby bills are sent electronically to third parties through electronic data interfacing (EDI). This not only accelerates the transmission of bills, but also provides an editing function that reduces the number of processing errors and subsequent audits, ultimately decreasing turnaround time.

Key Point

To achieve timely collection of billing, health care providers need to examine the areas of preadmission, billing, claims processing, management information systems, and follow-up.

Of course, the best way to avoid having money owed to a health care organization is to be paid ahead of time or at the point of service. This approach is taken by many physicians' offices, and it is a primary component of many capitation agreements that pay providers a per member per month (PMPM) fee in advance.

Collection Float

Collection Float: The time between when a bill is paid and the time the payment is deposited.

Collection float is the time between the issuance of the bill and the time funds are available for use by the health care organization. It has two components: mail float and processing float. **Mail float** refers to the time from when the patient or third-party payor sends in the payment to the time the health care provider receives the payment. Note that mail float begins *after* the patient or the third party has sent the bill. Improved clarity of who, where, by when and to whom to send payments helps to ensure timely delivery of payments. **Processing float** is the time it takes the facility to process the payment once received and to deposit it in the bank. Incidentally, there is another aspect to processing float: the time it takes the bank to process the transaction. Thus, processing float spans both collection float and transit float.

Key Point

The government typically requires that fiscal intermediaries, the insurance companies that process Medicare claims for the government, pay "clean" Medicare claims within 27 days of their receipt. Clean claims are those that require no further response or modification by the provider.

Of course, in cases where patients or their third parties do not pay in full or in a timely manner, collections policies and procedures should identify the steps in the process to follow up, including which accounts will be sent to collections agencies and when accounts will be written off as bad debt. For example, some facilities send out follow-up letters 40 days after discharge, make follow-up phone calls 60 days after discharge, employ a collection agency 150 days after discharge, and write off accounts 180 days after discharge.

Transit Float

Transit Float: The time between when a payment is deposited until the funds are accessible for use.

Transit float is the time involved to clear the check through the provider's bank until the funds are available to the provider. Techniques developed to reduce collection and transit float include:

- Decentralized collection centers and concentration banking.
- Lockboxes.
- Wire transfers.

Decentralized Collection Centers and Concentration Banking

Decentralized collection centers and **concentration banking** allow the health care provider to establish collection centers so that payors send their payment to a location near them (thus reducing mail float). These collection centers deposit the payments they have received in the provider's local bank. Finally, the funds are transferred to a concentration bank where the health care provider can draw on the cash for payments. This procedure is designed to help a health care provider reduce its mail and processing float, but there is a tradeoff between the number of collection centers and the savings they provide and the costs incurred to maintain accounts at a number of different financial institutions.

Key Point Decentralized Collection Center, Concentration Banking, Lockboxes, and Wire Transfers are methods to reduce collection and transit float.

Lockboxes

Under the **lockbox** form of collection, a payor sends payments to a post office box located near a Federal Reserve Bank or branch. The bank picks up the payments from the box, and at various times during the day deposits these funds into the health care provider's account, processes the checks, and sends the facility a list of the payors and payments. Having the bank perform these duties enables the facility to reduce its mail and processing time. The decision to invest in the lockbox approach depends upon whether the interest earned from the acceleration of funds exceeds the cost of having a lockbox. Lockboxes usually have a fixed fee and a variable rate based on a per check basis. To offset the costs to establish a lockbox, an organization may be able to save money by freeing up internal staff who perform some of the functions that the bank would be taking over.

Lockbox: A post office box located near a Federal Reserve Bank or branch, from which the bank will pick up and process checks quickly, but for a fee.

Wire Transfers

Wire transfers eliminate mail and transit float. They are generally operated two ways: 1) third parties electronically deposit payments in the health care organization's bank; and 2) banks of multi-provider systems electronically transfer cash from their local branches to the corporate headquarters' bank account, where all payments are made from. This minimizes the "excess cash" kept at subsidiaries and maximizes the amount at headquarters, which is responsible to invest all cash. However, this approach is often quite expensive, as banks often charge $2 to $4 per transfer. However, one large, central bank account may draw a better overall return than would several smaller accounts, and there is an increased likelihood that the central account would have adequate working capital funds available to meet all current expenses, with reduced likelihood of needing to borrow. Related techniques are zero-balance accounts and sweep accounts, whereby the bank automatically removes any excess cash from subsidiaries and places it in the account of the parent corporation.

Disbursement Float

Disbursement Float: The amount of time between when funds are available for disbursement and when they are actually released.

Remote Disbursement: The use of a bank situated far from the health care provider's vendors or suppliers to increase float.

Unlike the other types of float that are oriented toward reducing the time it takes to get money into the organization, **disbursement float** focuses on how long the organization can keep its money before it pays its bills. The options available to control cash going out of the organization are managing trade payables (also called trade credit or accounts payable) and remote disbursement (see Perspective 5–4). **Trade payables** refers to short-term debt that results from supplies purchased on credit for a given length of time. This allows an organization to use the supplier's money to pay for the purchase up until the time it pays the supplier the amount owed. **Remote disbursement** involves the use of a bank situated far from the health care provider's vendors or suppliers. By writing checks against this account, the health care provider increases its transit float or check-clearing process through the Federal Reserve System. Thus, the facility may earn an additional day in the use of its funds. For example, a facility located in a metropolitan area in the South may use a local bank for vendors located in the Midwest, but might use a bank in another part of the country to pay local vendors. However, in doing so, a facility may want to consider the importance of maintaining good relations with its vendors, because the vendors are playing the same game and want to receive their payments as quickly as possible.

 Key Point   Disbursement Float is the opposite of Collection Float. Disbursement Float focuses on how long an organization keeps its cash before it pays its bills.

Investing Cash on a Short-term Basis

After an organization has gone through the effort to reduce disbursement float, it wants to ensure that the money that has not yet been disbursed is invested appropriately to generate a favorable return. Myriad short-term investment instruments exist, including treasury bills, certificates of deposit, commercial paper, and money market mutual funds. Some of the key attributes of these short-term investments are summarized in Exhibit 5–10.

PERSPECTIVE 5–4

Processing Claims via the Internet

Seven large managed-care companies: Aetna Inc.; Anthem Inc.; Cigna Corp.; Health Net Inc.; Oxford Health Plans Inc.; PacifiCare Health Systems Inc.; and WellPoint Health Networks Inc. have implemented plans for an Internet-based system to accelerate the processing of health-care transactions. The health plans have come together to fund a closely held company called "MedUnite Inc.," based in San Diego, to create an interactive network to execute transactions, such as payment claims, patient referrals, and eligibility checks that are now handled mostly on paper or via private electronic networks. The health plans expect electronic transactions will reduce the costs, inefficiencies, and ill feeling that develop from the current paper-claims system.

MedUnite will concentrate on transactions, for example, by enabling the thousands of doctors who employ Medical Manager practice-management software, now owned by WebMD, to link to MedUnite's network. Presently, the majority of doctors hire staff to perform the often time-consuming transactions – such as submitting claims for payment, checking a patient's eligibility for treatment, and requesting authorization to refer a patient to another doctor – by paper or telephone, or via private electronic networks that don't use the Internet. Developing an interactive, Internet-based system can lower costs and speed handling, enabling doctors to receive payment faster, according to Mr Cox.

Another reason to create the electronic system is the federal Health Insurance Portability and Accountability Act, known as HIPAA, which requires the health-care industry to develop a standard format for electronic transactions in the next few years. Plans call for doctors' offices to pay a flat monthly subscription fee for unlimited transactions, and for health plans to pay fees on a per-transaction basis. Some critics are unconvinced that health plans truly want to accelerate payment of claims to doctors, since plans typically invest premiums that are paid to them up-front and earn interest on that money, known as the "float." But the company indicates that the savings available by eliminating errors in claims submissions – so they don't have to be resubmitted – far outweigh any benefit that the health plans get by sitting on their money.

Source: Ann Carrns "Health Plans Create a Rival for WebMD." Wall Street Journal, November 15, 2000, p. B8. Copyright © 2000, Dow Jones & Company, Inc.

Exhibit 5–10   Characteristics of Selected Short-term Investments

Investment	Denominations	Term	Where Purchased	Comments
T-bills	$10,000; $15,000; $50,000; $100,000; $500,000; $1,000,000	Usually 13/26/52 weeks	Banks; Government	1
CDs	Large: $100,000 to $1,000,000 + Small: $500 to $10,000	Usually 2 weeks to 18 months	Banks	2
Commercial Paper	$100,000 or more	1–270 days	Broker, Dealer, or Corporation	3
Money Market Mutual Funds	Varies; may be <$1,000	Varies (can be bought and sold on the market)	Mutual Fund, Broker, or Bank	4

[1] Most liquid and default free; purchased at a discount and redeemed at face value
[2] Higher risk and higher yield than T-bills; smaller amounts have lower returns than larger amounts
[3] Higher risk and higher yield than CDs
[4] Highly liquid; higher risk and higher yield than commercial paper

Treasury Bills (T-bills)

Treasury bills are financial instruments purchased for a short term. Normally, they have maturities of 13, 26, or 52 weeks and are sold in units of $10,000, $15,000, $50,000, $100,000, $500,000, and $1,000,000. Since they are issued by the government and are part of an active secondary market to buy and sell these securities, they are considered default-free and the most liquid short-term investment available. Instead of earning interest directly, T-bills are purchased at a discount and redeemed at face value when they mature. The discount represents the difference between the purchase price and the face value at time of maturity. Typically, the face value is presented on a $100 maturity value basis. If the discount price is $6.00, purchase price is $94.00.

Negotiable Certificates of Deposit (CDs)

CDs are issued by commercial banks as negotiable, interest-bearing, short-term certificates. In other words, when the deposit matures, the investor receives the interest earned plus the amount deposited. The maturities of CDs usually range from 14 days to 18 months. Small-value CDs are normally issued in $500 to $10,000 denominations. Large-value CDs are normally issued in $100,000 to $1,000,000 denominations. Because of their size, large-value CDs earn a higher return than do small-value CDs. "Negotiable" means the investor may sell the certificate to someone else before maturity. Non-negotiable CDs are offered in smaller denominations. CDs are not as liquid as T-bills and have a higher risk because they are issued by banks rather than the federal government. Because of their risk and illiquidity, investors demand a higher yield or return on CDs than they do on T-bills.

Commercial Paper

Commercial paper is a negotiable promissory note issued at a discount by large corporations (usually publicly traded) that need to raise internal capital. This instrument is issued for maturities of 1 to 270 days through a bank or a dealer that specializes in selling short-term securities. Commercial paper is sold in denominations of $100,000 or more. Because of the possibility of default from a major corporation, this security has a higher credit risk than do T-bills or CDs and, therefore, requires a higher yield.

Money Market Mutual Funds

These funds, which have a minimum investment of $1,000, represent a pooling of investors' funds for the purchase of a diversified portfolio of short-term financial instruments, such as CDs, T-bills, and commercial paper. This pooling of funds allows small investors, such as small health care facilities, to earn short-term money market rates on their investments. Furthermore, most money market funds offer an investor a high degree of liquidity by allowing withdrawals by check, telephone, and wire transfer.

 Key Point | Some of the primary instruments for health care organizations to invest in on a short-term basis are: Treasury Bills, Certificates of Deposit, Commercial Paper, and Money Market Funds.

Forecasting Cash Surpluses and Deficits – The Cash Budget

In order to minimize costs and plan ahead to finance deficits and invest excess cash, a health care organization needs to clearly identify the timing of its cash inflows and outflows. The main vehicle to project cash inflows and outflows is a cash budget. Depending on the decision at hand, it may show inflows on a daily, weekly, monthly, quarterly, semi-annual, annual, or multi-year basis. For instance, forecasts about weekly inflows and outflows are not needed for long-range planning, but monthly planning may require forecasting on a weekly or even daily basis. Much of the information about preparing the cash budget comes from the operating and capital budgets (see Chapter 10 on budgeting).

To illustrate cash inflows and outflows, a monthly cash budget for January through March, 20X1 for Community Health Organization (CHO) is illustrated in Exhibit 5–11.

Cash Inflows

Cash inflow estimates are generally derived from patient revenues, other operating revenues, proceeds from borrowing and/or stock issuances (for investor-owned organizations), and non-operating contributions. To estimate cash receipts from patient revenues for the month, CHO needs to estimate the amount of revenues and when they will be received in cash. Assume CHO forecasts the following revenues for 20X1 based upon 20X0 data:

Actual Patient Revenues 20X0		Estimated Patient Revenues 20X1	
October	$400,000	January	$500,000
November	$500,000	February	$600,000
December	$300,000	March	$700,000

From its historical records, CHO estimates that it will collect 50 percent of revenues earned in the month of service, 40 percent the following month, and 10 percent two months after service has been delivered. All other revenues, such as contributions, appropriations, cash from sale of investments and used equipment, and interest income, are expected to total $44,000, $55,000, and $52,000 in January, February, and March, respectively.

Based on this information, CHO can calculate cash inflows. For instance, February's cash inflows of $585,000 are composed of 50 percent of February's rev-

Exhibit 5–11   A Cash Budget for Three Months, Beginning January 20X1

Givens:

1 **Revenues:**

Actual Patient Revenues, 20X0		Estimated Patient Revenues, 20X1	
October	$400,000	January	$500,000
November	$500,000	February	$600,000
December	$300,000	March	$700,000

2 Funds are received as follows: 50% within the month of service, 40% one month after service, and 10% two months after service.
3 "Other Revenues" includes interest earned and are forecasted to be $44,000 in January, $55,000 in February, and $52,000 in March.
4 Cash outflows are forecasted to be $350,000, $450,000, $600,000, and $500,000 in January, February, March, and April, respectively.
5 "Cash Outflows" are for the current month.
6 The ending cash balance for December was $50,000.
7 CHO desires a required cash balance of 40% of the following month's forecasted cash outflows.

CHO Cash Budget For the Quarter Ending March 31, 20X1

	Item	Formula	January	February	March	Total
	Cash Inflows					
A	From October	[Givens 1,2]	$0	$0	$0	$0
B	From November	[Givens 1,2]	50,000	0	0	50,000
C	From December	[Givens 1,2]	120,000	30,000	0	150,000
D	From January	[Givens 1,2]	250,000	200,000	50,000	500,000
E	From February	[Givens 1,2]	0	300,000	240,000	540,000
F	From March	[Givens 1,2]	0	0	350,000	350,000
G	Other Revenues	[Given 3]	44,000	55,000	52,000	151,000
H	Net Cash Inflows	[Sum A:G]	464,000	585,000	692,000	1,741,000
I	Forecasted Cash Outflows	[Givens 4,5]	350,000	450,000	600,000	1,400,000
J	*Monthly/Quarterly Net Cash Flow*	[H–I]	114,000	135,000	92,000	341,000
K	Beginning Balance	[1]	50,000	180,000	240,000	50,000
L	*Cash Before Borrowing or Investing*	[J+K]	164,000	315,000	332,000	391,000
M	Required Cash Balance	[2]	180,000	240,000	200,000	200,000
N	Surplus (Deficit)	[L–M]	(16,000)	75,000	132,000	191,000
O	Investment of Surplus in ST Investments	[3]	0	(75,000)	(132,000)	(207,000)
P	Short-term Borrowing	[4]	16,000	0	0	16,000
Q	Ending Cash Balance	[M+N+O+P]	$180,000	$240,000	$200,000	$200,000

[1] January: [Given 6]; February/March: [Row Q], previous month.
[2] [Given 7] × [Row I], next month.
[3] [–Row N], but only if there is a surplus.
[4] [–Row N], but only if there is a deficit.

enue ($600,000 × 0.50 = $300,000), 40 percent of January's revenue ($500,000 × 0.40 = $200,000), 10 percent of December's revenue ($300,000 × 0.10 = $30,000), plus the other revenues for February ($55,000) given above.

 Key Point The cash budget is the major budgetary tool to forecast an organization's cash surplus and deficits over a given period of time.

Cash Outflows

Cash outflows are estimated at $350,000, $450,000, $600,000, and $1,400,000 for January, February, March, and Total, respectively (Exhibit 5–11, row I). These outflows include such operating items as salaries and benefits, supplies, interest, capital expenditure outflows for equipment and land, and debt payments.

Ending Cash Balance

By subtracting cash outflows from net cash inflows, CHO can derive its monthly net cash flow. To this amount, it adds the beginning cash balance to calculate the cash available before borrowing or investing. For instance, in January there were net cash inflows of $464,000 and cash outflows of $350,000 that resulted in a $114,000 net cash inflow for the month (row J). When this is added to the $50,000 available at the beginning of the month (row K), CHO had $164,000 in cash before borrowing or investing (row L).

> **Required Cash Balance:** The amount of cash an organization must have on hand at the end of the current period to ensure that it has enough cash to cover the expected outflows during the next forecasting period.

Though this number represents how much cash is available at the end of the month as a result of the normal cash flows during the month plus the beginning balance, many health care organizations are required to end a month (actually, begin the next month) with a certain minimum balance, called a **required cash balance**. If they are below this amount they must borrow money, and if they are above they invest the excess. In the case of CHO, the required cash balance is 40 percent of the next month's forecasted cash outflows (row M, January and row I, February: $180,000/$450,000 = 0.40).

To illustrate this process, CHO had $164,000 in January's cash before borrowing or investing (row L), but the required cash balance is $180,000 (0.40 × $450,000, February's cash outflows). Therefore, it must borrow $16,000 to make up the difference (row P). This results in an ending cash balance of $180,000 (row Q). If there had been a surplus, as in February (row N), CHO would have invested the excess funds (row O).

◄ACCOUNTS RECEIVABLE MANAGEMENT►

Accounts receivable, most of which comes through third-party payors, constitutes approximately 75 percent of a health care provider's current assets. Having a large dollar amount in accounts receivable means lost returns in other investment opportunities. Because third-party payors are volume purchasers of health care services, health care providers are confronted with the problem of trying to externally control the timely payment of accounts. In order to expedite collections, health care provider management does hold some degree of control with respect to processing payments internally. The earlier discussion introduced several ways to reduce float, including: preadmission and admission screenings, computerized information systems, electronic billing, and billing and collection policies and procedures. These methods also reduce receivables, since bringing cash in more quickly reduces the amount outstanding.

Methods to Monitor Accounts Receivable

Since not all money is collected in advance, it is important that an organization closely monitor its outstanding balances. The tracking of outstanding accounts is often carried out through an analysis similar to that presented in Exhibit 5–12.

Net accounts receivable (row A) presents the total amount of receivables outstanding, both in total and by month. Thus, at the end of the first quarter, there are $6.4 million in receivables outstanding, of which $3.6 million are aged 1–30 days (row B), $2.0 million are aged 31–60 days, and $0.8 million are aged 61–90 days. For simplicity, assume that each month has 30 days and that all accounts are written off as bad debt after 90 days.

Exhibit 5–12   Key Measures to Monitor Accounts Receivable

	Formula	QUARTER 1 (in '000) Month 1	Month 2	Month 3	Total
A Net Accounts Receivable	[Given]	$800	$2,000	$3,600	$6,400
B Days Old	[Given]	61–90	31–60	1–30	1–90
C Aging Schedule	[1]	12.5%	31.3%	56.3%	
D Net Patient Revenues	[Given]	$4,000	$5,000	$6,000	$15,000
E Average Daily Patient Revenue	[D/B]	$133	$167	$200	$167
F Days in Accounts Receivable	[A/E]				38.4
G Receivables as a Percentage of Revenue	[A/D]	20%	40%	60%	

[1] [Row A] (month)/[Row A] (quarter).

	Formula	QUARTER 2 (in '000) Month 1	Month 2	Month 3	Total
H Net Accounts Receivable	[Given]	$200	$1,000	$6,900	$8,100
I Days Old	[Given]	61–90	31–60	1–30	1–90
J Aging Schedule	[2]	2.5%	12.3%	85.2%	
K Net Patient Revenues	[Given]	$1,000	$2,500	$11,500	$15,000
L Average Daily Patient Revenue	[K/I]	$33	$83	$383	$167
M Days in Accounts Receivable	[H/L]				48.6
N Receivables as a Percentage of Revenue	[H/K]	20%	40%	60%	

[2] [Row H] (month)/[Row H] (quarter).

Using this information, it is possible to prepare an **aging schedule**, shown in row C. Thus, at the end of the first quarter, of the $6.4 million in receivables outstanding, 56.3 percent were generated in the third and most recent month ($3.6/$6.4), 31.3 percent in the second month ($2.0/$6.4) and 12.5 percent in the first month ($0.8/$6.4). Row D in each quarter shows the revenues recorded during each of the three months of the quarter and for the quarter as a whole. Row E is the average daily patient revenue (monthly revenue/30 days).

Aging Schedule: A table which shows the percentage of receivables outstanding by the month they were incurred.

The information combined from rows A, B, and D yields two new measures: days in accounts receivable for the quarter (row F) and monthly receivables as a percentage of revenue (row G). Days in accounts receivable is calculated by dividing the net accounts receivable (row A) by the average daily patient revenue for the quarter (row E). For the first quarter, the average daily net revenue was $15.0 million/90 days = $166,667 per day, whereas the net accounts receivable is $6.4 million; therefore, the days in accounts receivable (row F) at the end of the quarter is $6,400,000/$166,667 = 38.4 days. This same procedure can be applied to each month to show the number of days of outstanding receivables attributable to each month (using the quarter's average daily net revenue as the denominator).

The final item, receivables as a percentage of revenue (row G), is computed by dividing net accounts receivable (row A) for each 30-day period by its corresponding net patient revenue (row D). For example, at the end of the first quarter, 60 percent of the third month's revenues ($3.6/$6.0), 40 percent of the second month's revenues ($2.0/$5.0), and 20 percent of the first month's revenues ($0.8/$4.0) are all receivables outstanding (dollar figures expressed in millions). A similar analysis follows throughout for Quarter 2 (rows H–N).

Receivables as a percentage of revenues is probably a better measure than days in accounts receivable to judge management's success in collecting revenues, though many health care organizations continue to rely upon the latter as a key ratio to measure performance. In the example, it may appear as if collections are worsening, since days in accounts receivable rose from 38.4 days for the first quarter to 48.6 days for the second quarter. However, receivables as a percentage of revenue shows that collections as a percentage of revenue for each 30-day period remain the same for both quarters: 60 percent, 40 percent, and 20 percent. The reason for the discrepancy is that during the first quarter, a higher percentage of revenues came in the early months than did revenues in the second quarter, when most of the patient revenues occurred in the last month of the quarter. Thus, the reason that the days in accounts receivable went up is not because collection efforts have changed, but rather because the timing of the revenues varied (total revenues are $15,000,000 in each quarter). Because patient revenues are higher in the earlier months of the first quarter, more revenues have been collected by the end of the quarter. In turn, this outcome reduces the days in accounts receivable to 38.4 days as well as the percentage of receivables outstanding.

Key Point A common mistake is to infer that because days in accounts receivable is decreasing, collections are improving. This is not necessarily the case.

Methods to Finance Accounts Receivable

In addition to trying to improve its cash and receivables collections, an organization has two other options to bring funds in to meet cash needs: selling its accounts receivable, called "factoring," and using receivables as collateral.

Factoring

Factoring: Selling accounts receivable at a discount, usually to a financial institution. The latter then assumes the role of trying to collect upon the outstanding payment obligations.

Factoring is the selling of accounts receivable, usually to a bank, at a discount. There are two main reasons why a health care organization would decide to factor its accounts: 1) it needs the cash currently tied up in receivables before it can collect that money from patients and third parties; and 2) it predicts that the benefits of selling the receivables at a discount would outweigh the possible returns it would receive by holding on to the accounts and trying to manage the collections process.

Typical discounts involved in factoring transactions range from 5 to 10 percent. In addition, the financing institution may impose a factoring fee equal to 15–20 percent of the value of the receivables. Under this arrangement, the financing institution purchasing the receivables assumes the risk and control over the collection of the receivables from the health care provider. The more risky the collection of the accounts receivable, the higher the discount demanded by the bank and the higher the fees.

It is important to recognize that when a health care organization resorts to selling its receivables to acquire cash as quickly as possible (perhaps out of desperation), another institution is then involved in the collections process. The potential ill will which may be generated to collect these funds by this other organization which purchased the receivables should receive serious consideration before factoring is undertaken. Of note, *it is illegal to factor Medicaid accounts receivable*.

Pledging Receivables as Collateral

Collateral: A tangible asset which is pledged as a promise to repay a loan. If the loan is not paid, the lending institution as legal recourse may seize the pledged asset.

As noted earlier, health care organizations can negotiate a line of credit with a financial institution in order to cover temporary cash shortfalls. In such instances, the amount of receivables outstanding can be used as collateral. The cost of a line of credit is typically one to two percentage points above the prime rate, unless an organization has an excellent credit history, in which case it can negotiate for the prime rate or even slightly below it.

 Key Point

Factoring and using receivables as collateral are two ways to receive cash advances from outstanding accounts receivable.

◀Laws and Regulation for Billing Compliance▶

Hospitals and other health care organizations must comply with a multitude of laws and regulation restrictions that include areas such as patient billing, cost reporting, physician transactions, and occupational health and safety. Given the rise in health care fraud and abuse, Federal and State governments have a strong incentive to reduce any abusive practices in the area of patient billing. Likely, the most stringent restrictions are those passed down by the Centers for Medicare and Medicaid Services (CMS – called the Health Care Financing Administration, or HCFA, prior to June 1, 2001) for the billing of Medicare patients. An example of a billing practice likely to be considered fraud by Medicare is unbundling: where a hospital charges for multiple laboratory tests, when in reality a single battery of tests was done. Another example of Medicare fraud is when a health care provider submits claims for medical supplies that were never provided to the patient.

To ensure compliance with laws and regulations, health care providers need to implement and maintain an effective corporate compliance plan. The plan should ensure that corporate policies, practices, and culture promote the understanding and adherence to appropriate legal requirements. This means that health care providers must develop effective programs to detect and prevent violations of the law, which includes "whistle-blower" protections and hot-lines. Listed below are questions that will help health care providers to assess their billing compliance:

- Is there consistency in charging patients the same dollar amount for the same service, regardless of patient's payor and where the service was rendered?
- Are controls implemented to assure proper recording and billing of services?
- Do the medical records document that services billed were provided and record the results of the tests?
- Is there a practice in place that ensures that adjustments to patient accounts (bad debt, discounts, etc.) are allowed and performed only by designated and responsible individuals?
- Are overpayments received by Medicare and other federal government programs refunded in a timely manner?
- Are policies and procedures developed to collect copayments and deductibles from patients?
- Are the changes in billing codes completed in a timely manner?
- Are charges listed and bundled properly?

HIPAA

One of the major compliance regulations that hospitals face is the Health Insurance Portability and Accountability Act (HIPAA). HIPAA provides reform in several areas ranging from portability of health insurance, preventing fraud and abuse, information security, and administrative simplification. HIPAA regulations covering fraudulent activities are enforced under codes of criminal conduct. For example, individuals who

Corporate Compliance: Mandated legislation and regulations bestowed upon health care institutions to ensure fairness, accuracy, honesty, and quality in the provision of and billing for health care services.

Corporate Compliance Officer: The individual (or department) responsible for knowing the corporate compliance rules and regulations, and for ensuring that the organization strictly abides by them.

HIPAA: Health Insurance Portability and Accountability Act. A public law designed to improve efficiency in health care delivery by standardizing electronic data interchange, and protecting the confidentiality and security of health data through setting and enforcing standards.

knowingly defraud a health care benefit program by giving false statements or embezzling money can face personal fines, imprisonment, or both. Additionally, organizations must take important measures to ensure that patient-specific information is kept confidential, especially in the electronic age, and organizations can be held accountable if reasonably appropriate measures have not been put into place.

HIPAA also requires the adoption of industry standards for the electronic transmission of health information. According to the Department of Health and Human Services (DHHS), at the start of the new millennium there were about 400 formats for electronic health care claims processing in use nationwide. As a result, health care providers and health plans are unable to standardize their claims processing, which increases the expense to develop and maintain software and reduces their overall efficiency and savings in administrative transactions (see Perspective 5–5). Health care providers and health plans will need to achieve this standardization in the following administrative and financial health care transactions: health claims and equivalent encounter information, enrollment and disenrollment in a health plan, eligibility for a health plan, health care payment and remittance advice, health plan premium payments, health claim status, referral certification and authorization, and coordination of benefits. By meeting the HIPAA standards in the areas of content and format, health care providers and plans could save over $3–5 billion annually. However, there is a significant investment cost beforehand to become compliant.

To meet these standards, health care providers will need to do the following:

- Train personnel on the standards.
- Develop a management team that assesses the impact of these standards across the organization.
- Identify and select vendors that support complying software.
- Budget for the information system costs to adhere to these standards.

PERSPECTIVE 5–5

Report Predicts Huge HIPAA Price Tag

A rating analyst from the Fitch rating agency expects that healthcare providers will incur four times the costs of what they incurred on Y2K in following the HIPAA regulations. The rating analyst estimates that healthcare providers will spend about $25 billion nationwide, in contrast to the $8.2 billion cost of Y2K. As the analyst noted: "HIPAA is going to be all that, plus it will require ongoing monitoring, which will elevate costs. . . . Plus there will be changes in process, in security, in privacy, and in the culture of privacy within hospitals and healthcare."

Conversely, another analyst from a consulting firm that's monitoring HIPAA's effects on providers provides a lower estimation. This analyst predicts that "HIPAA will cost providers a little more than Y2K did, likely from $10 billion to $15 billion." The analyst also found from a recent survey that 20% of integrated delivery systems had done preliminary research on what HIPAA would cost them and found an estimated average compliance cost of $5 million per system.

Source: Barbara Kirchheimer, "Report Predicts Huge HIPAA Price Tag." *Modern Healthcare*, October 2, 2000, p. 48.

Health care providers face the obstacles of state variation in billing codes for government programs, health plans, and other commercial insurers, as well as local variation in clinical codes.

◄Summary►

Working capital refers to the current assets and current liabilities of a health care organization. Working capital is important because it turns the capacity of an organization (its long-term assets) into services and revenues. All health care organizations must ensure that it has sufficient working capital available at appropriate times to meet its day-to-day needs.

The management of working capital involves managing the working capital cycle: 1) obtaining cash; 2) purchasing resources and paying bills; 3) delivering services; and 4) billing and collecting for services rendered. There are two components to a working capital management strategy: determining asset mix and financing mix. Asset mix is the amount of working capital the organization keeps on hand relative to its potential working capital obligations. Financing mix is how the organization chooses to finance its working capital needs. To determine its level of working capital, a health care facility must evaluate the risk/return tradeoff between over-investment or under-investment in working capital. A conservative approach with a higher investment in working capital increases an organization's liquidity, but does so at the expense of lower returns. An aggressive approach with less investment in working capital decreases liquidity but frees funds to invest in higher returning fixed assets. The decision to select either option or some comfortable medium depends upon the health care provider's environment and financial condition.

A major component of current assets is cash and cash equivalents. There are three reasons to hold cash: daily operations, precautionary reasons, and speculative purposes. The sources of temporary cash are bank loans, trade credit and billing, collections, and disbursement policies and procedures. Types of bank loans include normal and revolving lines of credit and transaction notes. Lines of credit are usually pre-established and allow a health care organization to borrow money in a reasonably expeditious manner. Transaction notes are short-term, unsecured loans made for specific purposes, such as the purchase of supplies. Both of these borrowing methods may involve either a commitment fee or compensating balance.

A second important source of temporary cash is trade credit, which does not actually bring in cash, but instead slows its outflow. Although not commonly thought of in this way, it is a loan by a vendor to the health care organization, and vendors often provide discounts for early payment. It is normally beneficial for a health care organization to take the discount. To determine the approximate interest rate, the following formula is used:

Approximate Interest Rate = Discount%/(1 − Discount%) × (365/Net Period)

Another formula is the effective interest rate:

$$\text{Effective Interest Rate} = \frac{(\text{Interest Expense on Amount Borrowed} + \text{Total Fees})}{(\text{Amount Borrowed} - \text{Compensating Balance})}$$

Because the approximate interest rate declines the longer the payment is delayed, a prudent policy is to make the payment as close to the last day of the discount period as is operationally feasible or, if the discount is not taken, on the last day of the "net" period. Although interest costs decrease as the number of days increases after the last day for the discount in which the bill is not paid, at a certain point new costs are encountered. These costs include late fees, loss of discounts in the future, loss of priority status with this supplier, etc.

A third source of temporary cash is good billing, collections, and disbursement policies and procedures, all of which decrease the amount of float (time delays) existing in the working capital cycle. The principal types of float are: billing, collection, transit, and disbursement. Billing float is the delay in getting a bill to the patient or the third-party payor. Techniques to reduce billing float include preadmissions and admissions screening, accurate claims processing, utilization review, and effective billing policies and procedures.

There are several well used techniques to reduce collection float (the time between the issuance of a bill and the time the monies are available for use) and transit float (the time it takes for a check to clear the banking system). These techniques include using decentralized collection centers, lockboxes, and electronic deposit of funds. The tools to reduce disbursement float include taking suppliers' discounts and using remote disbursement accounts.

A major function of cash management is to ensure that any excess cash is earning a reasonable return at an acceptable level of risk. There are four primary vehicles for short-term investment of cash: treasury bills, certificates of deposit, commercial paper, and money market mutual funds. These financial vehicles may differ on degrees of risk, return, and initial outlay.

A well managed cash strategy is based on accurate forecasting of cash flow. The principal tool for this is the cash budget. A cash budget should forecast not only cash inflows and outflows, but also when excess cash will become available or when cash deficiencies that necessitate borrowing will occur.

In addition to managing cash, good working capital management involves managing accounts receivable. Most of the methods used to decrease accounts receivable are the same methods discussed under ways to speed up the inflows of cash. Managing receivables is based on good record keeping and periodic review. There are three main tools used to monitor receivables: creating an aging schedule, monitoring days in accounts receivable, and monitoring receivables as a percentage of revenues. Though days in accounts receivable is probably the most used ratio to monitor receivables, it may be overly sensitive to the timing of revenues. Therefore, receivables as a percentage of revenues is used to overcome this problem. Organizations can also do much for their bottom line simply by keeping a well trained staff, implementing good information systems, and maintaining good relations with payors. Finally, health care organizations need to develop a compliance program to ensure that their payroll, billing, and other financial transactions comply with governmental regulations.

◀KEY TERMS▶

AGING SCHEDULE	DISBURSEMENT FLOAT	REQUIRED CASH BALANCE
APPROXIMATE INTEREST RATE	EFFECTIVE INTEREST RATE	REVOLVING LINE OF CREDIT
ASSET MIX	FACTORING	TRADE CREDIT
BILLING FLOAT	FINANCING MIX	TRADE PAYABLES
COLLATERAL	FLOAT	TRANSACTION NOTE
COLLECTION FLOAT	HIPAA	TRANSIT FLOAT
COMMITMENT FEE	LIQUIDITY	WORKING CAPITAL
COMPENSATING BALANCE	LOCKBOX	WORKING CAPITAL STRATEGY
CORPORATE COMPLIANCE	NET WORKING CAPITAL	
CORPORATE COMPLIANCE OFFICER	NORMAL LINE OF CREDIT	

◀KEY EQUATIONS▶

Approximate Interest Rate = Discount%/(1 − Discount%) × (365/Net Period)

Effective Interest Rate = (Interest Expense on Amount Borrowed + Total Fees)/
(Amount Borrowed − Compensating Balance)

◀QUESTIONS AND PROBLEMS▶

1. **Definitions.** Define the following terms:
   a. Aging Schedule.
   b. Approximate Interest Rate.
   c. Asset Mix.
   d. Billing Float.
   e. Collateral.
   f. Collection Float.
   g. Commitment Fee.
   h. Compensating Balance.
   i. Corporate Compliance.
   j. Corporate Compliance Officer.
   k. Disbursement Float.
   l. Effective Interest Rate.
   m. Factoring.
   n. Financing Mix.
   o. Float.
   p. HIPAA.
   q. Liquidity.
   r. Lockbox.
   s. Net Working Capital.
   t. Normal Line of Credit.

    u. Required Cash Balance.

    v. Revolving Line of Credit.

    w. Trade Credit.

    x. Trade Payables.

    y. Transaction Note.

    z. Transit Float.

  aa. Working Capital.

  bb. Working Capital Strategy.

2. **Working Capital.** What is the function of working capital?

3. **Working Capital Cycle.** In terms of cash flow, what are the stages of the working capital cycle?

4. **Working Capital Management Strategy.** Describe the two components of a working capital management strategy.

5. **Asset Mix Strategies.** Compare aggressive and conservative asset mix strategies. The comparison should address goals, liquidity, and risk.

6. **Borrowing.** What is the difference between temporary and permanent working capital needs? What is the general rule about when to borrow long-term or short-term?

7. **Borrowing.** In terms of risk and return (profit), compare the advantages and disadvantages of short- and long-term borrowing to meet working capital needs.

8. **Cash.** State the three reasons why a health care facility holds cash.

9. **Cash.** What are the main sources of temporary cash?

10. **Loans.** What is an unsecured loan?

11. **Loans.** What are the two types of unsecured bank loans? Describe each.

12. **Compensating Balance.** Describe how compensating balances impact the "true" rate the borrower pays.

13. **Discounts.** What does "1.5/15 net 25" mean?

14. **Discounts.** What is the formula to determine the approximate annual interest cost for not taking a discount? When should discounts be taken?

15. **Collections.** What are the objectives of billing, credit, and collections policies?

16. **Float.** What is the purpose of cash disbursement policies?

17. **Float.** Define float. What are the major types of float?

18. **Float.** What is a hospital's objective regarding collection and disbursement float?

19. **Billings.** In the hospital's billing process, why is medical records a critical department?

20. **Float.** Describe the remote disbursement technique of disbursement float.

21. **Lockboxes.** Describe the lockbox technique of collection float.

22. **Float.** What is the purpose of preadmissions screening?

23. **Investments.** Identify the alternatives for investing cash on a short-term basis, and discuss the general characteristics of each.

24. **Accounts Receivable.** List three ways to measure accounts receivable performance.

25. **Accounts Receivable.** Two methods to monitor accounts receivable are as a percentage of net patient revenues, and as days in accounts receivable. What factor can cause the former to be a better measure than the latter with regard to collections activities?

26. **Accounts Receivable.** Identify and define two methods to finance accounts receivable.

27. **Trade Credit Discount.** Compute the annual approximate interest cost of not taking a discount using the following scenarios. What conclusion can be drawn from the calculations?
   a. 1/10 net 20
   b. 1/10 net 30
   c. 1/10 net 40
   d. 1/10 net 50
   e. 1/10 net 60

28. **Trade Credit Discount.** Compute the annual approximate interest cost of not taking a discount using the following scenarios. What conclusion can be drawn from the calculations?
   a. 2/10 net 20
   b. 2/10 net 30
   c. 2/10 net 40
   d. 2/10 net 50
   e. 2/10 net 60

29. **Trade Credit Discount.** Compute the annual approximate interest cost of not taking a discount using the following scenarios. What conclusion can be drawn from the calculations?
   a. 1/10 net 30
   b. 1/15 net 30
   c. 1/20 net 30
   d. 1/25 net 30

30. **Trade Credit Discount.** Compute the annual approximate interest cost of not taking a discount using the following scenarios. What conclusion can be drawn from the calculations?
   a. 2/10 net 30
   b. 2/15 net 30
   c. 2/20 net 30
   d. 2/25 net 30

31. **Trade Credit Discount.** Compute the annual approximate interest cost of not taking a discount using the following scenarios. What conclusion can be drawn from the calculations?
   a. 1/5 net 30
   b. 2/5 net 30
   c. 3/5 net 30
   d. 4/5 net 30

32. **Trade Credit Discount.** Compute the annual interest cost of not taking a discount using the following scenarios. What conclusion can be drawn from the calculations?
   a. 1/10 net 30
   b. 2/10 net 30
   c. 3/10 net 30
   d. 4/10 net 30

33. **Accounts Receivable Management.** Given the information below, compute the days in accounts receivable, aging schedule, and accounts receivable as a percentage of net patient revenues for Quarter 1 and Quarter 2, 20X1. Compare the two quarters to determine if the organization's collection procedure is improving.

Quarter 1, 20X1 (in '000)

Days Outstanding	Total	1–30	31–60	61–90
Net Accounts Receivable	$2,500	$200	$500	$1,800
Net Patient Revenue	$7,500	$500	$2,500	$4,500

Quarter 2, 20X1 (in '000)

Days Outstanding	Total	1–30	31–60	61–90
Net Accounts Receivable	$2,500	$800	$500	$1,200
Net Patient Revenue	$7,500	$2,000	$2,500	$3,000

34. **Accounts Receivable Management.** Given the information below, compute the days in accounts receivable, aging schedule, and accounts receivable as a percentage of net patient revenues for Quarter 1 and Quarter 2, 20X1. Compare the two quarters to determine if the organization's collection procedure is improving.

Quarter 1, 20X1 (in '000)

Days Outstanding	Total	1–30	31–60	61–90
Net Accounts Receivable	$5,000	$1,500	$500	$3,000
Net Patient Revenue	$15,000	$3,000	$2,500	$9,500

Quarter 2, 20X1 (in '000)

Days Outstanding	Total	1–30	31–60	61–90
Net Accounts Receivable	$5,000	$3,000	$500	$1,500
Net Patient Revenue	$15,000	$9,500	$2,500	$3,000

35. **Accounts Receivable Management.** Given the information below, compute the days in accounts receivable, aging schedule, and accounts receivable as a percentage of net patient revenues for Quarter 1 and Quarter 2, 20X1. Compare the two quarters to determine if the organization's collection procedure is improving.

Quarter 1, 20X1 (in '000)

Days Outstanding	Total	1–30	31–60	61–90
Net Accounts Receivable	$2,500	$200	$500	$1,800
Net Patient Revenue	$7,500	$500	$2,500	$4,500

Quarter 2, 20X1 (in '000)

Days Outstanding	Total	1–30	31–60	61–90
Net Accounts Receivable	$2,500	$1,800	$500	$200
Net Patient Revenue	$7,500	$2,000	$2,500	$3,000

36. **Accounts Receivable Management.** Given the information below, compute the days in accounts receivable, aging schedule, and accounts receivable as a percentage of net patient revenues for Quarter 1 and Quarter 2, 20X1. Compare the two quarters to determine if the organization's collection procedure is improving.

Quarter 1, 20X1 (in '000)

	Total	1–30	31–60	61–90
Days Outstanding				
Net Accounts Receivable	$9,990	$799	$1,998	$7,193
Net Patient Revenue	$30,000	$2,000	$10,000	$18,000

Quarter 2, 20X1 (in '000)

	Total	1–30	31–60	61–90
Days Outstanding				
Net Accounts Receivable	$9,990	$7,193	$1,998	$799
Net Patient Revenue	$30,000	$8,000	$10,000	$12,000

37. **Compensating Balance.** On January 2, 20X1, City Hospital established a line of credit with First Union National Bank. The terms of the line of credit called for a $200,000 maximum loan with an interest of 11 percent. The compensating balance requirement is 15 percent of the total line of credit (with no additional fees charged).
   a. What is the effective interest rate for City Hospital if 50 percent of the total amount were used during the year?
   b. What is the effective interest rate if only 25 percent of the total loan were used during the year?
   c. How would the answer to part a change if the additional fees were $500?
   d. How would the answer to part b change if the additional fees were $1,000?

38. **Compensating Balance.** Lawrence Hospital wishes to establish a line of credit with a bank. The first bank's terms call for a $300,000 maximum loan with an interest rate of 11 percent and a $1,000 fee. The second bank for the same line of credit charges an interest rate of 12 percent, but no fee. The compensating balance requirement is 15 percent of the total line of credit for either bank.
   a. What is the effective interest rate for Lawrence Hospital from the first bank if 50 percent of the total amount were used during the year?
   b. What is the effective interest rate for Lawrence Hospital from the first bank if 25 percent of the total amount were used during the year?
   c. What is the effective interest rate for Lawrence Hospital from the second bank if 50 percent of the total amount were used during the year?
   d. What is the effective interest rate for Lawrence Hospital from the second bank if 25 percent of the total amount were used during the year? Which bank would be the better choice for Lawrence Hospital?

39. **Cash Budget.** Jay Zeeman Clinic provided the following financial information in Exhibit 5–13. Prepare a cash budget for the quarter ending March, 20X1.

40. **Cash Budget.** Iowa Diagnostic Center provided the following financial information in Exhibit 5–14. Prepare a cash budget for the quarter ending March, 20X1.

41. **Cash Budget.** Stacie Zeeman Clinic provided the following financial information in Exhibit 5–15. Prepare a cash budget for the quarter ending March, 20X1.

Exhibit 5–13   Jay Zeeman Clinic

Revenues/Expenses:

Patient Revenues, 20X1		Estimated Patient Revenues, 20X1	
October	$1,500,000	January	$1,700,000
November	$1,600,000	February	$1,300,000
December	$1,700,000	March	$1,200,000

Other Revenues, 20X1		Estimated Cash Outflows, 20X1[1]	
January	$44,000	January	$1,199,000
February	$55,000	February	$1,263,800
March	$52,000	March	$1,390,600
		April	$855,000

Receipt of Payment for Patient Services		Ending Cash Balances	
Month earned	60%	December, 20X0	$200,000
2nd month	30%		
3rd month	10%	[2]	40%
4th+ months	0%		

[1] "Cash Outflows" within the given month.
[2] The ending balance for each month as a percentage of the estimated cash outflows for the next month.

Exhibit 5–14   Iowa Clinic

Revenues/Expenses:

Patient Revenues, 20X1		Estimated Patient Revenues, 20X1	
October	$1,000,000	January	$1,300,000
November	$1,200,000	February	$1,350,000
December	$1,300,000	March	$1,400,000

Other Revenues, 20X1		Estimated Cash Outflows, 20X1[1]	
January	$40,000	January	$1,250,000
February	$50,000	February	$1,300,000
March	$60,000	March	$1,350,000
		April	$1,400,000

Receipt of Payment for Patient Services		Ending Cash Balances	
Month earned	60%	December, 20X0	$150,000
2nd month	30%		
3rd month	10%		
4th+ months	0%	[2]	40%

[1] "Cash Outflows" within the given month.
[2] The ending balance for each month as a percentage of the estimated cash outflows for the next month.

Exhibit 5–15 Stacy Zeeman Clinic

Revenues:

Patient Revenues, 20X0		Patient Revenues, 20X0		Estimated Patient Revenues, 20X1	
July	$1,500,000	October	$1,420,000	January	$1,600,000
August	$1,350,000	November	$1,210,000	February	$1,350,000
September	$1,530,000	December	$1,800,000	March	$1,220,000

Other Revenues, 20X1		Receipt of Payment for Patient Services	
January	$44,000	Month earned	45%
February	$55,000	2nd month	25%
March	$52,000	3rd month	10%
		4–7 months	5%

Expenses[1]:

Supplies Purchases 20X0		Estimated Supply Purchases, 20X1		Other Estimated Expenses, 20X1[1]			
					Nursing	Admin.	Other
October	$400,000	January	$500,000	January	$500,000	$50,000	$145,000
November	$500,000	February	$600,000	February	$550,000	$50,000	$235,000
December	$300,000	March	$700,000	March	$600,000	$50,000	$175,000
		April	$100,000	April	$350,000	$50,000	$105,000

Timing of Cash Payment for Supplies Purchases		Ending Cash Balances	
0%	Month purchased	December, 20X0	$400,000
60%	+1 Month	[2]	50%
30%	+2 Months		
10%	+3 Months		

[1] All estimated expenses are cash outflows for the given month.
[2] The ending balance for each month as a percentage of the estimated cash outflows for the next month.

42. **Cash Budget.** Happy Valley Rehab Facility provided the following financial information in Exhibit 5–16. Prepare a cash budget for the quarter ending March, 20X1.

43. **Cash Budget.** How would the cash budget in Problem 41 change if new credit and collection policies were implemented such that collections resulted as follows:
    40% month earned
    30% + 1 month
    10% + 2 months
    5% + 3–6 months

44. **Cash Budget.** How would the cash budget in Problem 42 change if new credit and collection policies were implemented such that collections resulted as follows:
    40% month earned
    30% + 1 month

Exhibit 5–16   Happy Valley Rehab Facility

Revenues:

Patient Revenues, 20X0		Patient Revenues, 20X0		Estimated Patient Revenues, 20X1	
July	$2,200,000	October	$2,500,000	January	$2,600,000
August	$2,400,000	November	$2,550,000	February	$2,500,000
September	$2,500,000	December	$2,600,000	March	$2,500,000

Other Revenues, 20X1		Receipt of Payment for Patient Services	
January	$100,000	Month earned	45%
February	$110,000	2nd month	25%
March	$115,000	3rd month	10%
		4–7 months	5%

Expenses[1]:

Supplies Purchases 20X0		Estimated Supply Purchases, 20X1		Other Estimated Expenses, 20X1[1]			
					Nursing	Admin.	Other
October	$800,000	January	$900,000	January	$1,000,000	$100,000	$700,000
November	$850,000	February	$925,000	February	$1,100,000	$100,000	$675,000
December	$900,000	March	$950,000	March	$1,200,000	$100,000	$650,000
		April	$975,000	April	$1,300,000	$100,000	$525,000

Timing of Cash Payment for Supplies Purchases		Ending Cash Balances	
0%	Month purchased	December, 20X0	$500,000
60%	+1 Month	[2]	50%
30%	+2 Months		
10%	+3 Months		

[1] All estimated expenses are cash outflows for the given month.
[2] The ending balance for each month as a percentage of the estimated cash outflows for the next month.

        10% + 2 months
        5% + 3–6 months

45. **Discounts.** Stacie Zeeman Clinic in Exhibit 5–15 is going to take better advantage of credit terms offered by suppliers. The clinic has negotiated a 3 percent discount for all supplies purchases
beginning in 20X1, if paid in full during the month of service. How does this change the answer to Problem 41?

46. **Discounts.** Happy Valley Clinic in Exhibit 5–16 is going to take better advantage of credit terms offered by suppliers. The clinic has negotiated a 3 percent discount for all supplies purchases
beginning in 20X1, if paid in full during the month of service. How does this change the answer to Problem 42?

Chapter Six

THE TIME VALUE OF MONEY

LEARNING OBJECTIVES

After completing the material in this chapter, you will be able to:

▶ Explain why a dollar today is worth more than a dollar in the future.
▶ Define the terms **future value** and **present value**.
▶ Calculate the future value of an amount and annuity.

Chapter Outline

(Continues)

Chapter Outline (*Contd*)

◀INTRODUCTION▶

Is it better to receive $10,000 today or at the end of the year? The clear answer is today, for a variety of reasons:

> **Opportunity Cost:** Proceeds lost by forgoing other opportunities.

1. **Certainty.** A dollar in hand today is certain, whereas a dollar to be received sometime in the future is not.
2. **Inflation.** During inflationary periods, a dollar will purchase less in the future than it would today. Thus, because of inflation, the value of the dollar in the future is worth less than it is today.
3. **Opportunity Cost.** A dollar today can be used or invested elsewhere. The interest forgone by not having the dollar to invest now is an opportunity cost.

The concept of **interest** determines how much an amount of money invested today will be worth in the future (its **future value**). It can also be used to determine how much a dollar received at some point in the future would be worth today (its **present value**) (see Exhibit 6–1). *This chapter focuses on both future and present value, the basics of the time value of money, which is essential to making long-term decisions – the focus of Chapter 7.*

◀THE FUTURE VALUE OF A DOLLAR INVESTED TODAY▶

> **Time Value of Money:** The concept that a dollar received today is worth more than a dollar received in the future.

What a dollar invested today will be worth in the future depends on the length of the investment period, the method used to calculate interest, and the interest rate. There are two types of methods to calculate interest: the simple method, and compounding. When the **simple interest method** is used, the interest is calculated only on the *original principal* each year. When the **compound interest method** is used, interest is calculated on both the *original principal* and on any *accumulated interest* earned up to that point. Perspective 6–1 presents a review of how stock prices are affected by the time value of money.

> **Simple Interest Method:** A method which calculates interest only on the original principal. The principal is the amount invested.

Exhibit 6–2 part A uses the simple interest method to calculate how much $10,000 invested today at 10 percent interest would be worth in five years. Since the simple interest method calculates interest on the principal only, each year of investment would earn $1,000 interest (0.10 × $10,000). After five years, the net worth of the investment would be $15,000 ($10,000 plus $5,000 in interest).

Exhibit 6–1 Comparison of Future Value and Present Value Concepts

Future Value (FV) — The worth in the future of an amount invested today, or the worth in the future of a series of payments made over time.

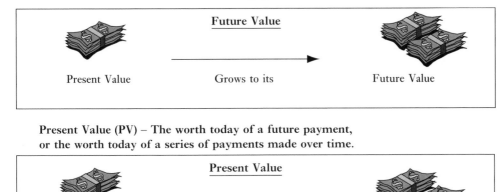

Present Value (PV) – The worth today of a future payment, or the worth today of a series of payments made over time.

Exhibit 6–2 part B uses the same scenario to illustrate the difference of compounded interest. In the first year, there is no difference between using the simple and compound interest methods, since no interest has yet been earned. However, in the second and all subsequent years, more interest is earned using the compound interest method, because 10 percent is earned on the original $10,000, *plus 10 percent on the total amount of interest previously accumulated.* Thus, the future value of $10,000 invested at 10 percent interest after five years is $16,105 using compound interest, compared to $15,000 using simple interest.

Compound Interest Method: A method which calculates interest on both the original principal and on all interest accumulated since the beginning of the investment time period.

PERSPECTIVE 6–1

The Time Value of Money in Stock Valuation

Understanding the time value of money is crucial to prudent investing in stocks and bonds. The price of a stock is the sum of its anticipated future earnings or cash flow, taking into account the time value of money.

The "cost of capital"; could be thought of as the investment hurdle or opportunity cost for similar risk investments; in other words, it is the minimum return an investor will accept to invest in a stock of similar risk. Typically, this rate is greater than the return on US Treasury Bonds. In January of 2000, Treasury bond rates were around 6.5%, which are guaranteed by the federal government. If an investor did not expect to achieve a return of at least 6.5% on a stock investment, then there would be no reason to take on the risk. However, over the past 70 years, most investors have received a premium of 7% above the bond rate to compensate for this risk. In other words, stocks have outpaced government bonds by 7%. Thus, the value of stock hinges upon two factors: the cost of capital, and the expected future earnings or cash flow streams.

Source: Shawn Tully, "Has the Market Gone Mad?" *Fortune,* January 24, 2000, pp. 81–2

Exhibit 6–2   Comparison of Investing $10,000 Over Five Years at 10 Percent Using Simple and Compound

A. The future value of investing $10,000 over five years at 10 percent *simple* interest:

A Year [Given]	B Total at Beginning of Year [D, Previous Year)	C Interest earned [$10,000 × 10%]	D Amount at End of Year[1] [B + C]
1	$10,000	$1,000	$11,000
2	$11,000	$1,000	$12,000
3	$12,000	$1,000	$13,000
4	$13,000	$1,000	$14,000
5	$14,000	$1,000	$15,000
Summary:			
Beginning Balance	$10,000		
Interest Earned		$5,000	
Ending Balance			**$15,000**

B. The future value of investing $10,000 over five years at 10 percent *compound* interest:

E Year [Given]	F Total at Beginning of Year [H, Previous Year]	G Interest earned [F × 10%]	H Amount at End of Year[1] [F + G]
1	$10,000	$1,000	$11,000
2	$11,000	$1,100	$12,100
3	$12,100	$1,210	$13,310
4	$13,310	$1,331	$14,641
5	$14,641	$1,464	$16,105
Summary:			
Beginning Balance	$10,000		
Interest Earned		$6,105	
Ending Balance			**$16,105**

[1] Also called *future value*.

Future Value (FV):
What an amount invested today (or a series of payments made over time) will be worth at a given time in the future using the compound interest method, which accounts for the time value of money. See also Present Value.

The difference between the two methods is considerable and increases with time. After 10 years, $10,000 invested at 10 percent simple interest would grow to $20,000, after 20 years it would be worth $30,000, and after 50 years it would grow to $60,000. The comparable numbers for compound interest are $25,937, $67,275 and $1,173,909, respectively. These differences are illustrated in Exhibit 6–3, which compares the constant rate of growth using simple interest to the increasing growth rate using compound interest.

Using a Formula to Calculate Future Value

One approach to calculating future value is to use the *formula*:

$$FV = PV \times (1 + i)^n$$

Exhibit 6–3 The Future Value of $10,000 Earning 10 Percent Using Simple and Compound Interest

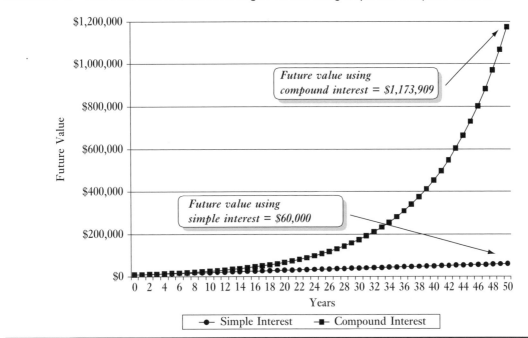

 Key Point Simple interest only calculates interest on the original principal, whereas compound interest calculates interest on both the principal and any accumulated interest. Thus, the value in the future using compound interest will always be higher than that using simple interest, except in the first period.

where: **PV** is the present value (initial investment amount), **i** is the interest rate, and **n** is the number of time periods of the investment. This formula says that an investment's worth in the future, **FV**, is equal to the investment's present worth today, **PV**, multiplied by a factor, $(1 + i)^n$, which takes into account the compounded growth in interest over the lifetime of the investment.

 Key Point As commonly used, the term *future value* implies using the compound interest method. It is used in this way throughout this text unless noted otherwise.

As an example, to calculate the future value of $10,000 in four years at 10 percent interest, the formula is set up as follows:

$$FV = PV \times (1 + i)^n$$

$$FV = \$10,000 \times (1 + 0.10)^4$$

$$FV = \$10,000 \times (1.4641)$$

$$FV = \$14,641$$

Similarly, to calculate the future value of $10,000 earning 10 percent interest over five years, the formula is set up as follows:

$$FV = PV \times (1 + i)^n$$

$$FV = \$10,000 \times (1 + 0.10)^5$$

$$FV = \$10,000 \times (1.6105)$$

$$FV = \$16,105$$

Notice that these are the same numbers derived in Exhibit 6–2 part B for four and five years, respectively.

Using Tables to Compute Future Value

An alternative to calculating the future value using the formula is to use a future value *table*. Table B–1, at the end of this chapter, contains a pre-calculated range of future value factors (FVF) using the future value formula, $(1 + i)^n$. Across the top of the table, the column headings list various interest rates. The leftmost column in the table, or the row headings, provides the number of compounding periods (annual, semi-annual, quarterly, etc.). The intersecting cell for a row/column combination contains the corresponding future value factor. For example, as shown in Exhibit 6–4, the FVF to invest $10,000 at 10 percent for five years (abbreviated as $FVF_{10,5}$), is found by following the 10 percent column down to the fifth row (five years), to the number 1.6105. This number is then used in the following formula to derive the future value

$$FV = PV \times FVF_{i,n}$$

Key Point	The future value factor (FVF): $(1 + i)^n$, where i is the interest rate and n is the number of periods.

Key Point	The formula to find the future value: Future value = Present value × Future value factor. It is abbreviated as $FV = PV \times FVF_{i,n}$ or $FV = PV(1 + i)^n$.

Exhibit 6–4   Example of How to Find the Future Value Factor at 10 Percent Interest for Five Years Using Table B–1

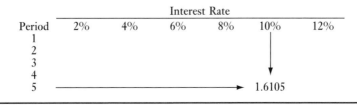

			Interest Rate			
Period	2%	4%	6%	8%	10%	12%
1						
2						
3						
4						
5						1.6105

in a manner similar to the last two steps in using the formula approach:

$$FV = \$10,000 \times (1.6105)$$

$$FV = \$16,105$$

This is the same result calculated earlier by using the formula, $FV = PV \times (1 + i)^n$. Table B–1 can be used to find the FVF for numbers up to 50 percent interest and 50 years.

Using a Spreadsheet to Calculate Future Value

Most spreadsheets have easy-to-use financial functions that can calculate future value. For example, to calculate the future value of $10,000 at 10 percent interest over five years using *Excel*, simply call up the future value function by clicking on "Insert," then "Function," then "Financial." On the right-hand side of the screen double-click on "FV." Enter the rate (10%), the number of periods (5), and the present value as a negative number (−10000), to represent the cash outflow of the investment. The future value, $16,105, is automatically calculated at the bottom (see Exhibit 6–5). Note that the future value is a positive number, because it represents a cash inflow of the principal and interest at a later point in time.

> **Present Value (PV):** The value today of a payment (or series of payments) to be received in the future, taking into account the cost of capital (sometimes called "discount rate"). It is calculated using the formula: Present Value = Future Value × Present Value Factor (PV = FV × PVF or PV = FV × $1/(1 + i)^n$).

◀THE PRESENT VALUE OF AN AMOUNT TO BE RECEIVED IN THE FUTURE▶

The focus until now has been on the future value of money that is invested today. The example showed that $10,000 invested by a clinic today will be worth $16,105 in five years at 10 percent interest each year. In this section, the question is turned around,

Exhibit 6–5   Using *Excel* to Calculate the Future Value for a Single Payment

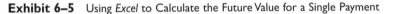

FV

Rate	10%		= 0.1
Nper	5		= 5
Pmt			= number
Pv	-10000		= -10000
Type			= number

= 16105.1

Returns the future value of an investment based on periodic, constant payments and a constant interest rate.

      Pv is the present value, or the lump-sum amount that a series of future payments is worth now. If omitted, Pv = 0.

Formula result = 16105.1   OK   Cancel

"How much is $16,105 to be received five years from now worth today?" The value today of a payment (or series of payments) to be received in the future taking into account the cost of capital is the *present value*. Taking future values back to the present is also called "discounting."

Key Point   The present value factor is the reciprocal of the future value factor and is calculated using the formula $1/(1 + i)^n$.

Key Point   The formula to find the present value: Present Value = Future Value × Present Value Factor. It is abbreviated as: $PV = FV \times PVF_{i,n}$ or $PV = FV \times 1/(1 + i)^n$.

Using a Formula to Calculate Present Value

Compounding:
Converting a present value into its future value taking into account the time value of money. See Compound Interest Method. It is the opposite of discounting.

Discounting:
Converting future cash flows into their present value taking into account the time value of money. It is the opposite of compounding.

Just as the present value is multiplied by a future value factor to determine the future value, the future value is multiplied by a present value factor to calculate present value. The **present value factor, $1/(1 + i)^n$,** is the inverse of the **future value factor, $(1 + i)^n$.**

Thus, using the formula, the present value of $16,105 at 10 percent interest for five years can be calculated as follows:

$$PV = FV \times 1/(1 + i)^n$$

$$PV = \$16,105 \times 1/(1 + 0.10)^5$$

$$PV = \$16,105 \times 1/(1.6105)$$

$$PV = \$16,105 \times (0.6209)$$

$$PV = \$10,000$$

The $1/(1.6105)$, which equals 0.6209, is the present value factor. It can be interpreted to mean that at 10 percent interest, a dollar received five years from now is worth only about 62 percent of its value in today's dollars. In the example, $16,105 received five years from now is only worth $10,000 in today's dollars.

Exhibit 6–6 illustrates the relationship between present value and future value. Just as $10,000 today grows to $16,105 over five years at 10 percent compound interest, $16,105 received five years from now is worth $10,000 today, assuming a 10 percent (discount) rate.

Key Point   To find future value, *compound*. To find present value, *discount*. Discounting is the opposite of compounding. *Compound* toward the future. *Discount* to the present.

Exhibit 6–6   The Relationship between Present Value and Future Value, 10 Percent, Five Periods

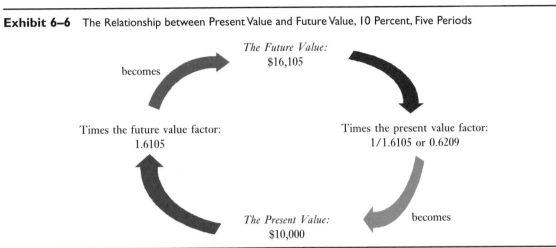

Using Tables to Compute Present Value

Just as Table B–1 contains a list of pre-calculated future value factors (FVF) based on the formula $(1 + i)^n$, Table B–3 contains a list of present value factors (PVF) based on the formula $1/(1 + i)^n$. (Tables B–2 and B–4 will be discussed shortly.) Finding a present value factor in Table B–3 is analogous to finding a future value factor in Table B–1. The process to locate the present value factor for five years at 10 percent interest is illustrated in Exhibit 6–7.

This present value factor can be used in the formula $PV = FV \times PVF_{i,n}$ to derive the present value of $16,105 at 10 percent interest for five years.

$$PV = FV \times PVF_{10,5}$$

$$PV = \$16,105 \times 0.6209$$

$$PV = \$10,000$$

This is the same result derived by using the formula. Table B–3 can also be used to find the PVF for a wide range of numbers up to 50 percent interest and 50 years.

Exhibit 6–7   Example of How to Find the Present Value Factor at 10 Percent Interest for Five Years Using Table B–3

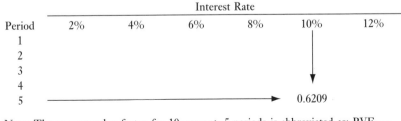

Note: The present value factor for 10 percent, 5 periods is abbreviated as: $PVF_{10,5}$

Exhibit 6–8   Using *Excel* to Calculate the Present Value for a Single Payment

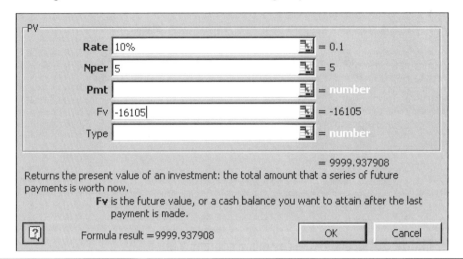

Using a Spreadsheet to Calculate Present Value

As with future value, most spreadsheets have basic financial functions that can calculate present value. For example, to calculate the present value of $16,105 at 10 percent interest for five years in *Excel* 7.0a, simply call up the present value function by clicking on "Insert," then "Function," then "Financial." On the right-hand side of the screen, double-click on "PV". Enter the rate, 10%, the number of periods, 5, and the future value as a negative number, −16,105. The present value, 9999.937908 ($10,000), is automatically calculated at the bottom (see Exhibit 6–8).

◄ANNUITIES►

The earlier discussion of present and future value shows how a *single* amount invested today grows over time, and how a *single* amount to be received in the future is discounted to today's dollars. But sometimes, instead of a single amount, there is a *series* of payments. This section deals with a particular kind of series of payments called an annuity. An **annuity** is a series of equal payments made or received at equally spaced (regular) time intervals.

The Future Value of an Ordinary Annuity

This section shows how to determine what an annuity to be received or invested will be worth at some future date. Suppose a donor were going to give $10,000 per year at the end of each year for the next three years. What would it be worth at the end of three years if it earned 10 percent interest each period? Based upon the

Annuity: A series of equal payments made or received at regular time intervals.

Future Value of an Annuity: What an equal series of payments will be worth at some future date using compound interest. See also Future Value Factor of an Annuity and Present Value of an Annuity.

information previously discussed, at the end of three years there would be $33,100, computed as shown in Exhibit 6–9.

Using Tables to Calculate the Future Value of an Ordinary Annuity

Rather than making three separate calculations (one for each year, as shown), a shortcut is to add the future value factors, which total 3.3100 (1.2100 + 1.1000 + 1.000), then multiply the sum by $10,000. In this case, 3.3100 × $10,000 = $33,100, the same value as seen in Exhibit 6–9. Rather than adding the factors for each of the three years, an alternative approach is to use a **future value factor of an annuity (FVFA)** table, such as Table B–2. Such tables contain the same figures as achieved by adding together the separate future value factors for each year. For example, in Table B–2, the future value factor of an annuity at 10 percent interest for three years, $\text{FVFA}_{10,3}$, is 3.3100. This is the same number derived by adding the future value factors for each of the three years in Exhibit 6–9. Thus, whenever a series of equal payments is to be made or received at the end of each period, the future value of an annuity table can be used rather than computing the future value of each year's cash flow and adding the results.

Using a Spreadsheet to Calculate the Future Value of an Ordinary Annuity

Most spreadsheets can easily calculate the future value of an ordinary annuity. For example, in *Excel* 7.0a, to calculate the future value of a series of $10,000 payments to be received at the end of each of three years, assuming a 10 percent interest rate, click on "Insert," then "Function," then "Financial." On the right-hand side of the screen, double-click on "FV." Enter the rate, 10%, the number of periods, 3, and the annu-

Future Value Factor of an Annuity (FVFA): A factor that when multiplied by a stream of equal payments equals the future value of that stream. See also Present Value Factor of an Annuity.

Ordinary Annuity: A series of equal annuity payments made or received at the end of each period.

$$\text{FV} = \text{Annuity} \times \text{FVFA10,3}$$

$$\text{FV} = \$10,000 \times 3.3100$$

$$\text{FV} = \$33,100$$

Incidentally, a series of payments made or received at the end of each period is called an ordinary annuity, while a series of payments made or received at the beginning of each period is called an annuity due (discussed shortly).

Key Point Whenever a series of payments is to be invested or received at the end of the year, an ordinary annuity table can be used to determine future value, rather than computing the future value of each year's cash flow.

Exhibit 6–9 Calculating the Future Value of $10,000 to Be Received at the End of Each of the Next Three Years, Assuming 10 Percent Interest

Year [Given]	A Amount to Be Received at the End of the Year [Given]	B Future Value Formula [Given]	C Future Value Factor [Table B–1]	D Future Value at End of Year 3 [A × C]
1	$10,000	$(1 + i)^2$	1.2100	$12,100
2	$10,000	$(1 + i)^1$	1.1000	$11,000
3	$10,000	$(1 + i)^0$	1.0000	$10,000
Total			3.3100	$33,100

ity or "pmt" input value as a negative number, −10,000. The future value is automatically calculated and appears at the bottom (see Exhibit 6–10).

The Future Value of an Annuity Due

Annuity Due: A series of equal annuity payments made or received at the beginning of each period.

The future value of an annuity table, such as Table B–2, is developed for ordinary annuities: cash flows which occur at the end of each period. Sometimes, however, a series of cash flows occurs at the beginning of each period, instead of at the end. Such an annuity is called an **annuity due**. The future value factor for an annuity due is equal to the factor from the future value of an ordinary annuity table for n + 1 years, less 1.

Suppose a lessee has agreed to pay an organization $10,000 today and at the beginning of each of the next four years, for a total of five $10,000 payments over five years. The organization thinks it can invest this money at 10 percent. To determine the future value of the investment after five years, the organization: 1) takes the future value factor for an ordinary annuity in Table B–2 at 10 percent interest for 5 + 1 = 6 years (7.7156); 2) subtracts 1 from this future value factor (7.7156 - 1 = 6.7156); and 3) multiplies this value by $10,000.

$$\text{FV annuity due} = (\text{FVFA}_{i,\,n+1} - 1) \times \text{Annuity}$$

$$\text{FV annuity due} = (\text{FVFA}_{10,\,5+1} - 1) \times \$10,000$$

$$\text{FV annuity due} = (7.7156 - 1) \times \$10,000$$

$$\text{FV annuity due} = 6.7156 \times \$10,000$$

$$\text{FV annuity due} = \$67,156$$

Exhibit 6–10 Using *Excel* to Calculate the Future Value for an Ordinary Annuity Payment

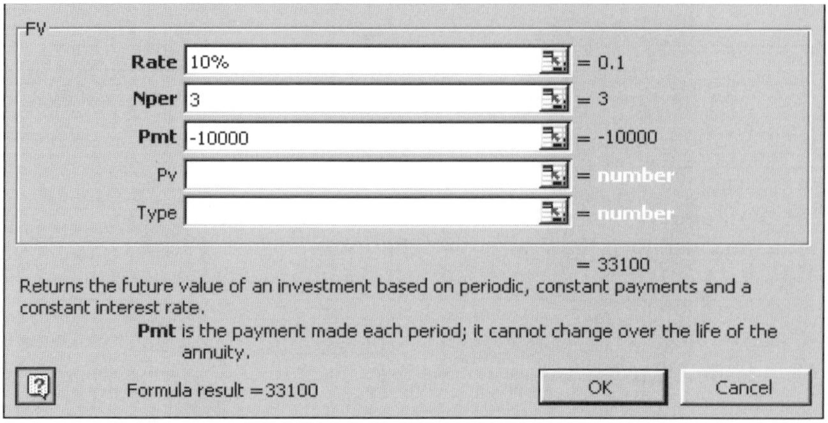

This procedure can also be performed on a spreadsheet using the future value function. In *Excel*, the function to find an ordinary annuity is used, but a "1" is entered in the space for "type" to indicate that this is an annuity due (see Exhibit 6–10).

The Present Value of an Ordinary Annuity

As with future value, it is possible to calculate the present value of an annuity, whether an ordinary annuity or an annuity due. Suppose a donor wants to give $10,000 per year at the end of each of the next three years. What is it worth today if the donations can earn 10 percent interest each period? One way to approach this problem is to calculate the present value of each year's cash flows and then add them, which equals $24,869 (see Exhibit 6–11).

Present Value of an Annuity: What a series of equal payments in the future is worth today taking into account the time value of money.

Using Tables to Calculate the Present Value of an Ordinary Annuity

The same result can be derived by first adding the three present value factors (0.9091 + 0.8264 + 0.7513 = 2.4869), and then multiplying the result times $10,000 (2.4869 × $10,000 = $24,869), as shown in Exhibit 6–11. A shortcut is to use a present value of an annuity table, such as Table B–4. Such tables contain the same numbers as would be derived by adding the separate present value factors for each year (differences due to rounding). For example, in Table B–4, the present value of an annuity factor for 10 percent interest for three years, $PVFA_{10,3}$, is 2.4869.

Key Point | Whenever a series of payments is to be received at the end of the year, an ordinary annuity table can be used to determine its present value rather than computing the present value of each year's cash flow. Each factor in the present value of an annuity table is the sum of each of the present value factors for each year of the annuity. *Present value annuity tables are set up as ordinary annuities.*

Exhibit 6–11 Calculating the Present Value of $10,000 to Be Received at the End of Each of the Next Three Years, Assuming 10 Percent Interest

Year [Given]	A Amount to Be Received at the End of the Year [Given]	B Present Value Formula [Given]	C Present Value Factor [Table B–3]	D Present Value at End of Year 3 [A × C]
1	$10,000	$1 / (1 + i)^1$	0.9091	$9,091
2	$10,000	$1 / (1 + i)^2$	0.8264	$8,264
3	$10,000	$1 / (1 + i)^3$	0.7513	$7,513
Total			2.4869	$24,869

$$PV = \text{Annuity} \times \text{PVFA}_{10,3}$$

$$PV = \$10,000 \times 2.4869$$

$$PV = \$24,869$$

Using a Spreadsheet to Calculate the Present Value of an Ordinary Annuity

Most spreadsheets easily calculate the present value of an ordinary annuity (in *Excel*, the function is called "PV"). Exhibit 6–12 shows the result of entering the numbers in the appropriate category to calculate the present value of a $10,000 annuity to be received at the end of each of the next three years, assuming 10 percent interest.

The Present Value of an Annuity Due

Table B–4, which shows the present value factors for an ordinary annuity, can be used to calculate the present value factor for an annuity due. This is done by finding the present value factor for n − 1 years, and then adding 1 to this factor.

Suppose a lessee has agreed to pay an organization $10,000 today and at the beginning of each of the next four years, for a total of five $10,000 payments over five years. To find the present value of this series of payments, assuming an interest rate of 10 percent, the organization: 1) determines the present value factor for an ordinary annuity from Table B–4 at 10 percent interest and 5 − 1 = 4 years (3.1699); 2) adds 1 to this factor to get the factor for an annuity due (3.1699 + 1 = 4.1699); and 3) multiplies this new factor by $10,000.

$$PV \text{ annuity due} = (\text{PVFA}_{i,\,n-1} + 1) \times \text{Annuity}$$

$$PV \text{ annuity due} = (\text{PVFA}_{10,\,5-1} + 1) \times \$10,000$$

Exhibit 6–12   Using *Excel* to Calculate the Present Value for an Ordinary Annuity Payment

PV

Rate	10%	= 0.1
Nper	3	= 3
Pmt	-10000	= -10000
Fv		= number
Type		= number

= 24868.51991

Returns the present value of an investment: the total amount that a series of future payments is worth now.

     Type is a logical value: payment at the beginning of the period = 1; payment at the end of the period = 0 or omitted.

Formula result =24868.51991   [OK]   [Cancel]

PV annuity due = $(3.1699 + 1) \times \$10,000$

PV annuity due = $4.1699 \times \$10,000$

PV annuity due = $\$41,699$

This procedure can also be performed on a spreadsheet using the present value function. In *Excel*, the function to find an ordinary annuity is used, but a "1" is entered in the space for "type" to indicate that this is an annuity due (see Exhibit 6–12).

◀SPECIAL SITUATIONS TO CALCULATE FUTURE OR PRESENT VALUE AND OTHER *EXCEL* FUNCTIONS▶

1. What if the interest rate is not expressed as an annual rate?

In the examples presented thus far, the interest rate has been expressed as an annual interest rate, and periods have been expressed in years. However, periods can also refer to other periods of time, such as months or days. If periods of time other than a year are being used, then the interest rate must be expressed for an equivalent period of time. For example, 12 percent annually is 1 percent a month.

Suppose an investment of $10,000 is invested at an interest rate of 12 percent and compounded semi-annually for ten years. Since interest rates are always annual unless stated otherwise, the formula must be adjusted to account for periods other than annual. The future value formula to compound at intervals more frequent than annual is:

$$FV = PV \times (1 + i/m)^{n \times m}$$

where i = annual interest rate, m = number of times during a year that compounding occurs (e.g. m = 4 for quarterly, m = 12 for monthly), and n = number of years.

Using the figures in the example:

$$FV = PV \times (1 + i/m)^{n \times m}$$

$$FV = \$10,000 \times (1 + 0.12/2)^{10 \times 2}$$

$$FV = \$10,000 \times (1 + 0.06)^{20}$$

$$FV = \$10,000 \times 3.2071$$

$$FV = \$32,071$$

Note that the final value, $32,071, is *higher* than it would have been had the same amount been invested and compounded annually rather than semi-annually. For example, had it been compounded annually using the standard formula $FV = PV \times FVF_{12,10}$, the future value factor would have been 3.1058, yielding a future value of $31,058 ($10,000 × 3.1058). This discrepancy is not a mistake (see Exhibit 6–13). It happens because compounding in the first instance is occurring twice during a year rather than once per year, so interest is growing upon interest more frequently. With quarterly compounding over the same 10-year time period (i.e. 3 percent per quarter for 40 quarters), the answer would be still higher, and with monthly compounding (i.e. 1 percent per month for 120 months), still higher yet. While the equation to calculate future value with continuous compounding is beyond the scope of this text, the key point is that the more frequent the compounding for any given interest level and time period, the higher the future value.

 Key Point The more frequent the compounding for any given interest level and time period, the higher the future value.

2. How to compute periodic loan payments using *Excel*

Excel can also calculate periodic loan payments with the PMT (payment) function. This function can only be used for loans which involve equal periodic payments over the length of the loan. Exhibit 6–14 provides an example of how to compute annual loan payments for a 10-year, $1,000,000 loan, which has an interest rate of 10 percent. Note that the present value, $1,000,000, is entered as a negative number to make the final result positive. This final result, $162,745, is interpreted to mean that by paying this annual amount under these conditions, the loan will be completely paid off at the end. This type of analysis is also called a **loan amortization**, which will be discussed in more detail in Chapter 8.

3. How to calculate the compounded growth rate

When examining data, researchers often like to present the compounded growth rate for numerical data, such as revenues, expenses, and earnings. Suppose Memorial Hospital would like to determine the compounded growth rate for patient revenues between 20X0 and 20X7, shown in Exhibit 6–15.

Exhibit 6–13   Effect of Compounding Using Various Compounding Periods

Givens:	
Initial Amount	$10,000
Annualized Interest Rate	12%
Time Horizon (Years)	10

Compounding Period	**Future Value**
Annual	$31,058
Semi-annual	$32,071
Quarterly	$32,620
Monthly	$33,004
Daily	$33,195
Continuously	$33,201

Exhibit 6–14   Using the *Excel* Payment Function to Compute Loan Payments

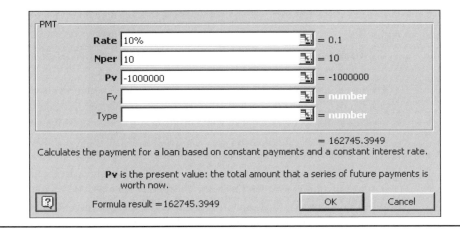

Exhibit 6–15   Patient Revenues for Memorial Hospital

Year	Patient Revenues
20X0	$2,123,000
20X1	$2,245,000
20X2	$2,555,000
20X3	$2,700,000
20X4	$2,889,000
20X5	$3,145,000
20X6	$3,496,000
20X7	$3,650,000

Solving this problem requires finding the compound growth rate (which is similar to compound interest) that causes 20X0 revenues to have a future value equal to 20X7 revenues (seven time periods into the future). To do this analysis:

Step 1: Solve for FVF in the equation, $FV = PV \times FVF_{i,n}$, where: $FV =$ 20X7 amount ($3,650,000); $PV =$ 20X0 amount ($2,123,000).

$$FV = PV \times FVF_{i,n}$$

$$\$3,650,000 = \$2,123,000 \times FVF_{i,7}$$

$$\$3,650,000 / \$2,123,000 = FVF_{i,7}$$

$$1.7192 = FVF_{i,7}$$

Step 2: Using Table B–1, Memorial then compares the calculated FVF, 1.7192, against all FVF factors in the row for seven time periods to find the factor closest to 1.7192. The appropriate interest rate is the rate given at the top of that column. In this case, 1.7138 is the closest number to 1.7192. Therefore the appropriate interest rate is approximately 8 percent, which also represents the average *compound* growth rate per year in sales from 20X0 to 20X7; however, year-to-year changes may be more or less than 8 percent.

4. How to calculate the present value of perpetual annuities

Perpetuity: An annuity for an infinite period of time. Also called a perpetual annuity.

All the annuities in the earlier sections of this chapter were calculated using a finite number of time periods, such as 10 years. In some instances, however, an organization needs to make an investment to generate an annuity (cash flow) for an infinite period of time. Such an annuity is called a **perpetual annuity**, or a **perpetuity**. For example, a donor may bequeath a large sum of money to a hospital under the condition that it generates a specified income every year for Alzheimer's research. Because there is no stipulation as to when this research funding should cease by allowing the funds to become depleted, the hospital would treat the donation as a perpetuity.

The concept of perpetuities and the calculations involved are actually quite simple. If $1,000,000 were reinvested each year forever at an annual 10 percent interest rate, $100,000 in interest income could be extracted every year ($1,000,000 × 10%) without ever depleting the principal. Every year after withdrawal of the interest income, the investment would still be worth $1,000,000 in real terms. Looked at another way, how much principal would need to be invested at 10 percent to earn $100,000 per year forever? The answer is obviously $1,000,000. This leads to the formula for a perpetuity:

$$\text{Amount of Perpetuity} = \text{Initial Investment} \times \text{Interest Rate}$$

Thus, using this formula, in order to generate a $100,000 perpetuity at a 10 percent interest rate, $100,000/0.10, or $1,000,000, would be needed.

Suppose that in her will, a wealthy donor leaves a $2,500,000 donation upon her death to her alma mater's university hospital. The funds are to be used solely to buy gifts for pediatric cancer patients and to subsidize hotel costs for visiting parents. The donor's only son died at age eight from leukemia, and she wished to give other children hope and happiness. She stipulates in her will that no less than $150,000 in gift monies be available every year from the donation. It is at the hospital's discretion to decide how to invest the money prudently. What rate of return must the investment generate after the donor's death in order to ensure that her wishes be granted?

The formula for a perpetuity can be rearranged to solve for rate of return, given the other two factors:

$$\text{Interest rate} = \text{Amount of Perpetuity}/\text{Initial Investment}$$

$$\text{Interest rate} = \$150,000/\$2,500,000$$

$$\text{Interest rate} = 0.06 = 6\%$$

Therefore, as long as the hospital can invest the $2,500,000 at a minimum 6 percent rate of return, the donor's wishes will be granted indefinitely.

5. How to solve for the interest rate of a loan with fixed loan payments

Assuming equal loan payments over the life of the loan, it is also possible to solve for the interest rate. If the present value of the loan, the annuity payments over time, and the length of the loan are given, the unknown interest rate of the loan, i, can be determined.

For example, suppose Mt Moriah Hospital needs to borrow $10,000 for a new computer system. The annual loan payments are $3,019 per year at the end of each year for the next four years. What is the interest rate of this loan? Using the present value formula for an ordinary annuity, solve for the interest rate, i:[1]

$$PV = Annuity \times PVFA_{i,4}$$

$$\$10,000 = \$3,019 \times PVFA_{i,4}$$

$$\$10,000/\$3,019 = PVFA_{i,4}$$

$$3.3124 = PVFA_{i,4}$$

$$3.3124 = PVFA_{8,4}$$

$$i = 8\%$$

Key Point

In the *Excel* "Rate" function, the PMT box or loan payment box must be a negative value.

This could also be done in a spreadsheet, such as by using the "Rate" function in *Excel*, as shown in Exhibit 6–16. This is a four-year, $10,000 loan with equal annual payments of $3,019. This "Rate" function can only be used for loan payments that are equal over the life of the loan. The loan payment value must be a negative value (cash outflow); otherwise, the rate function will give an incorrect value if both PMT and PV values are positive.

◀SUMMARY▶

Future value is used to determine the value of dollar payments in the future, whereas present value indicates the current value of future dollars. Either simple interest, where interest is only calculated on the principal, or compound interest, where the

Future Value Table: Table of factors which shows the future value of a single investment at a given interest rate.

---

[1] From Table B–4, the PVFA equal or closest to 3.3124 is found in the row for 4 time periods. At this PVFA, the interest rate of this column heading is 8%.

Exhibit 6–16   Using the *Excel* Rate Function to Compute a Loan Rate

---

Future Value of an Annuity Table: Table of factors which shows the future value of equal flows at the end of each period, given a particular interest rate.

Present Value Table: Table of factors which shows what a single amount to be received in the future is worth today at a given interest rate.

Present Value of an Annuity Table: Table of factors which shows the value today of equal flows at the end of each future period, given a particular interest rate.

---

interest is calculated on the principal *and* the interest, can be used to determine the future value of money. The compound interest method produces a larger sum of money in the future and is the standard method used.

The future value factor (FVF), or $(1 + i)^n$, where i is the interest rate and n is the number of periods of the investment, is part of the formula to determine how much an investment will be worth in the future. This entire formula to find future value is: **Future Value = Present Value × Future Value Factor**, abbreviated as **FV = PV × FVF$_{i,n}$** or **FV = PV$(1 + i)^n$**. The opposite formula calculates the present value: **Present Value = Future Value × Present Value Factor**, abbreviated as **PV = FV × PVF$_{i,n}$** or **PV = FV$/(1 + i)^n$**. Similar formulas are used to calculate the present value or future value of an annuity; all that changes is the factor. All these factors can be found in pre-calculated tables, which are known as future value tables and present value tables.

If a series of payments is to be paid or received at the end of each period, it is called an *ordinary annuity*. If the series of payments is to be paid or received at the beginning of each period, it is called an *annuity due*. The steps used to calculate each of these two types of annuities are somewhat different. An understanding of present and future values and annuities can be used to answer a number of key questions, such as, "How much will an investment today be worth in the future?" or "What is the rate of return for a loan?" Special situations and applications are described in the Appendices, and all calculations can be made either through the use of the accompanying tables, or with the aid of a spreadsheet.

◀KEY TERMS▶

ANNUITY	FUTURE VALUE OF AN ANNUITY	PRESENT VALUE FACTOR OF AN
ANNUITY DUE	FUTURE VALUE OF AN ANNUITY	ANNUITY
COMPOUND INTEREST METHOD	TABLE	PRESENT VALUE OF AN ANNUITY
COMPOUNDING	FUTURE VALUE TABLE	PRESENT VALUE OF AN ANNUITY
DISCOUNTING	OPPORTUNITY COST	TABLE
FUTURE VALUE	ORDINARY ANNUITY	PRESENT VALUE TABLE
FUTURE VALUE FACTOR	PERPETUITY	SIMPLE INTEREST METHOD
FUTURE VALUE FACTOR OF AN	PRESENT VALUE	TIME VALUE OF MONEY
ANNUITY	PRESENT VALUE FACTOR	

◀KEY EQUATIONS▶

Future Value Equation: $FV = PV \times (1 + i)^n$

Future Value Formula: $FV = PV \times FVF_{i,n}$

Future Value Formula, Annuity Due: $FV = \text{Annuity} \times (FVFA_{i,n+1} - 1)$

Future Value Formula, Ordinary Annuity: $FV = \text{Annuity} \times FVFA_{i,n}$

Future Value Formula, Period < 1 Year: $FV = PV \times (1 + i/m)^{n \times m}$

Perpetuity Formula: Amount of Perpetuity = Initial Investment × Interest Rate

Present Value Equation: $PV = FV \times 1/(1 + i)^n$

Present Value Formula: $PV = FV \times PVF_{i,n}$

Present Value Formula, Annuity Due: $PV = \text{Annuity} \times (PVFA_{i,n-1} + 1)$

Present Value Formula, Ordinary Annuity: $PV = \text{Annuity} \times PVFAi,n$

◀QUESTIONS AND PROBLEMS▶

1. **Definitions.** Define the following terms:
   a. Annuity.
   b. Annuity Due.
   c. Compound Interest Method.
   d. Compounding.
   e. Discounting.
   f. Future Value.

    g. Future Value Factor.

    h. Future Value Factor of an Annuity.

    i. Future Value of an Annuity.

    j. Future Value of an Annuity Table.

    k. Future Value Table.

    l. Opportunity Cost.

    m. Ordinary Annuity.

    n. Perpetuity.

    o. Present Value.

    p. Present Value Factor.

    q. Present Value Factor of an Annuity.

    r. Present Value of an Annuity.

    s. Present Value of an Annuity Table.

    t. Present Value Table.

    u. Simple Interest Method.

    v. Time Value of Money.

2. **Simple and Compound Interest.** What is the difference between simple interest and compound interest?

3. **Defining Future Value Equation Terms.** Write out the future value of an amount equation, and define each of the terms in it.

4. **Defining the exponent.** Does the n in the formula $(1 + i)^n$ always mean compounding on an annual basis?

5. **Multiple compounding periods in a year.** How should the future value equation be modified if compounding occurs more frequently than annually?

6. **Multiple compounding periods in a year (continued).** What is the future value of $10,000 with an interest rate of 16 percent and one annual period of compounding? With an annual interest rate of 16 percent and two semiannual periods of compounding? With an annual interest rate of 16 percent and four quarterly periods of compounding?

7. **Multiple compounding periods in a year (continued).** Based on the answer to Question 6, explain why the investment increases in value when the number of compounding periods increases.

8. **Present and Future Value Factors.** What is the relationship between the present value factor and the future value factor?

9. **Present Value Factor and Discount Rate.** What happens to the present value factor as the discount rate or interest rate increases for a given time period? If the discount rate or interest rate decreases?

10. **Relationship between Ordinary Annuity and Annuity Due.** Compare the results of the present value of a $6,000 ordinary annuity at 10 percent interest for 10 years with the present value of a $6,000 annuity due at 10 percent interest for 11 years. Explain the difference.

11. **Perpetuities.** How many years in a typical perpetuity?

12. **Factors.** What is the relationship between the future value factor for five years at 5 percent and the present value factor for five years at 5 percent.

13. **Future Value of an Annuity Table.** In the future value annuity table at any interest rate for one year, why is the future value interest factor of this annuity equal to 1.00?

14. **Present Value of an Amount and Present Value of an Annuity.** What is the relationship between the present value of a single dollar payment formula and the present value of an ordinary annuity formula for the same number of years and the same discount rate? Assume a discount rate of 10 percent and an *n* value of five periods. Explain with an example.

15. If a nurse deposits $1,000 today in a bank account and the interest is compounded annually at 12 percent, what will be the value of this investment:
    a. five years from now?
    b. ten years from now?
    c. fifteen years from now?
    d. twenty years from now?

16. If a nurse deposits $10,000 today in a bank account and the interest is compounded annually at 12 percent, what will be the value of this investment:
    a. three years from now?
    b. six years from now?
    c. nine years from now?
    d. twelve years from now?

17. If a business manager deposits $200 in a savings account at the end of each year for twenty years, what will be the value of her investment:
    a. at a compounded rate of 10 percent?
    b. at a compounded rate of 20 percent?
    What would the outcome be in both cases if the deposits were made at the beginning of each year?

18. If a business manager deposits $2,000 in a savings account at the end of each year for twenty years, what will be the value of her investment:
    a. at a compounded rate of 15 percent?
    b. at a compounded rate of 25 percent?
    What would the outcome be in both cases if the deposits were made at the beginning of each year?

19. The CFO of a home health agency needs to determine the present value of a $5,000 investment received at the end of year 10. What is the present value if the discount rate is:
    a. 5 percent?
    b. 10 percent?
    c. 15 percent?
    d. 20 percent?

20. The CFO of a home health agency needs to determine the present value of a $50,000 investment received at the end of year 15. What is the present value if the discount rate is:
    a. 4 percent?

    b. 8 percent?

    c. 12 percent?

    d. 16 percent?

21. If a hospital were to receive $4,000 in payments per year at the end of each year for the next 12 years from an uninsured patient who underwent an expensive operation, what would be the current value of these collection payments:

    a. at a 4 percent rate of return?

    b. at a 14 percent rate of return?

    If the funds were received at the beginning of the year, what would be the current value of these collection payments for each of the two rates of return?

22. If a hospital were to receive $14,000 in payments per year at the end of each year for the next 6 years from an uninsured patient who underwent an expensive operation, what would be the current value of these collection payments:

    a. at a 4 percent rate of return?

    b. at a 14 percent rate of return?

    If the funds were received at the beginning of the year, what would be the current value of these collection payments for each of the two rates of return?

23. After completing her residency, an obstetrician plans to invest $10,000 per year at the end of each year in a low-risk retirement account. She expects to earn five percent for 35 years. What will her retirement account be worth at the end of these 35 years?

24. After completing her residency, an oncologist plans to invest $15,000 per year at the end of each year in a high-risk retirement account. She expects to earn ten percent for 35 years. What will her retirement account be worth at the end of these 35 years?

25. Lincoln Memorial Hospital has just been informed that a private donor is willing to contribute $1,000 per year at the beginning of each year for 15 years. What is the current dollar value of this contribution if the discount rate is 8 percent?

26. Boulder City Hospital has just been informed that a private donor is willing to contribute $20,000 per year at the beginning of each year for 15 years. What is the current dollar value of this contribution if the discount rate is 16 percent?

27. If a community clinic invested $4,000 in excess cash today, what would be the value of its investment at the end of three years:

    a. at a 16 percent rate compounded semiannually?

    b. at a 16 percent rate compounded quarterly?

28. If a community hospital invested $8,000 in excess cash today, what would be the value of its investment at the end of three years:

    a. at a 32 percent rate compounded semiannually?

    b. at a 32 percent rate compounded quarterly?

29. Love Canal General Hospital wants to purchase a new blood analyzing device today. Its local bank is willing to lend it the money to buy the analyzer at a 2 percent monthly rate. The loan payments will start at the end of the month and will be $1,700 per month for the next 18 months. What is the purchase price of the device?

30. General Hospital wants to purchase a new MRI today. Its local bank is willing to lend it the money to buy the MRI at a 3 percent monthly rate. The loan payments will start at the end of the month and will be $5,000 per month for the next 30 months. What is the purchase price of the MRI?

31. Midstate Medical Center is starting an endowment fund to pay for the expenses of a medical research program. The expenses are $2,000,000 per year and the program is expected to last for ten years. Assuming payments are made at the end of each year and the interest rate is 9 percent per year, what should be the initial size of the endowment?

32. Seaside Medical Center is starting an endowment fund to pay for the expenses of a community outreach pediatric program. The expenses are $500,000 per year and the program is expected to last for five years. Assuming payments are made at the end of each year and the interest rate is 7 percent per year, what should be the size of the initial endowment?

33. In 2000, Lilliputian County Hospital's total patient revenues were $20 million. In 2008, patient revenues are expected to be $40 million. What is the compound growth rate in patient revenues over this time period?

34. In 2001, Wythe County Hospital's total patient revenues were $5 million. In 2010, patient revenues were expected to be $27.75 million. What was the compound growth rate in patient revenues over this time period?

35. Shawnee Valley Family Practice Center plans to invest $30,000 in a money market account at the beginning of each year for the next five years. The investment pays 12 percent annual interest. How much would this investment be worth after five years of investing?

36. Starting today, and every six months thereafter for the next ten years, St Luke's Hospital plans to invest $50,000 at 10 percent annual interest in an account. How much would this investment be worth after ten years of investing?

37. Dr Thomas plans to retire today and would like an income of $200,000 per year for the next 15 years with the income payments starting one year from today. He will be able to earn interest of 9 percent per year compounded annually from his investment account. What must he deposit today in his investment account to achieve this income of $200,000 per year?

38. Today, Williamson Hospital lends its Home Health Care Center $938,510. The center expects to repay them in quarterly installments for three years of $100,000 with the first payment starting one quarter from now. What annual interest rate is the hospital charging for this loan?

39. Goldfarb Cancer Research Institute just received a $1.2 million gift to cover the salary for a permanent scientific research position to study Hodgkin's

Disease. What would be the required rate of return on the investment if the position paid an annual salary of:

a. $60,000 per year?

b. $75,000 per year?

c. $100,000 per year?

40. Upon the untimely and tragic death of their wealthy aunt, the heirs wanted to memorialize her with a named donation to the local hospital. They offered the hospital a choice of $30,000 annual payments forever or a lump sum payment of $400,000 today.

    a. What should be the decision if the hospital thinks it could earn an average of 4 percent annually on this donation?

    b. What should be the decision if the hospital thinks it could earn an average of 8 percent annually on this donation?

    c. What should be the decision if the hospital thinks it could earn an average of 12 percent annually on this donation?

41. Stillwater Hospital is borrowing $2,000,000 for its medical office building. The annual interest rate is 6 percent. What will be the equal annual payments on the loan if the length of the loan is 4 years and payments occur at the end of each year?

42. Williamsburg Nursing Home is investing in a restricted fund for a new assisted-living home. How much do they need to invest each year in order to earn $5,000,000 after 15 years:

    a. If the expected rate of return on the investment is 10 percent, and the hospital invests at the end of each year?

    b. If the expected rate of return on the investment is 10 percent, and the hospital invests at the beginning of each year?

43. Carondelet Hospital is evaluating a lease arrangement for its ambulance fleet. The total value of the lease is $405,000. The hospital will be making equal monthly payments starting today.

    a. What is the monthly interest rate if the lease payments are $21,000 per month for 24 months?

    b. What is the monthly interest rate if the lease payments are $21,000 per month for 36 months?

    c. What is the monthly interest rate if the lease payments are $26,000 per month for 36 months?

44. A wealthy philanthropist has established the following endowment for a hospital. The details of the endowment include the following:

    a. A cash deposit of $10 million one year from now.

    b. An annual cash deposit of $3 million per year for the next 15 years. The first $3 million deposit will start today.

    c. At the end of year 15, the hospital will also receive a lump sum payment of $15 million.

    Assuming the cost of money is 5 percent, what is the value of this endowment in today's dollars?

Appendix B

Future and Present Value Tables

Appendix B presents pre-calculated tables to assist in determining future and present values, (FV) and (PV). Future value is used to determine the future value of dollar payments made earlier; present value indicates the current value of future dollars. Although the formulas to compute these values appear in Chapter 6, pre-calculated tables provide a quick and flexible reference for this information.

Appendix B presents this information in four ways. Table B–1 presents the future value of $1 (FV): what the future value of a single investment today will be worth at a future time at a given interest rate. Table B–2 reflects the future value of an annuity (FVFA): what the future value an annuity received or invested today will be worth at a future time, given the interest rate and number of periods involved. Table B–3 presents the present value of $1: how much a single, one time amount to be received in the future at a specified interest rate is worth today. Table B–4 reflects the present value of an annuity: the amount an annuity at a specified rate to be received at equal flows at the end of a specified number of periods, is worth today.

Table B–1 Future Value of $1

$$FVFi,n = PV(1 + i)^n; FV = PV(FVFi,n)$$

Period	1%	2%	3%	4%	5%	6%	7%	8%	9%	10%	11%	12%	13%	14%	15%
1	1.0100	1.0200	1.0300	1.0400	1.0500	1.0600	1.0700	1.0800	1.0900	1.1000	1.1100	1.1200	1.1300	1.1400	1.1500
2	1.0201	1.0404	1.0609	1.0816	1.1025	1.1236	1.1449	1.1664	1.1881	1.2100	1.2321	1.2544	1.2769	1.2996	1.3225
3	1.0303	1.0612	1.0927	1.1249	1.1576	1.1910	1.2250	1.2597	1.2950	1.3310	1.3676	1.4049	1.4429	1.4815	1.5209
4	1.0406	1.0824	1.1255	1.1699	1.2155	1.2625	1.3108	1.3605	1.4116	1.4641	1.5181	1.5735	1.6305	1.6890	1.7490
5	1.0510	1.1041	1.1593	1.2167	1.2763	1.3382	1.4026	1.4693	1.5386	1.6105	1.6851	1.7623	1.8424	1.9254	2.0114
6	1.0615	1.1262	1.1941	1.2653	1.3401	1.4185	1.5007	1.5869	1.6771	1.7716	1.8704	1.9738	2.0820	2.1950	2.3131
7	1.0721	1.1487	1.2299	1.3159	1.4071	1.5036	1.6058	1.7138	1.8280	1.9487	2.0762	2.2107	2.3526	2.5023	2.6600
8	1.0829	1.1717	1.2668	1.3686	1.4775	1.5938	1.7182	1.8509	1.9926	2.1436	2.3045	2.4760	2.6584	2.8526	3.0590
9	1.0937	1.1951	1.3048	1.4233	1.5513	1.6895	1.8385	1.9990	2.1719	2.3579	2.5580	2.7731	3.0040	3.2519	3.5179
10	1.1046	1.2190	1.3439	1.4802	1.6289	1.7908	1.9672	2.1589	2.3674	2.5937	2.8394	3.1058	3.3946	3.7072	4.0456
11	1.1157	1.2434	1.3842	1.5395	1.7103	1.8983	2.1049	2.3316	2.5804	2.8531	3.1518	3.4785	3.8359	4.2262	4.6524
12	1.1268	1.2682	1.4258	1.6010	1.7959	2.0122	2.2522	2.5182	2.8127	3.1384	3.4985	3.8960	4.3345	4.8179	5.3503
13	1.1381	1.2936	1.4685	1.6651	1.8856	2.1329	2.4098	2.7196	3.0658	3.4523	3.8833	4.3635	4.8980	5.4924	6.1528
14	1.1495	1.3195	1.5126	1.7317	1.9799	2.2609	2.5785	2.9372	3.3417	3.7975	4.3104	4.8871	5.5348	6.2613	7.0757
15	1.1610	1.3459	1.5580	1.8009	2.0789	2.3966	2.7590	3.1722	3.6425	4.1772	4.7846	5.4736	6.2543	7.1379	8.1371
16	1.1726	1.3728	1.6047	1.8730	2.1829	2.5404	2.9522	3.4259	3.9703	4.5950	5.3109	6.1304	7.0673	8.1372	9.3576
17	1.1843	1.4002	1.6528	1.9479	2.2920	2.6928	3.1588	3.7000	4.3276	5.0545	5.8951	6.8660	7.9861	9.2765	10.761
18	1.1961	1.4282	1.7024	2.0258	2.4066	2.8543	3.3799	3.9960	4.7171	5.5599	6.5436	7.6900	9.0243	10.575	12.375
19	1.2081	1.4568	1.7535	2.1068	2.5270	3.0256	3.6165	4.3157	5.1417	6.1159	7.2633	8.6128	10.197	12.056	14.232
20	1.2202	1.4859	1.8061	2.1911	2.6533	3.2071	3.8697	4.6610	5.6044	6.7275	8.0623	9.6463	11.523	13.743	16.367
21	1.2324	1.5157	1.8603	2.2788	2.7860	3.3996	4.1406	5.0338	6.1088	7.4002	8.9492	10.804	13.021	15.668	18.822
22	1.2447	1.5460	1.9161	2.3699	2.9253	3.6035	4.4304	5.4365	6.6586	8.1403	9.9336	12.100	14.714	17.861	21.645
23	1.2572	1.5769	1.9736	2.4647	3.0715	3.8197	4.7405	5.8715	7.2579	8.9543	11.026	13.552	16.627	20.362	24.891
24	1.2697	1.6084	2.0328	2.5633	3.2251	4.0489	5.0724	6.3412	7.9111	9.8497	12.239	15.179	18.788	23.212	28.625
25	1.2824	1.6406	2.0938	2.6658	3.3864	4.2919	5.4274	6.8485	8.6231	10.835	13.585	17.000	21.231	26.462	32.919
26	1.2953	1.6734	2.1566	2.7725	3.5557	4.5494	5.8074	7.3964	9.3992	11.918	15.080	19.040	23.991	30.167	37.857
27	1.3082	1.7069	2.2213	2.8834	3.7335	4.8223	6.2139	7.9881	10.245	13.110	16.739	21.325	27.109	34.390	43.535
28	1.3213	1.7410	2.2879	2.9987	3.9201	5.1117	6.6488	8.6271	11.167	14.421	18.580	23.884	30.633	39.204	50.066
29	1.3345	1.7758	2.3566	3.1187	4.1161	5.4184	7.1143	9.3173	12.172	15.863	20.624	26.750	34.616	44.693	57.575
30	1.3478	1.8114	2.4273	3.2434	4.3219	5.7435	7.6123	10.063	13.268	17.449	22.892	29.960	39.116	50.950	66.212
35	1.4166	1.9999	2.8139	3.9461	5.5160	7.6861	10.677	14.785	20.414	28.102	38.575	52.800	72.069	98.100	133.18
40	1.4889	2.2080	3.2620	4.8010	7.0400	10.286	14.974	21.725	31.409	45.259	65.001	93.051	132.78	188.88	267.86
45	1.5648	2.4379	3.7816	5.8412	8.9850	13.765	21.002	31.920	48.327	72.890	109.53	163.99	244.64	363.68	538.77
50	1.6446	2.6916	4.3839	7.1067	11.467	18.420	29.457	46.902	74.358	117.39	184.56	289.00	450.74	700.23	1,083.7

(Continues)

Table B-1 (*Contd*)

FVFi,n = PV(1 + i)ⁿ; FV = PV(FVFi,n)

$$FVF_{i,n} = PV(1 + i)^n; \quad FV = PV(FVF_{i,n})$$

Period	16%	17%	18%	19%	20%	21%	22%	23%	24%	25%	30%	35%	40%	45%	50%
1	1.1600	1.1700	1.1800	1.1900	1.2000	1.2100	1.2200	1.2300	1.2400	1.2500	1.3000	1.3500	1.4000	1.4500	1.5000
2	1.3456	1.3689	1.3924	1.4161	1.4400	1.4641	1.4884	1.5129	1.5376	1.5625	1.6900	1.8225	1.9600	2.1025	2.2500
3	1.5609	1.6016	1.6430	1.6852	1.7280	1.7716	1.8158	1.8609	1.9066	1.9531	2.1970	2.4604	2.7440	3.0486	3.3750
4	1.8106	1.8739	1.9388	2.0053	2.0736	2.1436	2.2153	2.2889	2.3642	2.4414	2.8561	3.3215	3.8416	4.4205	5.0625
5	2.1003	2.1924	2.2878	2.3864	2.4883	2.5937	2.7027	2.8153	2.9316	3.0518	3.7129	4.4840	5.3782	6.4097	7.5938
6	2.4364	2.5652	2.6996	2.8398	2.9860	3.1384	3.2973	3.4628	3.6352	3.8147	4.8268	6.0534	7.5295	9.2941	11.391
7	2.8262	3.0012	3.1855	3.3793	3.5832	3.7975	4.0227	4.2593	4.5077	4.7684	6.2749	8.1722	10.541	13.476	17.086
8	3.2784	3.5115	3.7589	4.0214	4.2998	4.5950	4.9077	5.2389	5.5895	5.9605	8.1573	11.032	14.758	19.541	25.629
9	3.8030	4.1084	4.4355	4.7854	5.1598	5.5599	5.9874	6.4439	6.9310	7.4506	10.604	14.894	20.661	28.334	38.443
10	4.4114	4.8068	5.2338	5.6947	6.1917	6.7275	7.3046	7.9259	8.5944	9.3132	13.786	20.107	28.925	41.085	57.665
11	5.1173	5.6240	6.1759	6.7767	7.4301	8.1403	8.9117	9.7489	10.657	11.642	17.922	27.144	40.496	59.573	86.498
12	5.9360	6.5801	7.2876	8.0642	8.9161	9.8497	10.872	11.991	13.215	14.552	23.298	36.644	56.694	86.381	129.75
13	6.8858	7.6987	8.5994	9.5964	10.699	11.918	13.264	14.749	16.386	18.190	30.288	49.470	79.371	125.25	194.62
14	7.9875	9.0075	10.147	11.420	12.839	14.421	16.182	18.141	20.319	22.737	39.374	66.784	111.12	181.62	291.93
15	9.2655	10.539	11.974	13.590	15.407	17.449	19.742	22.314	25.196	28.422	51.186	90.158	155.57	263.34	437.89
16	10.748	12.330	14.129	16.172	18.488	21.114	24.086	27.446	31.243	35.527	66.542	121.71	217.80	381.85	656.84
17	12.468	14.426	16.672	19.244	22.186	25.548	29.384	33.759	38.741	44.409	86.504	164.31	304.91	553.68	985.26
18	14.463	16.879	19.673	22.901	26.623	30.913	35.849	41.523	48.039	55.511	112.46	221.82	426.88	802.83	1,477.9
19	16.777	19.748	23.214	27.252	31.948	37.404	43.736	51.074	59.568	69.389	146.19	299.46	597.63	1,164.1	2,216.8
20	19.461	23.106	27.393	32.429	38.338	45.259	53.358	62.821	73.864	86.736	190.05	404.27	836.68	1,688.0	3,325.3
21	22.574	27.034	32.324	38.591	46.005	54.764	65.096	77.269	91.592	108.42	247.06	545.77	1,171.4	2,447.5	4,987.9
22	26.186	31.629	38.142	45.923	55.206	66.264	79.418	95.041	113.57	135.53	321.18	736.79	1,639.9	3,548.9	7,481.8
23	30.376	37.006	45.008	54.649	66.247	80.180	96.889	116.90	140.83	169.41	417.54	994.66	2,295.9	5,145.9	11,223
24	35.236	43.297	53.109	65.032	79.497	97.017	118.21	143.79	174.63	211.76	542.80	1,342.8	3,214.2	7,461.6	16,834
25	40.874	50.658	62.669	77.388	95.396	117.39	144.21	176.86	216.54	264.70	705.64	1,812.8	4,499.9	10,819	25,251
26	47.414	59.270	73.949	92.092	114.48	142.04	175.94	217.54	268.51	330.87	917.33	2,447.2	6,299.8	15,688	37,877
27	55.000	69.345	87.260	109.59	137.37	171.87	214.64	267.57	332.95	413.59	1,192.5	3,303.8	8,819.8	22,748	56,815
28	63.800	81.134	102.97	130.41	164.84	207.97	261.86	329.11	412.86	516.99	1,550.3	4,460.1	12,348	32,984	85,223
29	74.009	94.927	121.50	155.19	197.81	251.64	319.47	404.81	511.95	646.23	2,015.4	6,021.1	17,287	47,827	127,834
30	85.850	111.06	143.37	184.68	237.38	304.48	389.76	497.91	634.82	807.79	2,620.0	8,128.5	24,201	69,349	191,751
35	180.31	243.50	328.00	440.70	590.67	789.75	1,053.4	1,401.8	1,861.1	2,465.2	9,727.9	36,449	130,161	444,509	1,456,110
40	378.72	533.87	750.38	1,051.7	1,469.8	2,048.4	2,847.0	3,946.4	5,455.9	7,523.2	36,119	163,437	700,038	2,849,181	11,057,332
45	795.44	1,170.5	1,716.7	2,509.7	3,657.3	5,313.0	7,694.7	11,110	15,995	22,959	134,107	732,858	3,764,971	18,262,495	83,966,617
50	1,670.7	2,566.2	3,927.4	5,988.9	9,100.4	13,781	20,797	31,279	46,890	70,065	497,929	3,286,158	20,248,916	117,057,734	637,621,500

Table B-2 Future Value of an Annuity (FVFA)

Future Value of an Annuity of $1: FVIFAi, $n = [(1 + i)^n - 1] / i$

Period	1%	2%	3%	4%	5%	6%	7%	8%	9%	10%	11%	12%	13%	14%	15%
1	1.0000	1.0000	1.0000	1.0000	1.0000	1.0000	1.0000	1.0000	1.0000	1.0000	1.0000	1.0000	1.0000	1.0000	1.0000
2	2.0100	2.0200	2.0300	2.0400	2.0500	2.0600	2.0700	2.0800	2.0900	2.1000	2.1100	2.1200	2.1300	2.1400	2.1500
3	3.0301	3.0604	3.0909	3.1216	3.1525	3.1836	3.2149	3.2464	3.2781	3.3100	3.3421	3.3744	3.4069	3.4396	3.4725
4	4.0604	4.1216	4.1836	4.2465	4.3101	4.3746	4.4399	4.5061	4.5731	4.6410	4.7097	4.7793	4.8498	4.9211	4.9934
5	5.1010	5.2040	5.3091	5.4163	5.5256	5.6371	5.7507	5.8666	5.9847	6.1051	6.2278	6.3528	6.4803	6.6101	6.7424
6	6.1520	6.3081	6.4684	6.6330	6.8019	6.9753	7.1533	7.3359	7.5233	7.7156	7.9129	8.1152	8.3227	8.5355	8.7537
7	7.2135	7.4343	7.6625	7.8983	8.1420	8.3938	8.6540	8.9228	9.2004	9.4872	9.7833	10.089	10.405	10.730	11.067
8	8.2857	8.5830	8.8923	9.2142	9.5491	9.8975	10.260	10.637	11.028	11.436	11.859	12.300	12.757	13.233	13.727
9	9.3685	9.7546	10.159	10.583	11.027	11.491	11.978	12.488	13.021	13.579	14.164	14.776	15.416	16.085	16.786
10	10.462	10.950	11.464	12.006	12.578	13.181	13.816	14.487	15.193	15.937	16.722	17.549	18.420	19.337	20.304
11	11.567	12.169	12.808	13.486	14.207	14.972	15.784	16.645	17.560	18.531	19.561	20.655	21.814	23.045	24.349
12	12.683	13.412	14.192	15.026	15.917	16.870	17.888	18.977	20.141	21.384	22.713	24.133	25.650	27.271	29.002
13	13.809	14.680	15.618	16.627	17.713	18.882	20.141	21.495	22.953	24.523	26.212	28.029	29.985	32.089	34.352
14	14.947	15.974	17.086	18.292	19.599	21.015	22.550	24.215	26.019	27.975	30.095	32.393	34.883	37.581	40.505
15	16.097	17.293	18.599	20.024	21.579	23.276	25.129	27.152	29.361	31.772	34.405	37.280	40.417	43.842	47.580
16	17.258	18.639	20.157	21.825	23.657	25.673	27.888	30.324	33.003	35.950	39.190	42.753	46.672	50.980	55.717
17	18.430	20.012	21.762	23.698	25.840	28.213	30.840	33.750	36.974	40.545	44.501	48.884	53.739	59.118	65.075
18	19.615	21.412	23.414	25.645	28.132	30.906	33.999	37.450	41.301	45.599	50.396	55.750	61.725	68.394	75.836
19	20.811	22.841	25.117	27.671	30.539	33.760	37.379	41.446	46.018	51.159	56.939	63.440	70.749	78.969	88.212
20	22.019	24.297	26.870	29.778	33.066	36.786	40.995	45.762	51.160	57.275	64.203	72.052	80.947	91.025	102.44
21	23.239	25.783	28.676	31.969	35.719	39.993	44.865	50.423	56.765	64.002	72.265	81.699	92.470	104.77	118.81
22	24.472	27.299	30.537	34.248	38.505	43.392	49.006	55.457	62.873	71.403	81.214	92.503	105.49	120.44	137.63
23	25.716	28.845	32.453	36.618	41.430	46.996	53.436	60.893	69.532	79.543	91.148	104.60	120.20	138.30	159.28
24	26.973	30.422	34.426	39.083	44.502	50.816	58.177	66.765	76.790	88.497	102.17	118.16	136.83	158.66	184.17
25	28.243	32.030	36.459	41.646	47.727	54.865	63.249	73.106	84.701	98.347	114.41	133.33	155.62	181.87	212.79
26	29.526	33.671	38.553	44.312	51.113	59.156	68.676	79.954	93.324	109.18	128.00	150.33	176.85	208.33	245.71
27	30.821	35.344	40.710	47.084	54.669	63.706	74.484	87.351	102.72	121.10	143.08	169.37	200.84	238.50	283.57
28	32.129	37.051	42.931	49.968	58.403	68.528	80.698	95.339	112.97	134.21	159.82	190.70	227.95	272.89	327.10
29	33.450	38.792	45.219	52.966	62.323	73.640	87.347	103.97	124.14	148.63	178.40	214.58	258.58	312.09	377.17
30	34.785	40.568	47.575	56.085	66.439	79.058	94.461	113.28	136.31	164.49	199.02	241.33	293.20	356.79	434.75
35	41.660	49.994	60.462	73.652	90.320	111.43	138.24	172.32	215.71	271.02	341.59	431.66	546.68	693.57	881.17
40	48.886	60.402	75.401	95.026	120.80	154.76	199.64	259.06	337.88	442.59	581.83	767.09	1,013.7	1,342.0	1,779.1
45	56.481	71.893	92.720	121.03	159.70	212.74	285.75	386.51	525.86	718.90	986.64	1,358.2	1,874.2	2,590.6	3,585.1
50	64.463	84.579	112.80	152.67	209.35	290.34	406.53	573.77	815.08	1,163.9	1,668.8	2,400.0	3,459.5	4,994.5	7,217.7

(Continues)

Table B–2 (Contd)

Future Value of an Annuity of $1: $\text{FVIFA}_{i,n} = [(1 + i)^n - 1]/i$

Period	16%	17%	18%	19%	20%	21%	22%	23%	24%	25%	30%	35%	40%	45%	50%
1	1.0000	1.0000	1.0000	1.0000	1.0000	1.0000	1.0000	1.0000	1.0000	1.0000	1.0000	1.0000	1.0000	1.0000	1.0000
2	2.1600	2.1700	2.1800	2.1900	2.2000	2.2100	2.2200	2.2300	2.2400	2.2500	2.3000	2.3500	2.4000	2.4500	2.5000
3	3.5056	3.5389	3.5724	3.6061	3.6400	3.6741	3.7084	3.7429	3.7776	3.8125	3.9900	4.1725	4.3600	4.5525	4.7500
4	5.0665	5.1405	5.2154	5.2913	5.3680	5.4457	5.5242	5.6038	5.6842	5.7656	6.1870	6.6329	7.1040	7.6011	8.1250
5	6.8771	7.0144	7.1542	7.2966	7.4416	7.5892	7.7396	7.8926	8.0484	8.2070	9.0431	9.9544	10.946	12.022	13.188
6	8.9775	9.2068	9.4420	9.6830	9.9299	10.183	10.442	10.708	10.980	11.259	12.756	14.438	16.324	18.431	20.781
7	11.414	11.772	12.142	12.523	12.916	13.321	13.740	14.171	14.615	15.073	17.583	20.492	23.853	27.725	32.172
8	14.240	14.773	15.327	15.902	16.499	17.119	17.762	18.430	19.123	19.842	23.858	28.664	34.395	41.202	49.258
9	17.519	18.285	19.086	19.923	20.799	21.714	22.670	23.669	24.712	25.802	32.015	39.696	49.153	60.743	74.887
10	21.321	22.393	23.521	24.709	25.959	27.274	28.657	30.113	31.643	33.253	42.619	54.590	69.814	89.077	113.33
11	25.733	27.200	28.755	30.404	32.150	34.001	35.962	38.039	40.238	42.566	56.405	74.697	98.739	130.16	171.00
12	30.850	32.824	34.931	37.180	39.581	42.142	44.874	47.788	50.895	54.208	74.327	101.84	139.23	189.73	257.49
13	36.786	39.404	42.219	45.244	48.497	51.991	55.746	59.779	64.110	68.760	97.625	138.48	195.93	276.12	387.24
14	43.672	47.103	50.818	54.841	59.196	63.909	69.010	74.528	80.496	86.949	127.91	187.95	275.30	401.37	581.86
15	51.660	56.110	60.965	66.261	72.035	78.330	85.192	92.669	100.82	109.69	167.29	254.74	386.42	582.98	873.79
16	60.925	66.649	72.939	79.850	87.442	95.780	104.93	114.98	126.01	138.11	218.47	344.90	541.99	846.32	1,311.7
17	71.673	78.979	87.068	96.022	105.93	116.89	129.02	142.43	157.25	173.64	285.01	466.61	759.78	1,228.2	1,968.5
18	84.141	93.406	103.74	115.27	128.12	142.44	158.40	176.19	195.99	218.04	371.52	630.92	1,064.7	1,781.8	2,953.8
19	98.603	110.28	123.41	138.17	154.74	173.35	194.25	217.71	244.03	273.56	483.97	852.75	1,491.6	2,584.7	4,431.7
20	115.38	130.03	146.63	165.42	186.69	210.76	237.99	268.79	303.60	342.94	630.17	1,152.2	2,089.2	3,748.8	6,648.5
21	134.84	153.14	174.02	197.85	225.03	256.02	291.35	331.61	377.46	429.68	820.22	1,556.5	2,925.9	5,436.7	9,973.8
22	157.41	180.17	206.34	236.44	271.03	310.78	356.44	408.88	469.06	538.10	1,067.3	2,102.3	4,097.2	7,884.3	14,962
23	183.60	211.80	244.49	282.36	326.24	377.05	435.86	503.92	582.63	673.63	1,388.5	2,839.0	5,737.1	11,433	22,443
24	213.98	248.81	289.49	337.01	392.48	457.22	532.75	620.82	723.46	843.03	1,806.0	3,833.7	8,033.0	16,579	33,666
25	249.21	292.10	342.60	402.04	471.98	554.24	650.96	764.61	898.09	1,054.8	2,348.8	5,176.5	11,247	24,041	50,500
26	290.09	342.76	405.27	479.43	567.38	671.63	795.17	941.46	1,114.6	1,319.5	3,054.4	6,989.3	15,747	34,860	75,752
27	337.50	402.03	479.22	571.52	681.85	813.68	971.10	1,159.0	1,383.1	1,650.4	3,971.8	9,436.5	22,047	50,548	113,628
28	392.50	471.38	566.48	681.11	819.22	985.55	1,185.7	1,426.6	1,716.1	2,064.0	5,164.3	12,740	30,867	73,296	170,443
29	456.30	552.51	669.45	811.52	984.07	1,193.5	1,447.6	1,755.7	2,129.0	2,580.9	6,714.6	17,200	43,214	106,280	255,666
30	530.31	647.44	790.95	966.71	1,181.9	1,445.2	1,767.1	2,160.5	2,640.9	3,227.2	8,730.0	23,222	60,501	154,107	383,500
35	1,120.7	1,426.5	1,816.7	2,314.2	2,948.3	3,755.9	4,783.6	6,090.3	7,750.2	9,856.8	32,423	104,136	325,400	987,794	2,912,217
40	2,360.8	3,134.5	4,163.2	5,529.8	7,343.9	9,749.5	12,937	17,154	22,729	30,089	120,393	466,960	1,750,092	6,331,512	22,114,663
45	4,965.3	6,879.3	9,531.6	13,203	18,281	25,295	34,971	48,302	66,640	91,831	447,019	2,093,876	9,412,424	40,583,319	167,933,233
50	10,436	15,090	21,813	31,515	45,497	65,617	94,525	135,992	195,373	280,256	1,659,761	9,389,020	50,622,288	260,128,295	1,275,242,998

Table B–3 Present Value of $1

$PVF_{i,n} = 1/(1 + i)^n; PV = FV(PVF_{i,n})$

Period	1%	2%	3%	4%	5%	6%	7%	8%	9%	10%	11%	12%	13%	14%	15%
1	0.9901	0.9804	0.9709	0.9615	0.9524	0.9434	0.9346	0.9259	0.9174	0.9091	0.9009	0.8929	0.8850	0.8772	0.8696
2	0.9803	0.9612	0.9426	0.9246	0.9070	0.8900	0.8734	0.8573	0.8417	0.8264	0.8116	0.7972	0.7831	0.7695	0.7561
3	0.9706	0.9423	0.9151	0.8890	0.8638	0.8396	0.8163	0.7938	0.7722	0.7513	0.7312	0.7118	0.6931	0.6750	0.6575
4	0.9610	0.9238	0.8885	0.8548	0.8227	0.7921	0.7629	0.7350	0.7084	0.6830	0.6587	0.6355	0.6133	0.5921	0.5718
5	0.9515	0.9057	0.8626	0.8219	0.7835	0.7473	0.7130	0.6806	0.6499	0.6209	0.5935	0.5674	0.5428	0.5194	0.4972
6	0.9420	0.8880	0.8375	0.7903	0.7462	0.7050	0.6663	0.6302	0.5963	0.5645	0.5346	0.5066	0.4803	0.4556	0.4323
7	0.9327	0.8706	0.8131	0.7599	0.7107	0.6651	0.6227	0.5835	0.5470	0.5132	0.4817	0.4523	0.4251	0.3996	0.3759
8	0.9235	0.8535	0.7894	0.7307	0.6768	0.6274	0.5820	0.5403	0.5019	0.4665	0.4339	0.4039	0.3762	0.3506	0.3269
9	0.9143	0.8368	0.7664	0.7026	0.6446	0.5919	0.5439	0.5002	0.4604	0.4241	0.3909	0.3606	0.3329	0.3075	0.2843
10	0.9053	0.8203	0.7441	0.6756	0.6139	0.5584	0.5083	0.4632	0.4224	0.3855	0.3522	0.3220	0.2946	0.2697	0.2472
11	0.8963	0.8043	0.7224	0.6496	0.5847	0.5268	0.4751	0.4289	0.3875	0.3505	0.3173	0.2875	0.2607	0.2366	0.2149
12	0.8874	0.7885	0.7014	0.6246	0.5568	0.4970	0.4440	0.3971	0.3555	0.3186	0.2858	0.2567	0.2307	0.2076	0.1869
13	0.8787	0.7730	0.6810	0.6006	0.5303	0.4688	0.4150	0.3677	0.3262	0.2897	0.2575	0.2292	0.2042	0.1821	0.1625
14	0.8700	0.7579	0.6611	0.5775	0.5051	0.4423	0.3878	0.3405	0.2992	0.2633	0.2320	0.2046	0.1807	0.1597	0.1413
15	0.8613	0.7430	0.6419	0.5553	0.4810	0.4173	0.3624	0.3152	0.2745	0.2394	0.2090	0.1827	0.1599	0.1401	0.1229
16	0.8528	0.7284	0.6232	0.5339	0.4581	0.3936	0.3387	0.2919	0.2519	0.2176	0.1883	0.1631	0.1415	0.1229	0.1069
17	0.8444	0.7142	0.6050	0.5134	0.4363	0.3714	0.3166	0.2703	0.2311	0.1978	0.1696	0.1456	0.1252	0.1078	0.0929
18	0.8360	0.7002	0.5874	0.4936	0.4155	0.3503	0.2959	0.2502	0.2120	0.1799	0.1528	0.1300	0.1108	0.0946	0.0808
19	0.8277	0.6864	0.5703	0.4746	0.3957	0.3305	0.2765	0.2317	0.1945	0.1635	0.1377	0.1161	0.0981	0.0829	0.0703
20	0.8195	0.6730	0.5537	0.4564	0.3769	0.3118	0.2584	0.2145	0.1784	0.1486	0.1240	0.1037	0.0868	0.0728	0.0611
21	0.8114	0.6598	0.5375	0.4388	0.3589	0.2942	0.2415	0.1987	0.1637	0.1351	0.1117	0.0926	0.0768	0.0638	0.0531
22	0.8034	0.6468	0.5219	0.4220	0.3418	0.2775	0.2257	0.1839	0.1502	0.1228	0.1007	0.0826	0.0680	0.0560	0.0462
23	0.7954	0.6342	0.5067	0.4057	0.3256	0.2618	0.2109	0.1703	0.1378	0.1117	0.0907	0.0738	0.0601	0.0491	0.0402
24	0.7876	0.6217	0.4919	0.3901	0.3101	0.2470	0.1971	0.1577	0.1264	0.1015	0.0817	0.0659	0.0532	0.0431	0.0349
25	0.7798	0.6095	0.4776	0.3751	0.2953	0.2330	0.1842	0.1460	0.1160	0.0923	0.0736	0.0588	0.0471	0.0378	0.0304
26	0.7720	0.5976	0.4637	0.3607	0.2812	0.2198	0.1722	0.1352	0.1064	0.0839	0.0663	0.0525	0.0417	0.0331	0.0264
27	0.7644	0.5859	0.4502	0.3468	0.2678	0.2074	0.1609	0.1252	0.0976	0.0763	0.0597	0.0469	0.0369	0.0291	0.0230
28	0.7568	0.5744	0.4371	0.3335	0.2551	0.1956	0.1504	0.1159	0.0895	0.0693	0.0538	0.0419	0.0326	0.0255	0.0200
29	0.7493	0.5631	0.4243	0.3207	0.2429	0.1846	0.1406	0.1073	0.0822	0.0630	0.0485	0.0374	0.0289	0.0224	0.0174
30	0.7419	0.5521	0.4120	0.3083	0.2314	0.1741	0.1314	0.0994	0.0754	0.0573	0.0437	0.0334	0.0256	0.0196	0.0151
35	0.7059	0.5000	0.3554	0.2534	0.1813	0.1301	0.0937	0.0676	0.0490	0.0356	0.0259	0.0189	0.0139	0.0102	0.0075
40	0.6717	0.4529	0.3066	0.2083	0.1420	0.0972	0.0668	0.0460	0.0318	0.0221	0.0154	0.0107	0.0075	0.0053	0.0037
45	0.6391	0.4102	0.2644	0.1712	0.1113	0.0727	0.0476	0.0313	0.0207	0.0137	0.0091	0.0061	0.0041	0.0027	0.0019
50	0.6080	0.3715	0.2281	0.1407	0.0872	0.0543	0.0339	0.0213	0.0134	0.0085	0.0054	0.0035	0.0022	0.0014	0.0009

(Continues)

Table B-3 (*Contd*)

$PVF_{i,n} = 1/(1 + i)^n$; $PV = FV(PVF_{i,n})$

Period	16%	17%	18%	19%	20%	21%	22%	23%	24%	25%	30%	35%	40%	45%	50%
1	0.8621	0.8547	0.8475	0.8403	0.8333	0.8264	0.8197	0.8130	0.8065	0.8000	0.7692	0.7407	0.7143	0.6897	0.6667
2	0.7432	0.7305	0.7182	0.7062	0.6944	0.6830	0.6719	0.6610	0.6504	0.6400	0.5917	0.5487	0.5102	0.4756	0.4444
3	0.6407	0.6244	0.6086	0.5934	0.5787	0.5645	0.5507	0.5374	0.5245	0.5120	0.4552	0.4064	0.3644	0.3280	0.2963
4	0.5523	0.5337	0.5158	0.4987	0.4823	0.4665	0.4514	0.4369	0.4230	0.4096	0.3501	0.3011	0.2603	0.2262	0.1975
5	0.4761	0.4561	0.4371	0.4190	0.4019	0.3855	0.3700	0.3552	0.3411	0.3277	0.2693	0.2230	0.1859	0.1560	0.1317
6	0.4104	0.3898	0.3704	0.3521	0.3349	0.3186	0.3033	0.2888	0.2751	0.2621	0.2072	0.1652	0.1328	0.1076	0.0878
7	0.3538	0.3332	0.3139	0.2959	0.2791	0.2633	0.2486	0.2348	0.2218	0.2097	0.1594	0.1224	0.0949	0.0742	0.0585
8	0.3050	0.2848	0.2660	0.2487	0.2326	0.2176	0.2038	0.1909	0.1789	0.1678	0.1226	0.0906	0.0678	0.0512	0.0390
9	0.2630	0.2434	0.2255	0.2090	0.1938	0.1799	0.1670	0.1552	0.1443	0.1342	0.0943	0.0671	0.0484	0.0353	0.0260
10	0.2267	0.2080	0.1911	0.1756	0.1615	0.1486	0.1369	0.1262	0.1164	0.1074	0.0725	0.0497	0.0346	0.0243	0.0173
11	0.1954	0.1778	0.1619	0.1476	0.1346	0.1228	0.1122	0.1026	0.0938	0.0859	0.0558	0.0368	0.0247	0.0168	0.0116
12	0.1685	0.1520	0.1372	0.1240	0.1122	0.1015	0.0920	0.0834	0.0757	0.0687	0.0429	0.0273	0.0176	0.0116	0.0077
13	0.1452	0.1299	0.1163	0.1042	0.0935	0.0839	0.0754	0.0678	0.0610	0.0550	0.0330	0.0202	0.0126	0.0080	0.0051
14	0.1252	0.1110	0.0985	0.0876	0.0779	0.0693	0.0618	0.0551	0.0492	0.0440	0.0254	0.0150	0.0090	0.0055	0.0034
15	0.1079	0.0949	0.0835	0.0736	0.0649	0.0573	0.0507	0.0448	0.0397	0.0352	0.0195	0.0111	0.0064	0.0038	0.0023
16	0.0930	0.0811	0.0708	0.0618	0.0541	0.0474	0.0415	0.0364	0.0320	0.0281	0.0150	0.0082	0.0046	0.0026	0.0015
17	0.0802	0.0693	0.0600	0.0520	0.0451	0.0391	0.0340	0.0296	0.0258	0.0225	0.0116	0.0061	0.0033	0.0018	0.0010
18	0.0691	0.0592	0.0508	0.0437	0.0376	0.0323	0.0279	0.0241	0.0208	0.0180	0.0089	0.0045	0.0023	0.0012	0.0007
19	0.0596	0.0506	0.0431	0.0367	0.0313	0.0267	0.0229	0.0196	0.0168	0.0144	0.0068	0.0033	0.0017	0.0009	0.0005
20	0.0514	0.0433	0.0365	0.0308	0.0261	0.0221	0.0187	0.0159	0.0135	0.0115	0.0053	0.0025	0.0012	0.0006	0.0003
21	0.0443	0.0370	0.0309	0.0259	0.0217	0.0183	0.0154	0.0129	0.0109	0.0092	0.0040	0.0018	0.0009	0.0004	0.0002
22	0.0382	0.0316	0.0262	0.0218	0.0181	0.0151	0.0126	0.0105	0.0088	0.0074	0.0031	0.0014	0.0006	0.0003	0.0002
23	0.0329	0.0270	0.0222	0.0183	0.0151	0.0125	0.0103	0.0086	0.0071	0.0059	0.0024	0.0010	0.0004	0.0002	0.0001
24	0.0284	0.0231	0.0188	0.0154	0.0126	0.0103	0.0085	0.0070	0.0057	0.0047	0.0018	0.0007	0.0003	0.0001	0.0001
25	0.0245	0.0197	0.0160	0.0129	0.0105	0.0085	0.0069	0.0057	0.0046	0.0038	0.0014	0.0006	0.0002	0.0001	0.0001
26	0.0211	0.0169	0.0135	0.0109	0.0087	0.0070	0.0057	0.0046	0.0037	0.0030	0.0011	0.0004	0.0002	0.0001	0.0000
27	0.0182	0.0144	0.0115	0.0091	0.0073	0.0058	0.0047	0.0037	0.0030	0.0024	0.0008	0.0003	0.0001	0.0000	0.0000
28	0.0157	0.0123	0.0097	0.0077	0.0061	0.0048	0.0038	0.0030	0.0024	0.0019	0.0006	0.0002	0.0001	0.0000	0.0000
29	0.0135	0.0105	0.0082	0.0064	0.0051	0.0040	0.0031	0.0025	0.0020	0.0015	0.0005	0.0002	0.0001	0.0000	0.0000
30	0.0116	0.0090	0.0070	0.0054	0.0042	0.0033	0.0026	0.0020	0.0016	0.0012	0.0004	0.0001	0.0001	0.0000	0.0000
35	0.0055	0.0041	0.0030	0.0023	0.0017	0.0013	0.0009	0.0007	0.0005	0.0004	0.0001	0.0000	0.0000	0.0000	0.0000
40	0.0026	0.0019	0.0013	0.0010	0.0007	0.0005	0.0004	0.0003	0.0002	0.0001	0.0000	0.0000	0.0000	0.0000	0.0000
45	0.0013	0.0009	0.0006	0.0004	0.0003	0.0002	0.0001	0.0001	0.0001	0.0000	0.0000	0.0000	0.0000	0.0000	0.0000
50	0.0006	0.0004	0.0003	0.0002	0.0001	0.0001	0.0000	0.0000	0.0000	0.0000	0.0000	0.0000	0.0000	0.0000	0.0000

Table B-4 Present Value of an Annuity

$$PVA_{i,n} = [1 - 1/(1 + i)^n]/i; \quad PVA = PMT \text{ or Annuity} \times (PVA_{i,n})$$

Period	1%	2%	3%	4%	5%	6%	7%	8%	9%	10%	11%	12%	13%	14%	15%
1	0.9901	0.9804	0.9709	0.9615	0.9524	0.9434	0.9346	0.9259	0.9174	0.9091	0.9009	0.8929	0.8850	0.8772	0.8696
2	1.9704	1.9416	1.9135	1.8861	1.8594	1.8334	1.8080	1.7833	1.7591	1.7355	1.7125	1.6901	1.6681	1.6467	1.6257
3	2.9410	2.8839	2.8286	2.7751	2.7232	2.6730	2.6243	2.5771	2.5313	2.4869	2.4437	2.4018	2.3612	2.3216	2.2832
4	3.9020	3.8077	3.7171	3.6299	3.5460	3.4651	3.3872	3.3121	3.2397	3.1699	3.1024	3.0373	2.9745	2.9137	2.8550
5	4.8534	4.7135	4.5797	4.4518	4.3295	4.2124	4.1002	3.9927	3.8897	3.7908	3.6959	3.6048	3.5172	3.4331	3.3522
6	5.7955	5.6014	5.4172	5.2421	5.0757	4.9173	4.7665	4.6229	4.4859	4.3553	4.2305	4.1114	3.9975	3.8887	3.7845
7	6.7282	6.4720	6.2303	6.0021	5.7864	5.5824	5.3893	5.2064	5.0330	4.8684	4.7122	4.5638	4.4226	4.2883	4.1604
8	7.6517	7.3255	7.0197	6.7327	6.4632	6.2098	5.9713	5.7466	5.5348	5.3349	5.1461	4.9676	4.7988	4.6389	4.4873
9	8.5660	8.1622	7.7861	7.4353	7.1078	6.8017	6.5152	6.2469	5.9952	5.7590	5.5370	5.3282	5.1317	4.9464	4.7716
10	9.4713	8.9826	8.5302	8.1109	7.7217	7.3601	7.0236	6.7101	6.4177	6.1446	5.8892	5.6502	5.4262	5.2161	5.0188
11	10.368	9.7868	9.2526	8.7605	8.3064	7.8869	7.4987	7.1390	6.8052	6.4951	6.2065	5.9377	5.6869	5.4527	5.2337
12	11.255	10.575	9.9540	9.3851	8.8633	8.3838	7.9427	7.5361	7.1607	6.8137	6.4924	6.1944	5.9176	5.6603	5.4206
13	12.134	11.348	10.635	9.9856	9.3936	8.8527	8.3577	7.9038	7.4869	7.1034	6.7499	6.4235	6.1218	5.8424	5.5831
14	13.004	12.106	11.296	10.563	9.8986	9.2950	8.7455	8.2442	7.7862	7.3667	6.9819	6.6282	6.3025	6.0021	5.7245
15	13.865	12.849	11.938	11.118	10.380	9.7122	9.1079	8.5595	8.0607	7.6061	7.1909	6.8109	6.4624	6.1422	5.8474
16	14.718	13.578	12.561	11.652	10.838	10.106	9.4466	8.8514	8.3126	7.8237	7.3792	6.9740	6.6039	6.2651	5.9542
17	15.562	14.292	13.166	12.166	11.274	10.477	9.7632	9.1216	8.5436	8.0216	7.5488	7.1196	6.7291	6.3729	6.0472
18	16.398	14.992	13.754	12.659	11.690	10.828	10.059	9.3719	8.7556	8.2014	7.7016	7.2497	6.8399	6.4674	6.1280
19	17.226	15.678	14.324	13.134	12.085	11.158	10.336	9.6036	8.9501	8.3649	7.8393	7.3658	6.9380	6.5504	6.1982
20	18.046	16.351	14.877	13.590	12.462	11.470	10.594	9.8181	9.1285	8.5136	7.9633	7.4694	7.0248	6.6231	6.2593
21	18.857	17.011	15.415	14.029	12.821	11.764	10.836	10.017	9.2922	8.6487	8.0751	7.5620	7.1016	6.6870	6.3125
22	19.660	17.658	15.937	14.451	13.163	12.042	11.061	10.201	9.4424	8.7715	8.1757	7.6446	7.1695	6.7429	6.3587
23	20.456	18.292	16.444	14.857	13.489	12.303	11.272	10.371	9.5802	8.8832	8.2664	7.7184	7.2297	6.7921	6.3988
24	21.243	18.914	16.936	15.247	13.799	12.550	11.469	10.529	9.7066	8.9847	8.3481	7.7843	7.2829	6.8351	6.4338
25	22.023	19.523	17.413	15.622	14.094	12.783	11.654	10.675	9.8226	9.0770	8.4217	7.8431	7.3300	6.8729	6.4641
26	22.795	20.121	17.877	15.983	14.375	13.003	11.826	10.810	9.9290	9.1609	8.4881	7.8957	7.3717	6.9061	6.4906
27	23.560	20.707	18.327	16.330	14.643	13.211	11.987	10.935	10.027	9.2372	8.5478	7.9426	7.4086	6.9352	6.5135
28	24.316	21.281	18.764	16.663	14.898	13.406	12.137	11.051	10.116	9.3066	8.6016	7.9844	7.4412	6.9607	6.5335
29	25.066	21.844	19.188	16.984	15.141	13.591	12.278	11.158	10.198	9.3696	8.6501	8.0218	7.4701	6.9830	6.5509
30	25.808	22.396	19.600	17.292	15.372	13.765	12.409	11.258	10.274	9.4269	8.6938	8.0552	7.4957	7.0027	6.5660
35	29.409	24.999	21.487	18.665	16.374	14.498	12.948	11.655	10.567	9.6442	8.8552	8.1755	7.5856	7.0700	6.6166
40	32.835	27.355	23.115	19.793	17.159	15.046	13.332	11.925	10.757	9.7791	8.9511	8.2438	7.6344	7.1050	6.6418
45	36.095	29.490	24.519	20.720	17.774	15.456	13.606	12.108	10.881	9.8628	9.0079	8.2825	7.6609	7.1232	6.6543
50	39.196	31.424	25.730	21.482	18.256	15.762	13.801	12.233	10.962	9.9148	9.0417	8.3045	7.6752	7.1327	6.6605

(Continues)

Table B-4 (*Contd*)

$$PVA_{i,n} = [1 - 1/(1 + i)^n]/i; \quad PVA = PMT \text{ or Annuity} \times (PVAi,n)$$

Period	16%	17%	18%	19%	20%	21%	22%	23%	24%	25%	30%	35%	40%	45%	50%
1	0.8621	0.8547	0.8475	0.8403	0.8333	0.8264	0.8197	0.8130	0.8065	0.8000	0.7692	0.7407	0.7143	0.6897	0.6667
2	1.6052	1.5852	1.5656	1.5465	1.5278	1.5095	1.4915	1.4740	1.4568	1.4400	1.3609	1.2894	1.2245	1.1653	1.1111
3	2.2459	2.2096	2.1743	2.1399	2.1065	2.0739	2.0422	2.0114	1.9813	1.9520	1.8161	1.6959	1.5889	1.4933	1.4074
4	2.7982	2.7432	2.6901	2.6386	2.5887	2.5404	2.4936	2.4483	2.4043	2.3616	2.1662	1.9969	1.8492	1.7195	1.6049
5	3.2743	3.1993	3.1272	3.0576	2.9906	2.9260	2.8636	2.8035	2.7454	2.6893	2.4356	2.2200	2.0352	1.8755	1.7366
6	3.6847	3.5892	3.4976	3.4098	3.3255	3.2446	3.1669	3.0923	3.0205	2.9514	2.6427	2.3852	2.1680	1.9831	1.8244
7	4.0386	3.9224	3.8115	3.7057	3.6046	3.5079	3.4155	3.3270	3.2423	3.1611	2.8021	2.5075	2.2628	2.0573	1.8829
8	4.3436	4.2072	4.0776	3.9544	3.8372	3.7256	3.6193	3.5179	3.4212	3.3289	2.9247	2.5982	2.3306	2.1085	1.9220
9	4.6065	4.4506	4.3030	4.1633	4.0310	3.9054	3.7863	3.6731	3.5655	3.4631	3.0190	2.6653	2.3790	2.1438	1.9480
10	4.8332	4.6586	4.4941	4.3389	4.1925	4.0541	3.9232	3.7993	3.6819	3.5705	3.0915	2.7150	2.4136	2.1681	1.9653
11	5.0286	4.8364	4.6560	4.4865	4.3271	4.1769	4.0354	3.9018	3.7757	3.6564	3.1473	2.7519	2.4383	2.1849	1.9769
12	5.1971	4.9884	4.7932	4.6105	4.4392	4.2784	4.1274	3.9852	3.8514	3.7251	3.1903	2.7792	2.4559	2.1965	1.9846
13	5.3423	5.1183	4.9095	4.7147	4.5327	4.3624	4.2028	4.0530	3.9124	3.7801	3.2233	2.7994	2.4685	2.2045	1.9897
14	5.4675	5.2293	5.0081	4.8023	4.6106	4.4317	4.2646	4.1082	3.9616	3.8241	3.2487	2.8144	2.4775	2.2100	1.9931
15	5.5755	5.3242	5.0916	4.8759	4.6755	4.4890	4.3152	4.1530	4.0013	3.8593	3.2682	2.8255	2.4839	2.2138	1.9954
16	5.6685	5.4053	5.1624	4.9377	4.7296	4.5364	4.3567	4.1894	4.0333	3.8874	3.2832	2.8337	2.4885	2.2164	1.9970
17	5.7487	5.4746	5.2223	4.9896	4.7746	4.5755	4.3908	4.2190	4.0591	3.9099	3.2948	2.8398	2.4918	2.2182	1.9980
18	5.8178	5.5339	5.2732	5.0333	4.8122	4.6079	4.4187	4.2431	4.0799	3.9279	3.3037	2.8443	2.4941	2.2195	1.9986
19	5.8775	5.5845	5.3162	5.0700	4.8435	4.6346	4.4415	4.2627	4.0967	3.9424	3.3105	2.8476	2.4958	2.2203	1.9991
20	5.9288	5.6278	5.3527	5.1009	4.8696	4.6567	4.4603	4.2786	4.1103	3.9539	3.3158	2.8501	2.4970	2.2209	1.9994
21	5.9731	5.6648	5.3837	5.1268	4.8913	4.6750	4.4756	4.2916	4.1212	3.9631	3.3198	2.8519	2.4979	2.2213	1.9996
22	6.0113	5.6964	5.4099	5.1486	4.9094	4.6900	4.4882	4.3021	4.1300	3.9705	3.3230	2.8533	2.4985	2.2216	1.9997
23	6.0442	5.7234	5.4321	5.1668	4.9245	4.7025	4.4985	4.3106	4.1371	3.9764	3.3254	2.8543	2.4989	2.2218	1.9998
24	6.0726	5.7465	5.4509	5.1822	4.9371	4.7128	4.5070	4.3176	4.1428	3.9811	3.3272	2.8550	2.4992	2.2219	1.9999
25	6.0971	5.7662	5.4669	5.1951	4.9476	4.7213	4.5139	4.3232	4.1474	3.9849	3.3286	2.8556	2.4994	2.2220	1.9999
26	6.1182	5.7831	5.4804	5.2060	4.9563	4.7284	4.5196	4.3278	4.1511	3.9869	3.3297	2.8560	2.4996	2.2221	1.9999
27	6.1364	5.7975	5.4919	5.2151	4.9636	4.7342	4.5243	4.3316	4.1542	3.9903	3.3305	2.8563	2.4997	2.2221	1.9999
28	6.1520	5.8099	5.5016	5.2228	4.9697	4.7390	4.5281	4.3346	4.1566	3.9923	3.3312	2.8565	2.4998	2.2222	2.0000
29	6.1656	5.8204	5.5098	5.2292	4.9747	4.7430	4.5312	4.3371	4.1585	3.9938	3.3317	2.8567	2.4999	2.2222	2.0000
30	6.1772	5.8294	5.5168	5.2347	4.9789	4.7463	4.5338	4.3391	4.1601	3.9950	3.3321	2.8568	2.4999	2.2222	2.0000
35	6.2153	5.8582	5.5386	5.2512	4.9915	4.7559	4.5411	4.3447	4.1644	3.9984	3.3330	2.8571	2.5000	2.2222	2.0000
40	6.2335	5.8713	5.5482	5.2582	4.9966	4.7596	4.5439	4.3467	4.1659	3.9995	3.3332	2.8571	2.5000	2.2222	2.0000
45	6.2421	5.8773	5.5523	5.2611	4.9986	4.7610	4.5449	4.3474	4.1664	3.9998	3.3333	2.8571	2.5000	2.2222	2.0000
50	6.2463	5.8801	5.5541	5.2623	4.9995	4.7616	4.5452	4.3477	4.1666	3.9999	3.3333	2.8571	2.5000	2.2222	2.0000

Chapter Seven

THE INVESTMENT DECISION

LEARNING OBJECTIVES

After completing the material in this chapter, you will be able to:

▶ Explain the financial objectives of health care providers.
▶ Evaluate various capital investment alternatives.
▶ Calculate and interpret net present value (NPV).
▶ Calculate and interpret internal rate of return (IRR).

Chapter Outline

(Continues)

◀INTRODUCTION▶

Capital investment decisions involve major dollar investments that are expected to achieve long-term benefits for an organization. Such investments, quite common in health care, fall into three categories:

- **Strategic decisions:** Capital investment decisions designed to increase a health care organization's strategic (long-term) position (e.g. purchasing physician practices to increase horizontal integration).
- **Expansion decisions:** Capital investment decisions designed to increase the operational capability of a health care organization (e.g. increasing examination space in a group practice to accommodate increased volume).
- **Replacement decisions:** Capital investment decisions designed to replace older assets with newer, cost saving, ones (e.g. replacing a hospital's existing cost-accounting system with a newer, cost saving one).

A capital investment decision has two components: 1) determining if the investment is worthwhile; and 2) determining how to finance the investment. Although these two decisions are interrelated, they should be separated. This chapter focuses on the first component – determining whether a capital investment should be undertaken. It is organized around three factors related to analyzing capital investment decisions: 1) the objectives of capital investment analysis; 2) three techniques to analyze capital investment decisions; and 3) technical concerns related to capital budgeting. Chapter 8 focuses on capital financing alternatives. Perspectives 7–1 and 7–2 offer some examples of capital investments.

Capital Investment Decision: Decisions involving major dollar investments that are expected to achieve long-term benefits for an organization.

Expansion Decision: Capital investment decision designed to increase the operational capability of a health care organization.

Strategic Decision: Capital investment decision designed to increase a health care organization's strategic (long-term) position.

Caution

Although determining if an investment is worthwhile and how to finance the investment are interrelated, they should be considered separately.

PERSPECTIVE 7–1

Investment in Cancer Treatment Equipment

St Joseph Healthcare and Radiation Oncology Associates of Albuquerque, New Mexico, have collaborated for 11 years to provide radiation treatment for cancer. Their latest joint effort resulted in $2.2 million in state-of-the-art cancer treatment equipment. The investment in a new linear accelerator, a high-energy X-ray machine, was made possible by $1 million from Radiation Oncology Associates and a year of fund-raising by the nonprofit St Joseph Healthcare Foundation.

The nine-physician Radiation Oncology Associates, which built the $2.3 million cancer center in 1989, leases the building and equipment to St Joseph. "We needed a place to practice our trade," said Paul Anthony, who is a group member and St Joseph radiation oncology medical director. Physician groups in other cities often set up their own radiation treatment centers, but Radiation Oncology Associates wanted the stability of a hospital affiliation, Anthony said. The new equipment enhances the group's cancer treatment abilities as well as services available through St Joseph. That health-care organization reported $5 million in operating losses earlier this year and has since hired the Florida-based Hunter Group to find a way to reverse the decline in its financial fortunes.

The cancer center expansion "is financially viable whether the hospital does it or we do," Anthony said. Medicare still provides adequate reimbursement for radiation treatment, he added. "For the hospital to be in radiation therapy is good for the hospital." This is the center's second linear accelerator for radiation treatment of cancer. The new machine can handle about 30 percent more patients per day with more effective treatment and fewer side effects. A third accelerator, at St. Joseph's Downtown hospital, will be used for inpatient treatment. The Heights center will be able to treat 80 patients a day.

Source: Winthrop Quigley, "Doctors, St Joseph Gets New Tool." *Albuquerque Journal,* September 7, 2000, p. 1.

PERSPECTIVE 7–2

McKessonHBOC Announces Next-Generation, Integrated Clinical Solution to Improve Patient Safety and Reduce Cost of Care

The Information Technology Business of McKesson HBOC, Inc. (NYSE:MCK) recently announced a strategic relationship with Vanderbilt University Medical Center (Vanderbilt) in Nashville, Tenn., to offer a world-class solution for advanced clinical decision support and expert physician order entry. The solution, which has been in use at Vanderbilt for the past six years, will be known as Horizon Expert Orders.

Horizon Expert Orders assists physicians in decision-making by presenting clinically relevant information about a patient's condition along with treatment protocols and evidence-based guidelines agreed upon by the organization's physicians. Armed with this information, physicians and other clinicians can quickly enter orders with a few keystrokes or mouse clicks. Horizon Expert Orders also has financial implications. At Vanderbilt, system-driven results include a $5 million annual reduction in pharmacy costs – excluding the value of adverse drug event prevention. Vanderbilt also reduced its X-ray costs by more than $1.1 million.

Source: Jean Hodges, McKessonHBOC, Alpharetta (Information Technology Business), Atlanta, July 16, 2001.

◀THE OBJECTIVES OF CAPITAL INVESTMENT ANALYSIS▶

A capital investment is expected to achieve long-term benefits for the organization. Such benefits generally fall into three categories: non-financial benefits, financial returns, and the ability to attract more funds in the future (see Exhibit 7–1). Clearly, these three objectives are highly interrelated. In the following discussion, it is important to keep in mind that "investors" are not limited to those outside the organization. When an organization purchases new assets or starts a new program, it is also an investor – it is investing in itself.

Replacement Decision: Capital investment decision designed to replace older assets with newer, cost saving, ones.

Non-financial Benefits

A primary concern with many capital investment decisions is how well an investment enhances the survival of the organization and supports its mission, patients, employees, and the community. A particularly interesting movement in health care is the increasing number of governmental agencies with taxing authority asking for proof of community benefit. Community benefits include increased access to different types of care, higher quality of care, lower charges, the provision of charity care, and the employment of community members. Perspective 7–3 illustrates such an instance.

Financial Returns

Direct financial benefits are a primary concern not only to health care organizations, but also to many – if not all – investors who invest in health care organizations and their projects. Direct financial benefits to investors can take two forms. The first is periodic payments in the form of dividends to stockholders and/or interest to bondholders.

Exhibit 7–1   The Objectives of the Capital Investment Decision

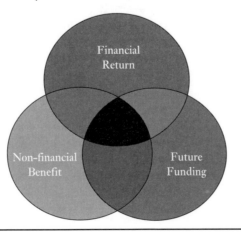

PERSPECTIVE 7–3

New Beckley Clinic to Help Thousands

Residents of Southern West Virginia who don't have health insurance will soon have a medical clinic dedicated to their care. Beckley Appalachian Regional Healthcare donated a building and will soon hire a nurse practitioner to see patients, said Joe Zager, community CEO for Beckley Appalachian Regional Hospital. The clinic is patterned after Helping Hands Health Right, a Charleston facility that offers medical care to the poor. "We have about 500 patients from Raleigh and Fayette counties who drive or hitchhike to get to our medical services in Charleston," said clinic administrator Pat White. "This facility in Beckley will make a tremendous difference for them, as well as for many other residents who are without access to health care." The Beckley clinic is supported by a team of ministers, health-care workers, and community leaders led by Jackie Snead, president of the board of directors of Helping Hands Health Right Inc.

House Speaker Bob Kiss, D-Raleigh, presented Snead with a $25,000 check to help with initial operating costs. An additional $5,000 was donated by Stanaford Missionary Baptist Church. Tom Williams, former director of Raleigh County Hospice Care, will serve as administrator of the clinic, which is expected to serve 6,000 to 9,000 patients during its first year.

Source: The Sunday Gazette Mail, Charleston, May 6, 2001, p. P7B.

Retained Earnings:
The portion of profits that an organization keeps in-house for itself to use in growth and support of its mission.

Capital Appreciation: Occurs whenever an asset is worth more when it is sold than when it was purchased. Common examples would be land, property, or stocks.

(Bonds are discussed in Chapter 8.) **Dividends** represent the portion of profit that an organization distributes to equity investors, whereas **interest** is a payment to creditors – those who have loaned the organization funds or otherwise extended credit.

The second type of benefit to an investor is in the form of **retained earnings,** the portion of the profits the organization keeps in-house to use in growth and support of its mission. This describes the plowing back or investing of funds (including retained earnings) into capital projects that appreciate in value. **Capital appreciation** takes place whenever an investment is worth more when it is sold than when it was purchased. For investor-owned organizations, this appreciation in value increases the value of their stock.

Though almost all organizations can make periodic payments to their investors in the form of interest, by law, only investor-owned health care organizations can distribute dividends outside the organization.

Ability to Attract Funds in the Future

Without new capital funds, many health care organizations would be unable to offer new services, support medical research, or subsidize unprofitable services. Therefore, another objective of capital investment is to invest in profitable projects or services that will attract debt (borrowing) and equity financing in the future. (Capital financing is discussed at length in Chapter 8. Capital financing includes funds from a variety of sources including government entities, foundations, and community-based organizations.)

◄ANALYTIC METHODS►

An investment decision involves many factors (see Perspectives 7–4 and 7–5). Three commonly used financial techniques to analyze capital investment decisions for health care organizations are:

- Payback.
- Net Present Value.
- Internal Rate of Return.

PERSPECTIVE 7–4

Carolinas HealthCare System (CHS) Gains $326,000 Profit for First Quarter

CHS is one of the Southeast's largest health-care systems, with dozens of hospitals, outpatient care centers, doctors' offices, and other medical services in the Carolinas. It's governed by a public hospital authority created by the General Assembly in1943. Like other hospitals, CHS has been hit by tightened reimbursements from government health insurance programs. CHS recently has been renegotiating its contracts with private insurers to try to increase revenues. "It's hard to say at this point" what effect those new contracts will have on CHS's bottom line, said Steven Graybill, a Charlotte-based health care consultant with William M. Mercer Inc.

In the meantime, CHS is working on other ways to raise revenues and cut expenses. On the revenue side, CHS opened Carolinas Integrative Health, a cash-only alternative medicine clinic in Dilworth that is expected to prove popular with people who seek massage, acupuncture, and nutritional supplements.

On the expense side, CHS continues to streamline its food services, contracting with a company that last month opened a $5.6 million central kitchen facility that now cooks the food for all the hospitals. The relationship with Morrison Healthcare Food Services is expected to save CHS $20 million over 10 years, a spokesman said.

Source: Mike Stobbe, *The Charlotte Observer,* June 20, 2001. Copyright 2001.

PERSPECTIVE 7–5

CEO of Nashville, Tenn.-Based Healthcare Company Defends Integrity

Dr Frist, HCA's chairman and CEO from 1987 to 1994, returned to that post in 1997. In his absence, the company then known as Columbia/HCA underwent explosive growth and ran afoul of the federal government. "I found it a far different company (in 1997) than the one I left," he said. "We had 67 hospitals when I left and 367 when I came back. We had to refocus the company, ask ourselves what markets we really wanted to be in." Dr Frist said HCA's roster now includes 200 hospitals, on which the company spends about $1.5 billion per year. The $36 million project at Parkridge includes expanded parking, renovation of patient rooms, and the hospital's emergency facility and construction of a cancer center. Frank Morgan, managing director and health care services analyst at the Nashville office of Jefferies and Co., said the Parkridge project is consistent with the track HCA has taken since Dr Frist's return. "They've downsized, paid down debt, and made major reinvestments in core markets," Mr Morgan said. "Why buy a hospital in a new market? Renovating and building replacement hospitals in markets you already know is viewed as less risky, and Chattanooga's been a very good market for them."

Source: Bob Gary Jr, "CEO of Nashville, Tenn.-Based Healthcare Company Defends Integrity." *Chattanooga Times/Free Press,* April 26, 2001. Copyright 2001.

Suppose Marquee Valley Hospital has $1,000,000 available to invest in a new business (Exhibit 7–2, rows 1, 3). After examining the marketplace, it has narrowed the possibilities to two promising options, each of which would require the full amount of money available: it could either buy a small existing physician practice, or it could build its own small satellite clinic. If it buys the physician practice, it would expect to generate new net cash inflows of $333,333 each year for six years (Exhibit 7–2, row 2). By investing in its own satellite clinic, Marquee Valley could expect to generate net cash flows of $200,000, $250,000, $300,000, $350,000, $450,000, and $650,000 over the next six years (Exhibit 7–2, row 4).

 Key Point   Until now, this book has stressed the accrual method of accounting. However, the techniques introduced in this chapter – payback, net present value (NPV), and the internal rate of return (IRR) – use only cash flows. Therefore, when only accrual information is available (such as information from financial statements), accrual items must be converted into cash flows. An example is shown in the discussion of net present value.

Payback Method: A method to evaluate the feasibility of an investment by determining how long it would take until the initial investment is recovered, disregarding the time value of money.

The Payback Method

One way to analyze these investments is to calculate the time it would take to recoup the investment. This is called the **payback method** and is illustrated in Exhibit 7–3, which builds on Exhibit 7–2.

Analysis

Exhibit 7–3 shows four rows for each investment: row A is the initial investment, row B is the beginning balance for each year, row C is the cash flow for each year, and row D is the cumulative cash flow for each year. Although the satellite clinic began the fourth year with a $250,000 deficit (row B), it had a cash flow of $350,000 during the year (row C); thus, its cumulative cash flow by the end of the fourth year was $100,000. From row D, it is apparent that during the fourth year, the hospital would have recouped its investment. Under either scenario, the hospital would be tying up its money for at least three years.

The actual month in which breakeven occurs can be obtained by dividing the amount of the deficit at the end of the year prior to breaking even by the average

Exhibit 7–2   Cash Flows for Two Alternative Project Investments

Givens:

Physician Practice	Years	0	1	2	3	4	5	6
1 Initial Investment		($1,000,000)						
2 Project's Cash Flows Each Year			$333,333	$333,333	$333,333	$333,333	$333,333	$333,333

Satellite Clinic	Years	0	1	2	3	4	5	6
3 Initial Investment		($1,000,000)						
4 Project's Cash Flows Each Year			$200,000	$250,000	$300,000	$350,000	$450,000	$650,000

Key Point

Formula to calculate the breakeven point in years if cash flows are equal each year:

Initial Investment/Annual Cash Flows

monthly inflow in the breakeven year. For example, the deficit at the end of the third year for the satellite clinic is $250,000, and the average monthly inflow during the fourth year is $29,167 ($350,000/12). Solving the equation, $250,000/$29,167 = 8.6 months. Thus, Marquee Valley would break even 6/10 of the way into month 9 (September) of the fourth year. If it bought the physician practice, it would break even at the end of year 3, since it ends year 3 with no deficit.

If net cash inflows are equal each year (as they are with the physician practice), then the number of years it takes to break even is simply the initial investment divided by the annual net cash inflows resulting from the investment, and use of a table such as in Exhibit 7–3 is unnecessary. Thus, the payback time for the physician practice would be $1,000,000/$333,333, which equals 3 years, the same answer derived in Exhibit 7–3.

Strengths and Weaknesses of the Payback Method

The strengths of the payback method are that it is: 1) simple to calculate; and 2) easy to understand (see Exhibit 7–4). There are three major weaknesses to the payback method, however: 1) it gives an answer in years, not dollars; 2) it disregards cash flows after the

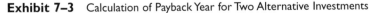

Exhibit 7–3   Calculation of Payback Year for Two Alternative Investments

Physician Practice	Years	0	1	2	3	4	5	6
A Initial Investment	[1]	($1,000,000)						
B Beginning of Year Balance	[2]		($1,000,000)	($666,667)	($333,333)	($0)	$333,333	$666,667
C Project's Cash Flows Each Year	[3]		$333,333	$333,333	$333,333	$333,333	$333,333	$333,333
D Cumulative Cash Flow	[A+B+C]	($1,000,000)	($666,667)	($333,333)	($0)	$333,333	$666,667	$1,000,000

[1] Exhibit 7–2, Row 1
[2] Balance from End of Previous Year, Row D
[3] Exhibit 7–2, Row 2
Breakeven year = Year 3

Satellite Clinic	Years	0	1	2	3	4	5	6
A Initial Investment	[4]	($1,000,000)						
B Beginning of Year Balance	[5]		($1,000,000)	($800,000)	($550,000)	($250,000)	$100,000	$550,000
C Project's Cash Flows Each Year	[6]		$200,000	$250,000	$300,000	$350,000	$450,000	$650,000
D Cumulative Cash Flow	[A+B+C]	($1,000,000)	($800,000)	($550,000)	($250,000)	$100,000	$550,000	$1,200,000

[4] Exhibit 7–2, Row 3
[5] Balance from End of Previous Year, Row D
[6] Exhibit 7–2, Row 4
Breakeven year = Year 4

Exhibit 7–4   Strengths and Weaknesses of the Payback Method

Strengths	Weaknesses
• Simple to calculate • Easy to understand	• Answers in years, not dollars • Disregards cash flows after payback • Does not account for the time value of money

payback time; and 3) it does not account for the time value of money. Each of these is discussed briefly in the next section.

1. **The payback is in years, not dollars.** Knowing that a project has a payback of three years does not provide key financial information such as the size of the dollar impact on the organization in future years.
2. **The payback method disregards cash flows after the payback time.** For example, the physician practice has equal annual cash inflows and a payback of three years, whereas the satellite clinic has unequal annual cash inflows and doesn't reach payback until year 4. Thus, the physician practice, with its shorter payback, would appear to be the better investment. However, the satellite clinic has better cash flows in later years, and by the end of year 6, it brings in $200,000 more than does the physician practice. Hence, in addition to time until payback, it is important to consider the cash flows after the payback date when making an investment.
3. **The payback method does not account for the time value of money.** Chapter 6 demonstrated that a dollar received sometime in the future is not worth the same as a dollar received today. The two evaluation methods discussed in the remainder of this chapter, net present value and internal rate of return, do take the time value of money into account, whereas the payback method does not.

Net Present Value:
The difference between the initial amount paid for an investment and the future cash flows that the investment brings in, adjusted for the cost of capital.

Discounted Cash Flows: Cash flows that have been adjusted to account for the cost of capital.

Cost of Capital: The rate of return required to undertake a project. The cost of capital accounts for both the time value of money and risk. Also called the hurdle rate or discount rate.

Net Present Value

Because of the deficiencies in using the payback method to analyze capital investments, a preferred alternative is a net present value analysis. **Net Present Value (NPV)** is the difference between the initial amount paid for an investment and the future cash flows the investment brings in over time after they have been adjusted (discounted) by the cost of capital. The cost of capital accounts for two costs: first, investors (bondholders and stockholders) are being asked to delay the consumption of their funds by investing in the project (time value of money); second, these investors face a risk that the investment may not generate the revenues and net cash flows anticipated, leaving them with an inadequate rate of return, or the project may fail altogether, leaving the investors with perhaps nothing other than a tax loss.

If the sum of the **discounted cash flows** resulting from the investment is greater than the initial investment itself, then the NPV is positive. Thus, from a purely financial standpoint, the project is acceptable, all else being equal. On the other hand, if the sum of the discounted cash flows resulting from the investment is less than the

 Key Point   The following terms are used interchangeably: *Cost of Capital, Discount Rate,* and *Hurdle Rate.*

investment itself, then the investment brings in less than was initially paid out, the NPV is negative, and the investment should be rejected.

NPV – Using the Satellite Clinic as an Example of an NPV Analysis

In the example used earlier (Exhibit 7–3), the annual cash flows were given, but in real-world situations, organizations may not always have such information readily available. Therefore, in the following example (see Exhibit 7–5), the same annual cash flows are used as in the previous example ($200,000, $250,000, $300,000, $350,000, $450,000, and $650,000), but these numbers are derived using additional information commonly found in a budget forecast (revenues, expenses, depreciation, etc.). With this in mind, the net present value of the satellite clinic alternative will be recalculated using the following steps:

Steps to Calculate Net Present Value of the Satellite Clinic Alternative

Step 1. Identify the initial cash outflow.
Step 2. Determine revenues and expenses (net income):
    a. Identify annual net revenues.
    b. Identify annual cash operating expenses and depreciation expense.
    c. Compute annual net income.
Step 3. Add back in depreciation expense to get net operating cash flows.
Step 4. Add (subtract) any non-annual cash flows.
Step 5. Adjust for working capital.
Step 6. Determine the present value of each year's cash flow.
Step 7. Sum the present values of all cash flows.
Step 8. Determine the net present value of the project.

1. **Identify the initial cash outflow (row A).** The initial investment in the satellite clinic is $1,000,000.
2. **Determine net income (rows B, C, D, E).**
    a. **Identify annual cash inflows (revenues).** Use net revenues rather than gross revenues to account for the fact that discounts and allowances will not be collected.
    b. **Identify annual cash operating expenses and depreciation expense.**
    c. **Compute annual net income.**
3. **Add back depreciation (rows F, G).** The annual expenses (Step 2b) include depreciation expenses. However, depreciation is an expense that does not require any cash outflow. Therefore, to calculate actual cash flows, an amount equal to depreciation expense is added back to net income. Depreciation is estimated at $145,000 annually. The end result is a higher cash flow.
4. **Add (subtract) any non-annual cash flows (rows H, I).** Some projects may have various non-annual cash flows that occur during the project. In this example, the only non-annual cash flow is a cash inflow in year 6 resulting from selling some assets of the investment project. The **salvage value** is estimated to be $130,000.

Salvage Value: The amount of cash to be received when an asset is sold, usually at the end of its useful life. Also called **terminal value, residual value,** and **scrap value.**

Exhibit 7-5 Computation of Net Present Value for the Satellite Clinic

Givens:	Years	0	1	2	3	4	5	6
1 Initial investment		($1,000,000)						
2 Net Revenue			$400,000	$550,000	$800,000	$900,000	$1,100,000	$1,370,000
3 Cash Operating Expense			$200,000	$300,000	$500,000	$550,000	$650,000	$850,000
4 Annual Depreciation			$145,000	$145,000	$145,000	$145,000	$145,000	$145,000
5 Salvage value (end of year 6)								$130,000
6 Cost of Capital	10%							

		Years	0	1	2	3	4	5	6
A Initial Investment	[Given 1]		($1,000,000)						
B Net Revenue	[Given 2]			$400,000	$550,000	$800,000	$900,000	$1,100,000	$1,370,000
C Less: Cash Operating Expenses	[Given 3]			$200,000	$300,000	$500,000	$550,000	$650,000	$850,000
D Less: Depreciation Expense	[Given 4]			$145,000	$145,000	$145,000	$145,000	$145,000	$145,000
E Net Operating Income	[B – C – D]			55,000	105,000	155,000	205,000	305,000	375,000
F Add: Depreciation Expense	[Given 4]			145,000	145,000	145,000	145,000	145,000	145,000
G Net Operating Cash Flows	[E + F]			200,000	250,000	300,000	350,000	450,000	520,000
H Add: Sale of Salvage Value	[Given 5]								130,000
I Project Cash Flows	[G + H]			$200,000	$250,000	$300,000	$350,000	$450,000	$650,000
J Cost of Capital	[Given 6]			10%	10%	10%	10%	10%	10%
K Present Value Interest Factors	$1/(1 + i)^n$			0.9091	0.8264	0.7513	0.6830	0.6209	0.5645
L Annual PV of Cash Flows[1]	[I × K]			$181,818	$206,612	$225,394	$239,055	$279,415	$366,908
M PV of Cash Flows	[Sum L]	$1,499,202							
N Net Present Value	[A + M]	$499,202							

[1] Present Value Interest Factors in the exhibit have been calculated by formula, but are necessarily rounded for presentation. Therefore, there may be a difference between the number displayed and that calculated manually.

5. **Adjust for working capital.** Some projects affect working capital, and to the extent that this effect is material, it must be considered. In this example, assume that there are no material working capital effects. Adjusting for working capital is discussed in Appendix D.

6. **Determine the present value of each year's cash flow (rows I, J, K, L).** Steps 1–5 estimate cash flows that will occur each year. Step 6 discounts these cash flows using the methods discussed in Chapter 6. A discount rate of 10 percent is assumed for the satellite clinic project.

   The $200,000 received at the end of year 1 (row I) is worth $181,818 in today's dollars (row L). The $250,000 received two years from now (row I) is worth only $206,612 today (row L). The cash flows received in years 3 through 6 are discounted similarly.

Key Point

In deriving the annual cash flows using pro forma operating statements that include depreciation expense, depreciation expense or any other non-cash expense (amortization of goodwill) is added back to the bottom line (operating income).

Key Point

Interest expense should not be included as a cash flow, since it is part of financing flows and is included in the discount rate. Therefore, if interest expense is included in the operating expenses, then for the non-taxpaying entity, it should be added back into revenue in excess of expenses or earnings.

---

7. **Sum the present values of all cash flows (row M).**

8. **Determine the net present value of the project (rows A, M, N).** The net present value of the project is the difference between the discounted annual cash flows and the initial investment. The net present value, $499,202, is computed by adding the initial investment, –$1,000,000, a cash outflow, to the present value of the annual cash flows, $1,499,202. If this were the only investment alternative, since the net present value is positive, this investment would be accepted based only on financial criteria.

> **Goodwill:** An amount paid above and beyond the book value of an asset (typically a business) when it is sold, representing the value of intangible factors such as brand reputation, customer or supplier relationships, employee competencies, etc.

It is also possible to calculate the NPV of the physician practice introduced in Exhibit 7–2. Since the cash flows from this investment are equal in both amount and timing, they can be treated as an ordinary annuity of $333,333 for six years at 10 percent. The present value factor for this ordinary annuity is 4.3553. Thus, the present value of the cash flows is $1,451,765 (4.3553 × $333,333) and the net present value of the physician practice is $451,765 ($1,451,765 – $1,000,000).

Key Point

The terms **present value** and **net present value** should not be confused. Whereas present value is the sum of discounted future cash flows, net present value is equal to the present value net (less) the cost of the initial investment. Hence, in Exhibit 7–5, whereas the present value of the cash flows is $1,499,202 (the sum of the cash flows for years 1–6), the net present value is only $499,202 (the cash flows from years 1–6 less the cost of the initial $1,000,000 investment).

Decision Rules Regarding NPV

As noted in Exhibit 7–5, the net present value of the satellite clinic investment, after adjusting for depreciation and salvage value, is $499,202.

- **The general decision rule regarding NPV is: If NPV > 0, accept the project; If NPV < 0, reject the project; If NPV = 0, then accept or reject.** Based on this rule, the satellite clinic should be purchased since it has a positive NPV of $499,202. This rule applies in most cases; however, the rule is modified for two other possible situations.
- **If more than one mutually exclusive project is being considered, the one with the higher/highest positive NPV should be chosen.** Thus, if a second project were being considered, such as the purchase of the physician practice, the satellite clinic alternative would be taken only if the physician practice's NPV were less than $499,202.
- **If more than one mutually exclusive project is being considered and one must be selected regardless of NPV, then the one with the higher/highest NPV should be chosen, even if its NPV is negative.** Suppose the organization was considering developing either a burn unit or a school-based education program. Upon analysis, it is determined that one project has a net present value of –$4,000,000, and the other has a net present value of –$1,500,000. If it has been decided in advance that one of the two projects will be undertaken, then the one with the higher NPV should be chosen. In this case, –$1,500,000 is the better choice.

Using Spreadsheets to Calculate NPV

Any popular spreadsheet is an ideal platform to calculate net present value, as most, if not all, have built-in functions that make determination of NPV simple. Exhibit 7–6 shows how the NPV function in *Excel* can be used to compute the present value, $1,499,202, of the annual cash flows in Exhibit 7–5. Note that all six years' cash flows are actually entered, although only the cash flows for the first four years are shown, *Excel*'s NPV function is similar to its PV function, but allows for the use of unequal cash flows. Finally, it is necessary to add the initial investment, –$1,000,000, to the outside of the NPV function formula, which computes the present value of the annual project cash flows, $1,499,202, to obtain the NPV of $499,202. (A common mistake among users of the NPV function is to include the initial investment as a value in the NPV function formula. The initial investment must be added outside the function and needs to represent the negative outflow for the initial investment.)

 Key Point   When using the *Excel* NPV function, the initial investment outlay must be added to the NPV function result, and not entered as a value within the function itself.

Exhibit 7–6   Using *Excel* to Calculate the Net Present Value of Unequal Annual Cash Flows, Assuming a 10 Percent Discount Rate

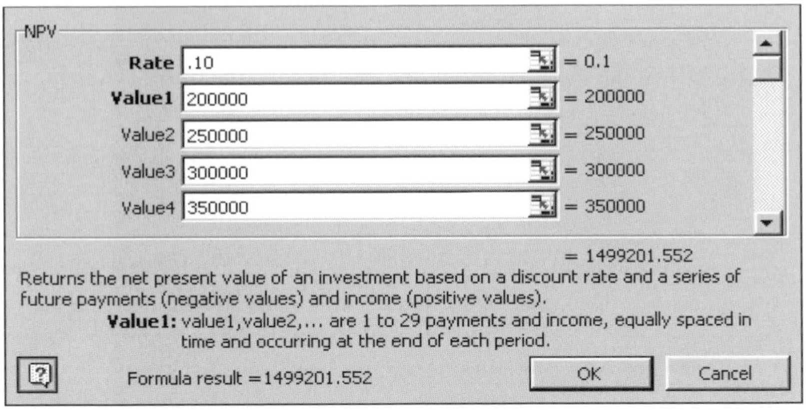

NPV		
Rate	.10	= 0.1
Value1	200000	= 200000
Value2	250000	= 250000
Value3	300000	= 300000
Value4	350000	= 350000

= 1499201.552

Returns the net present value of an investment based on a discount rate and a series of future payments (negative values) and income (positive values).

Value1: value1,value2,... are 1 to 29 payments and income, equally spaced in time and occurring at the end of each period.

Formula result = 1499201.552   OK   Cancel

Strengths and Weaknesses of the NPV Method

The NPV method has a number of strengths and weaknesses (see Exhibit 7–7). Its strengths are: 1) it provides an answer in dollars, not years; 2) it accounts for all cash flows in the project, including those beyond the payback period; and 3) it discounts the cash flows at the cost of capital. Its main difficulties are developing estimates of cash flows and the discount rate.

Conceptually, NPV is very strong because it accounts for all cash flows in a project and discounts at the cost of capital. However, the cost of capital can be difficult to determine, as discussed in Appendix C.

Internal Rate of Return (IRR)

The **internal rate of return (IRR)** on an investment can be defined and interpreted several ways. It is: 1) the discount rate at which the discounted cash flows over the life of the project exactly equal the initial investment; 2) the discount rate that results in a net

Exhibit 7–7   Strengths and Weaknesses of the NPV Analysis

Strengths

- Answers in dollars, not years
- Accounts for all the cash flows in the project
- Discounts at the cost of capital

Weaknesses

- Estimates may be difficult to develop
- Discount rate may be difficult to determine

Key Point

Internal Rate of Return: That rate of return on an investment which makes the net present value equal to $0, after all cash flows have been discounted at the same rate. It is also the discount rate at which the discounted cash flows over the life of the project exactly equal the initial investment

present value equal to zero; and 3) the percentage return on the investment. In contrast, NPV is the dollar return on the investment. The method to use to solve for the IRR depends on whether the cash flows are equal or unequal.

Equal Cash Flows

If the cash flows are equal each period, the IRR can be determined by first finding the present value factor for an annuity, and then converting the answer to a discount rate depending on the number of years. Since the physician practice example used earlier has equal cash flows each period, its IRR can be found by:

1. Computing the present value factor for an annuity (PVFA) (see Chapter 6):

$$PV = Annuity \times PVFA_{i,n}$$

$$\$1,000,000 = \$333,333 \times PVFA_{i,6}$$

$$PVFA_{i,6} = 3.0$$

2. Finding the interest rate that yields this PVFA factor. In the present value of an annuity table (Table B–4), in the row for 6 time periods (since the investment is over 6 years), the column heading for the number closest to 3.0 (the PVFA factor) is the IRR. In this case, the PVFA factor of 3.0 lies somewhere between the 24 percent and 25 percent columns; thus, the IRR is approximately 24.5 percent.

Unequal Cash Flows

Business calculators and computer programs make finding the IRR for unequal cash flows relatively easy. *Excel*'s function is called "IRR" (see Exhibit 7–8). All the operating cash flow values of the project, including the initial investment, are entered individually, or an array of cells is referenced (the initial investment must be a negative value in either case, because it is a cash outflow). As shown in Exhibit 7–8, the IRR appears at the bottom of the box.

Key Point

In contrast to *Excel*'s NPV function, the IRR function includes the initial investment as one of the entries in the function.

Exhibit 7–8   Using *Excel* to Calculate the Internal Rate of Return of a $1,000,000 Investment which Yields Unequal Operating Cash Flows to Be Received at the End of Each of Six Successive Years
Note : The values in the array A1 : A7 = − 1000000; 200000; 250000; 300000; 350000; 450000; 650000

```
┌─IRR─────────────────────────────────────────────────────────────────┐
│                                                                      │
│     Values │A1:A7│                         [⬚] = {-1000000;200000;2   │
│                                                                      │
│      Guess │                              │[⬚] = number              │
│                                                                      │
│                                            = 0.226362547             │
│   Returns the internal rate of return for a series of cash flows.    │
│                                                                      │
│        Values is an array or a reference to cells that contain numbers for which you │
│              want to calculate the internal rate of return.          │
│                                                                      │
│   [?]       Formula result =0.226362547          │  OK  │  │ Cancel │ │
└──────────────────────────────────────────────────────────────────────┘
```

Decision Rules with IRR

Required Rate of Return: An organization's minimally acceptable internal rate of return on any investment to justify an initial investment. Also called **Cost of Capital** or **Hurdle Rate.**

When an organization chooses a project according to the IRR method, its financial decision depends upon the value of the IRR relative to the **required rate of return** on the investment (which is also called the **cost of capital** or **hurdle rate**).

- If the IRR is greater than the required rate of return, the project should be accepted.
- If the IRR is less than the required rate of return, the project should be rejected.
- If the IRR is equal to the required rate of return, the facility should be indifferent about accepting or rejecting the project.

Strengths and Weaknesses of IRR Analysis

There are three major strengths to using IRR as a decision criterion: 1) it considers all the relevant cash flows related to the investment project; 2) it is a time value of money-based approach; and 3) managers are accustomed to evaluating projects by their respective rates of return. Similarly, there are three weaknesses to using internal rate of return as a decision criterion: 1) it assumes that proceeds are reinvested at the internal rate of return, which may or may not be equal to the cost of capital; 2) developing estimates of cash flows is difficult; and 3) internal rate of return sometimes generates multiple rates of return, if future cash flows are estimates. Still, this method is widely used in industry as the preferred way to make responsible investment decisions (see Exhibit 7–9).

Using an NPV Analysis for a Replacement Decision

The previous analyses have focused on situations in which an organization was interested in either expanding its existing services or offering a new service altogether.

Exhibit 7–9 Strengths and Weaknesses of the IRR Analysis

Strengths
• Considers all relevant cash flows of the investment project
• Time value of money-based approach
• Widely used by practitioners and easily understood

Weaknesses
• Assumes reinvestment of proceeds at the internal rate of return
• Estimates may be difficult to develop
• Can generate multiple rates of return

Replacement Decision: Capital investment decision designed to replace older assets with newer, cost saving ones.

However, a common and more complicated analysis is the **replacement decision**, which must be made by an organization when it contemplates replacing an older, existing asset with a newer, more cost-efficient one. There are two ways to undertake this problem, both using a net present value approach and both yielding the same result. The first approach is to compare the net present value of continuing as is to that of the replacement alternative, with the preferred investment alternative being the one yielding the higher net present value. The second approach is to perform a single net present value analysis using the *incremental differences* brought about by replacing an asset. If the single NPV is positive, then the replacement alternative is preferred.

Illustrative Example

Straight-line Depreciation: A method which depreciates an asset an equal amount each year until it reaches its salvage value at the end of its useful life.

Assume that a radiology laboratory in a not-for-profit organization is considering renovating its X-ray processing area with new equipment that is faster and produces better, more reliable images. The existing equipment was purchased five years ago for $1,150,000 and is being depreciated on a **straight-line** basis over a ten-year life to a $150,000 salvage value. The old equipment can be sold now for its current book value of $650,000 ($1,150,000 original cost less $500,000 in accumulated depreciation).

The new equipment can be purchased for $1,500,000 and is estimated to have a five-year life. It would be depreciated on a straight-line basis to a $750,000 salvage value. The radiology department is a revenue-producing center. Presently, 45 patients per day, 260 days/year, can be screened by one radiology technologist at an average reimbursement of $75 per test, but a significant portion of these patients must be given a second test at no additional charge because the first image is inconclusive. The new equipment, because it is not only faster but produces images of better quality, can process 60 patients per day. (In this example, the hospital believes that sufficient demand exists to fully utilize the higher capacity of the new equipment.) An in-depth discussion of how to estimate future cash flows is found in Appendix C.

The old equipment costs \$60,000 per year in utilities and maintenance. The new equipment would cost \$30,000 per year in utilities and maintenance. The annual labor expenses will not change because one radiology technologist is needed to operate either piece of equipment. Cost of capital for this organization is 9 percent.

Solution

Exhibits 7–10a and 7–10b present the *comparative approach* to solve this problem. This approach employs the same eight steps outlined in Exhibit 7–5. An NPV is calculated for each alternative, and then the NPVs are compared to determine which is higher. As an alternative method, Exhibit 7–11 uses the *incremental approach* to solve the same problem, whereby instead of calculating two NPVs and comparing them, it calculates a single NPV based upon marginal differences for each cash flow. The results are exactly the same.

Using the comparative approach, the net present value over the next five years for the new equipment, \$4,071,651 (Exhibit 7–10b, row N), is higher than that of the old equipment, \$3,277,280 (Exhibit 7–10a, row N). Therefore, the decision in this case would be to renovate the area with the new equipment. Similarly, using the incremental approach, the net present value is \$794,371 (Exhibit 7–11, row N). Thus, since the NPV is positive, the replacement decision should be made. Incidentally, note that the \$794,371 NPV using the incremental method is exactly the difference between the two alternatives (\$4,071,651 − \$3,277,280) using the comparative approach. Thus, the results are the same using either method; just the method of calculation differs.

Before a final decision is made, however, several issues must be considered: 1) the purchase of a new asset typically requires a large up-front expenditure, which may not always be feasible; 2) future cash flows are difficult to determine and may not always be accurate, especially the salvage value; 3) the exact cost of capital is difficult to determine; and 4) though not the case here, replacement of an old asset with a new asset may not make sense financially (i.e. $NPV_{New} < NPV_{Old}$), but replacement may be necessary for other reasons, such as to remain competitive by being able to offer the latest technology to consumers.

◄Summary►

This chapter introduces three methods to evaluate large dollar, multi-year investment decisions: payback, net present value, and internal rate of return. The payback method measures how long it takes to recover the initial investment. The strengths of the payback method are that it is simple to calculate and is easy to understand. Its major weaknesses are that it does not account for the time value of money, it provides an answer in years, not dollars, and it disregards cash flows after the payback.

The net present value (NPV) method overcomes the weaknesses of the payback method by accounting for cash flows after payback and discounting these cash flows

Exhibit 7–10a NPV Comparative Analysis of a Replacement Decision – Old Equipment

Cash flows with the Old Equipment

Givens:

1 Initial Investment	$0
2 Annual Revenues[1]	$877,500
3 Annual Cash Operating Expenses	$60,000
4 Annual Depreciation[2]	$100,000
5 Salvage Value at 10 Years (5 years hence)	$150,000
6 Cost of Capital	9%

[1] $75/Exam × 45 Exams/Day × 260 Operating Days/Year
[2] ($1,150,000 Initial Cost – $150,000 Salvage Value)/10 years

		Years	0	1	2	3	4	5
A	Initial Investment	[Given 1]	$0					
B	Net Revenues	[Given 2]		$877,500	$877,500	$877,500	$877,500	$877,500
C	Less: Cash Operating Expenses	[Given 3]		60,000	60,000	60,000	60,000	60,000
D	Less: Depreciation Expense	[Given 4]		100,000	100,000	100,000	100,000	100,000
E	Operating Income	[B – C – D]		717,500	717,500	717,500	717,500	717,500
F	Add: Depreciation Expense	[Given 4]		100,000	100,000	100,000	100,000	100,000
G	Net Operating Cash Flows	[E + F]		817,500	817,500	817,500	817,500	817,500
H	Add: Sale of Salvage	[Given 5]						150,000
I	Project Cash Flows	[G + H]		$817,500	$817,500	$817,500	$817,500	$967,500
J	Cost of Capital	[Given 6]		9%	9%	9%	9%	9%
K	Present Value Interest Factors	$1/(1 + i)^n$		0.9174	0.8417	0.7722	0.7084	0.6499
L	Annual PV of Cash Flows[3]	[I × K]		$750,000	$688,073	$631,260	$579,138	$628,809
M	PV of Cash Flows	[Sum L]	$3,277,280					
N	**Net Present Value**	[A + M]	**$3,277,280**					

[3] Present Value Interest Factors in the exhibit have been calculated by formula, but are necessarily rounded for presentation. Therefore, there may be a difference between the number displayed and that calculated manually.

Exhibit 7-10b NPV Comparative Analysis of a Replacement Decision – New Equipment

Cash flows with the New Equipment

Givens:

1 Initial Investment Amount[1]	$850,000
2 Annual Revenues[2]	$1,170,000
3 Annual Cash Operating Expenses	$30,000
4 Annual Depreciation[3]	$150,000
5 Salvage Value (5 years hence)	$750,000
6 Cost of Capital	9%

[1] $1,500,000 Initial Cost – $650,000 Sale of Old Equipment
[2] $75/Exam × 60 Exams/Day × 260 Operating Days/Year
[3] ($1,500,000 Initial Cost – $750,000 Salvage Value)/5 Years

	Years	0	1	2	3	4	5
A Initial Investment	[Given 1]	($850,000)					
B Net revenues	[Given 2]		$1,170,000	$1,170,000	$1,170,000	$1,170,000	$1,170,000
C Less: Cash Operating Expenses	[Given 3]		30,000	30,000	30,000	30,000	30,000
D Less: Depreciation Expense	[Given 4]		150,000	150,000	150,000	150,000	150,000
E Operating Income	[B – C – D]		990,000	990,000	990,000	990,000	990,000
F Add: Depreciation Expense	[Given 4]		150,000	150,000	150,000	150,000	150,000
G Net Operating Cash Flows	[E + F]		1,140,000	1,140,000	1,140,000	1,140,000	1,140,000
H Add: Sale of Salvage Value	[Given 5]						750,000
I Project Cash Flows	[G + H]		$1,140,000	$1,140,000	$1,140,000	$1,140,000	$1,890,000
J Cost of Capital	[Given 6]		9%	9%	9%	9%	9%
K Present Value Interest Factors	$1/(1 + i)^n$		0.9174	0.8417	0.7722	0.7084	0.6499
L Annual PV of Cash Flows[4]	[I × K]		$1,045,872	$959,515	$880,289	$807,605	$1,228,370
M PV of Cash Flows	[Sum L]	$4,921,651					
N Net Present Value	[A + M]	$4,071,651					

[4] Present Value Interest Factors in the exhibit have been calculated by formula, but are necessarily rounded for presentation. Therefore, there may be a difference between the number displayed and that calculated manually.

Exhibit 7-11 NPV Comparative Analysis of a Replacement Decision – The Incremental Approach

Cash Flows

Givens:	Old Equipment	New Equipment	Incremental Difference (New – Old)	Incremental = New – Old
1 Initial Investment		($850,000)	($850,000)	
2 Annual Revenues[1]	$877,500	$1,170,000	$292,500	Incremental Net Revenues
3 Annual Cash Operating Expenses	($60,000)	($30,000)	$30,000	Incremental Operating Cash Savings
4 Annual Depreciation[2]	$100,000	$150,000	$50,000	Incremental Depreciation Expenses
5 Salvage Value	$150,000	$750,000	$600,000	Incremental Salvage Value
6 Cost of Capital			9%	

[1] Old: $75/Exam × 45 Exams/Day × 260 Operating Days/Year   New: $75/Exam × 60 Exams/Day × 260 Operating Days/Year
[2] Old: ($1,150,000 Initial Cost – $150,000 Salvage Value)/10 Years   New: ($1,500,000 Initial Cost – $750,000 Salvage Value)/5 Years
The income statement below subtracts the $50,000 depreciation expense in row E.

	Years	0	1	2	3	4	5
A Initial Investment	[Given 1]	($850,000)					
B Incremental Net Revenues	[Given 2]		$292,500	$292,500	$292,500	$292,500	$292,500
C Incremental Operating Cash Savings	[Given 3]		30,000	30,000	30,000	30,000	30,000
D Incremental Depreciation Expenses	[Given 4]		50,000	50,000	50,000	50,000	50,000
E Incremental Net Operating Income	[(B + C) – D]		272,500	272,500	272,500	272,500	272,500
F Add: Incremental Depreciation	[Given 4]		50,000	50,000	50,000	50,000	50,000
G Incremental Net Operating Cash Flow	[E + F]		322,500	322,500	322,500	322,500	322,500
H Add: Incremental Salvage Value	[Given 5]						600,000
I Project Incremental Cash Flows	[G + H]		$322,500	$322,500	$322,500	$322,500	$922,500
J Cost of Capital	[Given 6]		9%	9%	9%	9%	9%
K Present Value Interest Factors	$1/(1+i)^n$		0.9174	0.8417	0.7722	0.7084	0.6499
L Annual PV of Incremental Cash Flows[3]	[I × K]		$295,872	$271,442	$249,029	$228,467	$599,562
M PV of Incremental Cash Flows	[Sum L]	$1,644,371					
N Net Present Value	[A + M]	$794,371					

[3] Present Value Interest Factors in the exhibit have been calculated by formula, but are necessarily rounded for presentation. Therefore, there may be a difference between the number displayed and that calculated manually.

by the project's cost of capital. The project's cost of capital is the rate of return that compensates investors for the time value of money and for the risk of the investment. *The net present value measures the difference between the present value of the operating cash flows generated by the investment and the initial cost of that investment.* The NPV technique measures the dollar return on the investment.

The general decision rule regarding NPV is: if NPV > 0, accept the project; if NPV < 0, reject the project; if NPV = 0, then accept or reject. If more than one mutually exclusive project is being considered, then the one with the higher/ highest positive NPV should be chosen. If more than one mutually exclusive project is being considered, and one must be undertaken regardless of NPV, then the one with the higher/highest NPV should be chosen, even if the NPV is negative.

The strengths of the NPV method of capital investment analysis are that it provides an answer in dollars, not years; it accounts for all cash flows from the project, including those beyond the payback period; and it discounts these cash flows at the cost of capital. The major weakness to the NPV method is that the discount rate is often difficult to determine and may be hard to justify. The calculation of an NPV can be accomplished in the eight steps presented in the chapter.

Step 1. Identify the initial cash outflow.
Step 2. Determine revenues and expenses (net income):
    a. Identify annual net revenues.
    b. Identify annual cash operating expenses and depreciation expense.
    c. Compute annual net income.
Step 3. Add back in depreciation expense to get net operating cash flows.
Step 4. Add (subtract) any non-annual cash flows.
Step 5. Adjust for working capital.
Step 6. Determine the present value of each year's cash flow.
Step 7. Sum the present values of all cash flows.
Step 8. Determine the net present value of the project.

The internal rate of return (IRR) method determines the actual percentage return on the investment. When an organization chooses a project according to the IRR method, its decision depends on the value of the IRR relative to the required rate of return on the investment (also called the cost of capital or hurdle rate).

- If the IRR is greater than the required rate of return, the project should be accepted.
- If the IRR is less than the required rate of return, the project should be rejected.
- If the IRR is equal to the required rate of return, the facility should be indifferent about accepting or rejecting the project.

◀KEY TERMS▶

CANNIBALIZATION

CAPITAL INVESTMENTS

CAPITAL INVESTMENT DECISIONS

CAPITAL APPRECIATION

COST OF CAPITAL

DISCOUNT RATE

DISCOUNTED CASH FLOWS

DIVIDENDS

EXPANSION DECISION

GOODWILL

HURDLE RATE

INCREMENTAL CASH FLOWS

INTEREST

INTERNAL RATE OF RETURN

INTERNAL RATE OF RETURN
   METHOD

NET PRESENT VALUE

NET PRESENT VALUE METHOD

NON-REGULAR CASH FLOWS

OPERATING CASH FLOWS

OPPORTUNITY COSTS

PAYBACK METHOD

REGULAR CASH FLOWS

REPLACEMENT DECISION

REQUIRED RATE OF RETURN

RESIDUAL VALUE

RETAINED EARNINGS

SALVAGE VALUE

SCRAP VALUE

STRAIGHT-LINE DEPRECIATION

STRATEGIC DECISION

SUNK COSTS

TERMINAL VALUE

◀KEY EQUATION▶

Payback in Years if Cash Flows are Equal Each Year:

Initial Investment/Annual Cash Flows

◀QUESTIONS AND PROBLEMS▶

Note that questions and problems include materials from the Appendices following this chapter.

1. Define the following terms:
    a. Cannibalization.
    b. Capital Appreciation.
    c. Cost of Capital.
    d. Discount Rate.
    e. Discounted Cash Flows.
    f. Dividends.
    g. Expansion Decisions.
    h. Goodwill.
    i. Hurdle Rate.
    j. Incremental Cash Flows.
    k. Interest.
    l. Internal Rate of Return.
    m. Internal Rate of Return Method.
    n. Net Present Value.
    o. Net Present Value Method.
    p. Non-regular Cash Flows.
    q. Operating Cash Flows.
    r. Opportunity Costs.
    s. Payback Method.

    t. Regular Cash Flows.
    u. Replacement Decisions.
    v. Required Rate of Return.
    w. Residual Value.
    x. Retained Earnings.
    y. Salvage Value.
    z. Scrap Value.
   aa. Straight-line Depreciation.
   bb. Strategic Decisions.
   cc. Sunk Costs.
   dd. Terminal Value.

2. Comment on the following statement. "When a not-for-profit facility receives a contribution from a member of the community, the cost of capital is inconsequential when deciding how to use this contribution, because it is, in effect, free money."

3. From a capital investment point of view, what are the goals of a health care facility?

4. What are the primary drawbacks of the payback method as a capital budgeting technique?

5. When using the IRR approach, when can the internal rate of return be determined simply by dividing the initial outlay by the cash flows?

6. Explain why pro forma income statements adjust for depreciation expense when developing projected cash flows for a project.

7. If a hospital were considering a new Women's Health Initiative, what spillover cash flows might result?

8. When performing a capital budgeting analysis, what costs should be included, and what costs should be excluded as part of the initial investment?

9. Why are financing flows such as interest expense and dividend payments excluded from the computation of cash flows?

10. Will a decision that is based upon NPV ever change if it were based upon IRR instead? Why or why not?

11. Marleboro Memorial Hospital is expecting its new cancer center to generate the following cash flows:

Year	0	1	2	3	4	5
Initial investment	($1,000,000)					
Net operating cash flows		$200,000	$300,000	$500,000	$300,000	$250,000

    a. Determine the payback for the new cancer center.
    b. Determine the net present value using a cost of capital of 12 percent.
    c. Determine the net present value at 16 percent and the internal rate of return.
    d. Based on net present value, should the project be accepted on a financial basis?

12. Buxton Community is expecting its new dialysis unit to generate the following cash flows:

Year	0	1	2	3	4	5
Initial investment	($5,000,000)					
Net operating cash flows		($150,000)	$800,000	$1,000,000	$4,000,000	$5,000,000

     a. Determine the payback for the new dialysis unit.
     b. Determine the net present value using a cost of capital of 11 percent.
     c. Determine the net present value at 20 percent and the internal rate of return.
     d. Based on net present value, should the project be accepted on a financial basis?

13. Letterman Hospital expects Projects A and B to generate the following cash flows:

Project A

Year	0	1	2	3	4	5
Initial investment	($500)					
Net operating cash flows		$900	$800	$300	$200	$100

Project B

Year	0	1	2	3	4	5
Initial investment	($500)					
Net operating cash flows		$100	$200	$300	$800	$900

     a. Determine the net present value for both projects using a cost of capital of 15 percent.
     b. Determine the net present value for both projects using a cost of capital of 5 percent.
     c. At a 5 percent discount rate, which project should be accepted? At a 15 percent discount rate, which project should be accepted? Explain.

14. Castle Rock Medical Center expects Projects X and Y to generate the following cash flows:

Project X

Year	0	1	2	3	4	5
Initial investment	($2,500)					
Net operating cash flows		$2,300	$1,500	$1,000	$800	$500

Project Y

Year	0	1	2	3	4	5
Initial investment	($2,500)					
Net operating cash flows		$500	$800	$1,000	$1,500	$2,300

   a. Determine the net present value for both projects using a cost of capital of 13 percent.

   b. Determine the net present value for both projects using a cost of capital of 8 percent.

   c. At an 8 percent discount rate, which project should be accepted? At a 13 percent discount rate, which project should be accepted? Explain.

15. Goodbar Practice expects Projects 1 and 2 to generate the following cash flows:

Project 1

Year	0	1	2	3	4	5
Initial investment	($3,755)					
Net operating cash flows		$900	$1,200	$1,300	$1,400	$1,450

Project 2

Year	0	1	2	3	4	5
Initial investment	($1,880)					
Net operating cash flows		$500	$500	$500	$500	$500

   a. Determine the payback for both projects.

   b. Determine the internal rate of return.

   c. Determine the net present value at a cost of capital of 12 percent.

16. Martin Medical expects Alpha Project and Beta Project to generate the following cash flows:

Alpha Project

Year	0	1	2	3	4	5
Initial investment	($8,000)					
Net operating cash flows		($4,000)	$2,500	$5,000	$7,000	$12,000

Beta Project

Year	0	1	2	3	4	5
Initial investment	($12,000)					
Net operating cash flows		$3,000	$3,000	$3,000	$3,000	$3,000

    a. Determine the payback for both projects.

    b. Determine the internal rate of return.

    c. Determine the net present value at a cost of capital of 14 percent.

17. Tin Man Memorial Hospital, a non-taxpaying entity, is starting a new heart center. The expected patient volume demands will generate $8,000,000 per year in revenues for the next five years. The expected operating expenses, excluding depreciation, will increase expenses by $3,000,000 per year for the next five years. The initial cost of building and equipment is $16,000,000. Straight-line depreciation is used to estimate depreciation expense and the building and equipment will be depreciated over a five-year life to their salvage value. The expected salvage value of the building and equipment at year five is $1,000,000. The cost of capital for this project is 8 percent.

    a. Compute the net present value and internal rate of return to determine the financial feasibility of this project.

    b. Compute the net present value and internal rate of return to determine the financial feasibility of this project if this were a taxpaying entity with a tax rate of 40 percent. (*Hint: see Appendix E*. Since the hospital is depreciating to the salvage value, there is no tax effect on the sale of the asset.)

18. Fall City Healthcare System, a non-taxpaying entity, is going to build a satellite ancillary facility. The tests will generate $15,000,000 per year in revenues for the next five years. The expected operating expenses, excluding depreciation, will increase expenses by $8,000,000 per year for the next five years. The initial cost for the building is $25,000,000, which will be depreciated on a straight-line basis to its salvage value. The salvage value at year 5 is $5,000,000. The cost of capital for this project is 9 percent.

    a. Compute the net present value and internal rate of return to determine the financial feasibility of this project.

    b. Compute the net present value and internal rate of return to determine the financial feasibility of this project if this were a taxpaying entity with a tax rate of 35 percent. (*Hint: see Appendix E*. Since the organization is depreciating to the salvage value, there is no tax effect on the sale of the asset.)

19. Due to rising fuel prices, Eastern Community Hospital wants to replace its existing fleet of ambulances with a more fuel-efficient fleet. The existing fleet was purchased three years ago for $150,000 and is being depreciated on a straight-line basis over an eight-year life to zero salvage value. Though the current book value for the existing fleet is $93,750, this fleet could only be sold for $80,000 today. The new fleet would cost $250,000 and would be depreciated on a straight-line basis over a five-year life to a zero salvage value. The new fleet would reduce fuel costs by $80,000 per year for five years and would not affect the level of net working capital. The economic life of the new fleet is five years and the required rate of return on the project is 5 percent.

    a. Should the existing fleet of ambulances be replaced? Use the incremental NPV approach to evaluate the decision under a non-profit assumption.

    b. If the facility were a taxpaying entity with a tax rate of 40 percent, should the existing fleet be replaced? Use the incremental NPV approach to evaluate the decision. (*Hint: see Appendix F*.)

20. Because of a rise in chart requests complicated by constant turnover within the Medical Records Department, Valley Regional wants to replace its existing medical records system with a labor saving optical disk version. The existing system, which has a current book value of $75,000, was purchased three years ago for $120,000 and is being depreciated on a straight-line basis over an eight-year life to zero salvage value. This system could be sold for $65,000 today. The new optical system would reduce the need for staff by three people per year for five years at a savings of $25,000 per person per year; however, it would require additional part-time programming costs to maintain the system at $15,000 per year. The project would not affect the level of net working capital. The new optical system would cost $300,000 and would be depreciated on a straight-line basis over a five-year life to a zero salvage value. The economic life of the new system is five years and the required rate of return on the project is 6 percent.

    a. Should the existing medical records system be replaced? Use the incremental NPV approach to evaluate the decision under a non-profit assumption.

    b. If the facility were a taxpaying entity with a tax rate of 40 percent, should the existing system be replaced? Use the incremental NPV approach to evaluate the decision. (*Hint: see Appendix F.*)

21. Washington Federal Hospital plans to invest in a new X-ray machine. The cost of the machine is $800,000. The machine has an economic life of seven years, and it will be depreciated over a seven-year life to a $100,000 salvage value. Additional revenues attributed to the new machine will amount to $600,000 per year for seven years. Additional operating costs, excluding depreciation expense, will amount to $400,000 per year for seven years. Over the life of the machine, net working capital will increase by $50,000 per year for seven years.

    a. Assuming Washington Federal is a non-taxpaying entity, what is the project's NPV at a discount rate of 7 percent, and what is the project's IRR?

    b. Assuming Washington Federal is a taxpaying entity and its tax rate is 40 percent, what is the project's NPV at a discount rate of 7 percent, and what is the project's IRR? (*Hint: see Appendices C, D, and E.*)

22. Lima Radiological Services has seen a growth in patient volume since its primary competitor decided to relocate to a different area of the city. To accommodate this growth, a consultant has advised that Lima invest in a new SPECT imaging system. The cost to implement the system would be $1,000,000. The useful life of this equipment is typically about seven years, and it will be depreciated over a seven-year life to a $160,000 salvage value. Additional patient volume will yield $1,200,000 in new revenues the first year, and revenues will increase by $50,000 each year thereafter, but the system is expensive to operate. Additional staff and variable costs, excluding depreciation expense, will come to $950,000 annually, but these expenses will rise by $60,000 every year. Over the life of the machine, net working capital will increase by $15,000 per year for seven years.

    a. Assuming Lima Radiological Services is a non-taxpaying entity, what is the project's NPV at a discount rate of 8 percent, and what is the project's IRR?

    b. Assuming Lima Radiological Services is a taxpaying entity and its tax rate is 35 percent, what is the project's NPV at a discount rate of 8 percent, and what is the project's IRR? (*Hint: see Appendices C, D and E.*)

23. Nimble Nursing Homes, Inc. owns an abandoned schoolhouse. The after tax value of the land is $600,000. The furniture and fixtures of the school have been fully depreciated to an after tax market value of $50,000. The two options Nimble faces are either to sell the land and furniture/fixtures, or to convert the building into a nursing home. To refurbish and renovate the facility would cost $30 million. The new building and equipment would be depreciated on a straight-line basis over a ten-year life to a $5 million salvage value. At the end of ten years, the land could be sold for an after tax value of $3 million. The new long-term care facility will have the pro forma income statement listed below for the next ten years. Net working capital will increase at a rate of $200,000 per year over the life of the project. Nimble Nursing Homes, Inc. has a 30 percent tax rate and has a required rate of return of 7 percent. Use both the NPV technique and IRR method to evaluate this project. (*Hint: see Appendices C, D and E.*)

Pro Forma Income Statement	Years 1–3	Years 4–10
Patient revenues	$5.0 million/year	$7.0 million/year
Operating expenses (includes depreciation expense)	$4.0 million/year	$5.0 million/year
Earnings before taxes	$1.0 million/year	$2.0 million/year
Less taxes (30%)	$0.3 million/year	$0.6 million/year
Earnings after taxes	$0.7 million/year	$1.4 million/year

24. Ridgewood Healthcare Enterprises is in possession of a non-operational 70-bed hospital. The after tax value of the land is $500,000. The equipment and the building are fully depreciated and have an after tax market value of $1,250,000. Ridgewood could either sell off its property or convert it into a fully functional nursing home for private-paying residents. An analysis of the market reveals that the facility could easily draw 100 patients per year, which is maximum capacity, at an initial reimbursement of $3,500 per resident per month for the first year, and increasing annually by $100 per month thereafter. Renovation costs to create a plush facility would be $20 million. The new facility would be depreciated on a straight-line basis over a ten-year life to a $2 million salvage value. At the end of ten years, the land is expected to be sold for an after tax value of $1.5 million. Net working capital will increase at a rate of $175,000 per year over the life of the project. Ridgewood has a 35 percent tax rate and has a required rate of return of 9 percent. The pro forma earnings before tax, which includes the deduction for depreciation expense, is projected to be $1,500,000 the first year and increase by $70,000 every year thereafter. Use the NPV technique and IRR method to evaluate this project. (*Hint: see Appendices C, D and E.*)

25. Faith Hospital, a tax-paying entity, wants to replace its current telemedicine system with a new version, which would cost $6 million. This new system has a five-year life and would be depreciated over a straight-line basis to a salvage of $900,000. The current telemedicine system was purchased five years ago for $8 million, has five years remaining on its useful life, and would be depreciated similarly to a salvage of $400,000. This current system could

be sold in the market place right now for $2 million. The new telemedicine system has annual labor operating costs of $25,000, while the current system has annual labor operating costs of $300,000. Neither system will change patient revenues. The hospital has a 40 percent tax rate and required rate of return of 6 percent. The financial analysis will be projected over a five-year period. Use the Net Present Value approach to determine if the new telemedicine system should be selected. (*Hint: see Appendix F.*)

26. Queen Victoria Hospital, a for-profit institution, wants to replace its CT scanner with a new model. The cost of the new CT scanner is $5 million. The current CT scanner was purchased three years ago for $3 million. The new scanner has a five-year life and will be depreciated over a straight-line basis to a salvage of $2 million. The current CT scanner has five years remaining on its life and will be depreciated over a straight-line basis to a salvage value of $1 million. The current scanner could be sold in the marketplace for $2.5 million. The new scanner is expected to generate annual cash labor savings of $500,000 per year relative to the current scanner. Neither system will change patient revenues. The hospital has a 40 percent tax rate and required rate of return of 5 percent. The financial analysis will project over a five-year period. Use the Net Present Value approach to determine if the new CT scanner should be selected. (*Hint: see Appendix F.*)

27. Alvin Hospital, a taxpaying entity, is considering a new pediatrics emergency room (ER). The building and equipment for the new pediatric ER will cost $10 million. The equipment and building will be depreciated on a straight-line basis over the project's five-year life to a $1 million salvage value. The pediatric ER projected net revenue and expenses are as follows. Net revenues are expected to be $4 million the first year and will grow by 12 percent each year thereafter. The operating expenses, which exclude interest and depreciation expenses, will be $2 million the first year and are expected to grow annually by 3 percent for every year after that. Interest expense will be $1 million per year, while principal payments on the loan will be $2.7 million a year. The new pediatric ER is expected to generate additional after tax cash flows of $0.5 million from radiology and other ancillary services, which will grow at an annual rate of 5 percent per year for every year after that. Starting in year 1, net working capital will increase by $1.5 million per year for the first four years, but during the last year of the project, net working capital will decrease by $1.5 million. The tax rate for the hospital is 40 percent and its cost of capital is 15 percent. Use the Net Present Value and IRR approach to determine if this project should be undertaken. (*Hint, see Appendix C and E.*)

28. Blackmoore Radiology, a taxpaying entity, is considering a new outpatient-imaging center. The building and equipment for the new center will cost $40 million. The equipment and building will be depreciated on a straight-line basis over its five-year life to a $10 million salvage value. The new imaging center's projected net revenue and expenses are listed below. The project will be financed partially by debt capital. Interest expense is expected to be $2 million per year while principal payments on the bank loan are expected to be $1.5 million per year for the first five years of the loan. The new outpatient-imaging center is expected to take after tax cash profits of $1 million per year away from

the inpatient imaging. The tax rate for the institution is 40 percent and its cost of capital is 10 percent. Two years ago, a $100,000 financial feasibility study was conducted and paid for. Pro forma working capital projections are listed below. These are the permanent account balances for inventory, accounts receivable and accounts payable. Use the net present value and internal rate of return approaches to determine if this project should be undertaken? (*Hint: see Appendices C and E.*)

Pro forma income statement before tax projections for outpatient-imaging center (in thousands):

Year	1	2	3	4	5
Net revenues	$12,000	$14,000	$19,000	$30,000	$40,000
Operating expenses	$5,000	$6,000	$7,000	$7,500	$8,000
Depreciation expense	$6,000	$6,000	$6,000	$6,000	$6,000
Interest expense	$2,000	$2,000	$2,000	$2,000	$2,000

Pro forma working capital for outpatient-imaging center (in thousands):

Year	1	2	3	4	5
Inventory/accounts receivable	$4,500	$9,000	$13,500	$11,500	$9,500
Accounts payable	$500	$1,000	$1,500	$2,000	$2,500

Appendix C

Technical Concerns Regarding Net Present Value

This appendix addresses three commonly asked questions about performing a net present value analysis: 1) determining the amount of the initial investment; 2) determining the annual cash flows; and 3) determining a discount rate.

Determining the Amount of the Initial Investment

Included Costs

Expenditures for plant, property, and equipment are usually the primary initial investment items in a capital project. The amount recorded for these items is the purchase price plus all costs related to making the investment "ready to go," including labor, renovation of space, rewiring, transportation, and any investment in working capital (cash, inventory).

Along with these relatively tangible costs, the initial investment should include any additional planning costs incurred specifically for the project *after* it has been selected. General planning costs to decide which capital project to undertake are not included, for they are **sunk costs** (those costs incurred *before* a specific project has been selected).

The final category of costs to include in the initial cost estimate is the **opportunity cost**, which are proceeds lost by forgoing other opportunities. For example, suppose a health care facility has a plot of land it is holding for investment purposes. It can either sell the land for $150,000 or use it to build a long-term care facility. If it builds on the land, it will be losing $150,000 from the new

Opportunity Costs: Lost proceeds by forgoing or delaying other opportunities.

facility: even though no cash is changing hands yet, losing the chance to collect $150,000 is a real cost to the organization. Thus, $150,000 would be included as part of the initial outlay as an opportunity cost or a cash outflow if the organization chose to build.

Excluded Costs

In an NPV analysis, several categories of costs should explicitly *not* be included as part of the initial investment costs. For example, though the purchase price of assets should be included in the initial cost, interest paid from borrowing money to finance those assets should not be included because interest costs are financing flows and are reflected in the cost of capital.

Sunk Costs: Costs incurred in the past. They should not be included in NPV-type analyses.

Costs that have already occurred in the past are sunk costs and should not be included in the analysis. For example, $50,000 *already* spent by the health care organization to renovate a building should not be included as part of the cost for a new project. The initial investment should only include the cost of plant, property, and equipment; investment in working capital; additional planning costs; and opportunity costs (see Exhibit C–1).

Determining the Annual Cash Flows

An NPV analysis is designed to analyze the relationship between an initial investment and the **incremental cash flows** resulting from that investment in the future. There are three types of incremental cash flows: operating, spillover, and non-regular.

Incremental Cash Flows: Cash flows that occur solely as a result of a particular action such as undertaking a project.

Operating Cash Flows

Incremental operating cash flows are the new, ongoing cash flows that occur solely as a result of undertaking a project. They include payments received for services rendered, and expenditures for such things as labor, materials, marketing, utilities, and taxes. Excluded from NPV analyses are principal and interest payments made on loans to finance the project, as well as any dividends that may result from the project. The purpose of maintaining this separation is to assess whether a project can generate enough positive cash flows from operations on its own merits to pay off its financing costs (interest, principal payments, and dividends) or costs of capital.

Key Point   Operating flows are kept separate from financing flows. Operating cash flows include: Revenues, Labor Expenses, Supply Expenses. Financing cash flows include: interest expenses, principal payments, dividends.

Key Point   If a facility is a for-profit organization, a project's positive net cash flows also entail tax payments according to the organization's tax rate. Therefore, operating cash flows are calculated *after tax*. Appendix E provides a detailed example of how to generate appropriate cash flows for taxable entities.

Exhibit C–1   Initial Costs of an investment

Included Costs

- Plant, property, and equipment, and related preparation costs
- Additional planning costs
- Opportunity costs

Excluded Costs

- Interest costs
- Sunk costs

To realize these flows under the cash basis of accounting, the revenue and expense accounts are converted to a cash basis by changes in net working capital. These adjustments are discussed under the example for computing cash flows in Appendix D.

Spillover Cash Flows

Cannibalization: When a new service decreases the revenues from other services or service lines. These are considered cash outflows.

Spillover cash flows, which can be classified into two types, are increases or decreases in cash flows that occur elsewhere in an organization if a project is undertaken. The first type occurs when a new service produces additional cash flows to other departments. For example, if a facility were expanding its emergency room department, additional revenues could be generated by ancillary support services, such as radiology or laboratory. The second type occurs when a new service diminishes cash flows elsewhere, sometimes called **cannibalization**. For example, if a facility were evaluating the development of an outpatient diagnostic center, it would have to consider the expected loss in cash flows for the existing inpatient diagnostic center. This loss in cash profits for inpatient services is a cash outflow.

Non-regular Cash Flows and Terminal Value Cash Flows

Operating Cash Flows: Cash flows that occur on a regular basis, oftentimes following implementation of a project. Also called regular cash flows.

As opposed to **operating cash flows**, which by definition occur on a regular basis, **non-regular cash flows** are incremental cash flows that typically occur on an irregular basis, typically at the end of the life of a project. One of the most common non-regular cash flows is salvage value, the money received from selling an asset at the termination of a project. Another typical cash flow at the end of project life is recovery of working capital, which is typically a cash inflow. Cash flows to be included or excluded are described in Exhibit C–2. The recovery of working capital is discussed in detail in Appendix D.

Accuracy of Cash Flow Estimates

Because cash flows occur at some point in the future, they cannot be measured precisely. Expected revenues or projected cost savings can only be estimated based upon a market analysis and the current operations of the organization. Unforeseeable events, such as new competition

Exhibit C–2 The Components of Incremental Cash Flow

Included Items	Excluded Items
Operating Cash Flows • Revenues in the form of payments (inflows) • Cash payments for labor, supplies, utilities, marketing, and taxes (outflows)	*Existing Cash Flows Not Affected by the Project Being Considered* • Revenues already being generated by an existing service
Spillover Cash Flows • Effects of a new service on other departments, such as ancillary services (inflows) • Effects of a new service's cannibalizing similar existing services (outflows)	*Financing-related Items* • Interest • Principal payments • Dividends
Non-regular Cash Flows (terminal value cash flows) • Salvage value of equipment that will be sold at the end of a project (inflow) • Recovery of working capital (inflow)	**Adjusted Items** *Accrual-based Items* • Revenues earned but not received in cash • Expenses recognized but no cash expended (i.e. depreciation, accrued expenses) *Other* • Changes in net working capital

or an unexpected rise in energy prices, could significantly cut back on positive cash inflows. On the other hand, an investment such as a convenient new visitor parking deck may be so popular that it draws in unexpected patient volume, which would increase revenues. Given that the future cash flows must be present in order to offset the cost of the initial investment, marked variation in these could alter the final net present value decision.

Non-regular Cash Flows: Cash flows that occur sporadically or on an irregular basis. A common non-regular cash flow is salvage value, receipt of funds following a one-time sale of an asset at the end of its useful life.

Determining a Discount Rate

Although commonly thought of as an adjustment for the time value of money, the discount rate also accounts for the effect of project risk. The discount rate or cost of capital is the required rate of return for investors who fund the project to compensate them for the risk of the investment opportunity and the temporary loss of funds to be used elsewhere. To estimate the required rate of return for investment projects with risk similar to the current risk of the health care organization, a facility can use its current cost of capital. This is the rate an organization currently pays for its use of debt and equity financing. However, it should adjust the cost of capital to a higher (lower) value if the risk of the project is higher (lower) than the overall risk of the health care organization. The determination of precise models to estimate cost of capital is technical and beyond the scope of this text.

Key Point

The **discount rate** is also called the **opportunity cost of capital** to the company undertaking the capital investment project. It is the cost of the next best alternative, those returns the company is forgoing by making this investment as opposed to another. From the lenders' or investors' points of view, it is the returns they forgo by investing their money in this project rather than alternative projects of similar risk. For example, if an investor-owned hospital chain were issuing stock to purchase a health insurance business, investors considering buying this stock would expect at least the return on the stocks of other publicly held health insurance companies, such as Cigna or Aetna.

Appendix D

Adjustments for Net Working Capital

To the extent that new projects impact working capital, adjustments in cash flows must be made. If working capital increases, then the organization has invested additional resources in working capital; that is, the project requires the organization to increase both current asset accounts, which result in cash outflows, and current liability accounts, which are cash inflows, since they delay the use of cash (example below). The difference between current assets and current liabilities is called **net working capital**, as discussed in Chapter 5. The effects of changes in net working capital, it must be accounted for each year. If there is an increase in net working capital, it is subtracted from net operating cash flows. Likewise, if there is a decrease, it is added to net operating cash flows.

An illustration of how to adjust for changes in net working capital is shown by continuing with the example of building a satellite hospital. Assume the organization had balance sheet results as shown in rows 7–9 of Exhibit D–1. As shown in row 9, its net working capital (current assets − current liabilities) is $1,000, $1,300, $1,800, $600, $400, and $300 in years 1–6, respectively.

The change in net working capital is the difference between the current year's net working capital and that from the previous year (row 10). For example, the change in net working capital the first year was $1,000 ($1,000 in Year 1 − $0 in Year 0). The second year's change in net working capital was $300 ($1,300 in Year 2 − $1,000 in Year 1). The same procedure is followed for Years 3–6. As noted earlier, if net working capital increased, then cash decreased, which

Exhibit D-1 Computation of Net Present Value for a Satellite Hospital, Including Working Capital Adjustments

Givens:	Years	0	1	2	3	4	5	6
1 Initial Investment		($1,000,000)						
2 Net Revenues			$400,000	$550,000	$800,000	$900,000	$1,100,000	$1,370,000
3 Cash Operating Expenses			200,000	300,000	500,000	550,000	650,000	850,000
4 Depreciation Expense			145,000	145,000	145,000	145,000	145,000	145,000
5 Sale of Assets								130,000
6 Cost of Capital	10%							
7 Current Assets			$2,200	$4,800	$7,400	$1,400	$1,300	$1,200
8 Current Liabilities			$1,200	$3,500	$5,600	$800	$900	$900
9 Net Working Capital	[Given 7 – Given 8]	$0	$1,000	$1,300	$1,800	$600	$400	$300
10 Change in Net Working Capital	[1]		$1,000	$300	$500	($1,200)	($200)	($100)

[1] Net Working Capital (Current Year) – Net Working Capital (Previous Year)

Net Present Value for Satellite Hospital, Adjusting for Depreciation, Working Capital and Salvage Value

	Years	0	1	2	3	4	5	6
A Initial Investment	[Given 1]	($1,000,000)						
B Net Revenues	[Given 2]		$400,000	$550,000	$800,000	$900,000	$1,100,000	$1,370,000
C Less: Cash Operating Expenses Before Depreciation	[Given 3]		200,000	300,000	500,000	550,000	650,000	850,000
D Less: Depreciation Expense	[Given 4]		145,000	145,000	145,000	145,000	145,000	145,000
E Operating Income	[B – C – D]		55,000	105,000	155,000	205,000	305,000	375,000
F Add: Depreciation Expense	[Given 4]		145,000	145,000	145,000	145,000	145,000	145,000
G Net Operating Cash Flows	[E + F]		200,000	250,000	300,000	350,000	450,000	520,000
H Add: Sale of Assets	[Given 5]							130,000
I Adjustments for changes in working capital	[– Given 10]		(1,000)	(300)	(500)	1,200	200	100
J Recapture of net working capital	[– Sum]		—	—	—	—	—	300
K Project Cash Flows	[G + H + I + J]		$199,000	$249,700	$299,500	$351,200	$450,200	$650,400
L Cost of Capital	[Given 6]		10%	10%	10%	10%	10%	10%
M Present Value Interest Factors	$1/(1 + I)^n$		0.9091	0.8264	0.7513	0.6830	0.6209	0.5645
N Annual PV of Cash Flows[2]	[K × M]		$180,909	$206,364	$225,019	$239,874	$279,539	$367,134
O PV of Cash Flows	[Sum N]	$1,498,838						
P Net Present Value	[A + O]	$498,838						

[2] Present Value Interest Factors in the exhibit have been calculated by formula, but are necessarily rounded for presentation. Therefore, there may be a difference between the number displayed and that calculated manually.

must be subtracted from the cash flows. If net working capital decreased, then cash increased, and that amount must be added to cash flows. Since net working capital increased by $1,000 in year 1 (row 10), $1,000 (row I) is subtracted from the net operating cash flows (row G). This process is continued for the remaining years.

In the first three years, cash outflows occurred and net working capital for the project increased (row 10). But in Year 4 and thereafter, the decreases in net working capital constitute cash inflows for the years. The facility is no longer investing cash in its current assets and liabilities. It is decreasing its investment in cash, collecting at a higher rate on its receivables, and/or reducing its outstanding payables.

Key Point   Increases in net working capital are cash *outflows*. Decreases in net working capital are cash *inflows*.

Key Point   Interest-bearing, short-term debt (notes payable) should be excluded from calculations of changes in net working capital because it represents financing flows and is accounted for in the cost of capital.

Once the changes in net working capital are calculated, they are entered into the NPV calculation to adjust for changes in cash flows due to changes in net working capital (rows I, J).

When a project ends, it is assumed that: 1) the total amount of net working capital investment is recaptured and is accounted for as a cash inflow; and 2) plant and equipment will be sold or disposed of. In regard to the recapture of net working capital, typically all project receivables are collected, all project inventory is sold, and all project payables are paid. The recapture of changes in net working capital is the sum of all the changes in net working capital during the life of the project, which, in the case of the satellite hospital, is –$300 [($1,000)+ ($300)+ ($500)+ $1,200+ $200+ $100]. The negative $300 indicates that there is an ending excess balance of $300 in net working capital to sell off; therefore, $300 in net working capital is a cash inflow that can be recaptured or recovered (see Exhibit D–1, row J).

Appendix E

Tax Implications for For-profits in a Capital Budgeting Decision, and the Adjustment for Interest Expense

This appendix introduces an NPV analysis for a for-profit entity. The total number of for-profit hospitals in the United States at the turn of the century represented less than 15 percent of the total number of short-term community hospitals. In contrast, there were more than 7,000 skilled and intermediate-care nursing homes nationwide, of which more than two-thirds were for-profit entities. Also, more than two-thirds of the managed-care insurers were taxpaying entities. Therefore, it is imperative to consider the tax effects that can take place in a for-profit investment analysis. Appendix C discussed the separation of financing flows from the operating cash flow analysis for an NPV analysis. When computing a cash flow analysis from a projected income statement, interest expense needs to be taken out to be able to adjust for the tax effect if the entity is for-profit. The following analysis shows the calculations had the satellite hospital project been a for-profit endeavor.

The two most important tax adjustments that must be made for for-profit entities are: 1) accounting for the effect of taxes on operating income; and 2) accounting for the tax effect from the gains/losses resulting from the sale of assets at the expected end of the project's life. This example focuses only on the first, since gains and losses, like most other tax effects, are complicated and only introduced in this text.

As evidenced in Exhibit E–1, the analysis is nearly identical to that for not-for-profit entities (Exhibit D–1), except for the tax expense and interest expense accounts, and the inclusion of a new line for payment of taxes (Exhibit E–1, row G, which assumes that the organization has a 40 percent tax rate on its net income). In Year 1, the organization had earnings before taxes of $30,000 (row F). Since the tax rate is 40 percent, it must pay an additional $12,000 in taxes ($30,000 × 0.40). In Year 2, it pays $32,000 in taxes on earnings before tax of $ 80,000 (rows F and G). A similar analysis is conducted for Years 3–6.

At this point, an adjustment must be made for interest, because interest expense affected net income (and thus the amount of taxes paid), but interest expense is not itself an operating cash flow. Thus, interest expense must be *added back* at the amount of (1 − tax rate) to determine true cash outflows. This is done in row J, where $15,000 is added back ($25,000 × (1 − 0.40)). In effect, the interest expense provided a *tax deduction* of $10,000 ($25,000 × 0.40 saved), which represents a cash inflow. Thus, the true cash outflow is only $15,000 ($25,000 − $10,000), which matches the value in row J. For non-profit entities with interest expense in the projected income statement, the full amount of the interest expense is added back in because the tax rate is zero. The remainder of the analysis remains the same. Overall, the net present value for the hospital as a taxpaying entity equals $181,116 (row T) versus $498,838 as a not-for-profit hospital (Exhibit D–1, row P), which is much less.

Appendix F

Comprehensive Capital Budgeting Replacement Cost Example

Assume that a cardiology laboratory is considering replacing its manual EKG (electrocardiogram) management information system with a new, more efficient one. The new system automatically stores EKG and stress records online. The existing system was purchased five years ago for $70,000 and is being depreciated over a ten-year life to a salvage value of $10,000. The old system can be sold now at a market price of $20,000 and has a book value of $40,000 ($70,000 original cost − $30,000 accumulated depreciation). The new system can be purchased for $100,000 and is estimated to have a five-year life. It can be depreciated to a salvage value of $20,000. Since the organization is paid on a capitated basis, there are no revenues directly associated with the EKG. Thus, the focus is on the cash savings in operational expenses. Labor expenses will drop from $50,000 for the old system to $15,000 with the new system, resulting in a labor cash savings of $35,000. Purchasing the new system will increase net working capital by $1,000 each year, compared to a $300 annual increase for the old system, starting in Year 1. The remainder of this appendix provides comparative and incremental NPV analyses of this situation, first assuming that the lab is not-for-profit, and then assuming that it is investor-owned. In both cases, the cost of capital is 5 percent.

Exhibit E-1 NPV Decision Assuming Satellite Hospital Is For-profit

Givens:	Years	0	1	2	3	4	5	6
1 Initial Investment		($1,000,000)						
2 Net Revenues			$400,000	$550,000	$800,000	$900,000	$1,100,000	$1,370,000
3 Cash Operating Expenses			$200,000	$300,000	$500,000	$550,000	$650,000	$850,000
4 Depreciation Expense			$145,000	$145,000	$145,000	$145,000	$145,000	$145,000
5 Interest Expense			$25,000	$25,000	$25,000	$25,000	$25,000	$25,000
6 Sale of Assets								$130,000
7 Cost of Capital	10%							
8 Tax Rate	40%							
9 Current Assets			$2,200	$4,800	$7,400	$1,400	$1,300	$1,200
10 Current Liabilities			$1,200	$3,500	$5,600	$800	$900	$900
11 Net Working Capital	[Given 9 – Given 10]	$0	$1,000	$1,300	$1,800	$600	$400	$300
12 Change in Net Working Capital	[1]		$1,000	$300	$500	($1,200)	($200)	($100)

[1] Net Working Capital (Current Year) – Net Working Capital (Previous Year)

(Continues)

Exhibit E-1 (Contd)

Net Present Value for Satellite Hospital, Adjusting for Depreciation, Interest, Working Capital and Salvage Value

	Years	0	1	2	3	4	5	6
A Initial Investment	[Given 1]	($1,000,000)						
B Net Revenues	[Given 2]		$400,000	$550,000	$800,000	$900,000	$1,100,000	$1,370,000
C Less: Cash Operating Expenses Before Dep. & Int.	[Given 3]		$200,000	$300,000	$500,000	$550,000	$650,000	$850,000
D Less: Depreciation Expense	[Given 4]		$145,000	$145,000	$145,000	$145,000	$145,000	$145,000
E Less: Interest Expense	[Given 5]		$25,000	$25,000	$25,000	$25,000	$25,000	$25,000
F Earnings Before Taxes	[B – C – D – E]		30,000	80,000	130,000	180,000	280,000	350,000
G Less: Tax Expense (40% Tax Rate)	[Given 8 × F]		12,000	32,000	52,000	72,000	112,000	140,000
H Earnings After Tax	[F – G]		18,000	48,000	78,000	108,000	168,000	210,000
I Add Depreciation Expense	[Given 4]		145,000	145,000	145,000	145,000	145,000	145,000
J Add Back Interest Expense at (1-Tax Rate)	[(1 – Given 8) × E]		15,000	15,000	15,000	15,000	15,000	15,000
K Net Operating Cash Flow	[H + I + J]		178,000	208,000	238,000	268,000	328,000	370,000
L Add: Sale Of Assets[2]	[Given 6]							130,000
M Adjustments For Changes In Working Capital	[– Given 12]		(1,000)	(300)	(500)	1,200	200	100
N Recapture Of Net Working Capital	[– Sum M]							300
O Project Cash Flows	[K + L + M + N]		$177,000	$207,700	$237,500	$269,200	$328,200	$500,400
P Cost Of Capital	[Given 7]		10%	10%	10%	10%	10%	10%
Q Present Value Interest Factors	$1/(1 + i)^n$		0.9091	0.8264	0.7513	0.6830	0.6209	0.5645
R Annual PV Of Cash Flows[3]	[O × Q]		$160,909	$171,653	$178,437	$183,867	$203,786	$282,463
S PV Of Cash Flows	[Sum R]	$1,181,116						
T Net Present Value	[A + S]	$181,116						

[2] There is no tax effect from selling the asset, because it was depreciated to the salvage value; therefore, salvage value equals book value.

[3] Present Value Interest Factors in the exhibit have been calculated by formula, but are necessarily rounded for presentation. Therefore, there may be a difference between the number displayed and that calculated manually.

Comparative Approach – Not-for-profit Analysis

As its name implies, the comparative approach compares the cash flows resulting from continuing with the existing alternative to those that would result if the equipment were replaced. It does this by separately calculating each of these cash flows and then comparing them (Exhibit F–1).

If the organization were to continue with the existing system, there would be no investment at Year 0 (it has already been made), and the operating loss would be $56,000 a year (row D), which includes operating expenses (row B) and depreciation (row C). However, since operating loss contains depreciation, and depreciation is an expense that does not require a cash outlay, depreciation must be added back in order to derive cash flows from operations. This is done in row F by adding $6,000 (row E) to the $56,000 operating loss (row D). Though the same result, $50,000 (row F), can be derived without first subtracting out and then adding back in depreciation expense, this approach is used to make it easier to compare the not-for-profit and for-profit analyses. In regard to the change in net working capital, since it increases by $300 each year, the resultant cash outflow must be accounted for (row G). However, as explained in Appendix D, assume that this is recovered at the end of the project (row I). The only other cash flow to account for would be the $10,000 salvage value that results in a cash inflow in Year 5 (row H). Finally, the cash flows are computed for each of the five years (row J), and then discounted using the cost of capital (rows K, L). This information forms the basis to calculate net present value of the cash flows attributable to the existing machine: –$208,762 (row O).

The initial outlay, expenses, depreciation, salvage value, and working capital effects differ for the purchase of the replacement system (Exhibit F–1, lower half). The initial outlay is computed in row A. Though the new equipment costs $100,000, the organization only has to pay $80,000 from its existing funds, since it can allocate $20,000 from the sale of the existing equipment.

Since net working capital increases by $1,000 each year, the resulting cash outflow must be accounted for (rows G, I). The remaining steps in the replacement analysis are the same as those in the previous analysis, and only the amounts differ. Using the comparative approach, the net present value of the replacement alternative is –$129,683 (row O). Thus, since the replacement alternative has a higher NPV (–$129,683 versus –$208,762), the replacement alternative should be undertaken.

Comparative Approach – For-profit Analysis

The for-profit analysis is exactly the same as that for the not-for-profit analysis with two exceptions (Exhibit F–2, rows E and F), which arise as a result of the effects of taxes on cash flows, and ultimately NPV. As in the not-for-profit analysis, earnings (loss) before tax is calculated in row D. Since earnings before tax is taxed at 40 percent, the resulting tax savings would be $22,400 for the existing alternative as compared to $12,400 for the replacement alternative, respectively (rows E, top and bottom). Because earnings before tax is negative, the organization is losing money but will not be incurring negative taxes. However, the tax expense becomes a positive value because this tax loss either can be carried forward to offset future income, or else carried back to offset prior income to result in a tax refund. This has the same effect as a cash inflow: for each additional $1.00 in expenses, the organization pays $0.40 *less* in taxes. Therefore, these tax savings get *added back* to the loss in row D. Taking into account the tax effects, the NPV of the existing alternative is -$111,782, and the NPV of the replacement alternative is –$67,998. Again, showing a smaller loss, or a saving of $43,784 (row R, bottom table), the replacement alternative should be undertaken, all other things being equal.

Exhibit F-1 Comparative Approach to Analyzing a Capital Budgeting Decision – Not-for-profit Entity

Existing Equipment

Givens:	Years	0	1	2	3	4	5
1 Initial Outlay		$0					
2 Operating Expenses			($50,000)	($50,000)	($50,000)	($50,000)	($50,000)
3 Depreciation Expense			($6,000)	($6,000)	($6,000)	($6,000)	($6,000)
4 Change in Net Working Capital			300	300	300	300	300
5 Salvage Value							$10,000
6 Cost of Capital	5%						

		Years	0	1	2	3	4	5
A Initial Outlay	[Given 1]		$0					
B Operating Expenses Before Depreciation	[Given 2]			($50,000)	($50,000)	($50,000)	($50,000)	($50,000)
C Depreciation Expense	[Given 3]			($6,000)	($6,000)	($6,000)	($6,000)	($6,000)
D Operating Income (loss)	[B + C]			(56,000)	(56,000)	(56,000)	(56,000)	(56,000)
E Add: Depreciation Expense	[− Given 3]			6,000	6,000	6,000	6,000	6,000
F Net Operating Cash Flow	[D + E]			(50,000)	(50,000)	(50,000)	(50,000)	(50,000)
G Change in Net Working Capital	[− Given 4]			(300)	(300)	(300)	(300)	(300)
Terminal Value Changes:								
H Salvage Value	[Given 5]							10,000
I Recovery of Net Working Capital	[− Sum G]							1,500
J Change in Net Cash Flow	[F + G + H + I]			($50,300)	($50,300)	($50,300)	($50,300)	($38,800)
K Cost of Capital	[Given 6]			5%	5%	5%	5%	5%
L Present Value Interest Factor	$1/(1 + i)^n$			0.9524	0.9070	0.8638	0.8227	0.7835
M Annual PV Of Cash Flows[1]	[J × L]			($47,905)	($45,624)	($43,451)	($41,382)	($30,401)
N Sum of PV of Cash Flows	[Sum M]	($208,762)						
O Net Present Value	[A + N]	($208,762)						

(Continues)

Exhibit F–1 (*Contd*)

Replacement Equipment

Givens:	Years	0	1	2	3	4	5
1 Initial Outlay[2]	[2]	($80,000)					
2 Operating Expenses			($15,000)	($15,000)	($15,000)	($15,000)	($15,000)
3 Depreciation Expense			($16,000)	($16,000)	($16,000)	($16,000)	($16,000)
4 Change in Net Working Capital			1,000	1,000	1,000	1,000	1,000
5 Salvage Value							$20,000
6 Cost of Capital	5%						

	Years	0	1	2	3	4	5
A Initial Outlay[2]	[Given 1]	($80,000)					
B Operating Expenses Before Depreciation	[Given 2]		($15,000)	($15,000)	($15,000)	($15,000)	($15,000)
C Depreciation Expense	[Given 3]		($16,000)	($16,000)	($16,000)	($16,000)	($16,000)
D Operating Income (loss)	[B + C]		(31,000)	(31,000)	(31,000)	(31,000)	(31,000)
E Add: Depreciation Expense	[– Given 3]		16,000	16,000	16,000	16,000	16,000
F Net Operating Cash Flow	[D + E]		(15,000)	(15,000)	(15,000)	(15,000)	(15,000)
G Change in Net Working Capital	[– Given 4]		(1,000)	(1,000)	(1,000)	(1,000)	(1,000)
Terminal Value Changes:							
H Salvage Value	[Given 5]						20,000
I Recovery of Net Working Capital	[– Sum G]						5,000
J Change in Net Cash Flow	[F + G + H + I]		($16,000)	($16,000)	($16,000)	($16,000)	$9,000
K Cost of Capital	[Given 6]		5%	5%	5%	5%	5%
L Present Value Interest Factor	$1/(1+i)^n$		0.9524	0.9070	0.8638	0.8227	0.7835
M Annual PV Of Cash Flows[1]	[J × L]		($15,238)	($14,512)	($13,821)	($13,163)	$7,052
N Sum of PV of Cash Flows	[Sum M]	($49,683)					
O Net Present Value	[A + N]	($129,683)					
P NPV Difference[3]	[3]	$79,079					

[1] Present Value Interest Factors in the exhibit have been calculated by formula, but are necessarily rounded for presentation. Therefore, there may be a difference between the number displayed and that calculated manually.

[2] – $100,000 purchase of new equipment + $20,000 sale of old equipment

[3] ($129,683) – ($208,762) = $79,079

Exhibit F-2 Comparative Approach to Analyzing a Capital Budgeting Decision – For-profit Entity

Existing Equipment

Givens:	Years	0	1	2	3	4	5
1 Initial Outlay		$0					
2 Operating Expenses			($50,000)	($50,000)	($50,000)	($50,000)	($50,000)
3 Depreciation Expense			($6,000)	($6,000)	($6,000)	($6,000)	($6,000)
4 Change in Not Working Capital			300	300	300	300	300
5 Salvage Value							$10,000
6 Cost of Capital	5%						
7 Tax Rate	40%						

Existing Equipment

		Years	0	1	2	3	4	5
A	Initial Outlay	[Given 1]	$0					
B	Operating Expenses Before Depreciation	[Given 2]		($50,000)	($50,000)	($50,000)	($50,000)	($50,000)
C	Depreciation Expense	[Given 3]		($6,000)	($6,000)	($6,000)	($6,000)	($6,000)
D	Earnings (Loss) Before Tax	[B + C]		($56,000)	($56,000)	($56,000)	($56,000)	($56,000)
E	Taxes at 40%	[Given 7 × D]		22,400	22,400	22,400	22,400	22,400
F	Earnings after Tax	[D + E]		(33,600)	(33,600)	(33,600)	(33,600)	(33,600)
G	Add: Depreciation Expense	[– Given 3]		6,000	6,000	6,000	6,000	6,000
H	Net Operating Cash Flow	[F + G]		(27,600)	(27,600)	(27,600)	(27,600)	(27,600)
I	Change in Net Working Capital	[– Given 4]		(300)	(300)	(300)	(300)	(300)
	Terminal Value Changes:							
J	Salvage Value	[Given 5]						10,000
K	Recovery of Net Working Capital	[–Sum I]						1,500
L	Change in Net Cash Flow	[H + I + J + K]		($27,900)	($27,900)	($27,900)	($27,900)	($16,400)
M	Cost of Capital	[Given 6]		5%	5%	5%	5%	5%
N	Present Value Interest Factor	$1/(1 + i)^n$		0.9524	0.9070	0.8638	0.8227	0.7835
O	Annual PV Of Cash Flows[1]	[L × N]		($26,571)	($25,306)	($24,101)	($22,953)	($12,850)
P	Sum of PV of Cash Flows	[Sum O]	($111,782)					
Q	Net Present Value	[A + P]	($111,782)					

(Continues)

Exhibit F–2 (Contd)

Replacement Equipment

Givens:	Years	0	1	2	3	4	5
1 Initial Outlay[2]	[2]	($72,000)					
2 Operating Expenses			($15,000)	($15,000)	($15,000)	($15,000)	($15,000)
3 Depreciation Expense			($16,000)	($16,000)	($16,000)	($16,000)	($16,000)
4 Change in Net Working Capital			$1,000	$1,000	$1,000	$1,000	$1,000
5 Salvage Value							$20,000
6 Cost of Capital	5%						
7 Tax Rate	40%						

Replacement Equipment

	Years	0	1	2	3	4	5
A Initial Outlay[2]	[Given 1]	($72,000)					
B Operating Expenses Before Depreciation	[Given 2]		($15,000)	($15,000)	($15,000)	($15,000)	($15,000)
C Depreciation Expense	[Given 3]		($16,000)	($16,000)	($16,000)	($16,000)	($16,000)
D Earnings Before Tax (Loss Before Tax)	[B + C]		(31,000)	(31,000)	(31,000)	(31,000)	(31,000)
E Taxes at 40%	[Given 7 × D]		12,400	12,400	12,400	12,400	12,400
F Net Income or Earnings after Tax	[D + E]		(18,600)	(18,600)	(18,600)	(18,600)	(18,600)
G Add: Depreciation Expense	[– Given 3]		16,000	16,000	16,000	16,000	16,000
H Net Operating Cash Flow	[F + G]		(2,600)	(2,600)	(2,600)	(2,600)	(2,600)
I Change in Net Working Capital	[– Given 4]		(1,000)	(1,000)	(1,000)	(1,000)	(1,000)
Terminal Value Changes:							
J Salvage Value	[Given 5]						20,000
K Recovery of Net Working Capital	[– Sum I]						5,000
L Change in Net Cash Flow	[H + I + J + K]		($3,600)	($3,600)	($3,600)	($3,600)	$21,400
M Cost of Capital	[Given 6]		5%	5%	5%	5%	5%
N Present Value Interest Factor	$1/(1 + i)^n$		0.9524	0.9070	0.8638	0.8227	0.7835
O Annual PV Of Cash Flows[1]	[L × N]		($3,429)	($3,265)	($3,110)	($2,962)	$16,767
P Sum of PV of Cash Flows	[Sum O]	$4,002					
Q Net Present Value	[A + P]	($67,998)					
R NPV Difference[3]	[3]	43,784					

[1] Present Value Interest Factors in the exhibit have been calculated by formula, but are necessarily rounded for presentation. Therefore, there may be a difference between the number displayed and that calculated manually.

[2] – $100,000 purchase of new equipment + $20,000 sale of old equipment + $8,000 in tax savings from loss on sale of existing equipment (0.40 Tax Rate × $20,000 loss)

[3] ($67,998) – ($111,782) = $43,784

Incremental Approach – Not-for-profit Analysis

Exhibit F–3 analyzes a replacement decision using the incremental approach. It looks at the savings for each item (or lack thereof) that would result if the decision were made to replace the old EKG with a new one. To make this decision, several aspects of cash flows must be taken into account.

To compute the initial outlay, though the new system cost $100,000, the facility received $20,000 for the old system. Thus, the initial outlay is -$80,000 (row A). The change in operating cash flows produced a net operating cash flow savings of $35,000 per year (row B: $15,000 replacement equipment versus $50,000 existing equipment).

As with the comparative analysis, in this non-taxpaying example, depreciation expense could be disregarded altogether, for it has no effect on cash flow. However, to compare the not-for-profit and for-profit examples, operating income is first computed (which is needed to compute taxes in the for-profit example) by subtracting the $10,000 in depreciation expense (row C) and then adding it back in, to show that net operating cash flows do not change as a result of depreciation (row E).

The effects of changes in working capital and the salvage value must be added to the analysis as well. Since net working capital increases by $700 annually, cash flows decrease by $700 each year (row G). In Year 5, the year in which the investment is assumed to end, there is an increase of $10,000 from the salvage value (row H, sale of assets), which equals the incremental difference between the salvage value of the new system, $20,000, and the salvage value of the old system, $10,000. Since the project is assumed to end at this time, it is also necessary to recapture $3,500 in net working capital (row I: 5 years × $700 per year).

To determine the net present value, the cash flows each year are discounted at 5 percent and summed (rows J through O), and then the initial outlay (row A) is added. Since the net present value is $79,079, which represents a positive return due to replacement, from a financial perspective, the new EKG system should be purchased.

Incremental Approach – For-profit Analysis

Exhibit F–4 presents a similar incremental analysis, but for a for-profit, taxpaying organization. In this case, the new initial outlay is still reduced from $100,000 to $80,000 by the additional $20,000 from the sale of the old system, but it is also reduced another $8,000 (to $72,000) by the tax effect of that sale (row 1). This tax benefit arises because the organization is selling a machine with a book value of $40,000 for $20,000, incurring a $20,000 loss. Assuming the tax rate is 40 percent, it will pay $8,000 less in taxes (0.40 × $20,000) than had it not sold the machine.

Taxes also affect operating income and represent a real cash outflow. Since the change in change in earnings before tax is $25,000 (row D), assuming a 40 percent tax rate, taxes will increase by $10,000 (row E), thereby reducing the change in net income to $15,000 (row F). However, reflected in this $15,000 net income is the $10,000 in depreciation expense that does not require a cash outflow. Therefore, it must be added back in, and cash flow becomes $25,000 (rows G, H). The remainder of the analysis remains the same as the not-for-profit analysis, adjusting for the change in net working capital and the terminal value.

After accounting for the sale of the new system at its termination date and discounting at the cost of capital, the decision to make this investment results in a positive net present value of $43,784. Since the NPV is positive, the investment should be made.

Exhibit F–3   Incremental Approach to Analyzing a Capital Budgeting Decision – Not-for-profit Entity

Givens:

1 Initial Outlay[1] ($80,000)
2 Cost of Capital 5%

Change in Annual Operating Expenses & Depreciation Expense:

	Old MIS	New MIS	Change (New–Old)
3 Operating Expenses (labor)	($50,000)	($15,000)	$35,000
4 Depreciation Expense[2]	($6,000)	($16,000)	($10,000)
5 Net Working Capital	($300)	($1,000)	($700)
6 Salvage Value	$10,000	$20,000	$10,000

[1] $100,000 Purchase of New Equipment + $20,000 Sale of Old Equipment
[2] Old MIS: ($70,000 – $10,000)/10 years = $6,000/year
New MIS: ($100,000 – $20,000)/5 years = $16,000/year

Years		0	1	2	3	4	5
A Initial Outlay	[Given 1]	($80,000)					
B Cash Savings Due to Decreased Operating Expenses	[Given 3]		$35,000	$35,000	$35,000	$35,000	$35,000
C Increase in Depreciation Expense	[Given 4]		(10,000)	(10,000)	(10,000)	(10,000)	(10,000)
D Change in Operating Income	[B + C]		25,000	25,000	25,000	25,000	25,000
E Add: Increase in Depreciation Expense	[– Given 4]		10,000	10,000	10,000	10,000	10,000
F Change in Net Operating Cash Flow	[D + E]		35,000	35,000	35,000	35,000	35,000
G Change in Net Working Capital	[Given 5]		(700)	(700)	(700)	(700)	(700)
Terminal Value Changes:							
H Salvage Value	[Given 6]						10,000
I Recovery of Net Working Capital	[– Sum G]						3,500
J Change in Net Cash Flow	[F + G + H + I]		$34,300	$34,300	$34,300	$34,300	$47,800
K Cost of Capital			5%	5%	5%	5%	5%
L Present Value Interest Factor	$1/(1+i)^n$		0.9524	0.9070	0.8638	0.8227	0.7835
M Annual PV of Cash Flows[3]	[J×L]		$32,667	$31,111	$29,630	$28,219	$37,453
N Sum of PV Cash Flows	[Sum M]	$159,079					
O Net Present Value	[A+N]	$79,079					

[3] Present Value Interest Factors in the exhibit have been calculated by formula, but are necessarily rounded for presentation. Therefore, there may be a difference between the number displayed and that calculated manually.

Exhibit F–4 Incremental Approach to Analyzing a Capital Budgeting Decision – For-profit Entity

Givens:

1 Initial Outlay[1]	($72,000)
2 Cost of Capital	5%
3 Tax Rate	40%

Change in Annual Operating Expenses & Depreciation Expense:

	Old MIS	New MIS	Change (New–Old)
4 Operating Expenses (labor)	($50,000)	($15,000)	$35,000
5 Depreciation Expense[2]	($6,000)	($16,000)	($10,000)
6 Net Working Capital	($300)	($1,000)	($700)
7 Salvage Value	$10,000	$20,000	$10,000

[1] ($100,000) purchase of new equipment + $20,000 sale of old equipment + $8,000 (0.40 × $20,000) tax savings due to sale at a loss
[2] Old MIS: ($70,000 – $10,000)/10 years = $6,000/year
New MIS: ($100,000 – $20,000)/5 years = $16,000/year

	Years	0	1	2	3	4	5
A Initial Outlay	[Given 1]	($72,000)					
B Cash Savings Due to Decreased Operating Expenses	[Given 4]		$35,000	$35,000	$35,000	$35,000	$35,000
C Increase in Depreciation Expense[3]	[Given 5]		(10,000)	(10,000)	(10,000)	(10,000)	(10,000)
D Change in Earnings Before Tax	[B + C]		25,000	25,000	25,000	25,000	25,000
E Less: Increased Tax Expense	[Given 3 × D]		10,000	10,000	10,000	10,000	10,000
F Increase in Net Income or Earnings after Tax	[D – E]		15,000	15,000	15,000	15,000	15,000
G Add: Increase in Depreciation Expense	[– Given 5]		10,000	10,000	10,000	10,000	10,000
H Change in Net Operating Cash Flow	[F + G]		25,000	25,000	25,000	25,000	25,000
I Change in Net Working Capital	[Given 6]		(700)	(700)	(700)	(700)	(700)
Terminal Value Changes:							
J Change in Salvage Value	[Given 7]						10,000
K Recovery of Net Working Capital	[– Sum I]						3,500
L Change in Net Cash Flow	[H + I + J + K]		$24,300	$24,300	$24,300	$24,300	$37,800
M Cost of Capital	[Given 2]		5%	5%	5%	5%	5%
N Present Value Interest Factor	$1/(1 + i)^n$		0.9524	0.9070	0.8638	0.8227	0.7835
O Annual PV of Cash Flows[4]	[L × N]		$23,143	$22,041	$20,991	$19,992	$29,617
P Sum of PV Cash Flows	[Sum O]	$115,784					
Q Net Present Value	[A + P]	$43,784					

[3] For Row C, Depreciation expense increased. However, it is an expense and must be deducted from cash savings.
[4] Present Value Interest Factors in the exhibit have been calculated by formula, but are necessarily rounded for presentation. Therefore, there may be a difference between the number displayed and that calculated manually.

Appendix Summary

This appendix provided both a comparative and an incremental NPV analysis of purchasing a new EKG system. The analysis was conducted for both a not-for-profit and a for-profit entity. The summary results are presented in Exhibit F–5, which show that the comparative and incremental approaches provide exactly the same answer. Thus, the method used depends only on preference, but has no effect upon the final result. It is also important to note that in this case, though tax effects are considerable, they do not change the decision.

Exhibit F–5 Results of the Comparative and Incremental NPV Analyses of Replacing an Existing EKG System

	Not-for-profit Institution	For-profit Institution
Replace Equipment	($129,683)[1]	($67,998)[2]
Keep Existing Equipment	($208,762)[1]	($111,782)[2]
Difference (Replace – Keep)	$79,079	$43,784
Incremental Approach	$79,079[3]	$43,784[4]

[1] Exhibit F-1, Comparative Approach
[2] Exhibit F-2, Comparative Approach
[3] Exhibit F-3, Incremental Approach
[4] Exhibit F-4, Incremental Approach

Chapter Eight

CAPITAL FINANCING FOR HEALTH CARE PROVIDERS

LEARNING OBJECTIVES

After completing this chapter, you will be able to:

▶ Describe the types of equity and debt financing.
▶ Define various bond terminology.
▶ Compare tax-exempt with taxable financing.
▶ Explain lease financing.

Chapter Outline

◄INTRODUCTION►

In Chapters 2 and 3, the basic accounting equation was defined as: Assets = Liabilities + Net Assets. Since liabilities are debts and net assets represent the community's equity in a not-for-profit health care organization, in terms of the sources of financing, the basic accounting equation can also be thought of as:

$$\text{Assets} = \text{Debt} + \text{Equity}$$

The equation shows that any increase in assets must be balanced by a similar increase in debt and/or equity. The structuring of debt relative to equity is called the **capital structure decision**, and is becoming increasingly important to both for-profit and not-for-profit providers. This has not always been the case. Until recently, the cost of capital was never a major concern for health care providers.

Like other operational costs, the costs of debt and equity financing were simply passed on to third-party payors. Hospitals had no trouble accessing capital markets because they were virtually guaranteed any income they needed to cover all their debts. Today's environment, however, is characterized by prospective and capitated payments, the increased use of managed care and outpatient services, and increasing cutbacks being forced by competition and cost-control. As a result, obtaining debt and equity financing has become more complicated and risky. Perspectives 8–1 and 8–2 offer additional opinions about equity financing issues and how too much debt can result in bankruptcy.

The first section of this chapter briefly examines equity financing. The remaining sections focus on the issuance of bonds, which is the main source of debt financing for many health care organizations.

> **Bond:** A form of long-term financing whereby an issuer receives cash from a lender (an investor), and in return issues a promissory note (a "bond") agreeing to make principal and/or interest payments on specific dates.

PERSPECTIVE 8–1

Ailing Stocks Land E-Health Companies in Sick Bay

In late 1990s, higher stock prices for growing internet companies enabled them to finance their purchase of other companies by using their stocks as currency for the acquisition. The "e-health" companies were using the Internet to reduce the paperwork among doctors, patients, hospitals, and insurers, and to acquire medical supplies and equipment. However, when stock prices plunged as they did in the year 2000, the acquisition plans of several "e-health" companies faced the possibility of being voted down by stockholders because of lower stock prices. From October 1999 until April 2000, the "e-health" companies of Healtheon/WebMD, TriZetto Group, MedicaLogic, and Neoforma.com saw their stock prices fall by 77%, 73%, 69%, and 82%, respectively. These companies all had several acquisition deals in the works: TriZetto had agreed to buy IMS Health; MedicaLogic had agreed to buy Medscape; Neoforma had agreed to buy Eclipsys; and Healtheon had agreed to buy several companies, including OnHealth Network, Medical Manager, and CareInsite. The reason behind these company mergers was to develop economies of scale and to enhance revenue growth.

Source: Robert McGough and Ann Carrns, *Wall Street Journal,* April 10, 2000, p. c1.

PERSPECTIVE 8–2

The Fall of the House of AHERF: The Allegheny Bankruptcy

On July 21, 1998, Allegheny Health, Education, and Research Foundation (AHERF) filed for bankruptcy in Philadelphia, PA. The Company listed total debt of $1.3 billion and outstanding claims from 65,000 creditors. The $1.3 billion was composed of the following claims: $200 million in loans from Pittsburgh; $497 million owed to suppliers, of which a bankruptcy court will determine how much if any the suppliers receive; and $605 million in bonds. 60 percent of these bonds were insured and will be paid off, while non-insured bonds will be decided upon in bankruptcy court.

The bankruptcy stems from several factors ranging from a lack of fiscal responsibility, poor management decisions, and overpayment of hospital and physician practices. In attempting to horizontally integrate, AHERF purchased hospitals with high capital demands and low profit margins. In attempting to vertically integrate, AHERF overpaid for 310 primary care practices in the Philadelphia area due to competition from other health systems.

To finance the expansions, AHERF used debt financing, but several factors contributed to the decline in cash flow to meet debt service requirements. Specifically: the competitive nature of the Philadelphia market from five major academic medical centers; reimbursement reductions from the Balanced Budget Act of 1997; and lower premium payments from managed care plans.

Source: L. R. Burns, J. Cacciamani, J. Clement, and W. Aquino, *Health Affairs*, Volume 19, number 1, January/ February 2000.

◀EQUITY FINANCING▶

The primary sources of equity financing for not-for-profit health care organizations are internally generated funds, philanthropy, and government grants, whereas the primary sources for for-profit organizations are internally generated funds and stock issuances. Unfortunately, internally generated funds – those funds retained from operations (retained earnings) – are shrinking. As discussed in Chapter 1, financial pressures have lowered revenues and eroded earnings for health care organizations, especially hospitals. However, these organizations still must be able to generate new sources of capital to be able to survive.

Because the equity account on the balance sheet represents the claim on assets, as earnings increase an organization builds its asset base. Typically, the health care organization uses its most liquid assets on the balance sheet (i.e. cash and marketable securities) to finance small capital purchases. But by doing so, an organization incurs an opportunity cost, which represents the lost financial returns from not putting these funds into short- and long-term investments. Assuming these funds are not invested in tax-exempt debt funds, the financial returns from these short and long-term investments are higher than the interest cost on tax-exempt debt. Since tax-exempt debt financing is a cheaper source of capital than equity financing, health care organizations try to minimize their cost of capital by utilizing more debt than equity in their financing decision.

Key Point   Equity financing for not-for-profits is derived from retained earnings, government grants, and contributions. Equity financing for for-profits comes from issuing stock as well as retained earnings.

The Tax Reform Act of 1986 was seen as a major setback for health care providers, because it lowered the tax deduction available to private individuals who wanted to make philanthropic donations. Nevertheless, charitable giving remains a major source of capital for certain health care providers. Although individuals who make contributions do not receive a direct monetary return, they expect non-monetary benefits for the community in terms of greater access to or increased quality of care. As health care providers reach their debt limits, equity financing becomes their only source of new funds. Besides externally generated equity, such as grants and appropriations, which are available to all health care organizations, for-profit organizations (commonly referred to as investor-owned) can also issue stock. Exhibit 8–1 lists selected advantages and disadvantages of issuing stock versus debt financing.

The stock markets generally require a higher rate of return on equity financing (issuing stock) relative to debt financing (issuing bonds). This is due to the greater uncertainty associated with equity relative to debt: organizations are legally required to pay back debt, but there is no legal obligation on the issuer's part to pay back the equity.

◀DEBT FINANCING▶

The major alternative to equity financing is debt financing: borrowing money from others at a cost. The remainder of this chapter describes several types of debt financing, and then describes the process to issue bonds. In the late 1980s hospitals were highly dependent on debt. Perspective 8–3 provides insight on how some non-profit hospital systems used debt financing in the year 2000. Recently, the uncertainty in the health care industry has reduced its access to debt financing.

Sources of Debt Financing by Maturity

The general rule of thumb is to borrow short-term for short-term needs and long-term for long-term needs. Short-term borrowing was discussed in the working cap-

Exhibit 8–1 Comparison of Stock and Debt Financing

	Stock	Debt Financing
Ownership	Gives up ownership to investors	No ownership rights given up
Tax Implications	Dividends are not tax deductible	Interest on debt is deductible
Set Payments	Dividends are not required to be paid	Debt service payments are legally required to be made
Amount of Payments	Dividend payment at the organization's discretion	Debt service payments are legally specified as to amount
Time Limit of Payments	No limit	Time limit is part of borrowing agreement
Restrictions on Other Actions	Indirect through giving up of ownership	May place restrictions on operations and capital acquisition

Key Point *Short-term financing* typically refers to a wide range of financing, from debt that must be paid back almost immediately, to debt that may not have to be paid off for a year. *Long-term financing* typically refers to debt that will be paid off in a period longer than one year.

Sinking Fund: A fund into which monies are set aside each year to ensure that a bond can be liquidated at maturity.

ital chapter. There are two important types of long-term financing: **term loans**, which typically must be paid off within ten years, and **bonds**, which typically can have a maturity of 20–35 years. Bonds are the primary source of long-term financing for tax-exempt health care entities. Term loans, such as bank loans, conventional mortgages, and FHA-issued mortgages, require the borrower to pay off or amortize the principal value of the loan over its life. The amortization of a loan requires equal periodic payments for principal and interest obligations. (Appendix G provides a detailed analysis on the computation and development of a loan amortization schedule.) In contrast, the payment of a bond can require the payment of the principal at maturity, at which time the bondholder receives the face value of the bond, and interest payments either can be paid periodically or else all at once at maturity, along with the principal.

As opposed to a bank, which lends funds, the issuer of a bond *receives* funds from the purchasers of the bond, typically the public. However, bond payments may be structured so that the issuer can make early repayments of the principal or equal pay-

PERSPECTIVE 8–3

Buying on Credit: Hospital Systems Post Modest Increase in Their Long-term Liabilities

Hospital acquisitions, medical office buildings, transportation systems, and equipment purchases all helped to increase the amount of long-term liabilities of the nation's healthcare systems in 2000. Hospital systems overall reported a 6% increase in long-term liabilities: $95 billion in the year 2000 as compared to $89.6 billion in 1999, according to Modern Healthcare's 25th annual Hospital Systems Survey. Not-for-profit systems reported a 3.3% increase; for-profit systems recorded an increase of 7.2%; and public systems reported the largest increase in long-term liabilities, 10.2%.

Long-term liabilities can include notes, mortgages, capital leases, bonds, and obligations under continuing-care contracts. The numbers seem to indicate that healthcare organizations took advantage of a favorable borrowing market in the year 2000 due to attractive long-term interest rates, a trend that has continued into 2001. Unlike for-profit chains, which can raise capital in the equity market without increasing debt, the not-for-profits are limited to borrowing in one way or another because they don't have investors, says Brian McGough, managing director at Banc One Capital Markets in Chicago. He says there were three main reasons why systems increased their long-term liabilities last year: not-for-profits borrowing to finance acquisitions of other not-for-profit facilities; not-for-profit systems buying hospitals divested by for-profit companies; and investments in technology, especially costs related to addressing the anticipated Y2K computer problems. "Considering those three variables . . . it's not surprising there has been a modest increase in debt," he says.

Source: Deanna Bellandi, *Modern Healthcare,* June 18, 2001, p. 94.

ments over the life of the bond through a **sinking fund**. In the latter case, the issuer makes payments to the bond trustee who then uses the funds to retire a portion of the debt.

Sources of Debt Financing by Type of Interest Rate: Fixed and Variable Interest

Fixed interest rate debt is a security whose rate does not change during the lifetime of the bond; conversely, variable interest rate debt is a security whose rate changes based on market conditions. Health care providers are attracted to fixed rate debt because of the predictability of future payments, but the generally higher cost of fixed rate debt may encourage a health care provider to borrow on a lower-cost, variable basis (see Exhibit 8–2).

The primary concern about variable interest rates is that interest rates may increase, which could cause an unanticipated demand for cash flow. However, health care providers may use variable rate debt if they have sufficient cash/investment accounts to hedge against changes in interest rates. The concept of **hedging** is that as variable rates increase and debt payments increase, so too will the returns on the facility's investments, thereby offsetting increased debt payments.

> **Hedging:** The art of offsetting high variable rate debt payments with returns from high-rate investments.

Selected Types of Health Care Debt Financing

This section discusses further several specific types of debt financing: bank loans, conventional mortgages, FHA program loans, and bonds.

Bank Term Loans

> **Term Loan:** A loan typically issued by a bank which has a maturity of 1 to 10 years.

Loans traditionally issued by banks with maturities of one to ten years are defined as term loans. These loans are usually paid off in equal or "level" amounts over the life of the loan.

Exhibit 8–2 Selected Advantages and Disadvantages of Fixed and Variable Rate Debt

	Advantages	Disadvantages
Fixed Rate Debt	1. Fixed debt service payments 2. Fixed interest rate	1. Higher up front or issurance expenses 2. Depending on market condition of variable debt, may pay higher interest cost over life of loan
Variable Rate Debt	1. Lower up front issuance costs 2. Lower initial interest rate	1. Higher interest costs if interest rates increase 2. Unstable debt service payments (interest rate risk) 3. Decline in cash flow if interest rates increase

Collateral: An asset with clear value (such as land or buildings) which is pledged against a loan to reduce risk to the lender. If the loan is not paid off satisfactorily, the lender has a legal claim to seize the pledged asset.

Conventional Mortgages

Under a conventional mortgage, the health care facility pledges its land or building(s) as collateral for a loan. Typical lenders include commercial banks, insurance companies, and savings and loan institutions. The term of a loan is normally 20 years. Unfortunately, the lender may allow the borrower to finance only a portion of the purchase, requiring a down-payment on the rest.

Pooled Equipment Financing

To create greater access to tax-exempt debt financing for less expensive loans, a program of pooled equipment financing was developed. Given the high fixed issuance costs of borrowing, pooled financing spreads these costs over a number of health care borrowers, who each receive a portion of the loan. State or regional hospital associations typically sponsor pooled equipment financing programs.

FHA Program Loans

To improve marketability and encourage lower interest rates, the government-sponsored Federal Housing Administration (FHA) provides mortgage insurance for health care facilities' loans. The insurance guarantees the principal and interest on a loan. The disadvantages are the fees charged and the time it takes to have a loan approved. Many FHA-insured loans can take a year or more to implement.

Bonds

A **bond** is a long-term contract whereby on specific dates a borrower agrees to make principal and/or interest payments to the holder of the bond who lent the funds. The section below describes key terms used in the rest of this chapter as they relate to bonds and the bond issuance process.

1. **Indenture** and **Covenant**. A legal document that states the conditions and terms of a bond is called an indenture. It usually is lengthy – often 100 pages or more – and covers the amount and timing of payments to be made to bondholders. It also lists the numerous covenants of the bond. A loan covenant is a legal provision stated in the bond that the issuer must follow, such as the security backing the bond, the amount of future debt that can be offered, and acceptable ranges for liquidity and debt service coverage ratios. Covenants protect the claims of bondholders on the facility's assets in case of default.

2. **Debenture.** A debenture is an unsecured bond; that is, it is not backed by specific assets of the organization.

3. **Subordinated Debenture.** A subordinated debenture is an unsecured bond that is junior to debenture bonds. In the case of default, debenture bondholders are paid first. A subordinated debenture is more risky to the investor and thus pays a higher interest rate.

4. **Par Value.** The par value of a bond is the security's face value, such as $1,000 or $5,000. This is the amount that a bondholder is paid at the time of the bond's maturity.

5. **Coupon Rate** and **Coupon Payment.** The coupon rate is the stated interest rate on the bond, as promised by the issuer. The coupon payment is the amount the holder of the coupon receives periodically, usually semi-annually. It equals the coupon rate times the face value of the bond payment. For example, if the coupon rate is 10 percent for a bond with a $1,000 par value, the coupon payment is $100 annually, or $50 semi-annually.

6. **Callable Bonds.** Callable bonds may be redeemed by the issuer before they mature. An issuer may call a bond if its coupon rate is higher than the presently prevailing interest rates for bonds, or if the issuer wants to eliminate restrictions caused by having the bond outstanding. In order to attract investors, most callable bonds guarantee a certain coupon payment for ten years (the *call protection period*), and contain a call price feature that equals par value plus a call premium, usually equal to one to two percent of the outstanding balance.

7. **Zero Coupon Bonds.** The term *coupon* refers to the amount of interest that will be paid by the issuer to the bondholders. Bonds issued with no coupon at all are called zero coupon bonds. The tradeoff to the issuer for not making any coupon payments over the lifetime of a bond is that the bond must be issued at a deep discount, i.e. less than face value, which means that the issuer receives less initially in bond proceeds. Investors are attracted to these bonds not only because of their bigger discount rates, but also because they need not concern themselves with managing and reinvesting coupon payments (although they still must pay annual taxes on portions of taxable bonds).

8. **Serial Bonds.** Bonds issued at various maturities and coupon rates are called serial bonds. Bonds of this nature allow the investor to purchase bonds with shorter maturities in addition to investing in bonds with longer maturities.

9. **Basis Points.** Security traders discuss the changes in a bond's interest rate by basis points. A basis point is 1/100th of 1 percent. Thus, 100 basis points is equal to 1 percent; one bond yielding 8.75 percent and one bond yielding 8.65 percent have a spread of 10 basis points. Traders also consider the basis point spread between different types of bonds. For example, the spread between taxable and tax-exempt bonds may be 300 basis points, or there may be a spread of 30 basis points between AAA and A-rated bonds (bond ratings are discussed more shortly).

10. **Sinking Fund.** As part of the bond contract, a covenant may establish that part of the principal be paid back each year, earmarked for the orderly retirement or the redemption of bonds before maturity. These funds, called sinking funds, are paid periodically to the trustee who maintains the fund for the health care provider. They are analogous to the principal repayment of a mortgage.

11. **Secondary Market.** Markets that deal in the buying and selling of bonds that have already been issued.

Tax-exempt Bonds

Tax-exempt bonds are bonds in which the interest payments to the investor have exempt status from the IRS; thus, the interest payments are typically lower than those from bonds, which do not have tax-exempt status. The lower interest payments of tax-exempt financing have made it the primary choice of debt financing for not-for-profit health care organizations. These bonds can only be issued by an organization which has received tax exemption as designated by the IRS, and the funds must be used for projects that qualify as "exempt uses." Rather than having assets as collateral, these bonds are usually backed by the organization's revenues; such issues are called **tax-exempt revenue bonds**.

Key Point   Tax-exempt bonds have lower interest rates than do taxable bonds because investors in tax-exempt bonds do not have to pay taxes on the interest income they receive.

An alternative to revenue bonds are **mortgage bonds**, which carry the health care provider's real property and equipment as security or collateral in the case of default. In today's market, health care providers with an A or higher bond rating normally are not required to pledge their assets as collateral; in the unlikely case of default, creditors are secured by the pledge of the health care provider's revenues. However, creditors can enhance their security indirectly by requiring a negative pledge on a health care provider's real estate. A **negative pledge** prohibits the health care provider from giving a lien (claim) on its real estate to any other creditor.

Another advantage to the issuer of tax-exempt bonds other than the lower interest rates is their long maturity to term, often 30–35 years, as compared to 20–25 years typical of taxable bonds. One disadvantage is the higher issuance cost due to documentation fees for the issuing authority, bond counsel fees, and other documentation required to achieve tax-exempt status on the issue. Slower issuance is another drawback. Since the facility must act through a governmental authority, the bureaucratic approval and issuance process increases the time it takes to bring the security to market.

Taxable Bonds

Taxable bonds differ from tax-exempt bonds primarily in that the coupon payments must be reported as taxable income by the investor. Taxable bonds typically have shorter maturity (20–25 years) and reduced marketability. To sell them, a health care facility must compete in the marketplace against such corporate giants as IBM and General Motors. Thus, to attract investors, the yields or coupon payments on these bonds have to be higher than those of bonds issued by the large, well established firms, because the investor faces greater risk buying bonds from a lesser-known organization. The major advantages that taxable bonds have over tax-exempt bonds are lack of restrictions as to use and quicker market turnaround time.

◀Bond Issuance Process▶

Before a bond can be issued, it must be sold under either public or private placement. Health care providers, whether they are issuing a taxable or a tax-exempt bond, must select between public or private placement. In a **public offering**, a bond is sold to the investing public through an **underwriter**, sometimes called an *investment banker*. **Private placements** are sold to a particular institution or group of institutions (banks, pension funds, or insurance companies), also with the assistance of an under-writer. Exhibit 8–3 introduces the key parties involved in the bond issuance process, which is discussed in more detail below.

Public versus Private Placement

The advantage of private over public placement is that the issuer avoids marketing and printing costs; moreover, depending on the requirements of the buyer, the seller may be able to lower issuance costs even further by forgoing the project's feasibility study and not having the bonds rated. The primary disadvantage of private placement

Exhibit 8–3   Parties Involved in a Tax-exempt Bond Issuance Process

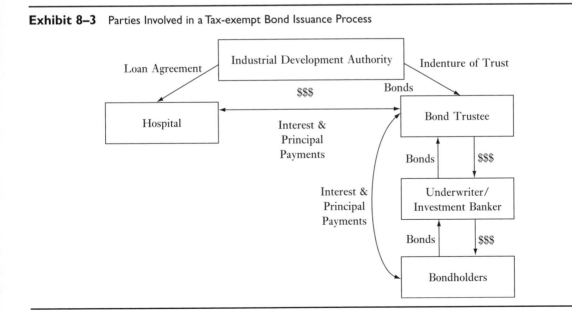

Feasibility Study: A study which examines market and management factors which affect the issuer's ability to generate the necessary cash flows to meet principal and interest requirements.

is that because of the bond's reduced liquidity in a narrower market, buyers demand higher interest rates. If the buyer desires to resell the bonds, there is no *public* secondary market, only other institutions. Other disadvantages of private placement are shorter maturity (leading to higher debt service payments) and increased bond restrictions. Most health care facilities select public placement because the lower interest cost differential over the lifetime of the bond offsets the front-end savings of a private placement.

Public offering of a bond by a tax-exempt health care institution requires an offering prospectus called an *Official Statement* (OS) and, due to a recent proposal by the Securities and Exchange Commission (SEC), also requires annual updates of financial statements to investors. In contrast, stock or bond issues by for-profit corporations require stiffer disclosure requirements for investors, registration with the SEC, and annual and quarterly reports to stockholders. The OS must fully disclose information about the issue, which includes the financial state of the facility (audited financial statements), operational background (medical and management staff, service area, services offered, sources of revenues), the terms of the issue, and, in some cases, a feasibility study of the project being financed.

The Steps in the Bond Issuance Process

Once an organization decides to use bonds as its source of capital, it must go through a long and arduous process before it actually receives any cash. The bond issuing process for not-for-profit organizations using public markets is described below, which can take 12–18 months before any cash is received.

1. The health care provider attempts to "get its house in order." Over a year before actually starting the bond issuance process, a health care agency needs to "get its house in order" to receive a high bond rating. For example, it may attempt to build up its cash reserves, decrease its receivables, and/or liquidate some of its existing debt. In addition, it may update its strategic plan and improve its information system or other parts of its infrastructure.

2. The health care agency is evaluated by a credit rating agency. When a lender evaluates a health care facility as a potential borrower, it considers a range of factors to evaluate risk, including financial, market, and management data. When issuing either tax-exempt or taxable bonds, health care providers turn to investment bankers and/or bond rating agencies to objectively evaluate their creditworthiness by universal standards. (For conventional mortgage loans, a commercial bank or insurance company performs the evaluation.) Regardless of the type of debt financing, lenders examine both financial and non-financial data thoroughly. The information is

 Key Point Debt Service Coverage ratio is one of the primary financial ratios used to evaluate a health care provider's ability to meet debt service payments.

often assembled as a financial feasibility study performed by a management-consulting firm. From the financial projections, the consultant determines whether the health care provider has sufficient funds to make principal and interest payments over the lifetime of the bonds in a timely manner.

Financial Evaluation

From a financial standpoint, the lender or rating agency is primarily interested in evaluating a health care provider's ability to pay. This can be measured by the debt service coverage ratio as discussed in Chapter 4:

$$\text{Debt Service Coverage} = \frac{\text{(Net income + Interest + Depreciation)}}{\text{Annual Debt Service Payments}}$$

The numerator represents the health care provider's cash flow before its interest payments and depreciation expense and is divided by the required annual loan payments of principal and interest. Lenders or rating agencies expect a minimum debt service coverage ratio of 2.0. They also measure ability to pay using several other financial ratios, such as days cash on hand or operating margin.

Market Evaluation

In this step, the lender or rating agency evaluates the demand for the investment project. A wide range of factors are considered in this step, including local demographics (population growth, income levels, unemployment rate in the market area), competition from other health care providers, penetration of managed care, and the industrial base of the local economy.

Physician and Management Evaluation

Because physicians are responsible for admissions, lenders pay particular attention to the characteristics of the staff including the number of medical staff members by specialties, their ages, the percentage of admissions by staff members, the number of board-certified physicians, and the recruitment and retention of staff.

The lender also examines the health care provider's management staff for such things as background and experience, how they are organized, and how they relate to the medical staff. Any recent turnover of management staff and its effect on the organization would be scrutinized closely.

3. **The bond is rated by a bond-rating agency.** Bond ratings assess the creditworthiness or the likelihood of default of a bond. The higher the rating, the lower the interest rate the organization has to pay (less risk to investors). The two primary rating agencies are Moody's and Standard & Poor's (S&P). The rating assigned to an issue affects the interest rate and marketability of the bond. Depending on the size and complexity of the issue, simply getting a rating can cost the issuer from $1,000 to

Key Point   Investment Grade bonds are at or above a S&P's BBB rating or Moody's Baa rating. Bonds below this rating in either category may be considered Junk Bonds.

$50,000. The assigned ratings for both agencies are listed in Exhibit 8–4. **Investment grade** ratings range from AAA to BBB (S&P), or Aaa to Baa (Moody's), of which the highest are called **quality** ratings. **Junk bonds** are rated BB and below by S&P and Ba and below by Moody's. Within the junk bond category are **substandard** and **speculative** bonds, both of which are considered very risky investments. Some providers may choose not to have their bonds rated because they are relatively small in size or they will receive a "below investment grade" rating.

A health care provider rarely achieves the top AAA or Aaa rating. Health care providers in the AA/Aa rating category not only have excellent financial strength, but also have strong management, large bed size, and a superior medical staff. These hospitals tend to rely less on Medicare and Medicaid revenues, exhibit low debt ratios, generate strong profits, and possess large cash reserves. Health care providers in the BBB/Baa and substandard categories are normally smaller facilities located in competitive or rural markets and serve a high proportion of Medicare and Medicaid patients. Furthermore, their cash reserves tend to be low and they possess a high amount of debt. Exhibit 8–5 lists three S&P ratings for not-for-profit hospitals in 2000 and offers a sample of their respective operating and financial measures. Perspective 8–4 lists some of the criteria that affect a hospital's rating.

A health care provider can strengthen its credit rating, and thereby lower its interest cost and increase marketability, through either bond insurance or a letter of credit. For a fee of 0.7–2 percent of the bond's total face value, a facility can obtain bond insurance that guarantees the timely payments of principal and interest to bondholders in the unlikely event of default by the issuer. The rating then attributed to the bond becomes a function of the credit strength of the bond insurance company. However, if an insurer's rating falls, so do the ratings of all its insured issues. The major insurers include AMBAC, MBIA, and FGIC.

Exhibit 8–4   Comparison of Moody's and Standard & Poor's Bond Ratings

Moody's Rating	S & P's Rating	Interpretation	Grade of the Bond
Aaa	AAA	Judged to be the best quality	Quality
Aa	AA	High quality, smaller amount of protection than AAA	Quality
A	A	Many favorable investment attributes	Investment Grade
Baa	BBB	Medium grade; neither highly protected nor poorly secured	Investment Grade
Ba	BB	Speculative elements; future cannot be considered as well assured	Substandard Junk Bonds
B	B	Generally lack characteristics of desirable investment	Substandard Junk Bonds
Caa	CCC	Poor standing; may be in default or have elements of danger	Speculative Junk Bonds
Ca, C	CC, C	Very speculative; often in default; very poor prospects	Speculative Junk Bonds
DDD	D	Bond in default	Speculative Junk Bonds

Exhibit 8–5 Selected Not-for-Profit Hospital Industry Bond Ratings and Medians: 2000

Measure	Bond Rating		
	AA	A	BBB
Average Daily Census	580	149	69
Net Patient Revenue ($000s)	601,458	125,217	48,419
Earnings Before Interest & Depreciation ($000s)	89,704	19,150	5,889
Bad Debt Expense to Operating Revenues	4.2%	3.3%	4.6%
Debt Service Coverage Ratio	4.4	3.3	2.4
Operating Margin	0.5%	1.4%	0.7%
Total Profit Margin	4.7%	4.0%	3.4%
Non-operating Revenue to Total Revenue	4.6%	2.7%	2.1%
Age of Plant (Years)	8.2	8.6	9.2
Days Cash on Hand	213	161	116
Days in Accounts Receivable	75.3	67.3	66.4
Average Payment Period (Days)	68.7	65.8	64.4
Long-term Debt to Total Capital	27.1%	32.7%	39.1%
Cash Flow to Total Debt	20.4%	19.2%	15.1%

Source: Standard & Poor's Median Health Care Ratios, October 19, 2000.

PERSPECTIVE 8–4

Health Care Rating Process

Moody's, a bond rating agency, uses both qualitative and quantitative factors to rate a hospital bond. These factors include service area characteristics such as medical staff, governance, services and service area, competition, and financial resources. Moody's looks for board members with knowledge of national and local health care issues, and it assesses a board's ability to balance opportunities with prudent financial performance. Moody's reviews the size of the medical staff, average age, number of board certified physicians, top-revenue producing physicians, and turnover. In terms of competition, Moody's evaluates: all the hospital competitors, specifically other hospitals, physicians, and surgery centers; the types and levels of services with respect to how they affect the hospital's competitive and financial position; and how well the hospital can influence or control a profitable patient population compared to its competitors. The rating agency also assesses its contracting clout with managed care companies. Last, Moody's places emphasis on cash flow generated from core operations, and it focuses on ratios that incorporate cash flow, and those ratios which are key to an organization's ability to repay its debt.

Source: Moody's Rating Methodology Handbook, Public Finance, November 2000.

A **letter of credit** through a bank is another option to enhance the rating of the issuer's bond. The cost is an initial fee plus an ongoing percentage of the outstanding amount remaining on the issue each year. Again, the bond's rating is dependent upon the strength of the bank.

The rating of a bond traded in the marketplace, called an **outstanding issue**, is reviewed on a periodic basis and could be either upgraded or downgraded depending on the issuer's present financial or operational conditions. For example, in the 1990s,

Letter of Credit:
Offered through a bank, this can be used to enhance the creditworthiness of an institution, and hence, a bond's rating.

**Outstanding Bond
Issue:** A bond that
trades in the
marketplace.

Moody's lowered the rating of National Healthcare Inc.'s subordinated debenture from B to Caa *after* it had already gone to market. The agency cited increased financial leverage and expectations for minimum profits as the cause for the downgrade. Recently, the pressures of competition and the constraints on reimbursement have resulted in more downgrades than upgrades. In 1999, the ratio of downgrades to upgrades stabilized at 5:1. See Perspective 8–5 for additional information on the factors affecting the downgrading of bonds.

4. The health care provider enters into a loan agreement with the governmental authority, the issuer of the bonds, via a trustee. The amount of the loan agreement is equivalent to the bond payments. The health care provider must ensure that the bond issuance process satisfies all federal regulations, which are designed to help protect the investors. At the same time, since the health care provider is engaging in a legally binding contract, it needs to ensure that the stated conditions are customized appropriately and are not simply generic guidelines. By doing so, the health care agency gives itself sufficient leverage and flexibility to pay off its debt should conditions change.

5. The governmental authority delivers the bonds to the underwriters. The governmental authority, sometimes called an industrial development authority, issues the bonds to one or more underwriters, sometimes called investment bankers. By playing the role of intermediary, the government is able to keep the transactions publicly recorded. Some bond issuances can be worth hundreds of millions of dollars,

---

PERSPECTIVE 8–5

Credit Rating Downgrade of Hospital Bonds

After downgrading much of the not-for-profit hospital industry during the past two years, two leading credit-rating agencies said the carnage might be winding down. But they haven't put away the ax. Last week, Moody's Investors Service predicted that not-for-profit hospital credit ratings will stabilize by the end of 2001. Its announcement followed a report with similar conclusions issued by competitor Standard & Poor's earlier this month. Both agencies, which rate a total of about 1,000 hospital credits, said they still expect downgrades to exceed upgrades this year, but at a smaller ratio than in the past. "We expect that the number of upgrades and downgrades will equalize toward the end of the year," said Bruce Gordon, a senior vice president at Moody's.

In another positive sign, Moody's last week changed its outlook for the for-profit hospital sector from negative to stable. It said the credit quality of for-profits has benefited from a more stable Medicare environment, growth in same-facility admissions, and organizations' ability to leverage market share to win better managed-care contracts. In the not-for-profit sector, downgrades have outpaced upgrades by about 5-to-1 in the past 24 months as rating agencies have reacted to financial pressures on the industry from the impact of the Balanced Budget Act of 1997, managed care, and failed business ventures. Last year, 1 in 10 hospitals with rated debt saw their ratings sink.

The for-profit sector still does face credit concerns including rising labor costs and the threat of less-favorable managed-care rates, Moody's said. To meet earnings targets, companies may turn to debt-financed acquisitions or stock buybacks.

Source: Mary Chris Jaklevic, Modern Healthcare, January 29, 2001, p. 17.

and it is crucial that the health care provider, the underwriter, and the investor are fully protected and are abiding by all the regulations.

6. The underwriters sell the bonds to bondholders at the public offering price, and the trustee provides the health care provider with the net proceeds. A pricing process actually begins several weeks before the true opening day sale of the bonds, when the underwriters issue a preliminary OS to prospective buyers called a *red herring*. At that time, underwriters construct a pre-pricing scale of interest rates for various maturities. Their objective is to achieve an equilibrium price that ensures marketability, yet avoids over-subscription of the issue. If over-subscription occurs, this indicates the bond price is too favorable to investors and, thus, unfavorable to the health care provider. In this case, the underwriter will either price the bond higher or lower the interest rate. Though this will decrease the number of bond orders, it makes the price fairer to the health care provider. Once the final price has been set, an agreement is signed by the issuer and the leading underwriter. Shortly thereafter, the underwriter purchases the bonds, sells them to investors at the predetermined price, and then transfers the proceeds to the health care provider via the governmental authority and then trustee. In short, the pricing period allows the underwriter to obtain commitments from buyers to reduce its own risk before buying the bonds.

Red Herring: A preliminary OS offered to prospective buyers of a bond by the underwriters to help determine a fair market price for the bond.

Net Proceeds from a Bond Issuance: Gross proceeds less the underwriter's and others' issuance fees.

After the issuance process has been completed, the health care provider makes its interest and principal payments to the trustee, who in turn pays the investors/bondholders. The health care facility is obliged to guarantee against bankruptcy for tax-exempt bonds.

Selected Roles of Underwriters and Trustees

Underwriters, sometimes referred to as investment bankers, help health care facilities issue bonds. Specifically, they advise management on the terms of the structure of the bonds (i.e. size, length, interest rate, loan restrictions, bond insurance, etc.). They also may buy the bonds themselves from the issuer at a discount and in turn try to sell them in the marketplace. In so doing, the investment banker incurs a major risk: a potential decline in bond prices (rise in interest rates) from when the bonds were originally purchased. This would result in reselling the bonds to investors at less profit, if not a loss.

To spread the risk, the leading investment banker will **syndicate** with other investment bankers to sell the bonds. The syndicate may consist of local investment banking firms (in order to enhance marketability), or national investment banking firms such as Prudential Securities, Smith Barney, Merrill Lynch, and Paine Webber.

On the other hand, the investment banker may avoid all risk by acting solely as an agent for the health care facility to help sell the bonds. In this case, the risk shifts back to the issuer, as all unsold bonds are returned to it.

The **trustee**, typically a bank, acts as an agent for the bondholders and performs two important functions. First, the trustee makes the principal and interest payments to the bondholders. Second, the trustee ensures that the health care provider complies with the legal covenants of the bond. For example, if the health care provider were required to maintain a debt service coverage ratio above 2.5 and debt to total capital less than 50 percent, the trustee would monitor its performance with respect to these ratios. If the health care provider did not comply, it would be in default of the bond.

◄LEASE FINANCING►

Trustee: An agent for bondholders who ensures that the health care facility is making timely principal and interest payments to the bondholders and complies with legal covenants of the bond.

As health care facilities find it more difficult to acquire capital to finance equipment, many consider lease arrangements as a necessary and viable alternative. Leasing now accounts for 20–25 percent of all health care provider equipment spending. A lease involves two parties: the **lessor**, who owns the asset, and the **lessee**, who pays the lessor for the use of the asset but does not own it. Some reasons why a health care provider may decide to enter into a lease arrangement are:

Lessor: An entity who owns an asset, which is then leased out.

1. **To avoid the bureaucratic delays of capital budget requests.** Because of the longer, closer scrutiny given capital budgeting requests by top management and the board, an administrator may find it more convenient to lease a piece of medical equipment rather than to request it in the capital budget. This is especially true for state- or city-owned facilities whose capital purchases require governmental approval.

Lessee: An entity who negotiates the use of another's asset via a lease.

2. **To avoid technological obsolescence.** Given the rapid changes in health care technology, lessees can avoid paying for high-tech equipment that may be outdated shortly. By leasing, a facility can continually upgrade its equipment; the risk of technological obsolescence then shifts to the lessor.

3. **To receive better maintenance services.** Most full-service leases include maintenance for the equipment. Some believe that since the lessor owns the equipment, maintenance is better.

4. **To allow for convenience.** If an asset is to be used for only a short time, leasing is less time-consuming and costly than buying and selling shortly thereafter. Since leasing constitutes 100 percent financing, leasing companies advertise that it frees cash for other purposes. A facility could also avoid a cash down payment by borrowing enough to cover the full cost of the lease, which is less than buying the asset outright. Thus, from a financial perspective, lease financing appears equivalent to debt financing; the only major difference being that a facility never actually owns a leased asset.

The two major types of leases are operating leases and capital leases.

Key Point | Lessor owns the asset while the lessee makes lease payments to the lessor for the use of the asset.

Operating Lease

An **operating lease** is for service equipment leased for periods shorter than the equipment's economic life, usually between a few days and a year. The lessor's aim is to lease for less than the equipment's full cost, but to recover the cost by leasing the asset many times over its economic life. The usual types of assets covered by operating leases are computers, copier machines, and vehicles. The lessor incurs all the ownership costs of maintenance, service, and insurance on the leased equipment.

Another characteristic of operating leases is a cancellation clause, giving the lessee the option to return the leased asset to the lessor with little or no penalty at any time during the life of the lease.

Operating Lease: A lease that lasts shorter than the useful life of the leased asset, typically one year or less. This type of leasing arrangement can be canceled at any time without penalty, but there is no option to purchase the asset once the lease has expired.

Capital Lease

In a **capital lease**, also called a **financial lease**, the lessor aims to lease the asset for virtually all of its economic life. In return, the lessee is committed to lease payments for the entire lease period. The lessee does not have the option to cancel a capital lease immediately without a substantial penalty but does have an option to buy the leased asset at the end of the lease agreement. The latter option tends to be more expensive than if the facility had initially bought the equipment outright, because the lessor always operates with a margin for profit.

One type of capital lease used by the health care industry is the **sale/leaseback arrangement**, whereby a health care provider sells an owned asset (such as a clinic) to a third party and simultaneously leases it back from the purchaser. By selling the owned asset, the facility is able to obtain immediate capital, though it still retains use of the asset.

From a financial management perspective, a capital lease has implications similar to buying an asset and financing it with debt. Buying through borrowing and negotiating a capital lease are similar in that both require contractual payments (debt or lease payments) over the life of the asset, and both options incur the costs of operating the asset. The primary difference occurs at the end of the asset's life, when the leasing arrangement requires the asset to be returned to the lessor (the owner), unless the contract stipulated an option to buy or renew. In contrast, under the buy/borrow option, the owner may either sell or continue to use an asset at any point.

Capital Lease: A lease that lasts for an extended period of time, up to the life of the leased asset. This type of lease cannot be canceled without penalty, and at the end of the lease period, the lessee may have the option to purchase the asset. Also called a *financial lease*.

Financial Lease: See *capital lease.*

Analysis of the Lease versus Purchase Decision

One of the most common financial decisions made by a health care organization is whether to buy or lease a needed asset. The usual approach is to compare the present value cost of a buy decision with the present value cost of a lease decision over a specified time period. From a purely financial standpoint, the option with the lower present value cost is preferable. In making this assessment, several factors must be considered. Taxpaying entities realize either an effective lower net lease payment from

Sale/Leaseback Arrangement: A type of capital lease whereby an institution sells an owned asset and then simultaneously leases it back from the purchaser. The selling institution retains rights to use the asset, but benefits from the immediate acquisition of cash from the sale.

Tax Shield: An investment, which reduces the amount of income tax, which has to be paid, often because interest and depreciation expenses are tax deductible.

the tax deduction of the lease payment, or an interest and depreciation tax shield from buying the asset. The cost of ownership includes the outflow of cash to maintain the asset offset by the inflow of cash from its salvage value. Interest and depreciation expenses act as **tax shields** because they are tax-deductible expenses, which reduce the taxes paid to the government. Last, the cash flows under the lease option are discounted back at the after-tax cost of debt rather than at the cost of capital.

Suppose Five-Star General Hospital is undecided about purchasing a $10 million piece of equipment or leasing it. If it decides to buy the asset, it can borrow the full amount from its local bank at a rate of 10 percent; the equipment would be depreciated at a rate of $2 million per year over its five-year life to a zero salvage value. Under the lease arrangement, the gross lease payments would be $3 million per year, starting one year from now. Assume the organization is a taxpaying entity with a 30 percent tax rate.

Exhibit 8–6 presents the analysis of this purchasing versus leasing decision. Because the present value sum of the financing flows for purchasing is the higher of the two options,– $7,540,000 versus – $8,610,000, purchasing the asset is the desired alternative to leasing.

- A loan amortization schedule similar to the one in Exhibit G–3 is presented in Columns A through D in the top section. The loan amortization amount ($2,638,000, row 1) is calculated using the present value factor for an annuity at 10 percent interest for five years (3.7908). Column A represents the only cash outflows, which are the loan payments.

- Columns E and F present cash inflows from interest and depreciation expense tax shields. The interest expense tax shield was computed by multiplying the interest expense in Column B by the same tax rate of 30 percent (row 4). The depreciation tax shield inflow ($600,000) was computed by multiplying the annual depreciation expense, $2 million, by the tax rate, 30 percent (rows 3 and 4).

- The net cash outflow, Column G, equals the annual loan payment from Column A less the tax shield amounts. Finally, the net cash outflow is discounted back at the net after tax cost of debt: 10 percent × (1 − 0.3) = 7 percent. Since the cash flows are net of taxes, the calculations should be based on the net after tax cost of debt as well. Column H gives the present value factors at 7 percent, while Column I shows the net present value of the decision to purchase the asset, − $7,540,000.

- The lower section shows the calculations for the leasing alternative. Cash outflows, Column L, are also examined net of taxes; thus, the net payment only equals $2.1 million per year [$3 million × (1 − 0.30)]. These payments are also discounted back at the same net after tax cost of debt rate of 7 percent. Column N shows the present value of the leasing decision, − $8,610,000.

If Five-Star General were a non-taxpaying entity, there would be no tax shield benefits. In this case, the analysis would be simplified by comparing only the

Exhibit 8–6 Comparison of Purchasing Arrangement to Leasing Arrangement for Five-Star General Hospital

General Hospital

Givens:

1	Annual Annuity Payment[1]	$2,638
2	Interest Rate	10%
3	Annual Depreciation Expense[2]	$2,000
4	Tax Rate	30%
5	Depreciation Expense Tax Shield[3]	$600
6	After Tax Cost of Debt[4]	7%
7	Before Tax Lease Payments	$3,000

[1]PVFA Formula: $10,000 Initial Investment; i = 10%; n = 5 Years
[2]$10,000 Purchase Price/5 Years Useful Life = $2,000 Depreciation Expense per Year
[3]$2,000 Depreciation Expense per Year × 30% Tax Rate = $600 Tax Shield per Year
[4](Interest Rate) × (1 − Tax Rate) = 10% × (1 − 30%) = 7%

Purchasing Arrangement

	A	B	C	D	E	F	G	H	I
	Annuity Payment	Interest Expense	Principal Payment	Remaining Balance	Interest Expense Tax Shield	Depreciation Expense Tax Shield	Net Cash Outflow (if owned)	PV Factor from	PV of Net Cash Outflows (if owned)
Year	[Given 1]	[D* × Given 2]	[A − B]	[D* − C]	[B × Given 4]	[Given 5]	[A − (E + F)]	[Given 6]	[G × H]
0			$10,000						
1	$2,638	$1,000	$1,638	8,362	$300	$600	$1,738	0.9346	$1,624
2	2,638	836	1,802	6,560	251	600	1,787	0.8734	1,561
3	2,638	656	1,982	4,578	197	600	1,841	0.8163	1,503
4	2,638	458	2,180	2,398	137	600	1,901	0.7629	1,450
5	2,638	240	2,398	0	72	600	1,966	0.7130	1,402
Total									$7,540

Note: D* is the previous year's Column D value.

(Continues)

Exhibit 8–6 (Contd)

Leasing Arrangement

	J	K	L	M	N
					PV of Net
	Before Tax	Lease Tax	Net After	PV Factor	Cash Outflows
	Lease Payments	Shield	Lease Payments	from	(if leased)
Year	[Given 7]	[J × Given 4]	[J – K]	[Given 6]	[L × M]
0					
1	$3,000	$900	$2,100	0.9346	$1,963
2	3,000	900	2,100	0.8734	1,834
3	3,000	900	2,100	0.8163	1,714
4	3,000	900	2,100	0.7629	1,602
5	3,000	900	2,100	0.7130	1,497
Total					$8,610

Note: All figures expressed in '000

present value of the loan payments to the present value of the lease payments, but the cost of debt would be 10 percent, not 7 percent. Though normally it would be necessary to go through these calculations if the payments differed each year, it can easily be seen here that with flat payments every year under both options ($2.638 million borrowing versus $3.0 million leasing), purchasing would be less costly than leasing. Therefore, the present value of the loan of $10,000,000 would be less than the present value of the lease, and the decision should be to borrow the funds and buy the asset.

Caution

Salvage or residual value of an asset should also be considered in the buy/borrow analysis evaluation. Residual values are a cash inflow. Since the cash flow of the residual value is less certain than the debt and lease cash flows, some financial analysts may use a higher rate than the after-tax cost of debt to discount this cash flow.

◀Summary▶

There are three ways to finance assets: using debt (liabilities), equity, or a combination of the two.

Assets = Debt + Equity

Any increase in assets must be balanced by a similar increase in debt and/or equity. The structuring of debt relative to equity is called the capital structure decision, and is increasingly important to both for-profit and not-for-profit providers. In today's environment, characterized by prospective and capitated payments, the increased use of managed care and outpatient services, and increasing cutbacks being forced by competition, obtaining debt and equity financing is a much more complicated undertaking. Both types of financing have advantages and disadvantages.

The primary sources of equity financing for not-for-profit health care organizations are internally generated funds, philanthropy, and government grants, whereas for-profit facilities primarily rely on internally generated funds and stock issuances. Unfortunately, internally generated funds – those funds retained from operations (retained earnings) – are shrinking.

A general rule of thumb is to borrow short-term for short-term needs and long-term for long-term needs. Short-term financing typically refers to a wide range of financing, from debt that must be paid back almost immediately to debt that may not have to be paid off for up to a year. Long-term financing typically refers to debt that must be paid off in a period longer than a year. The two major types of long-term financing are term loans, which must be paid off in one to ten years, and bonds, which may have a final maturity of up to 20 to 35 years. Bonds are the primary source of long-term financing for tax-exempt health care entities.

Types of debt financing available to not-for-profit health care organizations include bank term loans, conventional mortgages, Federal Housing Administration (FHA) insured mortgages, tax-exempt financing (available *only* to not-for-profit organizations), and taxable bonds.

Organizations that decide to issue bonds generally go through a series of six steps:

> Step 1. The health care provider attempts to "get its house in order."
> Step 2. The health care agency gets evaluated by a credit rating agency.
> Step 3. The bond is rated by a bond-rating agency.
> Step 4. The health care provider provides a note or lease to the governmental authority via a trustee.
> Step 5. The governmental authority delivers the bonds to one or more investment banking firms.
> Step 6. The investment banking firms sell the bonds to investors at the public offering price, and the trustee provides the health care provider with the net proceeds.

Bonds can be issued with either fixed interest or variable rate interest, each of which has advantages and disadvantages.

An alternative to traditional equity and debt financing is leasing. Leasing is undertaken for four reasons: 1) to avoid the bureaucratic delays of capital budget requests, 2) to avoid technological obsolescence, 3) to receive better maintenance services, and 4) to allow for convenience.

There are two types of leases: operating and capital. An operating lease is for service equipment leased for periods shorter than the equipment's economic life, usually between a few days and a year. Under a capital lease, also called a financial lease, the lessor aims to lease the asset for virtually all of its economic life. In return, the lessee is committed to lease payments for the entire lease period.

◄Key Terms►

Amortization	Lessee	Premium
Bond	Lessor	Red Herring
Capital Lease	Letter of Credit	Required Market Rate
Collateral	Market Value	Sale/Leaseback Arrangement
Discount	Net Proceeds from a Bond	Sinking Fund
Feasibility Study	Issuance	Tax Shield
Financial Lease	Operating Lease	Term Loan
Fixed Income Security	Outstanding Bond Issue	Trustee
Hedging	Par Value	Yield to Maturity

◄Key Equations►

Bond Valuation (Annual Coupon Payments):

Market Value = (Coupon Payment) × PVFA(k,n) + (Par Value) × PVF(k,n)

Bond Valuation (Other Semi-annual Periods for Coupon Payments):

Market Value = (Coupon Payment/2) × PVFA(k/2,n × 2) + (Par Value) × PVF(k/2, n × 2)

◄Questions and Problems►

1. **Definitions.** Define the following terms:
   a. Amortization.
   b. Bond.
   c. Capital Lease.
   d. Collateral.
   e. Discount.
   f. Feasibility Study.
   g. Financial Lease.
   h. Fixed Income Security.
   i. Hedging.
   j. Lessee.
   k. Lessor.
   l. Letter of Credit.
   m. Market Value.
   n. Net Proceeds from a Bond Issuance.
   o. Operating Lease.
   p. Outstanding Bond Issue.
   q. Par Value.
   r. Premium.
   s. Red Herring.

t. Required Market Rate.

u. Sale/Leaseback Arrangement.

v. Sinking Fund.

w. Tax Shield.

x. Term Loan.

y. Trustee.

z. Yield to Maturity.

2. **Equity Position.** What avenues are available for for-profit and not-for-profit health care providers to increase their equity position?

3. **Debt versus Equity Financing.** What are the advantages and disadvantages to a taxpaying entity in issuing debt as opposed to equity?

4. **Debt Financing.** Does adding debt increase or decrease the flexibility of a health care provider? Why?

5. **Basis Points.** How much is a basis point? How many basis points between $6\frac{5}{8}$ percent and $6\frac{3}{4}$ percent?.

6. **Debentures.** Explain the difference between subordinated debentures and debentures.

7. **Bonds.** Name at least two factors that might cause a facility to call in its bond.

8. **Bonds.** What are the advantages and disadvantages of a taxable bond relative to a tax-exempt bond? Who is the issuer of tax-exempt bonds?

9. **Bonds.** What party acts on the behalf of bondholders to insure that the issuing facility not only is complying with the covenants of the bond, but also is making timely principal and interest payments to the bondholders?

10. **Investment Bankers.** Why would an investment banker syndicate a bond issue with other investment bankers?

11. **Bonds.** Compare private placement bond issues with public placement bond issues.

12. **Credit Ratings.** Identify two ways that a health care provider can strengthen its credit rating. What are some of the ramifications of these options?

13. **Credit Ratings.** What can cause a health care provider's credit rating to be downgraded?

14. **Market Rates.** What impact do required market rate changes have on bonds of longer maturities?

15. **Leasing.** What are the two types of leasing arrangements and their primary differences?

16. **Leasing.** Why might an organization enter into a leasing arrangement?

17. **Bond Valuation.** If a $1,000 zero coupon bond with a 20-year maturity has a market price of $311.80, what is its rate of return?

18. **Bond Valuation.** If a $1,000 zero coupon bond with a 15-year maturity has a market price of $481.80, what is its rate of return?

19. **Bond Valuation.** A tax-exempt bond was recently issued at an annual 8 percent coupon rate and matures 20 years from today. The par value of the bond is $1,000.

a. If required market rates are 8 percent, what is the market price of the bond?

b. If required market rates fall to 5 percent, what is the market price of the bond?

    c. If required market rates rise to 15 percent, what is the market price of the bond?

    d. At what required market rate (5, 8, or 15 percent) does the above bond sell at a discount? At a premium?

20. **Bond Valuation.** A tax-exempt bond was recently issued at an annual 7 percent coupon rate and matures 30 years from today. The par value of the bond is $5,000.

    a. If required market rates are 7 percent, what is the market price of the bond?

    b. If required market rates fall to 4 percent, what is the market price of the bond?

    c. If required market rates rise to 14 percent, what is the market price of the bond?

    d. At what required market rate (4, 7, or 14 percent) does the above bond sell at a discount? At a premium?

21. **Bond Valuation.** Assuming that the bond in Problem 19 matures in five years, what would be the market prices under the various required market interest rate changes?

22. **Bond Valuation.** Assuming that the bond in Problem 20 matures in ten years, what would be the market prices under the various required market interest rate changes?

23. **Bond Valuation.** Charles City Hospital plans on issuing a tax-exempt bond at annual coupon rate of 6 percent with a maturity of 30 years. The par value of the bond is $1,000.

    a. If required market rates are 6 percent, what is the value of the bond?

    b. If required market rates fall to 3 percent, what is the value of the bond?

    c. If required market rates fall to 12 percent what is the value of the bond?

    d. At what required market rate (3, 6, or 12 percent) does the above bond sell at a discount? At a premium?

24. **Bond Valuation.** Assuming that the bond in problem 23 matures in ten years, what would be the market prices under the various required interest rate changes?

25. **Bond Valuation.** A $5,000 par value bond with an annual 8 percent coupon rate will mature in six years. Coupon payments are made semiannually. What is its market price if the required market rate is 6 percent?

26. **Bond Valuation.** A $1,000 par value bond with annual 7 percent coupon rate will mature in eight years. Coupon payments are made semi-annually. What is the market price if the required market rate is 4 percent?

27. **Bond Valuation.** Currently, Boston Common Community Hospital's tax-exempt bond is selling for $847.48 per bond and has a remaining maturity of 15 years. If the par value is $1,000 and the coupon rate is 8 percent, what is the yield to maturity?

28. **Bond Valuation.** Haven Hospital's tax-exempt bond is currently selling for $659.32 and has a remaining maturity of 12 years. If the par value is $1,000 and the coupon rate is 5 percent, what is the yield to maturity?

29. **Loan Amortization.** Dinglewood Hospital needs to borrow $1,000,000 to purchase an MRI. The interest rate for the loan is 6 percent. Principal and

interest payments are equal debt service payments, made on an annual basis. The length of the loan is five years. The CEO of Dinglewood wants to develop a loan amortization schedule for this debt borrowing for tomorrow morning's meeting. Prepare such a schedule.

30. **Loan Amortization.** Petersville Hospital needs to borrow $40 million dollars to finance its new facility. The interest rate is 11 percent for the loan. Principal and interest payments are equal debt service payments, made on an annual basis. The length of the loan is ten years. The CFO would like to develop a loan amortization schedule for this debt issuance.

31. **Purchase versus Lease.** Mercy Medical Mega Center, a taxpaying entity, has made the decision to purchase a new laser surgical device. The device costs $400,000 and will be depreciated on a straight-line basis over five years to a zero salvage value. Mercy Medical could borrow the full amount at a 15 percent rate for five years. The after-tax cost of debt equals 9 percent. Alternatively, it could lease the device for five years. The before-tax lease payments per year would be $80,000. The tax rate for this MegaCenter is 40 percent. From a financial perspective, should Mercy lease the surgical device or borrow the money to purchase it?

32. **Purchase versus Lease.** New Health Hospital Systems either wants to borrow money to purchase a hospital or else enter into a lease agreement with the City of Chesterville. The purchase price of the hospital is $15 million. Assuming 100 percent financing, the interest rate is 12 percent for the loan with an after tax cost of debt of 8 percent. The length of the loan is five years. The before tax lease payments are expected to be $3 million per year. The tax rate is 40 percent for New Health System. Should New Health System lease or borrow the money to purchase the hospital?

33. **Purchase versus Lease.** Carolina Ancillary Services for Hospitals (CASH), a taxpaying entity, is considering the purchase of a CT scanner. The cost of the scanner is $1 million. The scanner would be depreciated over ten years on a straight-line basis to a zero salvage value. At the end of five years, the scanner could be sold for its book value, $500,000. The tax rate is 40 percent. The financing options include either borrowing for the full cost of the scanner and selling it at the end of Year 5, or leasing one. The lease option is a five-year lease with equal before-tax lease payments of $320,000 per year. The borrowing alternative is a five-year loan covering the entire cost of the scanner at an interest rate of 12 percent. The after-tax cost of debt is 7 percent. Should CASH lease the scanner or borrow the full amount to purchase it?

34. **Purchase versus Lease.** Tidewater Hospital, a taxpaying entity, is considering leasing its ambulance fleet. The fleet of ambulances costs $125,000 and will be depreciated over a ten year life to a salvage value of $25,000. Tidewater could finance the entire fleet with equal annual debt and principal payments at a before tax cost of debt of 14 percent and an after tax cost of debt at 9 percent for ten years. Alternatively, it could lease the device for ten years. The before tax lease payments are $25,000 per year for

ten years. Tidewater's tax rate is 40 percent. From a financial perspective, should Tidewater lease or borrow the money to buy the ambulances?

Appendix G

Bond Valuation and Loan Amortization

A facility plans to market bonds at the lowest possible interest rate, but to do so, it first must carefully scrutinize the current market's relationship between bond prices and yield to maturity. Since many bonds have a call feature as well, the facility must also examine how this will affect interest rates. The facility must understand the process of paying off its debt.

Bond Valuation in Terms of Yield to Maturity

Fixed Income Security:
A bond which pays fixed amounts of interest at regular periodic intervals, usually semi-annually.

Market Value: What a bond would sell for in today's open market.

Par Value: The face value amount of a bond. It is the amount the bondholder is paid at maturity. It does not include any coupon payments.

Yield to Maturity: The rate at which the market value of a bond is equal to the bond's present value of future coupon payments plus par value.

Required Market Rate: The market interest rate on similar risk bonds.

Most bonds are **fixed income securities**, which mean the investor receives a fixed amount of interest periodically, usually semi-annually, over the lifetime of the bond. With fixed interest rate securities, the coupon payment does not change from year to year, even though the market interest rate may change. A bond's **market value** is the price at which a bond can be bought or sold today in the open market. While market value should not be confused with **par value**, a bond's face value, a bond may be issued with an equal market value and par value.

The **yield to maturity (YTM)**, or **required market rate** of a bond, is used by analysts to determine the return on the bond. YTM is the rate at which the market value of a bond is equal to the bond's present value of future coupon payments plus par value. The **bond valuation formula** is defined as:

$$MV = \left[\sum_{t=1}^{n} CP_t/(1+k)^t \right] + PV/(1+k)^n$$

where:

MV	=	Market value (price) of the bond
CP	=	Coupon payment on the bond
PV	=	Par value of the bond
n	=	Number of periods to maturity
t	=	1, 2, 3, . . . , n periods
k	=	Yield to Maturity (required market rate)

Fortunately, it is not necessary to use this formula in its present form, which can get quite lengthy and complicated. In fact, the first part of the formula after the summation sign is simply the calculation for the present value of an annuity; the latter part of the formula reduces to a basic present value term. In line with the terms discussed in Chapter 6, the formula can be simplified to:

$$\text{Market Value} = (\text{Coupon Payment}) \times PVFA(k,n) + (\text{Par Value}) \times PVF(k,n)$$

Exhibit G–1 shows how to use the formula by proving that when the coupon rate equals the required market rate, market value equals par value. Suppose a hospital wants to issue $100,000

Exhibit G–1 Example of How to Use the Bond Valuation Formula Where Coupon Rate Equals Required Market Rate

Givens:	
1 Par Value	$5,000
2 Market Rate (k)	8%
3 Time Horizon in Years (n)	20
4 Coupon Rate	8%
5 Coupon Payment[1]	$400

[1]Coupon Payment = (Coupon Rate) × (Par Value)

Market Value = (Coupon Payment) × PVFA(k,n) + (Par Value) × PVF(k,n)
Market Value = $400 × PVFA(0.08, 20) + $5,000 × PVF(0.08, 20)
Market Value = $400 × 9.8181 + $5,000 × 0.2145
Market Value = $3,927 + $1,073
Market Value = $5,000

worth of bonds with a 20-year maturity date. The present market interest rate is 8 percent, and the hospital sets its coupon rate at 8 percent to equal the required market rate. Bonds are sold in denominations of $1,000 or $5,000 each, which is the par value.

As with the techniques for finding the internal rate of return, trial and error is used to find yield to maturity, k. For example, if the coupon rate is 9 percent, par value is $1,000, market price is $1,200, and the time to maturity is 20 years, what is the yield to maturity? Solving for k through trial and error yields a value of about 7 percent:

$$\$1,200 = \$90 \times PVFA(k,20) + \$1,000 \times PVF(k,20)$$

$$\$1,200 = \$90 \times 10.594 + \$1,000 \times 0.258 \text{ when } k = \text{exactly } 0.07$$

Bond Valuation in Terms of Market Price

The formula can also be used to solve for the market value of a bond. It shows that market value equals the present value of the cash flows in the form of principal and interest payments, discounted back at the required market rate. The required market rate is estimated by examining market rates from publicly traded bonds of similar risk and maturity. This market rate is also how the market perceives the issuer's financial condition, the loan covenants, and a bond's collateral. (A more complete discussion of how market rates change is in the next section.)

There is an inverse relationship between market value and required market rate: when the required market rate is higher than a bond's coupon rate, the market value is less than par value; when the required market rate is lower, the required market value is higher. And, as stated before, when the coupon rate and the required market rate are equal, the market value will be equal to the par value.

When the required market rate is higher than the coupon rate, a bond is selling at a **discount** from its par value. The reason lies with the action of the market: no one will pay par value for a bond with 9 percent coupon payments if the market rate is 10 percent. Consequently, the

Discount: When the market rate is higher than the coupon rate, a bond is said to be selling at a discount from its par value. See also Premium.

Premium: When the market rate is lower than the coupon rate, a bond is said to be selling at a premium. See also Discount.

price of the outstanding bond must fall to a point that produces an effective market rate of 10 percent with the same coupon payment.

On the other hand, when the required market rate is lower than the coupon rate, a bond is said to be selling at a **premium**. Market factors again are the reason for this: if the present market rate is only 8 percent, but the coupon payments are at 9 percent, investors will be willing to pay more for the bonds than their par value, which pushes the market price up.

Though the focus to this point has been on the effect of changing interest rates in the marketplace, no mention has been given to the impact of maturity dates. In fact, if the required market rate equals the coupon rate, then regardless of the maturity date, market value will always be equal to par value. It is only when these two rates differ that maturity date has an effect. If a bond is selling at a discount (determined by interest rates), longer maturity bonds sell at a lesser price than do bonds of shorter maturities. Conversely, if a bond is selling at a premium, the longer maturity bonds sell for more than those of shorter maturity. Exhibit G–2 shows the impact of both required market rates and maturity on the market value for a $1,000 bond with 9 percent annual coupon payments.

Longer maturity makes bond prices more sensitive to changes in required market interest rates. Thus, in response to interest rate changes, the prices of longer maturity bonds change more than do those of shorter maturity bonds. When the coupon rate and the market rate are equal, the market price of a bond equals its face value, regardless of maturity.

Bond Valuation for Other Payment Periods

Many bonds pay interest semi-annually – in some cases quarterly. If so, the bond valuation formula can be adjusted to account for any number of payment periods within a year, q, using the following formula:

$$MV = [\sum_{t=1}^{n} CP_t/q \times (1+k/q)^t] + PV/(1+k/q)^{n \times q}$$

where:

MV = Market value (price) of the bond
CP = Coupon payment on the bond
PV = Par value of the bond
n = Number of periods to maturity
t = 1, 2, 3, . . . , n periods
k = Yield to maturity (required market rate)
q = Number of payment periods per year

Exhibit G-2   Effect of Market Rates and Maturity on a Bond's Market Value

	$k = 0.08$	$k = 0.09$	$k = 0.10$
Maturity = 10 years	$1,067	$1,000	$939
Maturity = 20 years	$1,099	$1,000	$915
Maturity = 30 years	$1,112	$1,000	$905

k = market interest rate

For example, suppose the previously described bond, which had an annual coupon rate of 9 percent, made its payments semi-annually instead of annually. If the term or maturity of the bond were 15 years, required market rate 8 percent, and the par value $1,000, the market value of the bond would be computed as follows:

$$\text{Market Value} = (\text{Coupon Payment}/2) \times \text{PVFA}(k/2, n \times 2) + (\text{Par Value}) \times \text{PVF}(k/2, n \times 2)$$

$$\text{MV} = (\$90/2) \times \text{PVFA}(0.08/2, 15 \times 2) + \$1,000 \times \text{PVF}(0.08/2, 15 \times 2)$$

$$\text{MV} = \$45 \times \text{PVFA}(0.04, 30) + \$1,000 \times \text{PVF}(0.04, 30)$$

$$\text{MV} = \$45 \times 17.292 + \$1,000 \times 0.308 = \$1,086.14$$

Amortization of a Term Loan

The **amortization** of a term loan is the gradual process of paying off debt through a series of equal periodic payments. Each payment covers a portion of the principal plus current interest. The periodic payments are equal over the lifetime of the loan, but the proportion going toward the principal gradually increases. For most long-term debt, health care providers opt for this form of level debt service. This option usually is not available for short-term financing. Some short-term debt loans require equal interest payments over the life of the loan and a total principal payment at the end of the loan.

To illustrate how an issuer computes its level debt service requirement, assume a health care provider borrows $1,000,000 at an interest rate of 10 percent for ten years. The first step is to determine the periodic debt service requirements, which equate to the present value of an annuity:

$$\$1,000,000 = (\text{Annuity Payment}) \times \text{PVFA}(0.10, 10)$$

The present value interest factor for an annuity at 10 percent for ten years is 6.1446.

$$\$1,000,000 = \text{Annuity Payment} \times 6.1446$$

$$\$1,000,000/6.1446 = \text{Annual Payment}$$

$$\$162,745 = \text{Annual Payment}$$

Thus, the annual loan payment amount from the health care provider is $162,745 for ten years. Also, one could use the *Excel* PMT function to arrive at annual payments, which was discussed in Chapter 6. As noted earlier, each payment is composed of both principal and interest. The loan amortization schedule for this example is given in Exhibit G–3.

> **Amortization:** The gradual process of paying off debt through a series of equal periodic payments. Each payment covers a portion of the principal plus current interest. The periodic payments are equal over the lifetime of the loan, but the proportion going toward the principal gradually increases. The amount of a payment can be determined by using the formula to calculate the present value of an annuity.

Exhibit G–3   Loan Amortization Schedule for a $1,000,000 Loan at 10 Percent Interest over 10 Years

	Givens:			
1	Annuity Payment	$162,745		
2	Interest Rate	10%		

Year	[A] Annuity Payment [Given 1]	[B] Interest Expense [Given 2 × D]	[C] Principal Payments [A – B]	[D] Remaining Balance[1,2] [D – C]
0				$1,000,000
1	$162,745	$100,000	$62,745	937,255
2	162,745	93,725	69,020	868,235
3	162,745	86,823	75,922	792,313
4	162,745	79,231	83,514	708,799
5	162,745	70,880	91,866	616,933
6	162,745	61,693	101,052	515,881
7	162,745	51,588	111,157	404,724
8	162,745	40,472	122,273	282,451
9	162,745	28,245	134,500	147,950
10	$162,745	$14,795	$147,950	$0

[1] D* is the previous year's value of D
[2] Columns may not total due to rounding

Chapter Nine

USING COST INFORMATION TO MAKE SPECIAL DECISIONS

LEARNING OBJECTIVES

After completing this chapter, you will be able to:

▶ Define fixed and variable costs.
▶ Compute price, fixed cost, variable cost per unit, or quantity, given the others.
▶ Construct and interpret a breakeven chart.
▶ Apply the concepts of contribution margin and product margin to the following types of decisions: make/buy, adding/dropping a service, and expanding/reducing a service.

Chapter Outline

◀INTRODUCTION▶

From time to time administrators face such decisions as:

- Should we offer a particular service or group of services?
- What volume of services do we need to provide in order to break even?
- How much must we charge or be reimbursed for a service to be financially viable?
- Should we offer a service in-house or should we contract with another organization?
- Should we replace equipment?

Questions such as these are called **special decisions** because they are made on an "as needed" basis as opposed to a standard schedule. This chapter provides tools to help answer these and similar questions. It begins with a discussion of breakeven analysis and the role of fixed and variable costs in decision-making. It then turns to the related topics of the breakeven chart, contribution margin, and product margin.

Key Point When the special decisions discussed in this chapter involve multi-year periods, the time value of money must be considered, as discussed in Chapters 6 and 7.

Although this chapter focuses primarily on financial concerns, non-financial criteria must also be considered when making special decisions. In certain cases, non-financial criteria may even outweigh the results of a financial analysis. For instance, though a financial analysis shows that a project meets the financial criteria, such as breaking even, management may decide not to undertake the project because it does not sufficiently meet its community service goals. As shown in Exhibit 9–1, the course of action is clear only when it meets or fails to meet both financial and non-financial criteria.

Exhibit 9–1   The Relationship between Meeting Financial and Non-financial Criteria

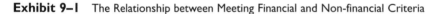

Meets Non-financial Criteria	Meets Financial Criteria	
	Yes	*No*
Yes	Proceed	?
No	?	Don't Proceed

◀BREAKEVEN ANALYSIS▶

One of the most fundamental financial criteria used to make special decisions is whether or not, in the future, a service's revenues will be sufficient to cover its costs. In attempting to answer such a question, management must understand the relationship of revenues, costs, and volume. **Breakeven analysis**, also called Cost-Volume-Profit (CVP) analysis, provides tools to study these relationships. The remainder of this section explores breakeven analysis and how it can be used to help answer numerous questions facing health care organizations.

Breakeven Analysis: A technique to analyze the relationship among revenues, costs, and volume. It is also called Cost-Volume-Profit or CVP analysis.

Using the Breakeven Approach to Determine Prices, Charges, and Reimbursement

Suppose a home health director wants to know how much her agency must be reimbursed per visit for her commercial home health service line to break even. Assuming for the moment that the only costs for this service line are $200,000 for staffing (two RNs and three nursing assistants), then to break even, revenues must also equal $200,000.

$$\text{Revenues} = \text{Costs}$$

$$\$200,000 = \$200,000$$

Though knowing that $200,000 is necessary to cover costs is useful information, the director still does not know how much she must be reimbursed *for each visit* to reach her $200,000 target. The fewer the number of visits, the higher the reimbursement needs to be; conversely, the higher the number of visits, the lower that reimbursement needs to be to earn the $200,000. Thus, in order to determine the necessary per visit reimbursement to break even, she must know the number of visits.

Key Point | Formula to determine total revenue when price and quantity are known: Total Revenue = Price × Quantity.

As shown in Exhibit 9–2, if only 1,000 visits were made, she would have to receive $200 (Column D, $200,000/1,000) for each visit. However, if there were 5,000 visits, she would have to receive only $40 per visit ($200,000/5,000). This inverse relationship between price and volume to obtain a specified amount of revenue (i.e. $200,000) is summarized in the equation:

Key Point | The terms *quantity*, *volume*, and *activity* are often used interchangeably when referring to the number of visits, number of patients, number of services, or the activities of providers and patients related to the delivery or receipt of health care goods and services.

Exhibit 9–2 Illustration of the Inverse Relationship Between Volume and Both Price and Fixed Cost per Visit, Holding Total Revenue and Total Fixed Costs Constant

A Number of Visits [Given]	B Total Revenues [Given]	C Total Fixed Costs [Given]	D Price/Visit [B/A]	E Fixed Cost/Visit [C/A]
1,000	$200,000	$200,000	$200	$200
2,000	$200,000	$200,000	$100	$100
3,000	$200,000	$200,000	$67	$67
4,000	$200,000	$200,000	$50	$50
5,000	$200,000	$200,000	$40	$40

$$\textbf{Total Revenue} = \textbf{Price} \times \textbf{Quantity}$$

where quantity is used generically to stand for such things as number of visits, number of patients, number of services, etc. Since price times quantity equals total revenue, and total revenues equal total costs, the basic breakeven formula can be restated as:

$$\textbf{(Price} \times \textbf{Quantity)} = \textbf{Total Costs}$$

This is shown in Modification I in Exhibit 9–3.

Caution

For simplification purposes, the terms price and reimbursement are used interchangeably in the following discussion. To the extent they differ in any particular situation, an adjustment should be made.

Breakeven Analysis: The Role of Fixed Costs

Just as price per visit varies inversely with volume, if total revenue remains constant average fixed cost per visit is also inversely related to volume as long as total fixed cost remains constant (Exhibit 9–2, column E). If the fixed costs remain at $200,000 and only 1,000 visits are delivered, the average fixed cost per visit is $200 ($200,000/1,000 visits). But at 5,000 visits, the average fixed cost per visit drops to $40 ($200,000/5,000 visits).

This example illustrates the two major attributes of fixed costs:

1. Fixed costs stay the same in total as volume increases (in Exhibit 9–2 they remained at $200,000).
2. Fixed costs per unit change inversely with volume (in Exhibit 9–2 they decreased from an average of $200 per visit to $40 per visit as volume increased from 1,000 to 5,000 visits).

Exhibit 9–3   Using the Concept of Breakeven to Develop the Breakeven Equation

The Basic Breakeven Concept	*Total Revenues = Total Costs*
Modification I to Recognize: a. Revenues = Price × Volume	Price × Volume = Total Costs
Modification II to Recognize: a. Revenues = Price × Volume b. Total Costs = Fixed Costs + Variable Costs	Price × Volume = Fixed Costs + Variable Costs
Modification III to Recognize[1]: a. Revenues = Price × Volume b. Total Costs = Fixed Costs + Variable Costs c. Variable Costs = Variable Cost Per Unit × Volume	Price × Volume = Fixed Costs + (Variable Cost Per Unit × Volume)

[1] Modification III is commonly referred to as the Breakeven Equation

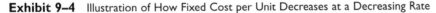

Key Point   The term *cost per unit* is shorthand for *average cost per unit*. Thus, the terms *average fixed cost per unit* and *fixed cost per unit* are used interchangeably. Similarly, the terms *average variable cost per unit* and *variable cost per unit* are used interchangeably. Note: variable costs will be discussed shortly.

Although fixed cost per unit decreases as volume increases, it does so at a decreasing rate. Exhibit 9–4 shows that cost per visit drops quickly at first, but as the number of visits increases towards capacity, the less each additional visit decreases the per unit visit cost. In other words, fixed assets provide the capacity to provide service, and if these assets are being used inefficiently (low volume relative to capacity), considerable gains can be made in per unit cost by increasing volume. However, if these assets are already being used efficiently (high volume relative to capacity), the less per unit cost decreases for each additional unit of service provided. Perspective 9–1 illustrates how an e-commerce health care organization has been forced to cut its fixed costs.

Exhibit 9–4   Illustration of How Fixed Cost per Unit Decreases at a Decreasing Rate

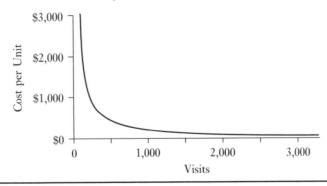

PERSPECTIVE 9–1

Drkoop.com Lays Off Third of Work Force

AUSTIN, Texas – Online health company drkoop.com Inc. has slashed its work force for the second time in three months, saying the layoffs are part of a new corporate restructuring plan aimed at cutting costs.

Late Tuesday, the Austin-based company said it was cutting 50 positions, about one-third of its current work force. The move came on the heels of an announcement Monday that drkoop.com had secured $27.5 million in new financing and revamped its management team. "We said from the beginning that we were going to run this company like a real business," said Ed Cespedes, the company's newly appointed president. "There are real people behind these layoffs and these were not easy decisions. However, we are ready to put the past behind us and move forward with our plans to rebuild this company and maximize shareholder value."

Source: The Boston Globe, August 31, 2000.
© Copyright 2000 Globe Newspaper Company.

The Relevant Range:
The range of activity over which *total fixed costs* and/or *per unit variable cost* do not vary.

Fixed Costs: Costs that stay the same in total over the relevant range, but change inversely on a per unit basis as activity changes.

Of course, at some point, the capacity of the assets is reached and there is a need to expand (for instance, by buying new equipment or hiring new staff). In such a case, fixed costs would no longer remain fixed at $200,000, but would step up to a new level. When the lower or upper limits of capacity are reached, and it becomes necessary to add or drop capacity (e.g. full-time staff), the organization is said to be going beyond the **relevant range** of its **fixed costs**. However, within the relevant range, fixed costs remain fixed.

Exhibit 9–5 shows that the fixed costs of $200,000 in labor are considered fixed up to 5,000 visits (Relevant Range 1). Then, assuming an additional full-time RN is needed if volume extends past 5,000 visits, the fixed costs would take a step up to $250,000 (assuming that each new RN costs $50,000). The fixed costs then remain at this level (Relevant Range 2) until visits reach 7,500, at which point they step up to $300,000 (Relevant Range 3), when another full-time RN again has to be hired. To the extent that there are **step-fixed costs**, the breakeven formula can become complicated. Thus, it is strongly suggested that breakeven analyses with step-fixed costs be done on electronic spreadsheets.

Exhibit 9–5   Step-Fixed Costs Occurring at 5,000 and 7,500 Visits

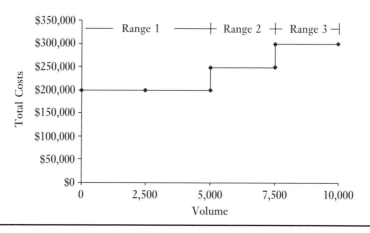

Caution. There are two major errors that must be avoided when using fixed cost information to make decisions: 1) Assuming that cost per unit does not change when volume changes; and 2) Using fixed cost per unit derived at one level to forecast total fixed costs at another level. How fixed cost per unit costs changes with a change in volume was just illustrated. In regard to the second type of error: suppose that the home health agency, which has $200,000 in fixed costs, made 4,000 visits this year (Exhibit 9–6, second row). Using this information, the administrator correctly calculates the average fixed cost per visit to be $50 ($200,000/4,000 visits). The next year the agency plans to make 5,000 visits (third row). The administrator would be making an error if she assumed that the average fixed cost per visit would remain at $50. Since volume increases from 4,000 visits to 5,000, and total fixed cost remains at $200,000 (it's fixed!), the average fixed cost per visit decreases from $50 per visit ($200,000/4,000 visits) to $40 per visit ($200,000/5,000 visits). Thus, if the administrator were trying to set her price to cover her fixed cost, she may set it too high ($50) instead of recognizing that cost has decreased (to $40) because of increased volume. Conversely, as shown in Exhibit 9–6, if the administrator were using the $50 per visit derived at 4,000 visits to estimate her fixed cost at 3,000 visits, her estimate would be too low.

> **Step-Fixed Costs:** Costs that increase in total over wide, discrete steps.

Breakeven Analysis: The Role of Variable Costs

Thus far, it has been assumed that all costs are fixed or step-fixed. However, a home health visit does not require just labor; each visit also requires certain items particular to that visit (supplies, transportation, etc.). If these other costs average $25 a visit, then 100 visits would cost $2,500 (100 × $25). For 1,000 or 10,000 visits, costs would increase to $25,000 (1,000 × $25) and $250,000 (10,000 × $25), respectively. Because total cost varies *directly* with activity (in this case volume), these costs are called **variable costs**, though the cost per unit remains the same, $25.

Thus, the two major characteristics of variable costs have been identified, and they are just the opposite of those for fixed costs:

> **Variable Costs:** Costs that stay the same per unit but change directly in total with a change in activity over the relevant range. Total Variable Cost = Variable Cost Per Unit × Number of Units of Activity.

Exhibit 9–6 Illustration of the Error of Using Fixed Cost per Unit Derived at One Level of Activity to Calculate Total Fixed Cost at Another Level

A Volume [Estimated]	B Assumed per Unit Fixed Cost[1] [Given]	C Estimated Total Fixed Cost [A × B]	D Actual Fixed Cost [Given]	E Over (Under) Estimate [C − D]
3,000	$50	$150,000	$200,000	($50,000)[2]
4,000	$50	$200,000	$200,000	($0)[3]
5,000	$50	$250,000	$200,000	$50,000[4]

[1] All three examples use the unit cost derived at 4,000 units to estimate total fixed cost.
[2] If the unit fixed cost is originally derived at a higher volume, the total fixed cost estimated will be too low.
[3] If the unit fixed cost is originally derived at the same volume, the total fixed cost estimated will be just right
[4] If the unit fixed cost is originally derived at a lower volume, the total fixed cost estimated will be too high.

1. **Total variable cost** changes directly with a change in activity; and

2. **Variable cost per unit** stays the same with a change in activity.

The formula that describes the relationship between variable cost and activity is:

**Total Variable Cost = Variable Cost Per Unit
× Number of Units of Activity**

As discussed earlier, when total fixed costs go beyond the relevant range, they often take the form of step-fixed costs, though it is possible to substitute variable costs for fixed costs (e.g. paying a home health nurse by the visit rather than hiring another full-time nurse). When variable costs per unit go beyond the relevant range, it is possible to have either an increase or decrease in cost per unit. For instance, if volume increases significantly, an organization may be able to obtain a volume discount on supplies. It would no longer be $25, but a lower amount. Of course, if volume dropped, the opposite effect may occur – the loss of discounts and an increase in variable cost per unit. As with fixed costs, as volume goes beyond the relevant range, it becomes difficult to use the breakeven formula to solve breakeven problems with variable costs, and using a spreadsheet model is recommended.

 Key Point By convention, when the terms *fixed* and *variable costs* are used, it is understood that they remain constant in total (fixed costs) or on a per unit basis (variable costs), respectively, *only within a relevant range.*

Exhibit 9–7 summarizes and compares the major characteristics of fixed and variable costs in relation to volume within a relevant range. Fixed costs stay the same in total but change per unit as volume changes, whereas variable costs change in total but remain constant per unit with changes in volume. A method using physician education to control costs is shown in Perspective 9–2, while Perspective 9–3 illustrates the complex interaction between cost and inpatient care.

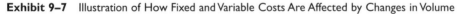

Exhibit 9–7   Illustration of How Fixed and Variable Costs Are Affected by Changes in Volume

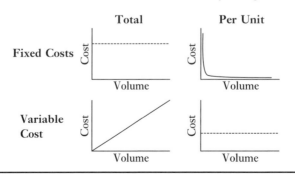

PERSPECTIVE 9–2

Targeting Disease Treatment Could Save States Thousands in Medicaid Costs and Improve Health Outcomes for Patients with Asthma

Virginia Program Results Could Be Duplicated Nationwide

Washington, DC – The Virginia Health Outcomes Partnership (VHOP), a model disease management program, conducted in eight Virginia counties and metropolitan Richmond between 1995 and 1997, saved thousands of dollars in Medicaid costs for the treatment of asthma in fiscal year 1997, according to a peer-reviewed article appearing today in the economics journal *Inquiry*. At the same time, rates of urgent care visits for patients with asthma in the pilot area were reduced.

The study, the first of its kind in a Medicaid population, estimated annual savings of over $1 million if the program was implemented statewide. . . . The program's goals were to educate physicians to help them improve their communications skills and their ability to educate patients on how to manage their asthma. . . . The dispensing of drugs recommended by the guidelines for asthma also rose significantly during the study period in the intervention communities. In some cases this increase was as much as 25 percent. "Asthma drugs can be very effective at keeping people out of the emergency room when used properly," said Rossiter. "The VHOP program was designed specifically to help the low-income Medicaid population and their physicians and pharmacists tap into the potential cost savings and health benefits of better adherence to treatment regimens."

Source: AHA News, August 28, 2000

PERSPECTIVE 9–3

Study: Reducing Hospital LOS by One Day Saves Little

Length of Stay's Effect on Hospital Admission Cost Is Minimal

Cost containment and cost reduction in hospitals remain a focus of all sectors of the healthcare delivery industry. It has been generally accepted that reducing the length of stay (LOS) for hospital inpatient admissions is one of the best ways to reduce costs. A study published in the August 2000 Journal of the American College of Surgeons, however, questions the veracity of this financial sacred cow.

The researchers reviewed the cost-accounting records of all surviving patients (n = 12,365) discharged from University of Michigan Health System (UMHS) during fiscal year 1998 with LOS of four days or more. . . . Individual patient costs were broken out on a per-day basis and further subdivided into variable-direct, fixed-direct, and indirect costs. Then, the incremental resource cost of the last full day of the inpatient stay versus the total cost for the entire stay was determined. The data also were stratified by LOS and by surgical costs. . . .

The researchers found that the average incremental costs incurred on the last full day of an inpatient stay was $420, or just 2.4 percent of the $17,734 mean total cost per stay for all 12,365 patients. Mean end-of-stay costs represented only a slightly higher percentage of total costs when the LOS was short (6.8 percent for patients with an LOS of four days). Even when the data focused only on patients without major operations, the average last-day, variable-direct cost of $432 was only 3.4 percent of the $12,631 average total cost of care.

The researchers focused on the trauma center to help explain this result. The variable-direct costs for the trauma center accounted for 42 percent of the mean total cost per stay of $22,067. The remaining 58 percent comprised fixed and indirect hospital overhead costs. The median variable-direct cost on the first day of a trauma center admission was $1,246, and the median variable-direct cost on discharge was $304. Approximately 40 percent of the variable costs were incurred during the first three days of admission.

(Continues)

Perspective 9–3 (*Contd*)

The researchers concluded that for most patients, the costs directly attributable to the last day of a hospital stay are an economically insignificant component of total costs. Reducing LOS by as much as one full day reduces the total cost of care an average of 3 percent or less. The researchers suggest that physicians and administrators should deemphasize reducing LOS and focus instead on process changes that make better use of capacity and resources during the early stages of admission.

Source: P. A. Taheri, D. A. Butz, and L. J. Greenfield, *Journal of the American College of Surgery*, Volume 191, Number 2, August 2000, pp. 123–30.

Using the Breakeven Equation

The breakeven formula can now be expanded and modified to include variable costs (see Exhibit 9–3, Modification II):

$$\text{Price} \times \text{Volume} = \text{Fixed Cost} + \text{Variable Cost}$$

Expanding this equation based on the above discussion yields the basic breakeven equation:

$$\text{Price} \times \text{Volume} = \text{Fixed Costs} + (\text{Variable Cost Per Unit} \times \text{Volume})$$

as shown in Modification III in Exhibit 9–3.

Exhibit 9–8 illustrates how the breakeven formula can be used to find the price, quantity (volume), fixed cost, or variable cost per unit needed to break even, if each of the other factors is known. In Situation 1 of Exhibit 9–8, *price* is unknown; in Situation 2, *quantity* (volume) is unknown; in Situation 3, *total fixed cost* is unknown; and in Situation 4, *variable cost per unit* is unknown.

Expanding the Breakeven Equation to Include Indirect Costs and Required Profit

Up to this point, the example has looked at situations where revenues exactly match only those costs which the organization can directly associate with a service, those of the two RNs and three nursing assistants, and miscellaneous variable costs such as supplies and transportation. However, in many cases it is often desirable that revenues cover other costs, such as overhead, and, perhaps, provide a margin (profit). As discussed in more detail in Chapter 12, *direct costs* are those that an organization can measure or trace to a particular patient or service (e.g. the time a nurse or nursing assistant spends with a client), while *indirect costs* are those which the organization is not able to associate with a particular patient or service (e.g. the cost of the billing clerk or computer system). Exhibit 9–9 extends the breakeven equation in Exhibit 9–3 to account for indirect costs and profit, while Exhibit 9–10 expands the example from Exhibit 9–8 to illustrate how to use the extended equation. Since it is usually the case,

Exhibit 9–8   Applying the Breakeven Formula

Givens.	[A] Situation	[B] Price	[C] Quantity[1]	[D] Total Fixed Cost	[E] Variable Cost per Unit[2]
	Situation 1	?	4,000	$200,000	$25
	Situation 2	$100	?	$200,000	$25
	Situation 3	$100	4,000	?	$25
	Situation 4	$100	4,000	$200,000	?

[1] E.g. number of visits.
[2] E.g. cost of supplies per visit.

Situation 1.   Finding the breakeven *price*, given quantity, total fixed cost, and variable cost per unit.

		Total Fixed	Variable Cost
Setup:	(Price × Quantity) =	Cost	+ (Per Unit × Quantity)
Solution:	(Price × 4,000) =	$200,000	+ ($25 × 4,000)
	(Price × 4,000) =	$200,000	+ $100,000
	(Price × 4,000) =	$300,000	
	Price =	$75	

Situation 2.   Finding the breakeven *quantity*, given price, total fixed cost, and variable cost per unit.

		Total Fixed	Variable Cost
Setup:	(Price × Quantity) =	Cost	+ (Per Unit × Quantity)
Solution:	($100 × Quantity) =	$200,000	+ ($25 × Quantity)
	($75 × Quantity) =	$200,000	
	Quantity =	2,667	

Situation 3.   Finding the breakeven *total fixed cost*, given price, quantity, and variable cost per unit.

		Total Fixed	Variable Cost
Setup:	(Price × Quantity) = Cost		+ (Per Unit × Quantity)
Solution:	($100 × 4,000) = TFC		+ ($25 × 4,000)
	$400,000 = TFC		+ $100,000
	$300,000 = Total Fixed Cost		

Situation 4.   Finding the breakeven *variable cost per unit*, given price, quantity, and total fixed cost.

		Total Fixed	Variable Cost
Setup:	(Price × Quantity) = Cost		+ (Per Unit × Quantity)
Solution:	($100 × 4,000) = $200,000		+ (VCu × 4,000)
	$400,000 = $200,000		+ (VCu × 4,000)
	$200,000 =		VCu × 4,000)
	$50 = Variable Cost Per Unit		

Exhibit 9–9   Expanding the Breakeven Equation to Include Indirect Costs and Desired Profit

---

The Basic Breakeven Equation[1]   Price × Volume = Fixed Costs + (Variable Cost per Unit × Volume)
The Basic Breakeven Equation Modified
  to include Indirect Costs and Desired
    Profit   Price × Volume = Direct Costs + Indirect Costs[2] + Desired Profit[2]

Direct Fixed Costs + (Direct Variable Cost per Unit × Volume)

---

[1] From Exhibit 9–3, Modification III.
[2] Indirect Costs and Desired Profits usually are given as an amount, though they could also be broken down into their fixed and variable components, as are Direct Costs.

---

these examples assume that both indirect costs and profits are fixed amounts, though the equation can be modified to account for other instances.

In Situations 1–3 of Exhibit 9–10, *price* is unknown and various combinations of indirect costs and desired profit are added to the information originally provided in Exhibit 9–8. Such analyses would be used when an organization is trying to determine if the reimbursement it will receive is sufficient to cover its costs and desired profit for a particular service. For example, in Situation 3, if the organization were not reimbursed at least $111 per visit, management could conclude that the reimbursement would be insufficient to cover its direct and indirect costs and desired margin and perhaps decide not to provide the service at this rate, or try to renegotiate a higher rate.

In Situation 4 of Exhibit 9–10, all of the factors are given except for fixed costs. A situation such as this occurs when an organization is given a set price (reimbursement) and must control its costs in order to ensure that its costs don't exceed that reimbursement. In this case, given the indirect costs and desired profit, the organization must ensure that its direct fixed costs do not exceed $156,000. Such an approach, called **target costing**, is quite common in health care, where the government is the price-setter and the provider is the price-taker. Perspective 9–4 shows how rather than cutting back, a number of hospitals are attempting to increase both volume and profits through aggressive marketing. Perspective 9–5 illustrates a wide number of tools available to group practices to both control costs and increase revenues. Several of these are discussed in chapters 10, 11 and 12 of this book. Finally, Perspective 9–6 illustrates how one organization is attempting to control its supply costs by managing its supply chain.

Target Costing:
Controlling costs and/or decreasing profit margins in order to meet or beat a predetermined price or reimbursement rate.

The Breakeven Chart

A breakeven chart graphically displays the relationships in the breakeven equation. For instance, Exhibits 9–11a, b, and c present different ways to graph the data in Exhibit 9–8, where the revenue per visit is $100, fixed costs are $200,000, and variable cost is $25 per visit. Exhibit 9–11a presents this information in the traditional breakeven chart format, but with considerable annotation. The three lines represent fixed cost, total cost, and total revenues. The *total revenue line* begins at $0 (the

Exhibit 9–10   Applying the Breakeven Formula to Situations with Indirect Costs and/or Desired Profit

Situation	Price	Quantity[1]	Total Fixed Cost	Variable Cost Per Unit[2]	Indirect Costs	Desired Profit
Situation 1	?	4,000	$200,000	$50	$24,000	$0
Situation 2	?	4,000	$200,000	$50	$0	$20,000
Situation 3	?	4,000	$200,000	$50	$24,000	$20,000
Situation 4	$100	4,000	?	$50	$24,000	$20,000

[1] E.g. number of visits.
[2] E.g. cost of supplies per visit.

Situation 1.   Finding the breakeven *price*, given quantity, total fixed cost, variable cost per unit, and indirect costs.

			Total Fixed Cost	Variable Cost		
Setup:	(Price × Quantity)	=	Cost	+ (Per Unit × Quantity)	+ Indirect Costs +	Desired Profit
Solution:	(Price × 4,000)	=	$200,000	+ ($50 × 4,000)	+ $24,000	+ $0
	(Price × 4,000)	=	$200,000	+ $200,000	+ $24,000	
	(Price × 4,000)	=	$424,000			
	Price	=	$106			

Situation 2.   Finding the breakeven *price*, given quantity, total fixed cost, variable cost per unit, and desired profit

			Total Fixed Cost	Variable Cost		
Setup:	(Price × Quantity)	=	Cost	+ (Per Unit × Quantity)	+ Indirect Costs +	Desired Profit
Solution:	(Price × 4,000)	=	$200,000	+ ($50 × 4,000)	+ $0	+ $20,000
	(Price × 4,000)	=	$200,000	+ $200,000		+ $20,000
	(Price × 4,000)	=	$420,000			
	Price	=	$105			

Situation 3.   Finding the breakeven *price*, given quantity, total fixed cost, variable cost per unit, indirect costs, and desired profit.

			Total Fixed Cost	Variable Cost		
Setup:	(Price × Quantity)	=	Cost	+ (Per Unit × Quantity)	+ Indirect Costs +	Desired Profit
Solution:	(Price × 4,000)	=	$200,000	+ ($50 × 4,000)	+ $24,000	+ $20,000
	(Price × 4,000)	=	$200,000	+ $200,000	+ $44,000	
	(Price × 4,000)	=	$444,000			
	Price	=	$111			

Situation 4.   Finding the breakeven *total fixed cost*, given price, quantity, variable cost per unit, indirect costs and desired profit.

			Total Fixed Cost	Variable Cost		
Setup:	(Price × Quantity)	=	Cost	+ (Per Unit × Quantity)	+ Indirect Costs +	Desired Profit
Solution:	($100 × 4,000)	=	TFC	+ ($50 × 4,000)	+ $24,000	+ $20,000
	($100 × 4,000)	=	TFC	+ $200,000	+ $44,000	
	$400,000	=	TFC	+ $244,000		
	$156,000	=	Total Fixed Cost			

PERSPECTIVE 9–4

M. D. Anderson Works to Build Ties With the HMOs It Once Combated

Houston – Five years ago, battered by the onslaught of managed care, M. D. Anderson Cancer Center seemed headed for the intensive-care unit.

No matter that the half-century-old hospital had a reputation for saving patients told by others to begin planning their funerals, or that it consistently scored at the top of national quality surveys. M. D. Anderson's patient load was dropping precipitously, as health-maintenance organizations began steering patients to lower-cost community hospitals.

Consultants prognosticated that by the millennium, overnight stays would drop by a third, and the cancer hospital would be forced to shutter many of its facilities. "The consultants painted a doom-and-gloom picture," remembers Harry Holmes, the hospital's vice president of governmental affairs, "with graphs sloping down like a slide."

As it turned out, the graphs did slope steeply – but in the other direction. Revenue for the current fiscal year, which ends Thursday, is expected to be $1.07 billion, up 85% from five years ago. The average number of patients who stay each night at M. D. Anderson, a not-for-profit arm of the University of Texas, has risen 16% since the low in 1996. And instead of shutting buildings, the hospital is expanding on a grand scale with a new research building, more beds, and new rooms at the campus hotel.

M. D. Anderson's turnaround is due in part to its savvy, aggressive effort to recruit patients from across the US through the Internet and a heart-wrenching advertising campaign. The hospital also has gradually made its peace with managed care, cutting some costs to please HMOs while simultaneously fighting those that refuse to send their members to M. D. Anderson for the latest treatments. Its recent success is also due in part to demographics: As baby boomers reach the age at which cancer often begins, the oncology business is picking up.

M. D. Anderson's resurgence spotlights a striking development in American health care: Contrary to predictions, the high-priced, top-tier hospital business is alive and well. Even as many prestigious hospitals struggle with federal cutbacks, some of the best are figuring out how to thrive handsomely.

The University of California at Los Angeles has succeeded in funneling patients to its academic research hospital with an aggressive strategy for setting up primary-care clinics in the surrounding community. Other hospitals, aided by the draw of their national reputations, have capitalized on a growing pool of Internet-literate patients willing to travel anywhere for care.

Memorial Sloan-Kettering Cancer Center in New York, after eliminating beds during a slump in the mid-1990s, has now added back many of the beds it cut, and is building a giant new outpatient clinic to handle the influx of patients. The Mayo Clinic of Rochester, Minn., unable to handle its burgeoning patient load, is building a giant $400 million extension that it had postponed years back amid falling patient visits and anxiety over the Clinton administration's health-care plan.

Source: Laura Johannes, *Wall Street Journal*, August 29, 2000.

PERSPECTIVE 9–5

Practices with the Best Practices

With many doc groups losing money, MGMA study shows what makes a "better performer."

The Medical Group Management Association's annual cost survey has been a mainstay of its member benefits for 50 years, offering detailed revenue and expense data on practices nationwide. . . .

Through interviews with practice managers and industry experts, the report also discusses the ingredients that drive success. According to the report, there's no magic formula but rather a blend of good practices.

(Continues)

Perspective 9–5 (Contd)

For example, medical groups traditionally have placed more emphasis on generating revenues than controlling costs, according to the report. But better-performing groups do both. The report identifies seven common tools:

- Detailed cost accounting. Cost accounting systems enable practices to determine the cost of and revenues generated by each procedure, allowing effective resource allocation.
- Transaction costing. Knowing the true cost of delivering a unit of care improves a group's negotiating position with third-party payers and avoids money-losing contracts.
- Zero-based budgeting. Better performers start each budget from scratch rather than applying a uniform inflation factor to last year's numbers.
- Physician incentives. Better performers compensate physicians for controlling costs. They commonly measure the types and numbers of support staff a physician uses as well as adherence to practice protocols. Top performers also use lower-cost supplies.
- Effective managed-care contracting. Better performers have sophisticated methods of negotiating and monitoring managed-care agreements, including contract review committees that develop checklists of parameters for each contract.
- Effective coding. On the whole, medical groups "undercode" an estimated 50% to 60% of the time, meaning they lose revenues they're entitled to, according to the report. To enhance accuracy, better performers emphasize coding training, develop explicit coding processes and undergo outside assessments of their coding.
- Improved service delivery. Better performers invest in computerized scheduling systems, maintain sufficient support staff and often allocate three or more exam rooms per primary-care physician. E-mail consultations and telephone triage are common.

Source: Mary Chris Jaklevic, *Modern Healthcare*, February 8, 1999, pp. 64–5.

PERSPECTIVE 9–6

Mission to Stop Restocking Ambulances: Pardee, Park Ridge Hope to Continue

Bandages, endotracheal tubes and cold packs – necessities of Emergency Medical Services work – will continue to move from hospital shelves to ambulances trying to make quick turn-arounds, hospital officials hope. Pardee and Park Ridge hospitals hope to continue supplying ambulances with these and other types of equipment despite a decision by Mission St Joseph's Health System in Asheville to cut off the flow of such supplies by Aug. 1. Mission St Joseph's, under pressure from the Office of the Inspector General, the federal organization responsible for enforcing Medicare fraud rules, said it will no longer swap out supplies used by ambulances on a one-for-one basis.

The hospital now passes on the costs of the supplies by bundling them with hospital bills. In August, however, patients will pay for those costs at the front end with their ambulance bills, rather than the back end with their hospital bills. The cost of ambulance service could increase by $100 as a result, Buncombe County EMS personnel have said.

The move came after the Office of the Inspector General determined hospitals might be using supply trade-outs as enticements to draw ambulances and therefore patients to their doors. Because of this, the practice may violate anti-kickback legislation, the OIG said.

Henderson County-affiliated Pardee Hospital, however, uses a different system. The hospital allows ambulances to restock but keeps accounts and sends out bills, emergency room manager Ruby Icamina said.

Source: Joel Burgess, *Hendersonville News*, July 20, 2000.

Exhibit 9–11a   A Traditional Breakeven Chart with Annotation

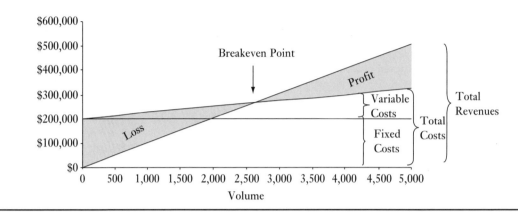

amount of revenue earned if no services are offered) and increases by $100 for each home health visit made. Since by definition fixed costs do not change with volume, the *fixed cost line* begins at $200,000 and remains at that level. Since total cost is made up of fixed cost plus variable cost, the *total cost line* begins at $200,000 (the level of fixed cost at zero units of service) and grows by $25 (the variable cost per unit) for each unit of service provided.

At 2,667 visits the total revenue and total cost lines cross. Before 2,667 visits net income is negative, whereas after 2,667 visits, it is positive. Thus, the **breakeven point**, the point at which total revenues equal total costs, is 2,667 visits. Before the breakeven point, the size of the space between the *total revenue* line and the *total cost* line equals the amount of loss. After the breakeven point, the size of the space between the *total revenue* line and the *total cost* line equals the amount of profit. Exhibit 9–11b presents the breakeven chart from Exhibit 9–11a in its traditional format; that is, without much of the annotation.

Since it is so difficult to visually determine how much the actual loss or profit is by using the traditional version, increasingly a newer version is being used (see Exhibit 9–11c). In addition to the information typically presented in Exhibit 9–11b, the newer version presents net income, total revenues less total costs. Note that in all three charts, breakeven is achieved at 2,667 visits. In general, the old version should be used where detailed cost information is important, and the new version should be used in cases where the amount of profit is the essential concern.

Breakeven Point: The point where total revenues equal total costs.

Contribution Margin per Unit: Per unit revenue minus per unit variable cost.

Incremental costs: Additional costs incurred solely as a result of an action or activity or a particular set of actions or activities.

A Shortcut to Calculating Breakeven: The Contribution Margin

Per unit revenue minus per unit variable cost is called **contribution margin per unit**, because after covering **incremental (variable) costs**, this is the amount left to contribute toward covering all other costs and desired profit. If the contribution margin is known and all other costs are fixed, a shortcut formula to calculate breakeven can be used:

Breakeven Volume = Fixed Costs/Contribution Margin per Unit

Exhibit 9–11b   A Traditional Breakeven Chart

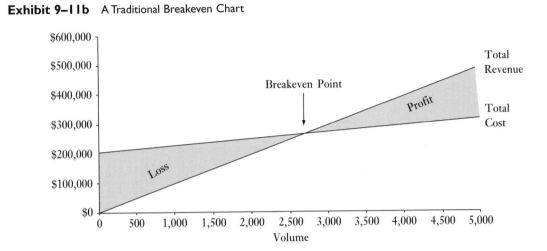

Note: Some presenters will include the fixed cost line. However, it is not absolutely necessary as it is equal to the amount where the total cost line crosses the Y axis: $200,000.

Exhibit 9–11c   A Breakeven Chart Emphasizing Net income

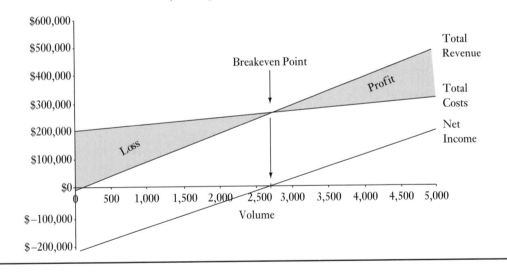

Assume that total fixed costs are $200,000, revenue per visit is $100, and variable cost is $25 per visit. Thus, contribution margin per unit is $75 ($100 – $25), which means that the organization makes $75 more on each visit than the incremental cost of that visit. Thus, using the above formula, to cover the $200,000 in fixed costs, there must be 2,667 visits ($200,000/$75; see Exhibit 9–12). This is the same answer that was derived using the longer formula in Exhibit 9–8, Situation 2.

Total Contribution Margin: Total revenues minus total variable costs.

Exhibit 9–12   The Breakeven Equation Using the Contribution Margin Approach

Given: Revenue per Visit $100
        Variable Cost per Visit $25
        Contribution Margin per Visit $75
        Fixed Cost $200,000

To determine the breakeven quantity using the contribution margin approach:

$$\frac{\text{Fixed Cost}}{\text{Contribution Margin per Unit}} = \frac{\$200,000}{\$75} = \textbf{2,667 Visits}$$

Contribution Margin Rule: If the contribution margin per unit is positive and no other additional costs will be incurred, then it is in the best financial interest of the organization to continue to provide additional units of that service, even if the organization is not fully covering all of its other costs. On the other hand, if the contribution margin is negative, it is not in the best interest of the organization to continue to provide additional units of service.

Finally, notice that even if the organization does not reach breakeven, each unit of service it delivers contributes $75 toward covering its fixed costs and overhead. This leads to the **Contribution Margin Rule**: if the contribution margin per unit is positive and no other additional costs will be incurred, then it is in the best financial interest of the organization to continue to provide additional units of that service, even if the organization is not fully covering all of its other costs. On the other hand, if the contribution margin is negative, it is not in the best interest of the organization to continue to provide additional units of service.

Key Point

Contribution Margin can be determined on a total or a per unit basis. Total Contribution Margin = *Total Revenue – Total Variable Cost*. Contribution Margin per Unit = *Revenue per Unit – Variable Cost per Unit*. It is the amount of profit made on each additional unit produced if all other costs remain the same.

Effects of Capitation on Breakeven Analysis

With an increasing emphasis on cost control, various managed care companies have turned to capitation as their preferred method of payment. As capitated payment systems are discussed in detail in Chapter 13, the focus here is on how breakeven analysis can be used with capitation. Briefly, under full capitation, the insurer prepays a health care provider an agreed-upon amount per member that covers a designated set of services for the insured population over a defined time period. Typically, these payments are made on a *per member per month (PMPM)* basis. If there are no terms to the contrary, in return for the capitated payments, the provider agrees to bear all the risk for the costs of services provided. If the provider's costs are below the global capitation amount, the provider can keep the difference. If the provider's costs are more than the capitation, the provider is at risk for the difference. Obviously, negotiations on both the capitated amount and any particulars of the contract (e.g. services not covered, and arrangements which limit the financial risk of the provider) are critical to the provider, who must estimate the volume and type of services that may have to be performed, and the amount of money needed to cover them. The following example shows a breakeven analysis for a health care provider under a capitated system.

Hospital A, which has a capitation arrangement with a managed care organization, wants to negotiate a capitated contract with a multi-specialty group practice to provide a major portion of the medical services that Hospital A is obligated to provide. This type of arrangement is commonly called a *subcapitation arrangement*. The population covered under this subcapitation arrangement consists of 1,400 covered lives with no Medicare or Medicaid beneficiaries.

The director of managed care contracts for the clinic is under pressure to bring in new business. In weighing this opportunity, he must balance many factors, some of which will not be known until the contract is actually in effect, including: 1) the per member per month rate; 2) the expected proportion of members needing services; and 3) the average cost of the services that the members will actually receive. Exhibit 9–13 offers three separate scenarios, each varying one of these three factors while holding the other two constant.

In keeping with the same example used throughout the chapter, assume that fixed costs equal $200,000, and that the variable cost per unit equals $25. However, the fixed cost figure represents the *annual* amount, whereas capitation is being paid here on a *monthly* basis (PMPM). Thus, annual fixed costs must be converted into equivalent monthly amounts, or $16,667 ($200,000/12 months). Variable costs remain the same and do not need to be converted.

In the first scenario (Exhibit 9–13), only the capitation rate is unknown. The clinic either gains or loses depending upon whether the capitation amount is above or below $14.40 PMPM. Note that in this scenario, *total costs remain constant* (columns H, I, J), regardless of the capitation amount, but *total revenues vary* based on the capitation rate to be paid (column A). While Exhibit 9–13 uses a spreadsheet approach to solving scenario 1, another way to solve this problem is to set it up as an equation:

$$\text{PMPM} \times \text{Enrollees} = (\text{Enrollees} \times \text{Utilization Rate} \times \text{Variable Cost/Unit}) + \text{Fixed Cost}$$

$$\text{PMPM} \times 1,400 = (1,400 \times 0.10 \times 25) + 16,667$$

$$1,400 \text{ PMPM} = 20,167$$

$$\text{PMPM} = \sim \$14.40$$

In the second scenario, the percentage of members each month receiving services is unknown, but capitation is held to $15 PMPM. As expected, the lower the percentage of members receiving services, the greater the net income for the clinic. Note that in this scenario, *total revenues remain constant* (column F), but *total costs vary* (columns I, J). As with the previous scenario, scenario 2 can also be set up as an equation:

$$\text{PMPM} \times \text{Enrollees} = (\text{Enrollees} \times \text{Utilization Rate} \times \text{Variable Cost/Unit}) + \text{Fixed Cost}$$

$$15 \times 1,400 = (1,400 \times \text{Utilization Rate} \times 25) + 16,667$$

$$4,333 = 35,000 \times \text{Utilization Rate}$$

$$\text{Utilization Rate} = 0.1238$$

In the final scenario, capitation and percentage of members receiving services are held constant, but average cost per member receiving services is unknown. As average cost per member rises (column C), net income falls for the clinic (column K), as would

Exhibit 9–13 An Example of How to Perform a Breakeven Analysis under a Capitated Arrangement

Givens	Number of Members	Total Fixed Cost	PMPM	Utilization Rate	Variable Cost/Unit
Scenario 1	1,400	$16,667	?	10%	$25
Scenario 2	1,400	$16,667	$15	?	$25
Scenario 3	1,400	$16,667	$15	10%	?

Scenario 1: Using the breakeven equation to determine breakeven *PMPM subcapitation rate*, given service cost and utilization rates.

[A] Monthly Capitation Amount (PMPM)   ?
[B] Fixed Costs per Month $16,667
[C] Average Costs of Services per Member Receiving $25
[D] Percentage of Members Receiving Services Each Month   10%
[E] Total Number of HMO Capitated Members   1,400

[A] Monthly Capitation [Estimate]	[F] Revenues [A × E]	[G] Members w/Services [D × E]	[H] Fixed Costs [B]	[I] Variable Costs [C × G]	[J] Total Costs [H + I]	[K] Net Income [F − J]
$5.00	$7,000	140	$16,667	$3,500	$20,167	($13,167)
$10.00	$14,000	140	$16,667	$3,500	$20,167	($6,167)
$14.40	**$20,167**	**140**	**$16,667**	**$3,500**	**$20,167**	**$0**
$15.00	$21,000	140	$16,667	$3,500	$20,167	$833
$20.00	$28,000	140	$16,667	$3,500	$20,167	$7,833
$25.00	$35,000	140	$16,667	$3,500	$20,167	$14,833

Scenario 2: Using the breakeven equation to determine breakeven *utilization rates*, given service cost and PMPM subcapitation rates.

[A] Monthly Capitation Amount $15
[B] Fixed Costs per Month $16,667
[C] Average Costs of Services per Member Receiving $25
[D] Percentage of Members Receiving Services Each Month   ?
[E] Total Number of HMO Capitated Members   1,400

[D] Average Util Rate [Estimate]	[F] Revenues [A × E]	[G] Members w/Services [D × E]	[H] Fixed Costs [B]	[I] Variable Costs [C × G]	[J] Total Costs [H + I]	[K] Net Income [F − J]
5.00%	$21,000	70	$16,667	$1,750	$18,417	$2,583
10.00%	$21,000	140	$16,667	$3,500	$20,167	$833
12.38%	**$21,000**	**173**	**$16,667**	**$4,333**	**$21,000**	**$0**
15.00%	$21,000	210	$16,667	$5,250	$21,917	($917)
20.00%	$21,000	280	$16,667	$7,000	$23,667	($2,667)
25.00%	$21,000	350	$16,667	$8,750	$25,417	($4,417)

(Continues)

Exhibit 9–13 (Contd)

Scenario 3: Using the breakeven equation to determine breakeven *service cost*, given PMPM subcapitation rates and utilization rate.

[A] Monthly Capitation Amount	$15
[B] Fixed Costs per Month	$16,667
[C] Average Costs of Services per Member Receiving	?
[D] Percentage of Members Receiving Services Each Month	10%
[E] Total Number of HMO Capitated Members	1,400

[C] Service Costs [Estimate]	[F] Revenues [A × E]	[G] Members w/Services [D × E]	[H] Fixed Costs [B]	[I] Variable Costs [C × G]	[J] Total Costs [H + I]	[K] Net Income [F − J]
$15.00	$21,000	140	$16,667	$2,100	$18,767	$2,233
$20.00	$21,000	140	$16,667	$2,800	$19,467	$1,533
$25.00	$21,000	140	$16,667	$3,500	$20,167	$833
$30.00	$21,000	140	$16,667	$4,200	$20,867	$133
$30.95	**$21,000**	**140**	**$16,667**	**$4,333**	**$21,000**	**$0**
$35.00	$21,000	140	$16,667	$4,900	$21,567	($567)

be expected. Note that in this third scenario, like the one before it, *total revenues remain constant*, but *total costs vary*. As with the previous scenarios, scenario 3 can also be set up as an equation:

$$\text{PMPM} \times \text{Enrollees} = (\text{Enrollees} \times \text{Utilization Rate} \times \text{Variable Cost/Unit}) + \text{Fixed Cost}$$

$$15 \times 1,400 = (1,400 \times 0.10 \times \text{Variable Cost/Unit}) + 16,667$$

$$4,333 = 140 \times \text{Variable Cost/Unit}$$

Variable Cost/Unit = $30.95

As with non-capitated payments, a breakeven chart can also be constructed under a capitated payment environment. Exhibit 9–14 provides an illustration of this using the same cost structure as in Exhibit 9–11 (FC = $16,667 and VC = $25/visit), but revenue remains constant at $21,000 (PMPM = $15 × 1,400 patients). As opposed to the non-capitated situation where net income increases as volume increases, the more services provided here, the *lower* the net income. This is because revenues remain constant, but costs increase at $25/visit.

The examples given in this chapter illustrate how a Cost-Volume-Profit analysis can be used in both non-capitated and capitated environments. However, as the factors being considered increase, a more thorough analysis is suggested. Such an approach is presented in Chapter 10, where such things as acuity level, payor mix, productivity, and labor force distribution are taken into account.

◄PRODUCT MARGIN►

While the above discussion dealt with breaking even regarding a single service, health care delivery is often quite complex. The next section of this chapter introduces tools

Exhibit 9–14   A Traditional Breakeven Chart with Capitated Payments

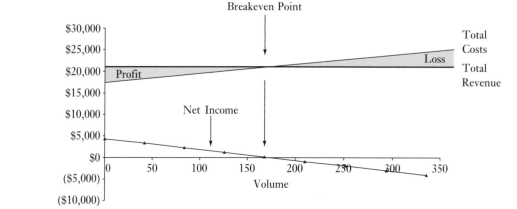

and concepts applicable to situations involving multiple services. For instance, a home health agency might offer the following services: nursing assistant services, infusion therapy, physical therapy, registered dietitian services, and occupational therapy. Later, the situation is expanded to cases where there are multiple payors.

Multiple Services

Avoidable Fixed Cost: A fixed cost that is avoided if a service is not performed. *Example:* full-time nursing costs saved if a service were closed.

In instances where multiple services are being offered, both organizational fixed costs and service-specific fixed costs must be considered. Fixed costs present only because a service is being provided, and not otherwise, are called **avoidable fixed costs**. For instance, continuing with the home health example, assume that of the $200,000 in fixed costs, $50,000 is to be paid for a full-time RN for just one particular service (Exhibit 9–15, row D), and, if the service were not delivered, this position would be eliminated (and not just transferred to another service). In regard to the decision of whether or not to drop the service, the cost of this position, $50,000, is an avoidable fixed cost.

Non-avoidable Fixed Costs: A fixed cost that will remain even if a particular service is discontinued. *Example:* full-time nursing costs in an organization that will continue, even though one of several services is dropped.

Assume the other $150,000 of the original $200,000 of the home health agency's fixed costs will remain and must be covered regardless of whether or not the particular service is dropped (Exhibit 9–15, row E). Since these costs cannot be eliminated, they are called **non-avoidable fixed costs**. Assume in the case of the home health agency that $100,000 of the $150,000 in non-avoidable fixed costs is for salaries and benefits and $50,000 is for overhead (Exhibit 9–15, rows E1 and E2). Incidentally, overhead (i.e. rent, administration, insurance, etc.) is a type of common cost: a cost that is not attributable to any particular service, but must be covered by all of them. **Common costs** are also called **joint costs**.

 Caution

Note that even if an organization drops a service, if the employees are transferred within the organization, their costs are considered non-avoidable.

Exhibit 9–15 An Illustration of the Product Margin Rule

Given:	A	Net Revenue Per Visit	$100		
	B	Variable Cost Per Visit	$25		
	C	Contribution Margin Per Visit [A − B]	$75		
	D	Avoidable Fixed Costs	$50,000		
	E	Other Fixed Costs	$150,000		
		E1 Salaries and Benefits		$100,000	
		E2 Overhead Costs		$50,000	

F	G	H	I	J	K	L	M	N
		Total	Total					
	Total	Variable	Contribution	Avoidable	Product	Salaries &	Overhead	Net
Volume	Revenues	Costs	Margin	Fixed Costs	Margin	Benefits	Costs	Income
[Estimate]	[A × F]	[B × F]	[G − H]	[D]	[I − J]	[E1]	[E2]	[K − L − M]
2,000	$200,000	$50,000	$150,000	$50,000	$100,000	$100,000	$50,000	($50,000)
2,500	$250,000	$62,500	$187,500	$50,000	$137,500	$100,000	$50,000	($12,500)
2,667	**$266,700**	**$66,675**	**$200,025**	**$50,000**	**$150,025**	**$100,000**	**$50,000**	**$25**
3,000	$300,000	$75,000	$225,000	$50,000	$175,000	$100,000	$50,000	$25,000
3,500	$350,000	$87,500	$262,500	$50,000	$212,500	$100,000	$50,000	$62,500

Just as subtracting total variable cost from total revenue yields the total contribution margin, subtracting avoidable fixed cost from the total contribution margin yields the **product margin**. The **product margin decision rule** is: if a service's product margin is positive, the organization will be better off financially if it continues with the service, *ceteris paribus*.[1] Conversely, if a service's product margin is negative, the organization will be better off financially if it discontinues the service, *ceteris paribus*. It represents the amount which a service contributes toward covering all other costs after it has covered those costs which are there solely because the service is offered (its total variable cost and avoidable fixed cost) and would not be there if the service were dropped. As shown in Exhibit 9–15, if an organization violates this rule and closes a service with a positive product margin (column K), the organization increases its loss by the amount of the product margin that it forgoes. Note that this rule holds for any particular service, but does not work for all services taken together since common costs would not be covered.

Presume the home health agency is trying to decide whether or not to continue this service next year, and it forecasts it will make 2,000 visits (Exhibit 9–15, column F). If the home health agency made its decision on the basis of net income, it would conclude that it should drop the service, because it would conclude that it is losing $50,000 (column N). However, if it drops the service, it will be $100,000 worse off (the amount of the product margin, column K) than if it provided the 2,000 visits. Since the product margin is the amount left over after the service has covered all of its own costs, if the service were dropped, the home health agency would lose the $100,000 to

Common Costs:
Costs that benefit a number of services and whose costs are shared by all. *Examples:* rent, utilities, and billing. Also called joint costs.

Product Margin:
Total Contribution Margin - Avoidable Fixed Costs. It represents the amount which a service contributes toward covering all other costs after it has covered those costs which are there solely because the service is offered (its total variable cost and avoidable fixed costs) and would not be there if the service were dropped.

---

1. *Ceteris paribus:* with all else being the same.

help defray its other costs (rows E1 and E2). Note also, if they dropped the service, net income would drop from −$50,000 to −$150,000.

Multiple Payors

It is possible to extend the analysis presented in Exhibit 9–15 from one payor to multiple payors. The previous example assumed that revenues were $100 per visit, but in fact, this is really an average of $100. Three scenarios are shown in Exhibit 9–16. Scenario 1 presents the basic conditions of four payors paying different rates, with a weighted average revenue of $100 ("Total" row, columns F/E). Scenario 2 explores the effect on the product margin of increasing the rate for Payor 1 by 10 percent (from $110 to $121) with a corresponding drop in volume of 10 percent (from 300 visits to 270 visits). The result is that the product margin increases from $0 to $1,170 (column J). Scenario 3 shows the effect on the original conditions if all patients in Payor Category 1 are on a flat fee contract fixed at $33,000, and volume increases by 10 percent. Since there are no additional revenues for these patients, the cost increases but there is no change in revenue. Therefore, the product margin decreases from $0 to −$1,500. This same paradigm can be used to judge the effects of similar changes occurring with any of the four payors.

◀Applying the Product Margin Paradigm to Making Special Decisions▶

The product margin paradigm presented in Exhibits 9–15 and 9–16 can be used to address a number of special decisions, commonly categorized as: 1) Make/Buy; 2) Add/Drop; and 3) Expand/Reduce.

Make-or-buy Decisions

Decision rule: After comparing the product margins between the make and buy alternatives, the alternative with the higher product margin should be chosen.

Example: Zacharias Community Clinic (ZCC) is deciding whether to produce a portion of its non-urgent laboratory tests in-house, or purchase them from a reference lab. ZCC has $100,000 in fixed costs for the lab (primarily for facilities, equipment, and staffing), all of which would remain even if ZCC purchased the tests from a reference lab. Variable cost (primarily for reagents and other supplies) is $3 per test. The reference lab has offered to do the tests for a price of $9 each. Zacharias currently receives $15 per test. If there are 10,000 tests to be performed, is ZCC better off producing them in-house or contracting with the outside lab?

    The solution is shown in Exhibit 9–17, solution 1. The product margin of the buy alternative is $60,000 less than that of the make alternative (line K). Therefore the *make* alternative is preferred. Notice that fixed costs do not have to be included in the analy-

Exhibit 9–16   Expansion of the Product Margin Concept to Multiple Payors

Scenario 1: Original Conditions

Payor	A Payment/Unit
1	$110
2	$105
3	$101
4	$85

B Variable Cost/Unit   = $50
C Avoidable Fixed Costs   = $50,000

D Payor Category [Given]	E Volume [Given]	F Total Revenues [A × E]	G Total Variable Costs [B × E]	H Total Contrib. Margin [F – G]	I Avoidable Fixed Costs [C]	J Product Margin [H – I]
1	300	$33,000	$15,000	$18,000		
2	175	$18,375	$8,750	$9,625		
3	250	$25,250	$12,500	$12,750		
4	275	$23,375	$13,750	$9,625		
Total	1,000	$100,000	$50,000	$50,000	$50,000	$0

Scenario 2: Original conditions with rate for Payor 1 patients increased by 10%, while Payor 1 volume is decreased by 10%.

Payor	A Payment/Unit
1	$121
2	$105
3	$101
4	$85

B Variable Cost/Unit = $50
C Avoidable Fixed Costs = $50,000

D Payor Category [Given]	E Volume [Given]	F Total Revenues [A × E]	G Total Variable Costs [B × E]	H Total Contrib. Margin [F – G]	I Avoidable Fixed Costs [C]	J Product Margin [H - I]
1	270	$32,670	$13,500	$19,170		
2	175	$18,375	$8,750	$9,625		
3	250	$25,250	$12,500	$12,750		
4	275	$23,375	$13,750	$9,625		
Total	970	$99,670	$48,500	$51,170	$50,000	$1,170

Scenario 3: Original conditions with Payor 1 patients being covered under a flat fee contract in which the total payment remains $33,000, but Payor 1 volume is increased by 10%.

Payor	A Payment/Unit
1	$33,000
2	$105
3	$101
4	$85

B Variable Cost/Unit = $50
C Avoidable Fixed Costs = $50,000

D Payor Category [Given]	E Volume [Given]	F Total Revenues[1] [A × E]	G Total Variable Costs [B × E]	H Total Contrib. Margin [F – G]	I Avoidable Fixed Costs [C]	J Product Margin [H – I]
1	330	$33,000	$16,500	$16,500		
2	175	$18,375	$8,750	$9,625		
3	250	$25,250	$12,500	$12,750		
4	275	$23,375	$13,750	$9,625		
Total	1,030	$100,000	$51,500	$48,500	$50,000	($1,500)

[1] For Payor 1, this formula is not used, and Total Revenues equals the fixed $33,000.

sis, since they are the same for either alternative. However, if fixed costs do change between the two alternatives, then they have to be considered. For instance, if $80,000 of the fixed costs were avoidable, the analysis would be as shown in solution 2 of Exhibit 9–17, line J. As a result, the *buy* alternative becomes the preferred choice. Though it has a $60,000 lower total contribution margin (line I), it saves $80,000 in avoidable fixed costs, resulting in positive product margin of $20,000 (line K).

Adding-or-dropping a Service

Decision rules: 1) If a proposed new service is expected to have a positive product margin, it should be added; and 2) If an existing service has a negative product margin, it should be dropped.

Example: Geiser HMO asked Nathaniel Clinic, a pediatric group practice, to provide 3,000 well-baby visits. Nathaniel has excess capacity to see more patients, but would

Exhibit 9–17   Example of a Make/Buy Decision

			Alternative		Advantage (Disadvantage)
Givens:			Make[1]	Buy[2]	of Adding
A	Volume of Tests		10,000	10,000	
B	Revenue per Test		$15	$15	
C	Variable Cost per Test		$3	$9	
D	Contribution Margin per Test		$12	$6	
E1	Avoidable Fixed Cost Original		$0	$0	
E2	Avoidable Fixed Cost Modified		$80,000	$0	
Solution 1: No Avoidable Fixed Costs					
F	Volume	[A]	10,000	10,000	0[3]
G	Revenues	[A × B]	$150,000	$150,000	$0[4]
H	Variable Costs	[A × C]	$30,000	$90,000	($60,000)[5]
I	Total Contribution Margin	[G − H]	$120,000	$60,000	($60,000)[6]
J	Avoidable Fixed Cost	[E1]	$0	$0	$0[7]
K	Product Margin	[I − J]	$120,000	$60,000	($60,000)[8]
Solution 2: Avoidable Fixed Costs: $80,000					
F	Volume	[A]	10,000	10,000	0[3]
G	Revenues	[A × B]	$150,000	$150,000	$0[4]
H	Variable Costs	[A × C]	$30,000	$90,000	($60,000)[5]
I	Total Contribution Margin	[G − H]	$120,000	$60,000	($60,000)[6]
J	Avoidable Fixed Cost	[E2]	$80,000	$0	$80,000[7]
K	Product Margin	[I − J]	$40,000	$60,000	$20,000[8]

[1] Produce in-house.
[2] Purchase from vendor.
[3] Increase (decrease) in volume from choosing buy option.
[4] Amount saved (lost) in revenue from choosing buy option.
[5] Amount saved (lost) in variable costs by choosing buy option.
[6] Total Contribution Margin gained (lost) by choosing buy option.
[7] Amount saved (lost) in avoidable fixed costs from choosing buy option.
[8] Increase (decrease) in product margin from choosing buy option.

have to hire additional staff for $85,000. It estimates additional variable costs (such as disposable thermometers, linens, etc.) of $10 per visit. Geiser is willing to pay $65 per visit. Should Nathaniel contract with Geiser and provide the well-baby clinic?

The solution is shown in Exhibit 9–18a. Since the project has a positive product margin of $80,000, Nathaniel should agree to offer the service. But what happens now if Geiser changes the terms of the contract and will only pay $35 per visit? In this case, as shown in Exhibit 9–18b, Nathaniel would have a positive *total contribution margin*, $75,000 (line I), but a negative *product margin*, –$10,000 (line K). Nathaniel should not agree to offer the service at this price.

Expanding-or-reducing a Service

Decision rule: If only one alternative *will* or *must* be chosen, then the anticipated product margin of both alternatives should be compared. The alternative with the higher anticipated product margin should be chosen.

Example: Physicians Healthcare Group (PHG) is located in the greater Barnsboro metropolitan area. One of its major revenue centers, a radiology service, receives its revenues on a capitated basis: $55 per member per year to take care of all of their routine radiology needs. Assume that 20 percent of the 10,000 members will receive some routine radiological service each year, at an average cost of $50 per service.

Exhibit 9–18a Example of an Add/Drop Decision

Givens:		Alternative Don't Add[1]	Add[2]	Advantage (Disadvantage) of Adding
A Volume		0	3,000	
B Revenue per Visit		$0	$65	
C Cost per Visit		$0	$10	
D Contribution Margin per Visit		$0	$55	
E Avoidable Fixed Cost		$0	$85,000	
Solution:				
F Volume	[A]	0	3,000	3,000[3]
G Revenues	[A × B]	$0	$195,000	$195,000[4]
H Variable Costs	[A × C]	$0	$30,000	($30,000)[5]
I Total Contribution Margin	[G – H]	$0	$165,000	$165,000[6]
J Avoidable Fixed Costs	[E]	$0	$85,000	($85,000)[7]
K Product Margin	[I – J]	$0	$80,000	$80,000[8]

[1] Do not open new clinic.
[2] Open new clinic.
[3] Increase (decrease) in volume from choosing add option.
[4] Amount saved (lost) in revenue from choosing add option.
[5] Amount saved (lost) in variable costs by choosing add option.
[6] Total Contribution Margin gained (lost) by choosing add option.
[7] Amount saved (lost) in avoidable fixed costs by choosing add option.
[8] Increase (decrease) in product margin from choosing add option.

Exhibit 9–18b   Example of Add/Drop Decision

Givens:		Alternative Don't Add[1]	Alternative Add[2]	Advantage (Disadvantage) of Adding
A Volume		0	3,000	
B Revenue per Visit		$0	$35	
C Cost per Visit		$0	$10	
D Contribution Margin per Visit		$0	$25	
E Avoidable Fixed Cost		$0	$85,000	
Solution:				
F Volume	[A]	0	3,000	3,000[3]
G Revenues	[A × B]	$0	$105,000	$105,000[4]
H Variable Costs	[A × C]	$0	$30,000	($30,000)[5]
I Total Contribution Margin	[G – H]	$0	$75,000	$75,000[6]
J Avoidable Fixed Costs	[E]	$0	$85,000	($85,000)[7]
K Product Margin	[I – J]	$0	($10,000)	($10,000)[8]

[1] Do not new open clinic.
[2] Open new clinic.
[3] Increase (decrease) in volume from choosing add option.
[4] Amount saved (lost) in revenue from choosing add option.
[5] Amount saved (lost) in variable costs by choosing add option.
[6] Total Contribution Margin gained (lost) by choosing add option.
[7] Amount saved (lost) in avoidable fixed costs by choosing add option.
[8] Increase (decrease) in product margin from choosing add option

    PHG operates six satellite clinics that offer general and specialty medicine services to their customers. X-ray service is also available at every clinic so that patients can be examined on-site immediately. This has been a very successful marketing feature as shown by the annual patient satisfaction survey, but it has been costly. Stacy Helman, the new clinic manager, has suggested centralizing the radiology operations to two locations that could serve all six clinics. She feels this would help reduce the current fixed costs of the organization by $200,000. However, if the services were relocated, Ms. Helman predicts a 10 percent reduction in members, since they would probably change HMOs. The solution is shown in Exhibit 9–19.

Discussion: Given the product margin results (row K), it appears that PHG should centralize its radiology service. Even though 10 percent of the patient volume would be lost, there would be significant equipment cost savings with this option. PHG would be better off by $155,000 per year by centralizing.

    Though these examples illustrate the application of the product margin paradigm, it is important to understand that other financial analysis tools should also be employed when making these decisions. For instance, the impact of these decisions on the financial ratios of the organization should be considered (see Chapter 4). Similarly, to the extent that these decisions have multi-year implications, a more thorough analysis would discount future cash flows and assess the net present value of these decisions (see Chapters 6 and 7). Finally, these financial concerns must be weighed against non-financial concerns when making these decisions.

Exhibit 9-19 Example of an Expand/Reduce Decision

			Alternative		Advantage (Disadvantage) of Reducing
			Don't Reduce[1]	Reduce[2]	
Givens:					
A	Members		10,000	9,000	
B	Utilization Rate		20%	20%	
C	PMPY		$55	$55	
D	Cost per Test		$50	$50	
E	Avoidable Fixed Cost		$200,000	$0	
Solution:					
F	Members	[A]	10,000	9,000	$(1,000)^3$
G	Revenues	$[A \times C]$	$550,000	$495,000	$(\$55,000)^4$
H	Variable Costs	$[A \times B \times D]$	$100,000	$90,000	$\$10,000^5$
I	Total Contribution Margin	[G - H]	$450,000	$405,000	$(\$45,000)^6$
J	Avoidable Fixed Cost	[E]	$200,000	$0	$\$200,000^7$
K	Product Margin	[I - J]	$250,000	$405,000	$\$155,000^8$

[1] Don't centralize radiology service.
[2] Centralize radiology service.
[3] Increase (decrease) in volume from choosing reduce option.
[4] Amount saved (lost) in revenue by choosing reduce option.
[5] Amount saved (lost) in variable costs by choosing reduce option.
[6] Total Contribution Margin gained (lost) by choosing reduce option.
[7] Amount saved (lost) in avoidable fixed costs by choosing reduce option.
[8] Increase (decrease) in product margin from choosing reduce option.

◀SUMMARY▶

An understanding of fixed and variable costs provides a valuable tool to help make decisions of what price to charge, whether to add or drop a service, or whether to make or buy a service. Fixed costs are costs that do not vary in total but vary per unit over the relevant range. Variable costs vary in total but do not vary per unit over the relevant range. The relevant range is the range over which total fixed costs and/or per unit variable cost do not vary.

The breakeven equation can be used to determine price, volume, fixed costs, or variable cost per unit, if each of the other factors is known. The breakeven equation is: (Price × Volume) = Fixed Costs + (Variable Cost per Unit × Volume). The breakeven point is that volume where total revenues equal total costs. The results of a breakeven analysis are often presented on a breakeven chart, which illustrates fixed costs, total costs, total revenues, and volume. The distance between the total cost and total revenue lines represents the amount of profit or loss the service is experiencing at any particular volume of service. An alternative form of this chart shows the difference between the total cost and total revenue lines: net income.

The breakeven equation can be applied to capitated situations to determine capitation rates, utilization rates, or fixed or variable costs, given the others. The breakeven equation can also be extended to multi-payor and multi-service situations, though the latter is beyond the scope of this text. In conducting multi-payor analyses that include capitated and fixed-fee patients, it is important not to adjust revenues for changes in volume, though variable costs may change. This caveat also holds for fixed-fee patients, such as those who pay on the basis of DRGs.

Per unit contribution margin is calculated by subtracting per unit variable cost from per unit revenues. It is the amount of profit made on each additional unit provided all other costs (fixed costs and overhead) remain the same. It is also the amount of incremental income from an average unit of service that is available to cover all other costs. If the contribution margin is known, a shortcut formula to calculate breakeven can be used: Breakeven Volume = Total Fixed Costs/Contribution Margin per Unit. If 1) the decision has been made not to close down a service, 2) no other additional costs will be incurred, and 3) the contribution margin is positive, then it is in the best financial interest of the organization to continue to provide additional units of that service, even if it is not fully covering all of its other costs.

In instances where multiple services are offered, it is likely that there are both organizational fixed costs and service specific fixed costs. Fixed costs that are present just because the service is being provided and would not be there if the service were not offered are called avoidable fixed costs. Product margin is computed as follows: Total Revenues – Total Variable Costs – Avoidable Fixed Costs. The product margin decision rule states: if a service is covering its own variable and avoidable fixed costs, even if it does not fully cover its full share of other costs (non-avoidable fixed costs and common costs), the organization is better off delivering the service than not, all other things being equal (there are no better alternatives). If the organization violates this rule and closes a service with a positive product margin, the organization increases its loss by the amount of the product margin that it forgoes. The product margin concept is useful to help answer questions related to providing a service in-house or going outside (make-or-buy decision), adding or dropping a service, and expanding or reducing services. In all of these analyses, sunk costs should not be considered.

It is important to understand that other financial analysis tools should also be employed when making these decisions. For instance, the impact on the financial ratios of the organization should be considered. Also, decisions that have multi-year implications should include a more thorough analysis of future cash flows and net present value. Finally, as noted earlier, the financial concerns must be balanced with non-financial concerns to make these decisions.

◄Key Terms►

Avoidable Fixed Cost	Contribution Margin Per Unit	Product Margin
Breakeven Analysis	Contribution Margin Rule	Product Margin Decision Rule
Breakeven Point	Fixed Costs	Relevant Range
Capitation	Incremental costs	Step-Fixed Costs
Common Costs	Joint Costs	Target Costing
Contribution Margin	Non-avoidable Fixed Costs	Variable Costs

◄Key Equations►

Breakeven for capitation: PMPM × Enrollees = (Enrollees × Utilization rate × Variable Cost/Unit) + Fixed Cost

Breakeven volume: Fixed Costs/Contribution Margin per Unit

Breakeven volume: Price × Volume = Direct Cost + Indirect Costs + Profit. Where Direct Costs = Direct Fixed Costs + (Direct Variable Cost Per Unit × Volume)

Breakeven volume: Price × Volume = Fixed Costs + (Variable Cost Per Unit × Volume) + Desired Profit

Contribution margin per unit: Revenue Per Unit − Variable Cost Per Unit

Contribution margin: Total Revenue − Total Variable Cost

Product Margin: Total Contribution Margin − Avoidable Fixed Costs

◄Questions and Problems►

1. **Definitions:** Define the following terms:
   a. Avoidable Fixed Cost.
   b. Breakeven Analysis.
   c. Breakeven Point.
   d. Capitation.
   e. Common Costs.
   f. Contribution Margin.
   g. Contribution Margin Per Unit.
   h. Contribution Margin Rule.
   i. Fixed Costs.
   j. Incremental Costs.
   k. Joint Costs.
   l. Non-avoidable Fixed Costs.
   m. Product Margin.
   n. Product Margin Decision Rule.
   o. Relevant Range.
   p. Step Fixed Costs.
   q. Target Costing.
   r. Variable Costs.
2. **Breakeven Formulas.** What are the formulas for:
   a. The basic breakeven equation
   b. The basic breakeven equation expanded to include indirect costs and desired profit?
3. **Understanding Fixed and Variable Cost.** Briefly describe what happens to each of the following as volume increases:

    a. Total Fixed Cost

    b. Total Variable Cost

    c. Fixed Cost per Unit

    d. Variable Cost per Unit

4. **Step Fixed Cost and the Relevant Range.** Explain the relationship between step-fixed costs and the relevant range.

5. **Product Margin.** Based on the product margin, when is it in the best interests of an organization to continue or drop a service?

6. **Make-or-buy Decision and related analyses.**

    a. What is a make-or-buy decision?

    b. What other analyses are relevant to the types of decisions discussed in this chapter?

7. **Breakeven equation. Fill in the blank.** The following table contains selected data concerning several outpatient clinics in the new Ambulatory Care Center at Hope University Hospital. Fill in the missing information.

[A] Price per Visit	[B] Variable Cost/Unit	[C] Number of Visits	[D] Contribution Margin	[E] Fixed Costs	[F] Net Income
$85		3,000	$180,000		$80,000
$70	$20		$130,000	$90,000	
	$35	3,250		$78,000	$117,000
$65	$40	2,000		$60,000	

8. **Breakeven equation. Fill in the blank.** Instead of the information in problem 7, assume Ambulatory Care Center's data looked like this:

[A] Price per Visit	[B] Variable Cost/Unit	[C] Number of Visits	[D] Contribution Margin	[E] Fixed Costs	[F] Net Income
$90		4,000	$200,000		$90,000
$85	$35		$150,000	$75,000	
	$55	4,500		$78,000	$120,000
$50	$60	2,000		$60,000	

9. **Expand/Reduce Decision.** Laurie Vaden is a nurse practitioner with her own practice. She has developed contracts with several large employers to perform routine physicals, fitness for duty exams, and initial screening of on-the-job injuries. She currently sees 150 patients per month, charging $50 per visit. Her total costs are $7,500, of which $1,500 is for supplies. She has decided that she needs to increase profit, so she is considering raising her fee to $65. She expects to lose 10 percent of her business to competitors that charge an average of $60 per visit. Determine her current and predicted: 1) revenues, 2) variable costs, and 3) total contribution margin. What do you recommend she do? Why?

10. **Expand/Reduce Decision.** Janet Gilbert is director of labs. She has some extra capacity and has contracted with some small neighboring hospitals to run some of their lab tests. She has recently had a study conducted and has determined that her costs of these contracts are $10,000 of which $7,000 are for supplies and items related to each test. She currently charges an average of $10.00 per lab test. She is thinking of lowering her price by 20 percent in hopes of raising her current volume of 10,000 tests by 15 percent. Determine her current and predicted: 1) revenues, 2) variable costs, 3) total contribution margin, and 4) net income. What do you recommend she do? Why?

11. **Calculating Breakeven.** Ms Jasmine Gonzales, administrative director of Physicians Associates, a group practice, has been asked if the group should begin offering mammography screenings. The following are Ms Gonzales's projections:

Price per screening:	$90
Equipment[1]:	$60,000
Technicians' salaries:	$60,000
Operating costs per screening:	
Supplies:	$25
Developing:	$10

[1] Useful life of 10 years (assume straight-line depreciation)

   a. What annual volume must the unit operate at in order to break even on the service?
   b. How do breakeven projections change if the group practice required a $22,000 profit?
   c. Suppose reimbursement levels for mammography services provided only $65 per screening. How many screenings per year would the group practice have to perform to break even? (Assume no profit.)

12. **Calculating Breakeven.** Southern Regional Hospital is considering offering a new specialty service which will be provided out of its urgent care center. A pediatric cardiologist from the region's teaching hospital is willing to provide services 4 times a month to the facility. Not only will this add a needed service to SRH, it will also generate revenues from the echocardiograms performed on the children. The following represent the projections of the clinic:

Revenues per study:	$500
Echo cardiograph lease (per study)	$100
Physician salary (per day):	$750
Other expenses[1]:	$800

[1] Cost per month of high speed telephone line for transmission of digital data.

   a. At what volume per month does this service break even?
   b. What is the breakeven point if the clinic wants to make $800 profit?
   c. What is the breakeven if the revenue per study drops to $400 and the clinic wants to make $800 profit?

13. **Calculating Breakeven and Graphing.** San Juan Health Department's dental clinic projects the following costs and rates for the year 20XX.

Total fixed costs: $56,012
Variable costs: $48 per patient
Charges: $70 per patient

a. Using this information, determine the breakeven point in units.
b. Using this information, determine the breakeven point in dollars.
c. Graph this scenario in a breakeven chart using a range of 0 to 3,500 patients in 500 patient increments.
d. If the clinic decides it would like to make a profit of $5,500, what is the new breakeven point in units?
e. If the clinic decides it would like to make a profit of $5,500, what is the new breakeven point in dollars?

14. **Calculating Breakeven and Graphing.** The North Kingstown Cancer infusion therapy division expects tremendous growth over the next year and is projecting the following cost and rate structure for the service.

Revenue $750 per patient
Costs
Rent $3,600 per month
Staff $195,000 per month
Leases $10,000 per month
Other $20,000 per month
Pharmaceuticals $500 per patient
IV supplies $25 per patient
Other patient supplies $25 per patient

a. What volume of patients will it take for the Center to break even?
b. What is the breakeven point in dollars?
c. Graph the above scenario using a range of 0 to 2,500 patients in 500 patient increments.
d. If the clinic needs to make a profit of $75,000, what is the new breakeven point in volume and in dollars?

15. **Determining breakeven price in a reduce/expand decision.** QuickCare is a health care franchise that functions as a primary family health clinic, seeing unscheduled patients 24 hours a day. Several months after the grand opening, a corporate office management engineering study showed that the clinic was experiencing some dips in volume in the mid-afternoon hours. In order to increase volume, efficiency, and revenues, the clinic administrator contracted with the area high schools to provide after-school physicals for the sports teams. The initial agreement was that QuickCare would charge $75 per exam, the market average. With this increase, fixed costs remained at $30,000 and variable costs at $35 per physical. Though this strategy proved somewhat successful, gross profit margin lagged behind the corporate expectations. In order to improve margin, the clinic is considering increasing the exam price to $85. QuickCare's administrator projects that this price increase will cause the high

schools to send their athletes to other providers and that volume could drop by 33 percent. Last year, QuickCare performed 1,026 examinations. The administrator feels that if the program closes down, all $30,000 in fixed costs would be saved.

a. What should QuickCare's decision be assuming that this price increase will decrease the number of patients seen by one-third?

b. What price would QuickCare have to charge to make up for the loss of patients?

c. Using the information from part a, should QuickCare make the same decision if 40 percent of the fixed costs are avoidable? Would it be better or worse off? Why?

16. **Expand/Reduce.** The administrator of ABC Hospital, Mr Stevens, has just received the latest financial report and the news is not good. The hospital has been losing money for over a year, and if things don't improve, it may lose its AA bond rating. Mr Stevens has met with his VP Finance, Mr Sanger, and has asked him to identify areas for cutting costs, beginning with services that are operating at a loss. The following information is for services provided at ABC Hospital's ambulatory care clinic:

Annual volume (in patient visits):	10,000
Charge per visit:	$50
Variable cost per visit:	$30
Fixed costs:	$500,000

a. Suppose that all fixed costs are avoidable. What should Mr Sanger recommend to Mr Stevens regarding the clinic?

b. What if only $150,000 of the fixed costs were avoidable? Would this change his recommendation?

c. Are there any other considerations that should be taken into account when making this decision?

17. **Add/Drop Decision** The Ancome County Health Department is considering using 300 square feet of excess office space to provide a clinic for Healthchek visits. These visits are reimbursed at $67.30 under a Medicaid program. Variable costs per visit are $59, and providing the service requires an additional physician assistant and nurse with prorated salaries of $48,000 and $30,000, respectively. The state has mandated efforts to increase the utilization of Medicaid eligibility, so the Department of Social Services is conducting interventions to increase eligibility awareness in the community. As a result, the health department expects 10,000 Healthchek visits in the coming year. Unavoidable overhead costs for the Health Department are $300,000 per year and will be allocated to each program based on its proportional share of the Health Department's total office space of 2,700 square feet.

a. What are the total contribution margin and total product margin for a Healthchek visit?

b. Considering the total product margin, should the health department provide the service?

18. **Add/Drop Decision** The Midtown Women's Center offers bone densitometry scans in the office as a convenience to its patients. The clinic volume is expanding and Sam Loch, the Center's administrator, is considering dropping the bone densitometry service and converting the space to an exam room to allow for more outpatient visits. The following information has been gathered to help with the decision.

Number of scans per year	425
Reimbursement for bone densitometry scan	$65
Bone densitometry supply cost per scan	$15
Part-time, bone densitometry scan technician	$15,000
Reimbursement per office visit	$80
Supply cost per office visit	$20
Expected increase in outpatient volume if additional exam space is available	500

a. What is the contribution margin for the bone densitometry service per year?

b. Should this service continue as opposed to converting it to exam room space? Why or why not?

c. How many office visits would it take to replace the income from the bone densitometry service?

19. **Breakeven.** Sure Care Health Maintenance Organization is seeking a managed care contract with a local manufacturing plant. Sure Care estimates that the cost of providing care for the 300 employees will be $36,000 per month. The manufacturing company offered Sure Care a premium bid of $200 per employee per month.

a. If Sure Care accepts this bid and contracts with the manufacturing firm, will Sure Care earn a profit or loss for the year? How much?

b. What premium per employee per month does Sure Care need to break even?

c. If Sure Care wants to earn $100,000 in profit for the year, what is the required premium per employee per month?

d. What concerns do you have about this analysis?

20. **Breakeven.** Zack Millman Clinic is seeking to provide sports-related health care services to high schools in the are a. Zack Millman estimates that the cost to provide care would be $1,000 plus $12 per athlete per month on a nine-month basis. The high schools jointly offered to pay the clinic $10,000 for a nine-month contract to cover 75 athletes.

a. If Millman Clinic accepts this bid and contracts with the high schools, will it earn a profit or loss for the year? How much?

b. What would the contract price have to be for Millman to break even?

c. If Zack Millken wants to earn $5,000 in profit for the year, and the school system preferred to pay on a per athlete per month basis, what would the price have to be?

21. **Contribution Margin, Product Margin and Breakeven.** Dixon Pharmaceuticals, a drug manufacturing company, produces prescription medication for the treatment of respiratory infections. The company's leading product line is Cycladine. The wholesale price per tablet of Cycladine is $0.85. The

variable cost associated with the production of 1,000 tablets of Cycladine is $250. Other costs associated with the production include annual laboratory equipment rental of $100,000, annual salaries of employees who work in the Cycladine division of $180,000, and other miscellaneous fixed costs for the Cycladine division of $45,000 per year. The 45,000 square foot Cycladine division is located in a 136,364 square foot facility with several other product lines of Dixon Pharmaceuticals. Overhead totals $500,000 for the company and is allocated on the basis of the percent of the total square footage a division uses. Dixon Pharmaceuticals expects to sell 1,000,000 tablets of Cycladine in the upcoming year.

a. Determine the total contribution margin, total product margin, and net income for the Cycladine division of Dixon Pharmaceuticals.

b. Determine the net income breakeven point in tablets of Cycladine.

c. Determine the breakeven point for Dixon Pharmaceuticals to cover just its direct costs.

22. **Contribution Margin, Product Margin and Breakeven.** Capital Community Hospital is opening a new Radiation Oncology division within its Cancer Center. This service will add revenues while eliminating the costly travel and inconvenience to many patients that heretofore have to travel over 150 miles to receive this service. The new service plans to share waiting space, registration space, a full time medical director and a full time service line manger with the other existing Cancer Center Programs. There are no plans under foreseeable conditions that these positions would become part time. The following information is available:

Total waiting space (sq. ft)	1,000
Total allocated cost	$3,500
Space for radiation oncology (sq. ft)	400
Salary: Service Line Manager	$65,000
% Service Line Manager and Medical Director assigned to radiation oncology	30%
New space upfit cost (10 year useful life)	$550,000
Utilities/year	6,000
Lease for linear accelerator/year	$60,000
Film supplies/treatment	$14
Other supplies/treatment	$75
Medical Director salary	$166,667
Staffing for radiation oncology	$150,000
Revenue/treatment	$212
Treatments/patient	25
Total patients/year	150

a. Determine the Total Contribution Margin, Total Product Margin and Net Income for the new service.

b. Determine the breakeven point in number of patients.

c. Determine the breakeven point to cover the direct costs.

23. **Determining Charges for Private Pay Residents.** Shady Rest Nursing Home has 100 private pay residents. The administrator is concerned about

balancing the ratio of its private pay to non-private pay patients. Non-private pay sources reimburse an average of $100 per day whereas private pay residents pay on average 100 percent of full daily charges. The administrator estimates that variable cost per resident per day is $25 for supplies, food, and contracted services and annual fixed costs are $4,562,500.

    a. What is the daily contribution margin of each non-private pay resident?

    b. If 25 percent of the residents are non-private pay, what will Shady Rest charge the private pay patients in order to break even?

    c. What if non-private pay payors cover 50 percent of the residents?

    d. The owner of Shady Rest Nursing Home insists that the facility earn $80,000 in annual profits. How much must the administrator raise the per day charge for the privately insured residents if 25 percent of the residents are covered by non-private pay payors?

24. **Determining Charges for Private Pay Residents.** Shady Rest Nursing Home has 220 private pay residents. The administrator is concerned about balancing the ratio of its private pay to non-private pay patients. Non-private pay sources reimburse an average of $125 per day whereas private pay residents pay on average 90 percent of full daily charges. The administrator estimates that variable cost per resident per day is $45 for supplies, food, and contracted services and annual fixed costs are $6,000,000.

    a. What is the daily contribution margin of each non-private pay resident?

    b. If 25 percent of the residents are non-private pay, what will Shady Rest charge the private pay patients in order to break even?

    c. What if non-private pay payors cover 50 percent of the residents?

    d. The owner of Shady Rest Nursing Home insists that the facility earn $80,000 in annual profits. How much must the administrator raise the per day charge for the privately insured residents if 25 percent of the residents are covered by non-private pay payors?

25. **Add/Drop with Net Present Value Analysis (Builds on material in Chapters 6 and 7).** Franklin County Hospital, a non-profit hospital, bought and installed a new computer system last year for $65,000. The system is designed to relay information between labs and medical units. Charlene Walker, the hospital's new computer specialist, had a meeting with Lou Campbell, Vice President of Finance. She began: "Lou, today I read in a journal that a new computer system has just been introduced. It costs $42,000, but I believe that by replacing our old system, we could reduce operating and maintenance costs that are now being incurred." The following are Ms Walker's estimates:

Present System	New System	
Purchase and installment price	$65,000	$42,000
Useful life when purchased	6 years	5 years
Computer operating costs per year	$30,000	$20,000
Computer operating and maintenance costs per year	$20,000	$18,000
Depreciation expenses per year	$10,833	$18,000
Cost of capital	10%	10%

a. Based on an analysis, what advice do you recommend that Charlene give Lou?

b. At what price for the new computer system would Lou be indifferent?

c. Is this a typical make-or-buy decision? Why?

26. **Complex Make/Buy.** Dr Mike Roe is the Medical Director of the labs at Parkside Hospital, the acute care provider for the Sunstone HMO. The lab is looking to reduce its costs to remain competitive in the capitated market. One service that the laboratory offers is in-house cyclosporin (an anti-rejection drug) assays for immuno-compromised (low tolerance to infection) patients. This is a low-volume, fairly expensive procedure. Recently, Loache Laboratories, a reference lab, offered to perform these studies for Parkside. Loache has offered to produce the necessary results at a cost of $70 each. Parkside has projected the following data for the upcoming year to continue to perform the test in-house:

Volume:	960 tests or assays
Patient charges per lab test:	$75
Variable expenses per lab test:	$28.63
Annual expenses associated with Cyclosporin:	
Rent:	$10,000
Equipment rental:	$9,250
Laboratory technician salary:	$18,400
Allocated *overhead:*	$6,840

a. Should Parkside continue to perform the assays or purchase them from Loache?

b. Assume that it was highly likely that the volume would not reach 960 assays. At what volume should Dr Roe change his decision from the first question?

c. If Loache discounted the price by 10 percent for each test after the purchase of 900 assays, what should Dr Roe's decision be?

27. **Income statement and add/drop.** Lakespring Retirement Village is home to senior citizens who are fairly independent, but need assistance with basic health care and occasional meals. Jill Thompson, a licensed beautician, works on salary 16 hours a week at Lakespring. Funds at the retirement village have been getting quite tight, due to an increase in the number of Medicaid and other low-income residents. Carl Jones, Lakespring's administrator, told Ms Thompson that the hair salon might have to be closed. Mr Jones is sympathetic because he knows that it will be inconvenient for many residents to get this service elsewhere, and Ms Thompson's charges are about all the residents can afford, but he wonders how he can keep any unit open that does not break even. Mr Jones is looking for a way to save the hair salon and has provided you with the following information for your input:

Hair Cuts	Permanents	Brief Visits	
Charge per resident	$8.00	$14.00	$4.50
Variable costs per service performed			
Cleaning/styling/setting products	0.50	3.50	3.00
Variable water expense	0.15	0.25	0.25
Laundry expenses for towels, smocks, etc.	0.10	0.30	0.30

Jill is currently doing an average weekly business of 16 hair cuts, seven permanents, and four brief visits, which take half an hour, an hour, and 15 minutes, respectively. The hair salon is currently allocated rent of $150.00 per month and other upkeep expenses of $45.00 a month. Jill is paid $9 per hour, and she earned $576.00 last month.

a. Prepare a monthly income statement and determine the total contribution margin and total product margin for each service line. Determine net income for the service taken as a whole.

b. How would you advise Mr Jones: Should he close the hair salon? Why or why not?

c. Should Mr Jones try to persuade Jill to drop any service she now offers?

Chapter Ten
_____

BUDGETING

LEARNING OBJECTIVES

After completing this chapter, you will be able to:

▶ State the purposes of budgeting.
▶ Describe the planning/control cycle and list the five key dimensions of budgeting.
▶ List the major budgets and explain their relationship to each other and to the income statement and balance sheet.
▶ Construct each of the major budgets.

Chapter Outline

Strategic Planning: Identifying an organization's mission, goals, and strategy to best position itself for the future.

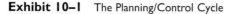

Planning: The process of identifying goals, objectives, tasks, activities, and resources necessary to carry out the strategic plan of the organization over the next time period, typically one year.

Mission Statement: A statement which guides the organization by identifying the unique attributes of the organization, why it exists, and what it hopes to achieve. Some organizations divide these attributes between a vision and a mission statement.

◀INTRODUCTION▶

The budget is one of the most important documents of a health care organization and is the central document of the planning/control cycle. The budget serves not only as a *planning* document that identifies the revenues and resources needed for an organization to achieve its goals and objectives, but also as a *control* document that allows an organization to monitor the actual revenues generated and its use of resources against what was planned.

The Planning/Control Cycle

As illustrated in Exhibit 10–1, the planning/control cycle has four major components: strategic planning, planning, implementing, and controlling. Budgeting is the central element that affects all these areas.

Strategic Planning and Planning

Strategic planning and planning activities provide the basis to develop the budget. The purpose of **strategic planning** is to identify the organization's vision, mission, goals, and strategy in order to position itself for the future. The purpose of **planning** is to identify the goals, objectives, tasks, activities, and resources necessary to carry out the strategic plan over a defined time period, commonly one year. The organization's mission is usually set forth in a mission statement, which is a broad, enduring statement of its vision and purpose. The **mission statement** guides the organization into the future by identifying the unique attributes of the organization, why it exists, and what it hopes to achieve (see Perspective 10–1).

Exhibit 10–1   The Planning/Control Cycle

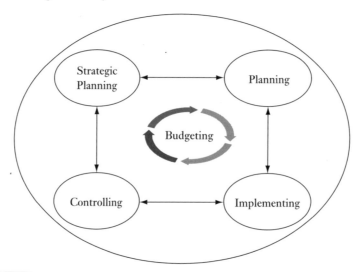

PERSPECTIVE 10–1

Mission Statement and Objectives of a Children's Hospital

The Shriners Hospitals' mission is to provide the highest quality care to children with neuro-musculoskeletal conditions, burn injuries and certain other special healthcare needs within a compassionate, family-centered and collaborative care environment. This mission is carried out without cost to the patient or family and without regard to race, color, creed or sex. And today Shriners operates the only health care system that is funded totally through philanthropy. The Chicago Shriners Hospital provides expert, family-centered medical care for children needing orthopedic, plastic and reconstructive surgery and spinal cord injury care.

Source: Shriners Hospitals for Children in Chicago (http://www.shrinerschicago.org/welcome.html)

A major activity of the strategic planning process is to assess the organization's external and internal environments. The external environment of most health care organizations is quite complex, and an environmental analysis must include surveying the local, regional, national, and international environments for changes that may occur in a variety of areas including the economy, regulation, technology, and health status of populations. Other areas of the external environment that must be examined are listed in the top part of Exhibit 10–2. Failing to thoroughly and correctly assess even one of these domains could lead to major problems for, or even the demise of, the organization. In addition to its external environment, a health care organization also has to examine its internal environment, which includes both *tangible factors*, such as financing, staff, services, and structure, and *intangible factors*, such as its history, reputation, and the strength of its Board.

An important outcome of the strategic planning process is to identify goals and objectives. In the past, goals and objectives for many health care organizations were fairly narrowly restricted to the nature and scope of services the organization hoped to provide. More recently, however, they have included population impacts (e.g. to reduce low-weight births in the covered population by 15 percent over the next five years); market penetration (e.g. to capture 25 percent of the HMO market within the next five years); and financial position (e.g. to increase return on assets by 10 percent over the next three years). The goals and objectives the organization chooses to pursue impact the revenues and resources the organization will need, and these in turn must be reflected in the budgets.

Whereas the organization's strategic planning process focuses on the long-term, the organization also develops shorter-term **plans** to help it achieve its short-term objectives. While the strategic plan is fairly general, short-term plans are more specific and identify short-term goals and objectives in more detail, primarily in regard to marketing/production, control, and financing the organization.

Short-term Plans: Specific plans which identify an organization's short-term goals and objectives in more detail, primarily in regard to marketing/production, control, and financing the organization.

Controlling Activities: Activities which provide guidance and feedback to keep the organization within its budget once it has been approved and is being implemented.

Controlling Activities

Planning activities provide input to develop a budget. Once the budget has been approved and implementation begins, **controlling activities** provide guidance

Exhibit 10–2   Relationship of Budgeting to Strategy, Tactics, and Operation

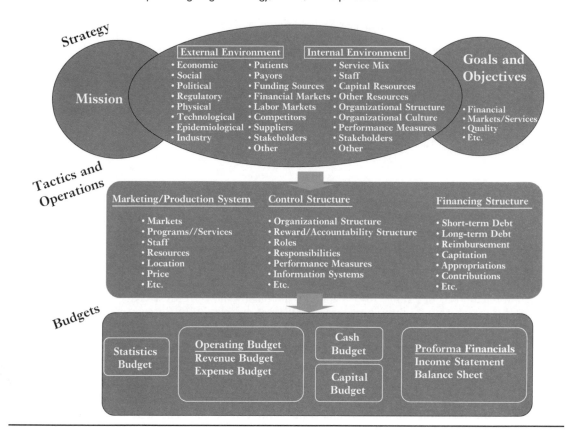

and feedback to keep the organization within its budget (see Exhibit 10–1). Control tools vary from organizational structure and information systems to financially related controlling activities such as monthly reports to department managers regarding their expenditures against budget, and mid-year bonuses based upon financial performance.

Organizational Approaches to Budgeting

Exhibit 10–3 lists five key dimensions over which organizations vary in regard to budgeting:

- Participation.
- Budget Model.
- Budget Detail.
- Budget Forecast.
- Budget Modifications.

Participation

The budgeting process can vary considerably from one organization to the next in terms of the roles and responsibilities of various positions in the organization. Under an authoritarian approach, the environmental assessment and planning of future activities are largely concentrated in a few hands at the top of the organization, and the budget is essentially dictated downward. The **authoritarian approach** is often called **top-down budgeting**. Perspective 10–2 illustrates a case where an outside authority dictates budget cuts. Perspective 10–3 illustrates a case where an inside, overriding authority dictates program cuts.

The opposite of the authoritarian approach is the **participatory approach**, in which the roles and responsibilities of the budgeting process are diffused throughout the organization. The participatory approach often begins with some general guidelines from the top, based on top management's knowledge of the environment. Within the restrictions of these general guidelines, department heads and service line managers (e.g. women's services, emergency services, outreach services) have great latitude to develop their own budgets to submit to upper management for approval. This approach is often called a **top-down/bottom-up approach**. The roles and responsibilities of various positions in the organization in the participatory approach are summarized in Exhibit 10–4.

The participatory approach to budgeting has a number of advantages beyond just forcing management to plan (see Exhibit 10–5). These advantages include:

- Developing a shared understanding of the goals and objectives of the organization by those who have participated in the budgeting process.
- Developing cooperation and coordination among the various departments.
- Clarifying roles and responsibilities throughout the organization (thus preventing overlap).

Authoritarian Approach: Budgeting and decision-making which are done by relatively few people concentrated in the highest level of the organizational structure. Opposite of the *participatory approach*.

Top-down Budgeting: See *Authoritarian Approach*.

Participatory Approach: A method of budgeting in which the roles and responsibilities of putting together a budget are diffused throughout the organization, typically originating at the department level. There are guidelines to follow, and approval must be secured by top management. Opposite to the *authoritarian approach*.

Exhibit 10–3   Key Budgeting Dimensions

Dimension	Approaches		
Participation	Authoritarian	◄───────►	Participatory
Budget Model	Incremental/ Decremental	◄───────►	Zero-based
Budget Detail	Line-item	◄─── Program ───►	Performance
Budget Forecast	Annual	◄───────►	Multi-year
	Static	◄───────►	Flexible
Budget Modifications	Controlled	◄───────►	Latitude

PERSPECTIVE 10–2

Services for Poor Put at Risk

Up to 50 jobs and a shopping cart of services could be gradually scrapped to accommodate $6.2 million in budget cuts that Wake County (North Carolina) Human Services must make.

At the Human Services board meeting Thursday, Director Maria Spaulding and board members lamented the political reality in which a prosperous county shunts aside its poorest.

Still, the bleak picture faced by Human Services is brighter now than it was. The agency originally was told to trim $9.6 million of its $400 million budget. But the actual cuts still took several board members by surprise. Spaulding, who has been mulling what to cut for weeks now, fairly bristled when board members complained about their nature.

"Don't talk to me about pain," she said, "because I can tell you a lot about it."

A seven-member committee representing various facets of the agency closeted itself away for nearly four days to draw up a list of potential cuts. Committee members went through each service provided and categorized it according to whether it was a mandated service and how closely it corresponded to the agency's 12 goals. Spaulding said she and other managers accepted 95 percent of the committee's recommendations.

Commissioner Linda Coleman said it may be time to aggressively pursue other funding sources, including a local sales tax option.

Those employees who find their jobs on the chopping block will be offered voluntary severance plans and retirement options, said Bob Sorrels, director of operations. Managers will try to find other positions within Human Services or county government for those employees who don't want to leave.

These are some of the Wake Human Services areas to be eliminated or reduced:

- Breast and cervical cancer prevention and mammography will be eliminated as a county service and possibly shift to Rex Healthcare.
- Adolescent/Women's Clinic, which serves more that 1,200 women a month, will revert to a family planning/pregnancy prevention clinic.
- Brentwood, a residential program for three to five severely mentally ill adults, will be eliminated.
- Dental Heal Promotion, which targets schoolchildren and some adults, will be discontinued.
- Crosby Clinic in downtown Raleigh, which examines children with attention deficit disorder, will be closed.
- Wake House and Garner Home, short- to medium-term residential care facilities for children – mainly those in the custody of the county – will be closed.
- WIC, a federal program that provides services to women, infants and children, will no longer be open after business hours, which have been paid for by the county.
- Cornerstone, which used federal dollars for health care to the homeless, will be transferred to another service provider.

- Motivating staff (by allowing them input into their roles, responsibilities, and accountability).
- Bringing about cost awareness as a result of being involved in resource allocation decisions.

Top-down/Bottom-up Approach: See *Participatory Approach.*

Although the participatory approach has many advantages, it has three important disadvantages:

- Participation may result in loss of control.

PERSPECTIVE 10–3

Beth Israel to Cut Back Services: Community Hospitals in Network to Assume Many Basic Functions

Dramatically altering the city's medical landscape, Beth Israel Deaconess Medical Center will close a range of services – including psychiatry, dermatology, and orthopedics – in a tough decision that will affect thousands of patients and medical residents but that executives hope ultimately will rescue the struggling Harvard teaching hospital.

The announcement yesterday that the hospital will eliminate or scale back seven clinical departments marks a significant departure for Beth Israel Deaconess, which instead of keeping with its tradition as a full-service hospital will focus on a few lucrative high-level specialties.

Community hospitals in the Beth Israel Deaconess network, called CareGroup, will position themselves to take over many of those services, a major shift in a city where patients visit expensive teaching hospitals far more often than the national average, even for basic care.

"This is the beginning of the rationalization of health care – deciding who gets what kind of care where – in Massachusetts," said Ellen Trager, head of the health-care consulting practice at Brown Rudnick and a consultant for New England Medical Center, a Beth Israel Deaconess competitor.

The turnaround plan, which CareGroup and the medical center will implement over four years, includes:

Moving certain services to other CareGroup hospitals, including general dermatology, ophthalmology, the pain management clinic, post-acute care, and rehabilitation services. The moves will occur over four years.

Dermatology, for example, educates one-quarter of all Harvard Medical School dermatology residents, doctors said.

Transferring elective orthopedic surgery and procedures to New England Baptist Hospital. Beth Israel Deaconess will continue to provide acute trauma services to patients with broken bones and other injuries.

Expanding core services including cardiology, cardiac surgery, organ transplantation, and cancer care.

"The Beth Israel Deaconess board has a real enthusiasm for what is believed to be a very strong plan," he [the CEO] said. "It will produce the kind of financial support to actually drive our mission on into the future. We have not had that kind of strong plan for the past couple of years." CareGroup lost $7 million to $8 million in July, about $2 million more than the organization predicted, CareGroup executives said earlier this month.

Physicians and staff were upset yesterday about possibly losing their jobs and the elimination of long-time services. Some felt the hospital network eventually would be taken over by its biggest competitor, Partners HealthCare System, another Harvard network headed by Brigham & Women's Hospital and Massachusetts General Hospital.

Source: Liz Kowalczyk, *Boston Globe*, September 27, 2000, p. E1.

- Participation is time-consuming and uses resources (mainly staff time) that could be devoted to other purposes.
- Participation may result in disappointment.

Budget Models

There are two basic budget models: incremental/decremental budgeting and zero-based budgeting (see Exhibit 10–3). The **incremental/decremental approach** begins with what exists and gives a slight increase, no change, or slight decrease to various line items, programs, or departments. In some cases, all programs may receive an equal increase or decrease. In other instances, management may differentially give increases or decreases.

Incremental/Decremental Approach: A method of budgeting which starts with an existing budget to plan future budgets.

Exhibit 10–4   The Participatory Approach to Budgeting

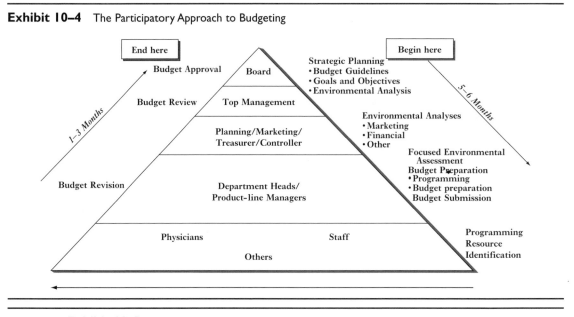

Exhibit 10–5   Advantages and Disadvantages of the Participatory Approach to Budgeting

Advantages	Disadvantages
Shared Understanding	Loss of Control
Cooperation and Competition	Time-consuming
Clarified Roles and Responsibilities	High Resource Use
Motivation	Potential Disappointment
Cost Awareness	

Where incremental/decremental budgeting begins by asking the question "How much of an increase or decrease should each program receive?," **zero-based budgeting (ZBB)** continually questions both the need for each program and its level of funding. It asks: "Why does this program or department exist in the first place?" and "What will happen by changing (increasing or decreasing) its level of funding?"

In preparation for the zero-based budgeting process, each budgeting unit (department, program, or service line) prepares a budget package that provides: 1) an overall justification for the program; and 2) a series of requests to show what the program would look like at various levels of funding. After receiving all budget packages from all budgeting units, management chooses from among them to find the best combination of programs and levels of programs to meet the goals of the organization within existing resource constraints.

The following scenario illustrates what a zero-based budgeting package might look like at the general level for a small rural hospital establishing a physician practice. In this instance, three alternative levels of service are proposed: minimum (level 1), adequate (level 2), and comprehensive (level 3). In addition to the information used in this example, most organizations would also require further detail of various line items. Such information can be found in the next section, Budget Detail.

Zero-based Budgeting (ZBB): An approach to budgeting that continually questions both the need for existing programs and their level of funding, as well as the need for new programs.

The Situation

San Maro is a rural town with a population of 20,000. The 125-bed local hospital provides comprehensive services except for obstetrics and pediatric care. Some of the local patients who need these services use the emergency room. This often results in a long wait and a frustrating experience for both patient and physicians. Many patients, unfortunately, leave the area and travel 50 miles to another facility.

In order to keep the majority of business at her hospital and to decompress the emergency room, the hospital administrator is proposing that the hospital board agree to create an in-house local obstetric and pediatric practice. According to estimates by the Chief Financial Officer, the hospital would gain substantial additional revenues from this new service, and patient satisfaction would improve.

Proposal to Create an In-house Obstetric and Pediatric Practice in San Maro

Purpose: To provide adequate primary care to pregnant women and children in San Maro.

Savings to the Hospital: Non-quantifiable decompression of emergency room. Last year 125 obstetric and 247 pediatric cases were seen in the emergency room. It is estimated that 75 percent of these cases were non-emergent.

Potential Revenue to the Hospital: The majority of women leave the local area to receive prenatal care and give birth because there is no local obstetrician. It is estimated that 300 babies are birthed annually by the local population. Only 23 babies were born at San Maro last year. A significant number of pediatric admissions also leave San Maro for their secondary care. It is estimated that up to 150 cases would receive their care at San Maro Hospital if there was an in-house pediatrics practice.

Three alternative levels of care are being proposed (see Exhibits 10–6a, 10–6b, 10–6c, and 10–6d). The incremental revenues that accrue to the hospital would be the result of increased inpatient volume. San Maro would receive no revenues from the physician

---

Exhibit 10–6a   Incremental Revenue and Cost Summary for Three Levels of Service

	Assumptions:	Level 1	Level 2	Level 3	
A	New Patient Days	450	700	1,320	
B	Incremental Hospital Revenues/day	$900	$900	$900	
C	Incremental Inpatient Costs/day	$290	$290	$290	
D	Incremental Practice Costs/Year	$261,000	$329,000	$782,500	
	Calculations:	**Formula**			
E	New Patient Days	[A]	450	700	1,320
F	Incremental Hospital Revenues	[A × B]	$405,000	$630,000	$1,188,000
G	Incremental Inpatient Costs	[A × C]	$130,500	$203,000	$382,800
H	Incremental Practice Costs	[D]	$261,000	$329,000	$782,500
I	Net Income	[F − G − H]	$13,500	$98,000	$22,700

Note: Details found in Exhibits 10–6b, c, and d, respectively.

Exhibit 10–6b   Zero-Based Budget Package: Level I

Package: Salary, Benefits, Capital, and Space Needs
Organization: Physician Practice
Purpose: To provide minimum primary obstetric care to the local population.
Methodology: Hospital must recruit 1 physician, 1 nurse, and 1 receptionist and arrange for backup coverage for weekends, vacation, sick leave, and holidays on a per diem basis from the local hospital. It must also lease, equip, and furnish office space for this practice.
Consequences of not approving this package: Were this practice not created, the local population either would have to visit the emergency room at the local hospital for its non-acute and routine care, or else travel outside the area (approximately 50 miles) to obtain primary obstetrical care. When patients use the emergency room for this coverage, oftentimes very long waits clog the flow in the ER area creating inefficiency that is both costly and frustrating. If patients leave the area, they are also more prone to obtain secondary and tertiary care elsewhere, which decreases market share for the local hospital. *Given this minimum obstetrical coverage, patients could receive primary obstetrical care at a physician's office locally during the week, only needing to visit the emergency room for acute needs.*

	Assumptions:		
A	New Patient Days		450
B	Incremental Hospital Revenues/day		$900
C	Incremental Inpatient Costs/day		$290
D	Incremental practice costs/year		$261,000
	Calculations:	**Formula**	
E	New Patient Days	[A]	450
F	Incremental Hospital Revenues	[A × B]	$405,000
G	Incremental Inpatient Costs	[A × C]	$130,500
H	Incremental practice costs	[D]	$261,000
I	*Net Income*	[F – G – H]	**$13,500**

practice itself. Exhibit 10–6a presents the incremental projections resulting from the three levels of care considered.

Staffing Concerns: Due to recent decreases in length of stay and shifts of patients to the outpatient area, the only additional cost is the variable daily care costs that total approximately $290 per day.

Recommendation: Level 3 practice with semi-annual review to assess need for additional resources. This will optimally decompress the emergency room and keep patients from leaving the area to receive these services elsewhere.

Concluding Remarks About Zero-based Budgeting

Zero-based budgeting was introduced and broadly used in the mid-1960s, but it soon dropped out of favor – primarily because it was such a laborious process. Many organizations felt that too much time was being spent preparing and reviewing budget packages, when in fact major changes rarely occurred. There are some signs, though, that zero-based budgeting is reemerging as health care organizations face an increasingly

Exhibit 10–6c   Zero-based Budget Package: Level 2

Package: Salary, Benefits, Capital, and Space Needs
Organization: Physician Practice
Purpose: To provide adequate primary obstetric practice and half-time pediatric coverage for the local population.
Methodology: Hospital must recruit 1.5 physicians, 1 nurse, and 1 receptionist and arrange for backup coverage for weekends, vacation, sick leave, and holidays on a per diem basis from the local hospital. It must also lease, equip, and furnish office space for this practice.
Consequences of not approving this package: Were this practice not created, the local population either would have to visit the emergency room at the local hospital for its non-acute and routine care, or else travel outside the area (approximately 50 miles) to obtain primary obstetrical care. When patients use the emergency room for this coverage, oftentimes very long waits clog the flow in the ER area creating inefficiency that is both costly and frustrating. If patients leave the area, they are also more prone to obtain secondary and tertiary care elsewhere, which decreases market share for the local hospital. *Given this adequate coverage, patients could receive primary obstetric and pediatric care at a physician's office locally during the week, only needing to visit the emergency room for acute needs.*

	Assumptions:		
A	New Patient Days		700
B	Incremental Hospital Revenues/day		$900
C	Incremental Inpatient Costs/day		$290
D	Incremental practice costs/year		$329,000
	Calculations:	**Formula**	
E	New Patient Days	[A]	700
F	Incremental Hospital Revenues	[A × B]	$630,000
G	Incremental Inpatient Costs	[A × C]	$203,000
H	Incremental practice costs	[D]	$329,000
I	*Net Income*	[F − G − H]	$98,000

competitive environment, seek to implement new revenue enhancement and cost avoidance activities, and try to capture new market niches.

Budget Detail

Based on the amount of detail they contain, budgets can be classified into three categories: line-item, program, and performance. A **line-item budget** has the least detail, merely listing revenues and expenses by category, such as labor, travel, and supplies. A line-item budget for the comprehensive level of care for the San Maro Medical Clinic is shown in Exhibit 10–7.

A **program budget** not only contains the line items, but also lists them by program. Exhibit 10–8 shows how the line-item budget for the comprehensive level of service for the San Maro physician practice would look as a program budget by providing detail about its four programs: general practice, prenatal care, well-baby care, and walk-in services.

Line-item Budget: The least detailed budget, showing only revenues and expenses by category, such as labor or supplies.

Program Budget: An extension of the line-item budget which shows revenues and expenses by program or service lines.

Exhibit 10–6d   Zero-based Budget Package: Level 3

Package: Salary, Benefits, Capital, and Space Needs

Organization: Physician Practice

Purpose: To provide comprehensive primary obstetric and pediatric physician coverage for the local population.

Methodology: Hospital must recruit 4 physicians, 1 nurse practitioner, 1.5 nurses, and 1 receptionist and arrange for backup coverage for weekends, vacation, sick leave, and holidays on a per diem basis from the local hospital. It must also lease, equip, and furnish office space for this practice.

Consequences of not approving this package: Were this practice not created, the local population either would have to visit the emergency room at the local hospital for its non-acute and routine care, or else travel outside the area (approximately 50 miles) to obtain primary obstetrical care. When patients use the emergency room for this coverage, oftentimes very long waits clog the flow in the ER area creating inefficiency that is both costly and frustrating. If patients leave the area, they are also more prone to obtain secondary and tertiary care elsewhere, which decreases market share for the local hospital. *Given this comprehensive coverage, patients could receive all obstetric and pediatric care at a local physician's office in expanded hours, including weekends.*

Assumptions:

A	New Patient Days	1,320
B	Incremental Hospital Revenues/day	$900
C	Incremental Inpatient Costs/day	$290
D	Incremental practice costs/year	$782,500

	Calculations:	**Formula**	
E	New Patient Days	[A]	1,320
F	Incremental Hospital Revenues	[A × B]	$1,188,000
G	Incremental Inpatient Costs	[A × C]	$382,800
H	Incremental practice costs	[D]	$782,500
I	*Net Income*	[F − G − H]	**$22,700**

Finally, a **performance budget** lists revenue and expenses by line item for each program or service covered by the budget like a program budget. In addition, it specifies performance objectives. Exhibit 10–9 shows how the line-item and program budgets for San Maro would look as performance budgets.

Exhibit 10–10 compares the level of detail shown in line-item, program, and performance budgets.

Though virtually all organizations have annual budgets, increasingly each is part of a **multi-year budget**. Rather than forecast revenues and expenses for just one year, organizations are finding it necessary to use multi-year budgets to forecast three to five years in advance. Since conditions change, many organizations use **rolling budgets**, which are regularly updated and extended multi-year forecasts. For example, the budget submitted for 20X1 would cover the years 20X1 through 20X5. When the 20X2 budget is prepared, it will cover the years 20X2 through 20X6. In this way, the budget is always forecasting five years ahead. Some organizations "roll forward" their budgets more often than every year, updating their multi-year forecasts on a semi-annual or even quarterly basis.

Exhibit 10–7 Line-Item Budget for a Proposed Physician Practice – Comprehensive Level of Care (Level 3)

Incremental Hospital Revenues				Total
New Patient Days	1,320			
Hospital Revenues/Day	$900			$1,188,000
Expenses				
Inpatient Costs/Day	$290			382,800
Costs associated with physician practice:				
Salaries and Benefits	# Units	Cost/Unit	Cost	
General Practitioners	2.0	$100,000	$200,000	
Pediatricians	2.0	$100,000	200,000	
Nurse Practitioner	1.0	$50,000	50,000	
Nurses	1.5	$40,000	60,000	
Receptionist	1.0	$20,000	20,000	
Subtotal				530,000
Fringe (as a % of Subtotal)	25%		132,500	
Malpractice Insurance			77,000	
Subtotal				209,500
Supplies and Equipment				
Medical			13,500	
Office			6,500	
Subtotal				20,000
Lease (Sq. Ft/Year)	2,300	$10		23,000
Total Costs for Physician Practice				782,500
Net Income				**$22,700**

Single year and multi-year budgets vary by the time horizon they forecast, whereas static and flexible budgets vary on the basis of volume projections. **Static budgets** forecast for a single level of activity and **flexible budgets** forecast revenues and expenses for various levels of activities. For example, whereas a static budget in an ambulatory care setting might forecast revenues and expenses for 15,000 visits, a flexible budget would forecast revenues and expenses for a range of visits between 14,000 and 16,000 visits. The use of flexible budgets is an important tool for controlling expenses, and is discussed in detail in Chapter 11.

Rolling Budget: A multiyear budget which is updated more frequently than annually, such as semi-annually or quarterly.

Static Budget: A budget which uses a single or fixed level of activity.

Budget Modifications

In most health care organizations, criteria are established beyond which managers must request permission to make changes to their budgets. The criteria are usually set as dollar amounts and/or a need to move funds from one category to another. For example, an administrator may be able to move amounts under $1,000 within a category (such as labor) without needing higher approval, but not from one category to another (such as from labor to equipment). Particularly dramatic examples of the need for budget revisions often occur during nursing shortages, when hospitals have to continually ask their boards to approve increases in nursing salaries or contract labor in the middle of the year.

Flexible Budget: A budget which accommodates a range or multiple levels of activities.

Exhibit 10-8 Program Budget for a Proposed Physician Practice – Comprehensive Level of Care (Level 3)

Incremental Hospital Revenues	Givens	Givens		General OB Practice	Well-Baby Care	Pediatric Walk-In	Subtotal	Total
New Patient Days		1,320						
Hospital Revenues/Day		$900						$1,188,000
Expenses								
Inpatient Costs/Day		$290						382,800
Costs associated with physician practice:								
Salaries and Benefits	# Units		Cost/Unit					
General Practitioners	2.0		$100,000	$200,000			$200,000	
Pediatricians	2.0		$100,000		$100,000	$100,000	200,000	
Nurse Practitioner	1.0		$50,000	25,000	25,000		50,000	
Nurses	1.5		$40,000	20,000	20,000	20,000	60,000	
Receptionist	1.0		$20,000	10,000	5,000	5,000	20,000	
Subtotal				255,000	150,000	125,000		530,000
Fringe (as a % of Subtotal)	25%			63,750	37,500	31,250	132,500	
Malpractice Insurance				62,000	8,000	7,000	77,000	
Subtotal				125,750	45,500	38,250		209,500
Supplies and Equipment								
Medical				9,500	2,000	2,000	13,500	
Office				5,000	500	1,000	6,500	
Subtotal				14,500	2,500	3,000		20,000
Lease (Sq. Ft/Year)	2,300		$10	12,000	11,000	0		23,000
Total Costs for Physician Practice				407,250	209,000	166,250		782,500
Net Income								**$22,700**

Exhibit 10-9 Performance Budget for a Proposed Physician Practice – Comprehensive Level of Care (Level 3)

Incremental Hospital Revenues	Givens	Givens	General OB Practice	Well-Baby Care	Pediatric Walk-in	Subtotal	Total
New Patient Days	1,320						$1,188,000
Hospital Revenues/Day	$900						
Expenses							
Inpatient Costs/Day	$290						382,800
Costs associated with physician practice:							
Salaries and Benefits	#Units	Cost/Unit					
General Practitioners	2.0	$100,000	$200,000			$200,000	
Pediatricians	2.0	$100,000		$100,000	$100,000	200,000	
Nurse Practitioner	1.0	$50,000	25,000	25,000		50,000	
Nurses	1.5	$40,000	20,000	20,000	20,000	60,000	
Receptionist	1.0	$20,000	10,000	5,000	5,000	20,000	
Subtotal			255,000	150,000	125,000		530,000
Fringe (as a % of Subtotal)	25%		63,750	37,500	31,250	132,500	
Malpractice Insurance			62,000	8,000	7,000	77,000	
Subtotal			125,750	45,500	38,250		209,500
Supplies and Equipment							
Medical			9,500	2,000	2,000	13,500	
Office			5,000	500	1,000	6,500	
Subtotal			14,500	2,500	3,000		20,000
Lease (Sq. Ft/Year)	2,300	$10	12,000	11,000	0		23,000
Total Costs for Physician Practice			$407,250	$209,000	$166,250		782,500
Net Income							$22,700

Performance Objectives

1) To assure that by the first year of operation, the practice is caring for 50% of the Obstetric and Pediatric patients in the community.
2) To assure that by the second year of operation, the practice is caring for 60% of the Obstetric and Pediatric patients in the community.
3) To assure that by the third year of operation, the practice is caring for 75% of the Obstetric and Pediatric patients in the community.

Performance Measures	20X1
Number of Obstetric Visits	2,700
Number of Well-Baby Visits	1,800
Number of Pediatric Visits	80
Total	4,580
Number of Inpatient Days	1,320

Exhibit 10–10   Major Characteristics of Three Types of Budgets by Level of Detail

Type of Budget	Budget by Line Item	Budget by Program	Performance Criteria
Line-item	X		
Program	X	X	
Performance	X	X	X

◀Types of Budgets▶

Although the term "the budget" is often used as if there were only one budget, most health care organizations develop four interrelated budgets: a statistics budget, an operating budget, a cash budget, and a capital budget. An overview of the relationship among these budgets is presented in Exhibit 10–11.

The Statistics Budget

The first budget to develop is the statistics budget. The **statistics budget** identifies the amount of services that will be provided, usually listed by payor type:

Exhibit 10–11   Overview of the Four Major Budgets

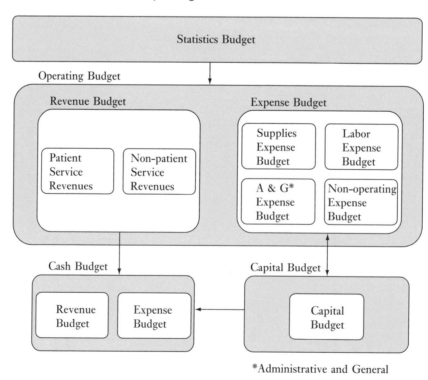

*Administrative and General

- **Charge-based payors** pay what is charged or some percentage of charges (such as 80 percent of charges).
- **Cost-based payors** pay based on an estimate of what it costs an organization to deliver the service for which they are paying. The cost is usually figured on a basis determined by the payor or a percentage of costs (such as 80 percent of average costs).
- **Flat fee payors** pay a predetermined fee per unit of service (such as a normal office visit, or a particular DRG), regardless of costs or charges.
- **Capitated payors** pay a fixed amount per enrollee for a fixed period of time, regardless of utilization, costs, or charges. The most common form of capitated payment is per member per month (PMPM).

> **Statistics Budget:** The first budget to be prepared. One of the four major types of budgets. It identifies the amount of services that will be provided, typically categorized by payor type.

Exhibit 10–12 presents the statistics budget for Walk-In Clinic. Note that these volume estimates are not stated in terms of the number of visits that will be made, but rather as weighted visits. Weighted visits take into account the amount of resources needed for various types of visits. This is necessary because not all visits consume equal resources. A patient who comes in complaining of a sore throat will likely consume far fewer resources than would a patient with a broken arm that must be X-rayed and put into a cast.

The Operating Budget

The **operating budget** (see Exhibit 10–13) is actually a combination of two budgets developed using the accrual basis of accounting: the revenue budget and the expense budget. Some organizations, especially those with relatively small non-operating items such as parking lot and gift shop revenues and expenses, include their non-operating budget with their operating budget.

> **Operating Budget:** One of the four major types of budgets, it is comprised of the revenue budget and the expense budget. The bottom line for this budget is net income.

The **revenue budget** is a forecast of the operating revenues that will be earned during the budget period (see Exhibit 10–13, rows A through E). It has two components: net patient revenues (row C) and non-patient revenues (row D). The **expense budget** lists all operating expenses that are expected to be incurred during the budget period (see Exhibit 10–13, rows F through G). Perspectives 10–4 and 10–5 illustrate some of the major concerns healthcare organizations face with one part of the expense budget, labor.

> **Revenue Budget:** A subset of the operating budget, which is a forecast of the operating revenues that will be earned during the current budget period.

Whether an item is classified as operating or non-operating is subject to interpretation by each organization. Though this matter has received considerable attention over the years by both the accounting and health care financial management professions, there remains a lack of standardization among health care organizations in classifying specific line items.

> **Expense Budget:** A subset of the operating budget, which is a forecast of the operating expenses that will be incurred during the current budget period.

 Caution Throughout this chapter, the numbers in the exhibits may be slightly different from those computed on a calculator and between exhibits due to the internal rounding rules used in the computer program upon which this example is based.

Exhibit 10–12 Statistics Budget for Walk-In Clinic

	JAN	FEB	MAR	APR	MAY	JUN	JUL	AUG	SEP	OCT	NOV	DEC	TOTAL
Charge-based	992	992	992	992	992	992	945	945	945	945	945	945	11,622
Cost-based	937	1,101	1,020	669	519	697	653	763	937	997	833	833	9,959
Flat-fee	223	112	112	112	112	112	112	268	246	112	112	112	1,745
Capitation	1,116	482	1,132	326	820	1,154	2,444	3,170	3,234	3,110	3,186	2,234	22,408
Total	3,268	2,687	3,256	2,099	2,443	2,955	4,154	5,146	5,362	5,164	5,076	4,124	45,734

Note: Numbers are weighted visits (RVUs). The large fluctuation in capitated patients reflects a dynamic pattern of the clinic's disengaging from managed care contracts and contracting new ones.

Exhibit 10–13 Operating Budget for Walk-In Clinic

		JAN	FEB	MAR	APR	MAY	JUN	JUL	AUG	SEP	OCT	NOV	DEC	TOTAL
A	Patient Revenues	$243,466	$200,182	$242,572	$156,376	$182,004	$220,148	$309,473	$383,377	$399,469	$384,718	$378,162	$307,238	$3,407,183
B	Deductions & Allowances	(57,503)	(6,284)	(52,738)	14,319	(19,206)	(46,931)	(125,335)	(197,990)	(203,062)	(185,253)	(180,281)	(113,240)	(1,173,503)
C	Net Patient Revenues	185,963	193,898	189,834	170,695	162,798	173,216	184,139	185,387	196,407	199,466	197,881	193,998	2,233,680
D	Non-Patient Revenues	2,914	3,271	3,945	3,890	4,418	4,600	4,703	5,069	5,128	5,122	5,585	5,886	54,531
E	Total Revenues	188,877	197,168	193,779	174,585	167,216	177,816	188,842	190,456	201,535	204,588	203,466	199,884	2,288,211
F	Operating Expenses													
	Labor	69,774	67,786	71,887	67,651	69,261	72,902	78,042	82,082	83,066	82,163	82,930	79,200	906,746
	Supplies	33,430	27,620	33,310	21,740	25,180	30,300	42,290	52,210	54,370	52,390	51,510	41,990	466,340
	A & G Expenses[1]													
	Interest	891	889	887	959	956	953	963	959	956	952	948	945	11,258
	Depreciation	1,498	1,498	1,498	1,498	1,656	1,656	1,656	1,669	1,669	1,669	1,669	1,669	19,305
	Utilities	12,000	12,000	12,000	12,000	12,000	12,000	12,000	12,000	12,000	12,000	12,000	12,000	144,000
	Rent	5,000	5,000	5,000	5,000	5,000	5,000	5,000	5,000	5,000	5,000	5,000	5,000	60,000
	Cleaning	500	500	500	500	500	500	500	500	500	500	500	500	6,000
	Telephone	600	600	600	600	600	600	600	600	600	600	600	600	7,200
	Travel	2,500	2,500	2,500	2,500	2,500	2,500	2,500	2,500	2,500	2,500	2,500	2,500	30,000
	Insurance	12,000	12,000	12,000	12,000	12,000	12,000	12,000	12,000	12,000	12,000	12,000	12,000	144,000
	Equipment Maintenance	150	150	150	150	150	150	150	150	150	150	150	150	1,800
	Bad Debt	4,083	4,358	4,223	3,634	3,383	3,681	3,488	3,673	3,964	4,065	3,790	3,790	46,132
	Total Operating Expenses	142,426	134,902	144,554	128,233	133,186	142,242	159,189	173,343	176,775	173,989	173,598	160,344	1,842,782
G	Non-Patient Care Expenses	97	97	97	97	97	97	97	97	97	97	97	97	1,164
H	Total Expenses	142,523	134,999	144,651	128,330	133,283	142,339	159,286	173,440	176,872	174,086	173,695	160,441	1,843,946
I	Excess of Revenues Over Expenses	$46,354	$62,170	$49,128	$46,255	$33,933	$35,477	$29,556	$17,015	$24,663	$30,501	$29,771	$39,443	$444,265

[1] Administrative and General

PERSPECTIVE 10-4

Hospital Makes Work Hour Cuts Voluntary

A mandatory 10 percent reduction in hours and pay for employees at Lexington Memorial Hospital has been lifted, effective with the payroll period that begins Sunday, according to hospital officials.

The cost reduction plan now is to be voluntary.

Budget deficits earlier in the fiscal year had led hospital administrators to require the mandatory cuts, but after learning of some "undue hardships" hospital employees were facing, the hospital's administrative council made the change to voluntary, said Kathy Sushereba, the hospital's community relations director. The administrative council is comprised of LMH President John Cashion and four vice presidents.

"All department managers are requested to continue scheduling as much time off as possible in their departments, along with sending employees home early, etc., as patient census or office workloads fluctuate," the announcement from the hospital administrative council states. "Department managers are also encouraged to take days off as scheduling permits."

The letter, which is addressed to hospital employees, medical staff, board of directors members and the hospital foundation's board of directors, also cautioned that overtime should be used only in emergency situations. The administrative council also plans to possibly reconsider the hiring freeze on a case-by-case basis as positions are vacated.

"We need to continue our reduction of the salaries and other expenses through the end of this fiscal year (Oct. 31)," the letter states.

The Dispatch received several calls from upset employees about the mandatory work hour cuts and hiring freeze in June.

The decision to cut employees' work hours came after a May review of the hospital financial report, which was released June 14. The May reports showed the hospital had experienced another month of over-budget salary expenditures.

Salary expense overages began in the fall of 1999, as employees worked overtime preparing for the hospital's Joint Commission Accreditation. Then, high numbers of patients in January, February and March resulted in the need for more overtime hours. In April, the hospital moved into its new business wing, resulting in additional payroll expenses.

The salary overages in May could not be justified, however, Cashion said, so the mandatory cutback was put in place in until the end of LMH's fiscal year on Sept. 30. He said last month the hospital wanted to avoid layoffs and continuing to go further over the $17 million budget allotted for salaries for the fiscal year.

All five of the hospital's nurse anesthetists resigned earlier this month. Callers to The Dispatch suggested that part of the reason for the mass departure was the hospital's mandatory 10 percent cut in work hours.

"As far as that having an impact on this change, I'm sure it was a consideration," Sushereba said. "Was it the primary reason for the change? I don't think so. It's a cumulative situation."

Source: Jill Doss-Raines, *The Dispatch*, July 26, 2000.

PERSPECTIVE 10-5

Shortage of Nurses Looming?

When a hospital doesn't have enough nurses, it can become a matter of life or death.

Such dramatic scenarios haven't occurred here yet, but medical professionals are concerned about the future. There is an acute shortage of people graduating from nursing programs, which has resulted in vacancies in the state and the nation – and, to a lesser degree, in Moore County.

(Continues)

Perspective 10–5 (Contd)

FirstHealth Moore Regional Hospital has been largely immune to the growing nationwide shortage so far. About 20, or 4 percent, of its 500 budgeted nursing positions are unfilled, according to Linda Wallace, director of nursing and other medical services at the hospital.

We see fewer people going into nursing, so there are fewer graduates for us to hire, Wallace said. The average age of the RN is older now, about 44, as they age out of the profession.

Patient surveys indicate they feel that the hospital's nurses are doing a good job providing care, Wallace said.

Wallace said nursing isn't attracting so many people now, partly because of other career opportunities. Nursing can take a toll on family life. It means working at nights, on weekends and on holidays. It is also taxing mentally and emotionally.

People are also a lot sicker now, when they are hospitalized, than they used to be, Wallace said. That creates additional stress on a profession that has become more and more of a highly specialized, high-tech field — one in which the nurturing side of nursing isn't as prominent anymore, some say.

FirstHealth does everything it can to keep nurses from being overloaded, which is the chief cause of burnout.

Compounding the national shortage, some say the profession has suffered because of managed care, which has shifted the decision-making on patient care from doctors and nurses to administrators. But that may be changing, some say.

Pay is also an issue. Earlier this year, a study showed that of most hospital personnel in the state and nation, nurses got smaller raises than the others did, according to the North Carolina Center for Nursing in Raleigh. All predictions are that by the year 2010 we'll have the worst nursing shortage we've ever had in the United States.

Source: Sara Lindau, *The Pilot LLC*, August 21, 2000. Copyright © 2000.

The Cash Budget

While the operating budget describes the expected revenues and the related resource flows, the **cash budget** (see Exhibit 10–14) represents the organization's cash inflows and outflows. The bottom line in the operating budget is the net income for the period; the bottom line in the cash budget is the amount of cash available at the end of the period. In addition to showing cash inflows and outflows, the cash budget also details when it is necessary to borrow to cover cash shortages and when excess funds are available to invest.

> **Cash Budget:** One of the four major types of budgets, it displays all of the organization's projected cash inflows and outflows. The bottom line for this budget is the amount of cash available at the end of the period.

 Key Point The operating budget is developed using the accrual basis of accounting. Cash inflows and outflows of each line item must be estimated to convert the operating budget to the cash budget.

The Capital Budget

The **capital budget** (see Exhibit 10–15) summarizes the anticipated purchases for the year. Capital budgets in outpatient facilities may be fairly small, but those for large systems with inpatient facilities may contain millions of dollars' worth of items.

> **Capital Budget:** One of the four major types of budgets, it summarizes the anticipated purchases for the year. Typically, to be included, all items in this budget must have a minimum purchase price, such as $500.

Exhibit 10–14 Cash Budget for Walk-in Clinic

	JAN	FEB	MAR	APR	MAY	JUN	JUL	AUG	SEP	OCT	NOV	DEC	SUMMARY
A Beginning Balance	$35,029	$11,000	$11,000	$11,000	$11,000	$11,000	$11,000	$11,000	$11,000	$11,000	$11,000	$11,000	$35,029
B Net Revenues	98,316	161,512	185,360	183,930	172,746	166,373	179,677	176,756	183,658	190,675	200,035	195,225	2,094,263
C Net Expenditures	(122,445)	(99,273)	(127,794)	(153,853)	(123,201)	(116,774)	(161,928)	(137,762)	(148,821)	(192,287)	(159,936)	(152,896)	(1,696,970)
Cash Available													
D Before Borrowing	10,900	73,239	68,567	41,076	60,545	60,598	28,750	49,994	45,837	9,388	51,099	53,329	432,322
E Cash Requirement	11,000	11,000	11,000	11,000	11,000	11,000	11,000	11,000	11,000	11,000	11,000	11,000	132,000
F Cash Shortage	(100)	0	0	0	0	0	0	0	0	(1,612)	0	0	(1,712)
G Cash Excess	0	62,239	57,567	30,076	49,545	49,598	17,750	38,994	34,837	0	40,099	42,329	423,034
H From S-T Investment	100	0	0	0	0	0	0	0	0	1,612	0	0	1,712
I Remaining Deficit	0	0	0	0	0	0	0	0	0	0	0	0	0
J From L-T Investment	0	0	0	0	0	0	0	0	0	0	0	0	0
K Remaining Deficit	0	0	0	0	0	0	0	0	0	0	0	0	0
L From Additional Debt	0	0	0	0	0	0	0	0	0	0	0	0	0
M Cash From All Sources	11,000	73,239	68,567	41,076	60,545	60,598	28,750	49,994	45,837	11,000	51,099	53,329	555,034
Less: Transfer of Excess to Short-term													
N Investments	0	(62,239)	(57,567)	(30,076)	(49,545)	(49,598)	(17,750)	(38,994)	(34,837)	0	(40,099)	(42,329)	(423,034)
O Ending Balance	$11,000	$11,000	$11,000	$11,000	$11,000	$11,000	$11,000	$11,000	$11,000	$11,000	$11,000	$11,000	$11,000

Exhibit 10–15 Capital Budget for Walk-in Clinic

Anticipated Purchases	Purchase Price	Life (Years)	Residual Value	Depreciable Base	Monthly Depreciation	Date of Purchase	Depreciation	Percent of Debt Financing	Percent Financed from Cash
Laboratory Equipment	$10,000	5	$500	$9,500	$158	1-Apr	N/A	100%	0%
Office Equipment	$2,000	8	$750	$1,250	$13	1-Jul	N/A	90%	10%
Total	$12,000								

Pro Forma Financial Statements and Ratios

Based on the information contained in these budgets, together with a small amount of additional information, an organization can develop pro forma financial statements. Pro forma financial statements are prepared to show what the organization's regular financial statements will look like if all budgets are met exactly as planned. The regular financial statements are prepared after the accounting period ends and present the actual results of the organization's activities during the period. As an example of the relationship between the budgets and financial statements, Walk-In Clinic's operating budget (see Exhibit 10–13) could serve as its statement of operations, with only a few modifications in format. Developing the balance sheet and statement of cash flows is not quite so straightforward, but it can be done with only a small amount of additional information.

Once the pro forma financial statements have been developed, they can be subjected to ratio analysis just as with regular financial statements. This process is reversed in strategic financial planning, where the organization first identifies its goals in terms of the various categories of ratios (liquidity, profitability, capitalization, and activity) and then develops its budgets, over time, to meet the targets it has set for itself.

◀An Extended Example of How to Develop a Budget▶

This section shows how to develop the numbers in a budget, using Walk-In Clinic as an example. The term "a budget" really is shorthand for four interrelated budgets: the statistics, operating, cash, and capital budgets.

The Statistics Budget

The statistics budget is created in two steps: 1) develop volume projections; and 2) convert volume projections into weighted visits. Incidentally, though an ambulatory setting is used for the example, the same principles are applied in inpatient settings.

Developing Volume Projections

The first step is to scan the environment and develop a projection of the number of visits classified by payor type. A common approach is to begin with the previous year's actual results and make adjustments for any anticipated changes. For charge-based, cost-based, and flat fee patients, projecting next year's visits is just a matter of estimating a percentage change from the previous year. However, this procedure must be revised slightly in the case of capitated patients. First, the number of enrollees for the next year is estimated, and then the percentage of these enrollees who will actually make a visit is forecasted (see Exhibit 10–16).

Exhibit 10–16 Calculation of Number of Visits by Payor Type

Payor Type	JAN	FEB	MAR	APR	MAY	JUN	JUL	AUG	SEP	OCT	NOV	DEC	TOTAL
Charge-based													
Projected This Year	350	350	350	350	350	350	350	350	350	350	350	350	4,200
Projected Growth	2.00%	2.00%	2.00%	2.00%	2.00%	2.00%	-3.00%	-3.00%	-3.00%	-3.00%	-3.00%	-3.00%	-0.43%
Projected Next Year	357	357	357	357	357	357	340	340	340	340	340	340	4182
Cost-based													
Projected This Year	386	454	421	276	214	287	278	324	398	423	354	354	4,169
Projected Growth	1.00%	1.00%	1.00%	1.00%	1.00%	1.00%	-2.00%	-2.00%	-2.00%	-2.00%	-2.00%	-2.00%	-0.50%
Projected Next Year	390	459	425	279	216	290	272	318	390	415	347	347	4148
Flat-fee													
Projected This Year	100	50	50	50	50	50	50	120	110	50	50	50	780
Projected Growth	12.00%	12.00%	12.00%	12.00%	12.00%	12.00%	12.00%	12.00%	12.00%	12.00%	12.00%	12.00%	11.92%
Projected Next Year	112	56	56	56	56	56	56	134	123	56	56	56	873
Capitated													
Last Month's Enrollment	6,010	6,130	6,171	6,213	6,256	6,300	6,343	7,830	7,172	7,320	7,476	8,165	6,010
Projected Growth	2.000%	0.663%	0.676%	0.692%	0.708%	0.686%	23.440%	-8.401%	2.061%	2.134%	9.221%	-4.329%	29.983%
20X1 enrollment	6130	6171	6213	6256	6300	6343	7830	7172	7320	7476	8165	7812	7,812
Visit Rate	7.0%	3.0%	7.0%	2.0%	5.0%	7.0%	12.0%	17.0%	17.0%	16.0%	15.0%	11.0%	10.3%
Projected Next Year	429	185	435	125	315	444	940	1,219	1,244	1,196	1,225	859	8,616
Total Visits	1,288	1,057	1,273	817	944	1,147	1,608	2,011	2,097	2,007	1,968	1,602	17,819

Historical information the organization has developed can provide the basis for many estimates used in the budgeting process. However, when new services are offered or when new patients are seen, estimation becomes a more difficult process. In such cases, the organization may try to draw on experiences of similar organizations with which it has a good relationship (perhaps elsewhere in its network), or it may turn to statistics that have been compiled by national professional associations, such as the Medical Group Management Association or the American Hospital Association.

Incidentally, although it is probably more common for health care organizations to develop their promotions by payor class (i.e. fee-for-service, cost-based, flat fee, and capitation), it is becoming increasingly necessary to project utilization by individual payor. For example, Walk-in Clinic might project its capitated visits for each managed care organization (Kaiser, Health Source, etc.).

Converting Visit Projections to Weighted Visits

Converting visit projections into weighted visits involves three steps: determining categories of visits and their relative resource consumption; estimating the percentage distribution by level by payor; and converting visits to weighted visits based upon the information developed in the first two steps.

Determining Categories of Visits and Their Relative Resource Consumption

Once a projection of the number of visits has been made as illustrated in Exhibit 10–16, the next step is to convert these visits into **weighted visits**, commonly called **relative value units (RVUs)**. Although theoretically any number of categories can be used, Walk-In Clinic uses three:

- **Brief visits** taking an average of 15 minutes each.
- **Routine visits** taking an average of 30 minutes and, thus, using twice the resources (mainly clinician time and supplies) as brief visits.
- **Complex visits** taking, on average, one hour and, thus, using an average of four times the amount of resources as brief visits.

In relative value unit terms, a routine visit consumes twice the resources of a brief visit, and a complex visit consumes four times the resources of a brief visit. Therefore, using a brief visit, which counts as one relative value unit, as the base, whenever Walk-In Clinic has a routine visit it counts as two relative value units, and each complex visit counts as four relative value units.

Estimating the Percentage Distribution by Level by Payor

Once the categories of visits and their relative levels of intensity have been developed, the next step is to determine the percentage distribution of visits by level by payor. For instance, Walk-In Clinic estimates that there will be considerable diversity by payor in the percentage of patients making brief, routine, and complex visits

Relative Value Units (RVUs): A standardized weighting applied to services which reflects the amount of resource consumption to provide that service. A service assigned two RVUs consumes twice the resources as does a service assigned one RVU.

Exhibit 10–17   Estimated Percent of Visits by Intensity Level and by Payor

	Charge-based	Cost-based	Flat-fee	Capitation
Brief (Level I)	6%	12%	10%	10%
Routine (Level II)	52%	62%	85%	55%
Complex (Level III)	42%	26%	5%	35%
Total	100%	100%	100%	100%

Exhibit 10–18   The Conversion of Visits into Weighted Visits

		Source	I	II	III	Total
A	Total Number of Capitated Visits Forecast in January	Exhibit 10–16				429
B	Percent of Visits by Level	Exhibit 10–17	10%	55%	35%	
C	Number of Visits by Level	[A × B]	43	236	150	
D	RVU Weight	[1]	1	2	4	
E	RVU-weighted Visits	[C × D]	43	472	601	1,115[2]

[1] Level I = Basic Visit. Levels II and III require 2 times and 4 times the resources as basic visits, respectively. These numbers would come from an internal study.

[2] Difference between the number derived here and appearing in Exhibit 10–12 for January is due to rounding in the computer model from which this example was derived.

(see Exhibit 10–17). Capitated patients are of particular interest in this step, for they may have different utilization patterns than do patients in other payor categories. For example, in addition to common life-cycle and gender-related visit patterns, first-time enrollees in an HMO tend to have higher utilization patterns.

Converting Visits to Weighted Visits

Converting visits to weighted visits is relatively straightforward and involves applying the information about intensity levels and visit distribution to the visit information developed in Step 1. Exhibit 10–18 shows how Walk-In Clinic converts its projected 429 capitated visits in January (see Exhibit 10–16) into the 1,116 RVU-weighted visits shown in the statistics budget for January (see Exhibit 10–12).

Walk-In Clinic began by estimating 429 capitated visits. After categorizing these visits by intensity of resources to be used per visit, it determined that these visits require the same resources as 1,115 brief visits. All the numbers in the statistics budget (see Exhibit 10–12) were derived similarly. Note that the difference between the number derived here (1,115) and that appearing in Exhibit 10–12 (1,116) is due to rounding.

Rounding differences aside, the importance of the accuracy of the numbers used in the statistics budget cannot be overemphasized. The utilization projections developed in the statistics budget serve as the foundation to project revenues, expenses, and cash flows.

The Operating Budget

As noted earlier, the operating budget (see Exhibit 10–13) comprises two budgets developed using the accrual basis of accounting: the revenue budget and the expense budget. Development of each of these budgets for Walk-In Clinic follows.

The Revenue Budget

The revenue budget has two primary parts: net patient revenues and non-patient revenues.

Net Patient Revenues

As discussed in Chapter 2, there is a difference between gross charges and net charges. **Gross charges** are the amount the organization would bill if everyone paid full charges. **Net charges** are the amount the organization bills after taking into account all discounts and allowances (except bad debt). Discounts and allowances include such items as contractual agreements between the health care provider and the payor, charity care, and sliding fee schedules.

Gross Charges: The amount that an organization would bill its patients if they all paid full charges.

Net Charges: The amount that an organization bills its patients after accounting for discounts and allowances.

Assume that Walk-In Clinic has the information about the different payors as shown in Exhibit 10–19. For Walk-In Clinic to determine gross patient charges, the number of RVUs for each payor is multiplied by the full charge. For example, as shown in the top half of Exhibit 10–20, January's total of $243,466 was calculated by multiplying 3,268 RVUs by $74.50 per RVU (rows A, B, and C, Total column).

The determination of net patient revenues is a little more complex. Walk-In Clinic determines net patient revenues as follows:

- As noted above, 15 percent of charge-based payors are considered charity patients. Therefore, only 85 percent of the charge-based RVUs are multiplied by the full charge. Net patient revenues for Walk-In Clinic in January ($62,818) are calculated as follows: $[(992 \text{ RVUs} \times 0.85) \times \$74.50]$ (see Exhibit 10–20).
- Since cost-based payors are paying 75 percent of charges, net patient revenues for these patients is calculated by multiplying the number of visits by 75 percent of charges. For Walk-In Clinic in January, the $52,355 in net patient revenues is

---

Exhibit 10–19 Walk-In Clinic's Basic Information About Various Payors

---

Full-charge Payors pay an average of $74.50 per RVU (15 percent of charge-based payors are considered charity patients).

Cost-based Payors pay an average of 75 percent of charges.

Flat-fee Payors have contracted to pay $30.00 per visit.

Capitated Payors pay an average of $11 PMPM.

Exhibit 10–20 Walk-In Clinic's Calculation of Gross and Net Charges for January

		Charge-based	Cost-based	Flat-fee	Capitated	Total
Determination of Gross Charges:						
A	Number of RVUs	992	937	223	1,116	3,268
		[Exhibit 10–12]				
B	Price per RVU	$74.50	$74.50	$74.50	$74.50	$74.50
		[Exhibit 10–19]				
C	Gross Charges	$73,904	$69,807	$16,614	$83,142	$243,466
		[A × B]				
Determination of Net Charges:						
D	Payment Basis	843 RVUs[1]	937 RVUs	112 Visits	6,130 Members[2]	
E	Payment Arrangement	$74.50 /RVU	$55.88 /RVU	$30.00 /Visit	$11.00 PMPM	
		[Exhibit 10–19]				
F	Net Charges	$62,818	$52,355	$3,360	$67,430	$185,963
		[D × E]				
G	Discounts and Allowances	$11,086	$17,452	$13,254	$15,712	$57,503
		[C − F]				

[1] There are 992 full-pay RVUs, of which 15% are charity care. Therefore, net revenues are based upon 85 percent of the 992 full-pay RVUs (992 × 85% = 843 RVUs).
[2] From Exhibit 10–16, January Capitated 20X1 Enrollment.

computed as follows: [($74.50 × 0.75) × 937 RVUs]. In this case it is assumed that cost-based payors have determined in advance what percentage of charges per RVU they will pay, based upon the payors' internal calculations of an appropriate ratio of Walk-in Clinic's cost to its charges.

- Flat fee net patient revenues are determined by multiplying the number of units on which payment is based by the price per unit. Assume Walk-In Clinic negotiated a contract to do physicals for $30.00 each. RVUs are ignored. To determine net charges, the number of physicals (visits) is multiplied by the price per visit. For January, this would be $3,360 (112 visits × $30.00/visit).

- Net patient revenues for capitated payors is determined by multiplying the PMPM fee by the number of enrollees. RVUs are ignored. Net patient revenues for Walk-In Clinic in January is determined as follows: 6,130 members (Exhibit 10–16) $11.00 PMPM = $67,430.

Using this information, the total net patient revenues for Walk-In Clinic for January is computed as follows (see Exhibit 10–20, row F):

Charge-based patients	$62,818
Cost-based patients	52,355
Flat fee patients	3,360
Capitated patients	67,430
Total net patient revenues	$185,963

The net patient revenues for the other months in Exhibit 10–13 were found in a similar manner. Note that the last line of Exhibit 10–20, discounts and allowances, shows that the difference between gross charges (the amount that Walk-In Clinic would bill if there were no discounts and allowances) and net charges (the amount Walk-In Clinic can actually bill after taking into account discounts and allowances) is $57,503 (differences due to rounding). Of this:

- $11,086 is due to charity care.
- $17,452 is due to cost-based payors paying an average of 75 percent of charges.
- $13,254 is due to a negotiated fee for physicals.
- $15,712 is due to receiving $11.00 PMPM from capitated payors.

Caution

In this situation, gross charges and gross revenues are used interchangeably.

Non-patient Revenues

In addition to patient service revenues, most organizations also have non-patient revenues. In the case of Walk-In Clinic, the non-patient revenues are interest and consulting fees. The estimate of interest earned is developed on a separate schedule related to the cash budget (not shown here). The estimate of consulting fees is based on a review of the organization's plans for this service. The calculation of the $54,531 of non-patient revenues in the operating budget (see Exhibit 10–13, Total column) is shown in Exhibit 10–21, Total column.

The Expense Budget

The second part of the operating budget (see Exhibit 10–13, rows F through H) is the expense budget. The expense budget itself is made up of three other budgets: the labor budget, supplies budget, and administrative and general budget (see Exhibit 10–22).

The Labor Budget

Labor Budget: A subset of the expense budget, this budget is composed of the fixed labor budget and the variable labor budget.

Note that the first item listed under expenses in the operating budget (see Exhibit 10–13) is labor, for it consumes the largest amount of the organization's resources. The amount listed for labor expense is developed in the **labor budget** (see Exhibit 10–23), which itself is composed of two budgets: the fixed labor budget and the variable labor budget. The **fixed labor budget** forecasts the costs of salaried personnel; the **variable labor budget** accounts for additional labor costs, which vary as additional part-time personnel or overtime hours are needed. Development of Walk-In Clinic's labor budget follows.

The Fixed Labor Budget

Fixed Labor Budget: A subset of the labor budget which forecasts the cost of salaried personnel.

The numbers on the fixed labor budget come from salary information, usually kept by position and/or person occupying the position. For example, the basic information used to construct Walk-In Clinic's fixed labor budget (see Exhibit 10–25) are found in Exhibit 10–24.

Exhibit 10–26 illustrates how the basic information in Exhibit 10–24 was converted to the fixed labor budget in Exhibit 10–25 (for example, see the case of Physician I for January).

The Variable Labor Budget

Variable Labor Budget: A subset of the labor budget which forecasts non-salary labor costs, such as part-time employees and overtime hours.

The second component of the labor budget is the variable labor budget, which accounts for wages of non-salaried employees and overtime. Health care organizations are increasingly turning to part-time employees because, often at less cost, they can meet flexible demands and cost less, as benefits do not need to be paid to these workers.

Because the number of part-time and overtime hours per month vary depending on the workload, it is not necessary to develop this budget by position as was done for the fixed labor budget. Instead, this budget is developed by: 1) estimating how many hours *will* be covered by full-time staff; 2) estimating how many hours *will not* be covered by full-time staff; 3) determining how many of these non-covered hours will be filled by overtime and how many will be filled by part-time personnel; and 4) applying the full-time and part-time rates to the full- and part-time hours to calculate full- and part-time wages.

Exhibit 10–21 Forecast of Non-Patient Revenues for Walk-In Clinic

	JAN	FEB	MAR	APR	MAY	JUN	JUL	AUG	SEP	OCT	NOV	DEC	TOTAL
Interest	$2,414	$2,771	$3,445	$3,390	$3,918	$4,100	$4,203	$4,569	$4,622	$4,628	$5,085	$5,386	$48,531
Consulting	500	500	500	500	500	500	500	500	500	500	500	500	6,000
Total	$2,914	$3,271	$3,945	$3,890	$4,418	$4,600	$4,703	$5,069	$5,122	$5,128	$5,585	$5,886	$54,531

Exhibit 10–22 Overview of the Operating Expense Budget

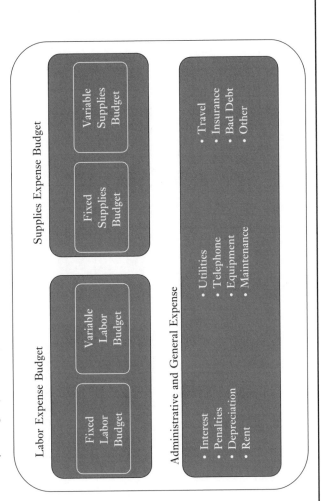

Labor Expense Budget

Fixed Labor Budget

Variable Labor Budget

Supplies Expense Budget

Fixed Supplies Budget

Variable Supplies Budget

Administrative and General Expense

- Interest
- Penalties
- Depreciation
- Rent

- Utilities
- Telephone
- Equipment
- Maintenance

- Travel
- Insurance
- Bad Debt
- Other

Exhibit 10–23 The Labor Budget

	JAN	FEB	MAR	APR	MAY	JUN	JUL	AUG	SEP	OCT	NOV	DEC	TOTAL
Fixed Salaries	$52,538	$52,704	$54,693	$54,783	$54,783	$56,557	$57,256	$57,256	$57,407	$57,407	$57,944	$57,944	$671,273
Fixed Benefits	7,881	7,906	8,204	8,217	8,217	8,484	8,588	8,588	8,611	8,611	8,692	8,692	100,691
Subtotal	60,419	60,610	62,897	63,000	63,000	65,041	65,845	65,845	66,018	66,018	66,635	66,635	771,963
Variable Wages	9,355	7,176	8,990	4,651	6,261	7,861	12,198	16,238	17,048	16,145	16,295	12,565	134,783
Total	$69,774	$67,786	$71,887	$67,651	$69,261	$72,902	$78,042	$82,082	$83,066	$82,163	$82,930	$79,200	$906,746

Exhibit 10–24 Data Used to Construct Walk-In Clinic's Fixed Labor Budget

	Annual Salary[1]	Benefits	Raise Date	% Raise
Physician I	$140,634	15%	Jan	5%
Physician II	$138,745	15%	Jul	5%
Physician's Assistant	$68,428	15%	Nov	5%
Physician's Assistant	$60,321	15%	Nov	5%
RN	$49,354	15%	Jan	5%
LPN I	$36,276	15%	Sep	5%
LPN II	$39,987	15%	Feb	5%
Nurse's Aide	$28,987	15%	Jul	5%
Office Manager	$35,000	15%	Jan	5%
Office Staff	$21,473	15%	Apr	5%
Office Staff	$23,864	15%	Mar[2]	N/A
Office Staff	$21,296	15%	Jun[2]	N/A

[1] All salaries and wages are paid twice monthly. The second payment is made on the last day of the month.
[2] To be hired on this date.

Exhibit 10–25 Walk-In Clinic's Fixed Labor Budget

Position	JAN	FEB	MAR	APR	MAY	JUN	JUL	AUG	SEP	OCT	NOV	DEC	TOTAL
Physician I	$14,151	$14,151	$14,151	$14,151	$14,151	$14,151	$14,151	$14,151	$14,151	$14,151	$14,151	$14,151	$169,816
Physician II	13,296	13,296	13,296	13,296	13,296	13,296	13,961	13,961	13,961	13,961	13,961	13,961	163,546
Physician's Assistant	6,558	6,558	6,558	6,558	6,558	6,558	6,558	6,558	6,558	6,558	6,886	6,886	79,348
Physician's Assistant	5,781	5,781	5,781	5,781	5,781	5,781	5,781	5,781	5,781	5,781	6,070	6,070	69,947
RN	4,966	4,966	4,966	4,966	4,966	4,966	4,966	4,966	4,966	4,966	4,966	4,966	59,595
LPN I	3,476	3,476	3,476	3,476	3,476	3,476	3,476	3,476	3,650	3,650	3,650	3,650	42,413
LPN II	3,832	4,024	4,024	4,024	4,024	4,024	4,024	4,024	4,024	4,024	4,024	4,024	48,093
Nurses Aide	2,778	2,778	2,778	2,778	2,778	2,778	2,917	2,917	2,917	2,917	2,917	2,917	34,168
Office Manager	3,522	3,522	3,522	3,522	3,522	3,522	3,522	3,522	3,522	3,522	3,522	3,522	42,263
Office Staff	2,058	2,058	2,058	2,161	2,161	2,161	2,161	2,161	2,161	2,161	2,161	2,161	25,620
Office Staff	0	0	2,287	2,287	2,287	2,287	2,287	2,287	2,287	2,287	2,287	2,287	22,870
Office Staff	0	0	0	0	0	2,041	2,041	2,041	2,041	2,041	2,041	2,041	14,286
Total	$60,419	$60,610	$62,897	$63,000	$63,000	$65,041	$65,845	$65,845	$66,018	$66,018	$66,635	$66,635	$771,963

Exhibit 10–26 Calculating Salaries and Benefits for Walk-In Clinic – Example of Physician 1

	Item	Source	Amount
A	Annual Base Salary	[Exhibit 10–24]	$140,634
B	Raise	[Exhibit 10–24]	5%
C	New Base Salary	[A × (1 + B)]	$147,666
D	Monthly Salary	[C/12]	$12,305
E	Benefits Percentage	[Exhibit 10–24]	15%
F	Benefits Amount	[D × E]	$1,846
G	Monthly Salary and Benefits	[D + F]	$14,151

1. **Estimate how many hours *will* be covered by full-time staff.** To calculate how many hours *will* be covered by full-time staff, the first step is to determine how many RVUs each LPN can serve per day. For Walk-In Clinic, the background information used to determine the number of RVUs per LPN per day is found in Exhibit 10–27. For January, an LPN spends an average of 22.5 minutes per RVU (row C). Of this time, 15 minutes is spent directly with the patient (row A), and an additional 7.5 minutes is spent in non-direct patient care activities such as meetings, phone calls, and paperwork (row B). Since it takes 22.5 minutes per RVU per LPN, one LPN can serve an average of 2.67 RVUs per hour (row D: 60 minutes per hour/22.5 minutes per RVU). If one LPN can serve 2.67 RVUs per hour, she can serve 21.33 RVUs per eight-hour day (row F: 2.67 RVUs/hour × 8 hours). As before, the numbers in the exhibits may be slightly different from those computed on a calculator due to computer rounding.

2. **Determine how many hours *will not* be covered by full-time staff.** That the LPN staff can serve 21.33 RVUs per day becomes the basis to determine how many additional staff are needed (see Exhibit 10–28). For Walk-in Clinic in January, if an LPN can serve 21.33 RVUs per day (row B), then he or she can serve almost 427 in 20 days (row C) and two LPNs can serve 853 RVUs (row E). From the information provided in the statistics budget, 3,268 RVUs are expected during this month (row F). Therefore, 2,415 RVUs will not be covered by the full-time LPN staff (row G). Since an LPN can serve 2.67 RVUs per hour (row H), it will take an additional 906 hours to serve the 2,415 unserved RVUs (row I).

3. **Determine how many of the non-covered hours will be filled by overtime and how many will be covered by part-time hours.** The two existing LPNs will only work 60 overtime hours each month (row J), leaving 846 hours to be covered by part-time personnel (row K).

4. **Apply the full-time and part-time rates to the full and part-time hours to calculate full and part-time wages.** Overtime wages are $15 per hour; part-time wages are $10 per hour (rows L, M). At $15 per hour, the overtime wages amount to $900 (row N) and the part-time wages are $8,455 (row O). Thus, Walk-In Clinic's non-fixed wages for January are $9,355 (row P).

The information from the *fixed labor budget* is added to the *variable labor budget* and placed in the labor budget. For Walk-In Clinic, fixed labor is $60,419 and variable labor is $9,355. Therefore, total labor for January is $69,774 (see Exhibit 10–23).

The Supplies Budget

The second expense item in the operating budget is supplies (see Exhibit 10–13). The information for this figure comes from the supplies budget (see Exhibit 10–29), which itself is made up of two budgets: a *variable supplies budget* and a *fixed supplies budget*. The **fixed supplies budget** covers items such as office supplies, which do not vary

Exhibit 10–27 Background Information for Walk-In Clinic's Variable Labor Budget

		JAN	FEB	MAR	APR	MAY	JUN	JUL	AUG	SEP	OCT	NOV	DEC
Number of RVUs/LPN/Day:													
A Direct Minutes/RVU/LPN	[Given]	15.00	15.00	15.00	15.00	15.00	15.00	15.00	15.00	15.00	15.00	15.00	15.00
B Indirect Minutes/RVU/LPN	[Given]	7.50	7.50	7.50	7.50	7.50	7.50	7.50	7.50	7.50	7.50	7.50	7.50
C Total Minutes/RVU/LPN	[A + B]	22.50	22.50	22.50	22.50	22.50	22.50	22.50	22.50	22.50	22.50	22.50	22.50
D RVUs/Hour/LPN	[60 min/C]	2.67	2.67	2.67	2.67	2.67	2.67	2.67	2.67	2.67	2.67	2.67	2.67
E Work Hours/LPN/Day	[Given]	8.00	8.00	8.00	8.00	8.00	8.00	8.00	8.00	8.00	8.00	8.00	8.00
F RVUs/LPN/Day	[D × E]	21.33	21.33	21.33	21.33	21.33	21.33	21.33	21.33	21.33	21.33	21.33	21.33
Other Information:													
G Full-Time LPNs		2.00	2.00	2.00	2.00	2.00	2.00	2.00	2.00	2.00	2.00	2.00	2.00
H Part-Time LPN Pay Rate Per Hour		$10.00	$10.00	$10.00	$10.00	$10.00	$10.00	$10.00	$10.00	$10.00	$10.00	$10.00	$10.00
I Overtime LPN Rate Per Hour		$15.00	$15.00	$15.00	$15.00	$15.00	$15.00	$15.00	$15.00	$15.00	$15.00	$15.00	$15.00
J Work Days Per Month		20.00	20.00	22.00	22.00	20.00	22.00	23.00	21.00	21.00	22.00	19.00	20.00
K Maximum LPN OT Hours/Month		60.00	60.00	60.00	60.00	60.00	60.00	60.00	60.00	60.00	60.00	60.00	60.00

Exhibit 10–28 Variable Labor Budget

		JAN	FEB	MAR	APR	MAY	JUN	JUL	AUG	SEP	OCT	NOV	DEC	TOTAL
A	Work Days/Month	20	20	22	22	20	22	23	21	21	22	19	20	252
B	RVUs/LPN/Day	21.33	21.33	21.33	21.33	21.33	21.33	21.33	21.33	21.33	21.33	21.33	21.33	21.33
C	Monthly RVU Capacity/LPN [A × B]	427	427	469	469	427	469	491	448	448	469	405	427	5,376
D	Fixed LPN FTEs	2	2	2	2	2	2	2	2	2	2	2	2	2
E	Monthly LPN RVU Capacity [C × D]	853	853	939	939	853	939	981	896	896	939	811	853	10,752
F	Budgeted RVUs This Month	3,268	2,687	3,256	2,099	2,443	2,955	4,154	5,146	5,362	5,164	5,076	4,124	45,734
G	Understaffed RVUs [F − E]	2,415	1,834	2,317	1,160	1,590	2,016	3,173	4,250	4,466	4,225	4,265	3,271	34,982
H	LPN RVUs/Hour	2.67	2.67	2.67	2.67	2.67	2.67	2.67	2.67	2.67	2.67	2.67	2.67	3.00
I	Excess LPN Hours Needed [G / H]	906	688	869	435	596	756	1,190	1,594	1,675	1,585	1,600	1,227	13,118
J	Maximum Overtime Hours /Month	60	60	60	60	60	60	60	60	60	60	60	60	60
K	Part-time Hours Needed [I − J]	846	628	809	375	536	696	1,130	1,534	1,615	1,525	1,540	1,167	12,398
L	Hourly Overtime Rate	$15	$15	$15	$15	$15	$15	$15	$15	$15	$15	$15	$15	$15
M	Hourly Part-time Rate	$10	$10	$10	$10	$10	$10	$10	$10	$10	$10	$10	$10	$10
N	Overtime Wages [J × L]	$900	$900	$900	$900	$900	$900	$900	$900	$900	$900	$900	$900	$10,800
O	Part-time Wages [K × M]	$8,455	$6,276	$8,090	$3,751	$5,361	$6,961	$11,298	$15,338	$16,148	$15,245	$15,395	$11,665	$123,983
P	Variable Wages [N + O]	$9,355	$7,176	$8,990	$4,651	$6,261	$7,861	$12,198	$16,238	$17,048	$16,145	$16,295	$12,565	$134,783

Note: The numbers in this exhibit may be slightly different from those computed on a calculator due to the internal rounding rules used in the computer program on which this example is based. For example, January's part-time wages, Row O, are $8,455. When calculated by hand, they are $8,460 ($10/hr ($10 × 846 hrs). Obviously, the computer was storing the 846 hours as 845.5 hours.

with the number of patients seen. The **variable supplies budget** includes those items that do vary with the number of patients seen, such as disposable syringes, disposable gloves, and X-ray film. The assumptions for compiling both the fixed and variable supplies budgets are in Exhibit 10–30.

The Fixed Supplies Budget

The fixed supplies budget (Exhibit 10–31) is composed mainly of items used in the office, such as office supplies and stamps. For Walk-In Clinic, the cost is estimated at $750 per month, as shown in the supplies budget assumptions (Exhibit 10–30, row 1).

The Variable Supplies Budget

The variable supplies budget for Walk-In Clinic, shown in Exhibit 10–32, is based on the following formula:

Opening Inventory + Purchases – Cost of Goods Used = Ending Inventory

Because accrual accounting is used, cost of goods used (COGU) is the only number to actually appear on the final supplies budget (see Exhibit 10–29, Variable Supplies, and Exhibit 10–32, Cost of Goods Used), for it represents the amount of resources consumed in providing service. However, the other items are necessary to derive cost of goods used. The components of Walk-In Clinic's variable supplies budget are as follows:

- *Opening Inventory:* For Walk-In Clinic in January, the opening inventory is $5,154 (Exhibit 10–32), which is also the ending inventory for December of the previous year (Exhibit 10–30, row 5).
- *Purchases:* The amount of supplies to be purchased in January is calculated based upon both the cost of goods used and the desired ending inventory at the end of the month. Walk-in Clinic is required to have its ending inventory for one month be 20 percent of the forecasted amount of cost of goods that will be used the next month (discussed further below).
- *Cost of Goods Used:* Cost of goods used is calculated by multiplying the number of RVUs provided during the month by the cost per RVU. In the case of Walk-In Clinic, the statistics budget shows that there are 3,268 RVUs to be provided in January (see Exhibit 10–12) and the cost of supplies per RVU is $10 each (see Exhibit 10–30, Total). Thus the cost of goods used is $32,680 (3,268 RVUs × $10/RVU).
- *Ending Inventory:* Since the ending inventory must equal 20 percent of the next month's COGU, the ending inventory for Walk-In Clinic in January, $5,374, is calculated by taking 20 percent of February's projected COGU (see Exhibit 10–32: $26,870 × 0.20).
- *Purchases (revisited):* Once the cost of goods used and the desired ending inventory for Walk-In Clinic have been calculated, the amount of purchases for January can be determined by using the formula presented earlier:

Fixed Supplies Budget: A subset of the supplies budget that covers those items which do not vary by patient volume.

Variable Supplies Budget: A subset of the supplies budget that includes those items which do vary based upon the volume of patients seen.

Exhibit 10–29 Supplies Budget for Walk-In Clinic

	JAN	FEB	MAR	APR	MAY	JUN	JUL	AUG	SEP	OCT	NOV	DEC	TOTAL
Variable Supplies	$32,680	$26,870	$32,560	$20,990	$24,430	$29,550	$41,540	$51,460	$53,620	$51,640	$50,760	$41,240	$457,340
Fixed Supplies	750	750	750	750	750	750	750	750	750	750	750	750	9,000
Total Supplies	$33,430	$27,620	$33,310	$21,740	$25,180	$30,300	$42,290	$52,210	$54,370	$52,390	$51,510	$41,990	$466,340

Exhibit 10–30 Supplies Budget Assumptions

1	Fixed Supply Purchases Each Month This Year and Last Year	$750
2	Supply Cost/RVU	$10
3	Desired Ending Inventory as a Percent of Next Month's COGU[1]	20%
4	Payment for Goods Purchased (made the following month)	
5	Ending Inventory, December of Previous Year	$5,154

[1] Cost of Goods Used.

Exhibit 10–31 Fixed Supplies Budget for Walk-In Clinic

	JAN	FEB	MAR	APR	MAY	JUN	JUL	AUG	SEP	OCT	NOV	DEC	TOTAL
Fixed Supplies	$750	$750	$750	$750	$750	$750	$750	$750	$750	$750	$750	$750	$9,000

Exhibit 10–32 Variable Supplies Budget for Walk-In Clinic

	JAN	FEB	MAR	APR	MAY	JUN	JUL	AUG	SEP	OCT	NOV	DEC	TOTAL
Opening Inventory	$5,154	$5,374	$6,512	$4,198	$4,886	$5,910	$8,308	$10,292	$10,724	$10,328	$10,152	$8,248	$5,154
Purchases	32,900	28,008	30,246	21,678	25,454	31,948	43,524	51,892	53,224	51,464	48,856	39,693	458,887
Goods Available	38,054	33,382	36,758	25,876	30,340	37,858	51,832	62,184	63,948	61,792	59,008	47,941	464,041
Cost of Goods Used	(32,680)	(26,870)	(32,560)	(20,990)	(24,430)	(29,550)	(41,540)	(51,460)	(53,620)	(51,640)	(50,760)	(41,240)	(457,340)
Ending Inventory	$5,374	$6,512	$4,198	$4,886	$5,910	$8,308	$10,292	$10,724	$10,328	$10,152	$8,248	$6,701	$6,701

Key Point The reason that COGU is used in the supplies budget rather than the cost of goods purchased is that accrual accounting is being used.

Beginning inventory	$5,154	(Exhibit 10–30)
+ Purchases	32,900	Derived by subtracting beginning inventory from goods available
Goods available	38,054	Derived by adding ending inventory and COGU
– COGU	32,680	Calculated by multiplying RVUs × Cost/RVU (Exhibits 10–12, 10–30)
Ending inventory	$5,374	Calculated as 20% of February's COGU (Exhibit 10–32)

The information from the fixed supplies budget and the COGU from the variable supplies budget is added and placed in the supplies budget. For January, Walk-In Clinic had fixed supplies of $750 and variable supplies of $32,680. Therefore, total supplies for January is $33,430 (see Exhibit 10–29).

The Administrative and General Expense Budget

The last part of the expense section of the operating budget (see Exhibit 10–13) is administrative and general (A & G) expenses, which are developed in the general and administrative budget (see Exhibit 10–33). They comprise the day-to-day expenses that are not contained in the labor or supplies budgets. The assumptions for the A & G expenses for Walk-In Clinic are listed in Exhibit 10–34. Incidentally, some organizations will consider interest and penalties as non-operating expenses.

The Cash Budget

As discussed in detail in Chapter 5, the *cash budget* is developed by determining when payments will be received from others and when payments will be made by the organization. Since it draws on information from the other budgets, the cash budget is the last budget to be developed.

The cash budget is organized into two sections. The first section determines how much cash is available before borrowing; the second section compares the cash available to the cash required and then determines if cash will be needed from other sources (there is a shortfall) or if cash will be invested (there is an excess of cash).

To determine cash available, the cash inflows (revenues) are added, and outflows (expenditures) are subtracted from the beginning balance (see Exhibit 10–14, rows A,

Exhibit 10–33 Administrative and General Expense Budget

	JAN	FEB	MAR	APR	MAY	JUN	JUL	AUG	SEP	OCT	NOV	DEC	TOTAL
Administrative & General													
Interest	$891	$889	$887	$959	$956	$953	$963	$959	$956	$952	$948	$945	$11,258
Penalties	0	0	0	0	0	0	0	0	0	0	0	0	0
Depreciation	1,498	1,498	1,498	1,498	1,656	1,656	1,656	1,669	1,669	1,669	1,669	1,669	19,305
Utilities	12,000	12,000	12,000	12,000	12,000	12,000	12,000	12,000	12,000	12,000	12,000	12,000	144,000
Rent	5,000	5,000	5,000	5,000	5,000	5,000	5,000	5,000	5,000	5,000	5,000	5,000	60,000
Cleaning	500	500	500	500	500	500	500	500	500	500	500	500	6,000
Telephone	600	600	600	600	600	600	600	600	600	600	600	600	7,200
Travel	2,500	2,500	2,500	2,500	2,500	2,500	2,500	2,500	2,500	2,500	2,500	2,500	30,000
Insurance	12,000	12,000	12,000	12,000	12,000	12,000	12,000	12,000	12,000	12,000	12,000	12,000	144,000
Equipment Maintenance	150	150	150	150	150	150	150	150	150	150	150	150	1,800
Bad Debt	4,083	4,358	4,223	3,634	3,383	3,681	3,488	3,673	3,964	4,065	3,790	3,790	46,132
Subtotal	$39,223	$39,495	$39,357	$38,842	$38,745	$39,040	$38,857	$39,051	$39,339	$39,436	$39,157	$39,154	$469,696

Exhibit 10–34 Information Used to Construct the Administrative and General Expense Budget

Item	Amount	Occurrence and Payment
Interest	Varies	Calculated on an amortization schedule[1]
Penalties	Varies	Calculated in the Cash Budget
Depreciation	Varies	Calculated on a depreciation schedule[1]
Utilities	$12,000	Per month, payable each month
Rent	$5,000	Per month, payable each month in advance
Cleaning	$500	Per month, payable each month
Telephone	$600	Per month, payable each month
Travel	$2,500	Per month, payable each month
Insurance	$12,000	Per month, payable each month
Equipment Maintenance	$150	Per month, payable each month
Bad Debt	Varies	4% of charge–based and 3% of cost–based net patient revenue

[1] Not included; assume the number as a given for this example

Exhibit 10-35   Converting Accrual Information into Cash Flows: Walk-In Clinic's Revenues for January

Janury's Net Revenues Using the Accrual Basis of Accounting – Full-charge Patients. Amount Collected in:	Percent to be Received by Month	Cash Inflow by Month[1]
January	31%	$19,474
February	56%	35,178
March	6%	3,769
April	3%	1,885
Written off	4%	2,513
Total	100%	$62,819

[1] Differences due to rounding.

B, C, and D). As how to determine these inflows and outflows was discussed in Chapter 5, the following shows how accrual data are converted into cash. As noted in Exhibit 10–20, row F, Walk-In Clinic earned $62,818 in January on its full-charge patients. Under the assumption that 31 percent will be collected in January, 56 percent in February, 6 percent in March, and 3 percent in April, and that the remaining 4 percent will be written off, the cash inflow pattern is shown in Exhibit 10–35.

The second part of the cash budget determines whether the organization has sufficient cash to begin the next month. Walk-in Clinic has decided that it should begin each month with $11,000 cash on hand. If it does not have $11,000, it would have to either obtain such funds from its own short-term or long-term investments (perhaps with some penalty for early withdrawal), or else borrow the funds from outside the organization. Fortunately, Walk-In Clinic does not find itself in such a position. If Walk-In Clinic has over $11,000, it invests the excess in short-term investments (see Exhibit 10–14, row N).

The Capital Budget

The capital budget was initially presented in Exhibit 10–15. Though the budget for Walk-In Clinic is relatively small, large organizations may have capital budgets totaling millions of dollars. The items that appear on the capital budget are likely to have been part of a much larger list of requests that various departments submitted.

◄SUMMARY►

The budget is one of the most important documents of a health care organization and is the central document of the planning/control cycle. It identifies the revenues and resources that are needed for an organization to achieve its goals and objectives and allows the organization to monitor the actual revenues generated and its use of resources against what was planned.

The planning/control cycle has four major components: strategic planning, planning, implementing, and controlling. The purpose of strategic planning is to identify the organization's mission and strategy in order to position the organization for the future. A primary activity of the strategic planning process is an assessment of the organization's external and internal environments. The organization also develops specific tactical and operational plans that identify short-term goals and objectives in marketing/production, control, and financing the organization.

Five key dimensions along which organizations vary in regard to budgeting are: participation, budget models, budget detail, budget forecasts, and budget modifications. Participation in the budgeting process varies from authoritarian to participative. The authoritarian approach is often called top-down budgeting, since the budget is essentially dictated to the rest of the organization. In the participatory approach, the roles and responsibilities of the budgeting process are diffused throughout the organization. Advantages of the participatory approach include developing a shared understanding of the goals and objectives of the organization, developing cooperation and coordination, clarifying roles and responsibilities, motivating staff, and bringing about cost awareness. Its disadvantages are loss of control and excessive use of time and resources.

There are two budget models: incremental/decremental budgeting and zero-based budgeting. The incremental/decremental approach begins with what exists and gives a slight increase, no change, or a slight decrease to various line items, programs, or departments. Zero-based budgeting continually questions both the need for each program and its level of funding. In zero-based budgeting, each budgeting unit provides: 1) an overall justification for its program; and 2) a series of requests to show what the program would look like at various levels of funding.

Based on the amount of detail they contain, budgets can be classified into three categories: line-item, program, and performance. A line-item budget has the least detail and merely lists revenues and expenses by category. A program budget not only lists the line items, but also lists them by program. A performance budget not only lists line items and programs, but also lists the performance goals that each program is expected to attain.

Since environmental conditions change, many organizations use rolling budgets, which are multi-year forecasts regularly updated and extended. Single-year and multi-year budgets vary by the time horizon they forecast; static and flexible budgets vary on the basis of volume projections. Static budgets forecast for a single level of activity; flexible budgets forecast revenues and expenses for various levels of activities.

Most health care organizations actually develop four interrelated budgets: a statistics budget, an operating budget, a cash budget, and a capital budget. The statistics budget identifies the amount of services that will be provided, usually by payor type.

The operating budget is a combination of two budgets developed using the accrual basis of accounting: the revenue budget and the expense budget. The revenue budget is a forecast of the operating revenues that will be earned during the budget period. It consists of net patient revenues and non-patient revenues. The expense budget lists all operating expenses that are expected to be incurred during the budget period, both fixed and variable.

The cash budget represents the organization's cash inflows and outflows. The bottom line of the cash budget is the amount of cash available at the end of the period. In addition to showing cash inflows and outflows, the cash budget also details when it is necessary to borrow when there are cash shortages, and when excess funds can be invested.

The capital budget summarizes the purchases to be made during the year. Capital budgets for outpatient facilities may be fairly small; those from large systems with inpatient facilities may contain millions of dollars' worth of items.

Based on the information contained in these budgets, plus small amount of additional information, the organization develops pro forma financial statements. Pro forma financial statements are prepared before the accounting period and present what the organization's financial statements will look like if all budgets are met exactly as planned. Once the pro forma financial statements have been developed, they can be subjected to ratio analysis just as with regular financial statements.

◄KEY TERMS►

AUTHORITARIAN APPROACH	LABOR BUDGET	REVENUE BUDGET
CAPITAL BUDGET	LINE-ITEM BUDGET	ROLLING BUDGET
CASH BUDGET	MISSION STATEMENT	SHORT-TERM PLANS
CONTROLLING ACTIVITIES	MULTI-YEAR BUDGET	STATIC BUDGET
EXPENSE BUDGET	NET CHARGES	STATISTICS BUDGET
FIXED LABOR BUDGET	OPERATING BUDGET	STRATEGIC PLANNING
FIXED SUPPLIES BUDGET	PARTICIPATORY APPROACH	TOP-DOWN BUDGETING
FLEXIBLE BUDGET	PERFORMANCE BUDGET	TOP-DOWN/BOTTOM-UP APPROACH
GROSS CHARGES	PLANNING	VARIABLE LABOR BUDGET
INCREMENTAL/DECREMENTAL	PROGRAM BUDGET	VARIABLE SUPPLIES BUDGET
APPROACH	RELATIVE VALUE UNITS (RVUs)	ZERO-BASED BUDGETING (ZBB)

◄KEY EQUATION►

Opening Inventory + Purchases − Cost of Goods Used = Ending Inventory

◄QUESTIONS AND PROBLEMS►

1. **Definitions.** Define the following terms:
   a. Authoritarian Approach.
   b. Capital Budget.
   c. Cash Budget.
   d. Controlling Activities.
   e. Expense Budget.
   f. Fixed Labor Budget.
   g. Fixed Supplies Budget.
   h. Flexible Budget.

   i. Gross Charges.

   j. Incremental/Decremental Approach.

   k. Labor Budget.

   l. Line-item Budget.

  m. Mission Statement.

   n. Multi-year Budget.

   o. Net Charges.

   p. Operating Budget.

   q. Participatory Approach.

   r. Performance Budget.

   s. Planning.

   t. Program Budget.

   u. Relative Value Units (RVUs).

   v. Revenue Budget.

  w. Rolling Budget.

   x. Short-term Plans.

   y. Static Budget.

   z. Statistics Budget.

  aa. Strategic Planning.

  bb. Top-down Budgeting.

  cc. Top-down/Bottom-up Approach.

  dd. Variable Labor Budget.

  ee. Variable Supplies Budget.

  ff. Zero-based Budgeting (ZBB).

2. What is the purpose of the budget? Why are requests for budget revisions necessary? When should a formal request for a budget revision be submitted?

3. What are the major components of the planning/control cycle?

4. Discuss the role of strategic planning in the budgeting process. How does it differ from short-term planning?

5. What are the advantages and disadvantages of the participatory approach to budgeting?

6. What are the four major budgets of a health care organization? Briefly discuss each.

7. Using Exhibits 10–6 through 10–8 as examples, construct line-item, program, and performance budgets for a service or program in a health care organization.

8. Using the data provided in Exhibit 10–16, explain the difference in predicting this year's visits for non-capitated and capitated patients.

9. **The Statistics Budget: Forecasting Visits.** Instead of its current forecast, Walk-In Clinic estimates that it will not obtain a major HMO contract, and its enrollment July—December will only go up 0.5 percent a month. Assuming these are the only changes to Exhibit 10–16, prepare a new forecast of the number of visits that will be made by capitated patients during the whole year.

10. **The Statistics Budget: Forecasting Visits.** Instead of its current forecast, Walk-In Clinic estimates that it will not obtain a major HMO contract, and its

enrollment July–December will only go up 6 percent a month. Assuming these are the only changes to Exhibit 10–16, prepare a new forecast of the number of visits that will be made by capitated patients during the whole year.

11. **The Statistics Budget: RVU Weighted Visits.** What are RVU weighted visits? Why is it necessary to weight visits by their intensity level?

12. **The Statistics Budget: Changing Intensity.** How would the statistics budget change if Walk-In Clinic used the following distribution instead of the distribution of visits by intensity shown in Exhibit 10–17.

	Charge-based	Cost-based	Flat Fee	Capitation
Brief (Level I)	10%	12%	10%	10%
Routine (Level II)	50%	62%	85%	55%
Complex (Level III)	40%	26%	5%	35%
Total	100%	100%	100%	100%

13. **The Statistics Budget: Changing Intensity.** How would the statistics budget change if Walk-In Clinic used the following distribution instead of the distribution of visits by intensity shown in Exhibit 10–17.

	Charge-based	Cost-based	Flat Fee	Capitation
Brief (Level I)	10%	15%	25%	15%
Routine (Level II)	40%	60%	60%	50%
Complex (Level III)	50%	25%	15%	35%
Total	100%	100%	100%	100%

14. **The Revenue Budget: Types of Payors.** What is the difference between charge-based, cost-based, flat fee, and capitated payors?

15. **The Revenue Budget: Calculating Gross Revenues.** Calculate Walk-In Clinic's January, February, and March gross revenues if it lowers its fee to $64.50 from $74.50 per RVU (assuming that cost-based payors continue to pay 75 percent of charges). (See Exhibits 10–19 and 10–20.)

16. **The Revenue Budget: Calculating Gross Revenues.** Calculate Walk-In Clinic's January, February, and March gross revenues if it lowers its fee to $70.00 from $74.50 per RVU (assuming that cost-based payors continue to pay 75 percent of charges). (See Exhibits 10–19 and 10–20.)

17. **The Revenue Budget: Gross and Net Charges.** What is the difference between gross charges and net charges?

18. **The Revenue Budget: Calculating Net Revenues.** Calculate Walk-In Clinic's January, February, and March net revenues if it lowers its fee to $64.50 from $74.50 per RVU. (See Exhibits 10–19 and 10–20.)

19. **The Revenue Budget: Calculating Net Revenues.** Calculate Walk-In Clinic's January, February, and March net revenues if it lowers its fee to $70.00 from $74.50 per RVU. (See Exhibits 10–19 and 10–20.)

20. **The Labor Budget: Fixed and Variable Labor.** What is the difference between a fixed and a variable labor budget?

21. **The Labor Budget: Calculating the Fixed Labor Budget.** Instead of the raises stated in Exhibit 10–24, assume that all benefits are 13 percent and all raises are 7 percent and calculate the fixed labor budget. Assume all the other assumptions in the exhibit remain the same. Explain why only LPN II's wages and benefits change from January to February.

22. **The Labor Budget: Calculating the Fixed Labor Budget.** Instead of the raises stated in Exhibit 10–24, assume that all benefits are 20 percent and all raises are 5 percent and calculate the fixed labor budget. Assume all the other assumptions in the exhibit remain the same. Explain why only LPN II's wages and benefits change from January to February.

23. **The Labor Budget: Variable Labor.** In the variable labor budget, why is it necessary to determine how many RVUs can be handled by full-time employees?

24. **The Variable Labor Budget: Direct and Indirect Time.** In the variable labor budget, what is the main difference between direct and indirect "minutes per RVU" per LPN?

25. **The Labor Budget (each part builds on the previous part).**
   a. Calculating the Effects of Changes in Indirect Time on RVU Capacity per LPN. How many RVUs per day could an LPN serve if the indirect time in Exhibit 10–27 were reduced to 6 minutes? All other information not dependent on indirect time in Exhibit 10–27 remains the same.
   b. Calculating the Effects of Changes in Indirect Time on Understaffed LPN Hours. If the indirect time in Exhibit 10–27 were cut to 6 minutes per RVU as in part a, how many understaffed hours would Walk-in Clinic have in January, February, and March? All other information not dependent on indirect time in Exhibit 10–27 remains the same.
   c. Calculating the Effects of Changes in Part-time and Overtime Wages on the Variable Labor Budget. Assume part-time wages change to $9 and overtime wages change to $14 per hour. If all other information in Exhibit 10–28 remains the same, what will Walk-in Clinic's variable labor budget be in January, February, and March?

26. **The labor budget. [Each part builds on the previous part.]**
   a. **Calculating the Effects of Changes in Indirect Time on RVU** Capacity per LPN. How many RVUs per day could an LPN serve if the indirect time in Exhibit 10–27 were reduced to 5.5 minutes? All other information not dependent on indirect time in Exhibit 10–27 remains the same.
   b. **Calculating the Effects of Changes in Indirect Time on Understaffed LPN Hours**. If the indirect time in Exhibit 10–27 were cut to 5.5 minutes per RVU as in part a, how many understaffed hours would Walk-in Clinic have in January, February, and March? All other information not dependent on indirect time in Exhibit 10–27 remains the same.
   c. **Calculating the Effects of Changes in Part-time and Overtime Wages on the Variable Labor Budget.** Assume part-time wages change to $12 and overtime wages change to $18 per hour. If all other information in

Exhibit 10–28 remains the same, what will Walk-in Clinic's variable labor budget be in January, February, and March?

27. **Calculating the Variable Supply Budget.** Calculate the variable supplies budget, assuming Walk-in Clinic changes its requirements so that ending inventory is 25 percent of next month's COGS. No other assumptions in Exhibit 10–30 change.

28. **Calculating the Variable Supply Budget.** Calculate the variable supplies budget, assuming Walk-in Clinic changes its requirements so that ending inventory is 15 percent of next month's COGS. No other assumptions in Exhibit 10–30 change.

Chapter Eleven

RESPONSIBILITY ACCOUNTING

LEARNING OBJECTIVES

After completing this chapter, you will be able to:

▶ Define decentralization and identify its major advantages and disadvantages.
▶ Identify the major types of responsibility centers found in health care organizations and describe their characteristics.
▶ Explain the relationship of responsibility, authority, and accountability in the performance measurement of responsibility centers.
▶ Compute volume and rate variances for revenues.
▶ Compute volume and cost variances for expenses.

Chapter Outline

(Continues)

Chapter Outline (Contd)

◀INTRODUCTION▶

Health care organizations have become increasingly complex over the past quarter century. One of the major changes is decentralization, which presents interesting problems when measuring financial performance. Whereas Chapter 4 dealt with measuring the financial performance of the organization as a whole, this chapter identifies the types of organizational units *within* a health care organization and measures their financial performance. These units may be as large as subsidiaries or as small as departments. This chapter begins with a discussion of decentralization, and then discusses the types of responsibility centers that exist in decentralized organizations. Next, the concepts of responsibility, authority, and accountability are explored. Finally, questions of how to measure the performance of responsibility centers are addressed.

◀DECENTRALIZATION▶

Decentralization: The degree of dispersion of responsibility within a health care organization.

Decentralization is the degree of dispersion of responsibility within an organization. Decentralization can evolve out of working arrangements and/or may be more formally prescribed in the organization's policies, procedures, and organizational structure. There are various advantages and disadvantages to decentralization, and each organization has to decide what level of decentralization is in its best interest.

Advantages of Decentralization

The advantages and disadvantages of decentralization are presented in Exhibit 11–1. The advantages (in no particular order) include: time, information relevance, quality, speed, talent, and motivation and allegiance.

Exhibit 11–1 Advantages and Disadvantages of Decentralization

Advantages	Disadvantages
Time	Loss of Control
Information Relevance	Decreased Goal Congruence
Quality	Increased Need for Coordination
Speed	and Formal Communication
Talent	Lack of Managerial Talent
Motivation and Allegiance	

Time

From the point of view of central management, a major advantage of decentralization is an increase in time available to devote to other tasks. Ideally, decentralization should relieve the central office of day-to-day operational decision-making, instead allowing it to concentrate more on tactical and strategic-level concerns.

Information Relevance

By spreading the responsibility for decision-making within the organization, the organization moves more toward a "need to know" environment, where information is filtered at each level, and only the information needed for decision-making at higher levels is passed on.

Quality

Those closer to a problem may be better suited to understand the specifics of the problem and be more responsive to the local context, thus leading to higher quality decisions.

Speed

Decentralized decision-making allows those closest to the problem to respond more quickly by shortening six time-consuming steps in communication. The person who identifies the problem must:

- *Communicate* the problem *up* the organization
- To those who must *receive* it. Then they
- Become aware of it,
- Decide a course of action, and
- *Communicate* their response *down* through the organization,
- Where it is ultimately *received* by the person authorized to respond.

Talent

A health care organization must ensure that it is developing the management capability to allow it to reach its objectives. Although occasionally it may want to look outside the organization for "new blood," this process can become expensive, intrusive, and time-consuming. It can also be demoralizing to those within the organization. Decentralization helps to draw upon and develop the expertise of existing staff.

Motivation and Allegiance

By delegating responsibility to others, a health care organization can develop increased motivation and allegiance. Increased involvement in the planning, implementation, and control process encourages buy-in by the staff, who may then experience an increased sense of ownership, belonging, and pride in their work.

Disadvantages of Decentralization

In considering what degree of decentralization to have, a health care organization has to balance the advantages of decentralization with its disadvantages, which include:

- Loss of control.
- Decreased goal congruence.
- Increased need for coordination and formal communication.
- Lack of managerial talent.

Loss of Control

By spreading responsibility throughout the organization, upper management loses direct control. For administrators who have an authoritarian style and for organizations that need top level management's expertise, this can be a significant problem. The specific ramifications of loss of control also appear in the other disadvantages of decentralization, which are all highly interrelated.

Decreased Goal Congruence

To the extent that responsibility is decentralized within the organization, organizational units tend to develop their own goals. To avoid this, considerable effort must be exerted to ensure that each division or unit is making consistent decisions that support the organization's strategic plan and are in the best interest of the organization as a whole, not just the division.

Increased Need for Coordination and Formal Communication

If responsibility is decentralized within the organization, there is an increased need to coordinate efforts among the various units and divisions. This results in the need for more formal communications, meetings, policies, and procedures.

Lack of Managerial Talent

If an organization decentralizes and does not have the talent available at lower levels to manage the new responsibilities, the organization as a whole could suffer greatly. This particular problem was all too common during the early stages of HMO development in the United States. Since no one in the organization had previous experience running HMOs, organizations placed people with experience running other health care entities in charge.

◀TYPES OF RESPONSIBILITY CENTERS▶

When responsibility is *formally* decentralized into organizational units, rather than *informally* to specific individuals, these units are called responsibility centers. A **responsibility center** is an organizational unit that has been formally given the responsibility to carry out one or more tasks and/or to achieve one or more outcomes. The four most common types of responsibility centers in health care are: service centers, cost centers, profit centers, and investment centers (see Exhibit 11–2).

Responsibility Center: An organizational unit that has been formally given the responsibility to carry out one or more tasks and/or to achieve one or more outcomes.

Service Centers

Service centers, the most basic type of responsibility center, are primarily responsible for ensuring that services are provided to a population in a manner that meets the volume and quality requirements of the organization. Since service centers have no budgetary control, their main responsibilities revolve around scheduling, directing, and monitoring the staff, and providing direct patient care. Although service centers

Exhibit 11–2 The Four Main Types of Responsibility Centers and Their Main Areas of Responsibility

Type of Center	Areas of Responsibility			
	Services	Costs	Profits	Investment
Service Center	X			
Cost Center	X	X		
Profit Center	X	X	X	
Investment Center	X	X	X	X

Service Centers:
Organizational units that are primarily responsible for ensuring that health care-related services are provided to a population in a manner that meets the volume and quality requirements of the organization. They have no direct budgetary control.

Cost Centers:
Organizational units responsible for providing services and controlling their costs.

Clinical Cost Centers:
Cost centers that provide health care-related services to clients, patients, or enrollees.

Administrative Cost Centers: Cost centers that support clinical cost centers and the organization as a whole. They are often considered the *infrastructure* of the organization.

Profit Centers:
Organizational units responsible for controlling costs and earning revenues.

use resources and thus affect costs, the actual budgetary control rests at a higher level in the organization. It is not unusual for nursing units to find themselves defined as service centers. They are responsible for patient care, but the budget is kept at the next higher level in the organization. Patient admitting and patient transportation are also often defined as service centers.

Cost Centers

Cost centers, the most common type of responsibility center in health care organizations, are responsible for providing services and controlling their costs. Ideally, they should be integrally involved in the planning, budgeting, and control process, for they are primarily responsible for resource utilization within the organization. Since payment cannot be *directly* tied to services under both flat fee (i.e. DRG) and capitated payment systems, a large number of responsibility centers are categorized as cost centers rather than profit centers.

There are two types of cost centers in health care organizations: clinical cost centers and administrative cost centers. **Clinical cost centers** provide health care-related services to clients, patients, or enrollees. Examples include nursing units, pharmacy, radiology, laboratory, and dietary services. **Administrative cost centers** support the clinical cost centers and the organization as a whole. Included in this category are general administration, the business office, information services, quality control, admitting, medical records, and housekeeping. Administrative cost centers are often considered the *infrastructure* of the organization. As with nursing, units that may be classified as cost centers in one organization may be considered service centers in another.

Profit Centers

Though many **profit centers** are responsible for service-related activities, all profit centers are responsible for controlling their costs and earning revenues. In some cases, the costs may be larger than the revenue they generate. For example, a pediatric screening program in a health department, which has to be offered, might be charged with earning sufficient revenues to cover just half of its $100,000 cost. Thus, although the pediatric screening program is considered a profit center by the health department, the amount of profit in this case is actually a loss of $50,000.

There are three types of profit centers in health care organizations: traditional profit centers, capitated profit centers, and administrative profit centers.

Traditional Profit Centers

Traditional profit centers are primarily responsible for providing health care services and earning a profit based on the health care services provided. Traditional profit centers have proliferated recently. Much of this growth can be traced back to the emergence of product-line management in health care in the later part of the twentieth century. Common product (or service) lines include cardiology, women's and children's services, and oncology. Traditional profit centers profit through a combination of markups on service and controlling costs in fee-for-service situations, as well as by controlling costs in flat fee arrangements such as the DRG payment system.

Capitated Profit Centers

Capitated profit centers earn revenues by agreeing to take care of the health care needs of a population for a per-member fee, often regardless of the amount of services needed by any particular patient. Such organizations are commonly called HMOs, PPOs, or managed care organizations. Interestingly enough, many managed care organizations purchase services from traditional profit centers. For example, an HMO may purchase its cardiology services from one health network and many of its oncology services from a different hospital system. Since it receives a set amount to cover the health care needs of a population, providers receiving capitation have considerable incentive to control costs through efficiency (the most service for any level of cost), economy (low costs), and prevention.

Administrative Profit Centers

There are two types of **administrative profit centers**: those that sell inside the organization and those that – although they do not deliver health services – are responsible for generating new revenues from outside the organization. Examples of administrative profit centers that *may* be required to sell their services inside the organization are legal services, computer services, and management engineering. The prices for these services that are charged internally to other organizational units are called **transfer prices**.

The setting of transfer prices is a very delicate matter, and if they are set too high there are several possible negative consequences. They may encourage potential users to buy these services outside the organization. If internal units (i.e. departments, subsidiary organizations) must use these resources, then they may suboptimize their use in order to cut costs and/or use the services, but be unhappy about it (causing morale problems).

Examples of administrative profit centers that are responsible for generating new revenues from outside the organization include development offices (whose primary function is to encourage donations and contributions to the organization), and field representatives for HMOs and PPOs, whose primary responsibility is to sign up markets for the organization. Other primary examples would be food services, gift shops, parking decks, and motel services. Incidentally, although their effects on profit are difficult to identify, marketing, advertising, and public relations may be considered

Traditional Profit Centers: Organizational units responsible for earning a profit by providing health care services. Revenues are earned either on a fee-for-service or a flat fee basis. Examples include cardiology, women's and children's services, and oncology.

Capitated Profit Centers: Organizational units responsible for earning a profit by agreeing to take care of the health care needs of a population for a per-member fee (which is not directly tied to services). Examples include HMOs, PPOs, and various managed care organizations.

Administrative Profit Centers: Organizational units that do not provide health care-related services, but are responsible for their profit. There are two types: those who sell their services internally, and those whose primary responsibility is to bring revenues into the organization.

Transfer Prices: The prices for products or services that are charged internally to other organizational units.

administrative profit centers in some organizations (others may consider them cost centers).

Investment Centers

Investment Centers:
Organizational units which not only have all the responsibilities of a traditional profit center, but also are responsible for making a certain return on investment.

In addition to having all the responsibilities of a traditional profit center, **investment centers** are responsible for making a certain return on investment. For example, where a profit center might be content with a simple $100,000 profit, an investment center might find this unacceptable if it does not provide the desired return on investment. An example of this is shown in Exhibit 11–3, where a surgi-center earns $100,000 in profit, but this is an insufficient amount of revenue to earn a required 15 percent return on investment. Perspective 11–1 provides an example of an investment center in a physician group that did not generate a promised return.

Investment centers have proliferated in the last few decades, and include all investor-owned health care entities that require their operating units to make a certain return. However, not all investment centers are investor-owned, for many not-for-profit health care organizations require various responsibility centers to make a certain return. It is not the ownership status that makes a responsibility center an investment center, it is the requirement that it make a certain return.

◀MEASURING THE PERFORMANCE OF RESPONSIBILITY CENTERS▶

The previous section categorized the different types of responsibility centers in terms of their increasing level of financial responsibility. However, measuring the performance of responsibility centers rests on the assumption that a responsibility center only be held accountable for those things over which it has control. Thus, responsibility is only one of three major attributes of a responsibility center. The other two are authority and accountability (see Exhibit 11–4).

Exhibit 11–3   An Example Evaluating an Investment on Its Profit and on Its Return

A	Investment in New Surgi-Center	[Given]	$1,000,000
B	Desired Return on Investment (ROI)	[Given]	15%
C	Desired ROI in Dollars	[A × B]	$150,000
	Actual Results:		
D	Net Revenues	[Given]	$500,000
E	Expenses	[Given]	$400,000
F	Net Income	[D – E]	$100,000
G	ROI	[F/A]	10%

Conclusion: Although the surgi-center made a profit of $100,000, it did not meet the desired ROI of 15%.

PERSPECTIVE 11–1

Wake County, NC, Hospital to Shed Its Network of Physician Groups

Rex Healthcare, Wake County's second-largest hospital, is getting out of the doctor business after seven years of trying – and failing – to make its network of physician practices profitable. Over the next year, the hospital plans to sell all but a few practices back to the doctors who work in them. Rex acquired the doctor groups in a buying spree beginning in 1994, hoping to ensure a steady stream of patients to its facility. The Rex network cares for about 250,000 patients in the region, but has never made money. "We think we've done an excellent job taking care of patients, but financially, it isn't the direction Rex needs to be going in," said David Coulter, Rex's vice president for operation. "We want these physicians to remain in the Rex family, but we think it works best for them and for us if they are in private practice."

Hospital management of physician practices has been generally acknowledged as a failed strategy. Hospitals across the country are selling their affiliated physician groups back into private practice. "I can't think of a single example of where it's worked," said Lendy Pridgen, president of the Raleigh consulting firm Capital Health Management. But it is clear that some doctors chafed under corporate management and constant pressure from Rex officials to boost the bottom line. "We felt we were working at maximum capacity, but there was always this undercurrent that we needed to be doing something to make the bottom line look better," said Dr Robert E. Littleton, whose OB/GYN practice reverted to private status Aug. 1.

Source: Jean P. Fisher, Business News, *The News & Observer*, Raleigh, North Carolina, August 16, 2001.

Exhibit 11–4   The Basic Attributes of a Responsibility Center

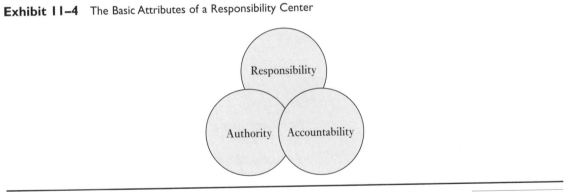

Responsibility, Authority, and Accountability

The relationship among responsibility, authority, and accountability is straightforward. Ideally, managers should be given the *authority* to carry out their *responsibilities*. To the extent that this occurs, managers should expect to be held *accountable* for the performance of their responsibility centers (see Perspectives 11–2 and 11–3).

Responsibility refers to the duties and obligations of a responsibility center, **authority** is the power to carry them out, and **accountability** means the sanctions, both positive and negative, attached to carrying out responsibilities. Exhibit 11–4 shows that these three attributes do not always coincide, and the larger the discrepancy, the more organizational problems and individual frustrations can be expected.

Responsibility: Duties and obligations of a responsibility center.

Authority: Power to carry out a given responsibility.

Accountability: Sanctions, both positive and negative, attached to carrying out responsibilities.

PERSPECTIVE 11–2

Reviving Ailing Hospitals: Turnaround Specialists Offer Antidote to Chronic Factors Afflicting Industry

Freeman Memorial Hospital in Inglewood, Calif., gave life to Catherine Fickes' healthcare career. Nearly 40 years later, she's come back to return the favor. Fickes, who trained as a nurse at the hospital in the mid-1960s, became Daniel Freeman's interim chief executive officer in October. She was part of a turnaround team that arrived at the hospital in early September. As CEO, she was given the task of reviving the 360-bed facility and its sister hospital, Daniel Freeman Marina Hospital in Marina del Rey, Calif. The hospitals were losing a combined $2 million per month before Fickes came on board with a mission to trim expenses and speed payment of collectibles, among other tasks. During an interview last month, Fickes estimated that the hospitals would break even this month. That's a far cry from just three months earlier, when there was talk in the local provider community that Daniel Freeman Memorial might soon close its doors. . . . When Fickes' work is done and the Daniel Freeman hospitals are back in the black, Carondelet plans to sell them to another operator, a common ending for turnarounds.

The factors creating a need for a turnaround firm can be extraordinarily varied, experts say. Not-for-profit institutions are more likely to need a turnaround because they tend to be more mission-focused and have fewer internal fiscal checks or have drained their on-hand capital. Although managed care and the budget law both have received a lot of the blame for healthcare's financial ailments, there are plenty of other factors. Experts specifically cite mismanagement, lack of governance or a combination of the two. Hospitals or healthcare systems can pursue business expansions that go sour and devour cash, such as when they purchase medical groups, or as in the case of UCSF-Stanford, fail to recognize economies of scale from a merger. Facilities can hire without care, and over a period of years become grossly overstaffed. Purchasing can lack standardization. Fear of fraud crackdowns often prompts overcautious coding, resulting in lost patient revenue. Bill collection isn't aggressively pursued. And just a few maverick physicians can do a lot of damage to a hospital's bottom line.

Source: Ron Shinkman, *Modern Healthcare*, April 9, 2001.

Performance Measures

Although responsibility centers should be held accountable for both financial and non-financial performance, this discussion is limited to an introduction to financial performance measures. Exhibit 11–5 shows that cost, profit, and investment centers, respectively, are held accountable for increasing levels of financial responsibility (note that service centers have no *direct* financial responsibilities). *Budget variances* are the most universal measure of financial performance.

◀BUDGET VARIANCES▶

Budget Variance: The difference between what was planned (budgeted) and what was achieved (actual).

A **budget variance** is the difference between what was budgeted and what actually occurred. Exhibit 11–6 shows an example of an ambulatory care clinic that originally budgeted to serve 25,000 enrollees of an HMO and predicted they would make 1,000 visits during the month. However, during the month, the clinic actually served 26,000 enrollees who made 1,200 visits. Their expected net income was $0, and their

PERSPECTIVE 11–3

Blue All Over: Novant Health Selling HMO Despite Plan's Profitability

In contrast to many other hospital systems, Novant Health, of Winston-Salem, NC, found running an HMO to be a profitable business. In the end, though, three years of profits at Partners National Health Plans, Novant's managed-care subsidiary, were not enough for Novant to justify keeping the HMO. Falling in line behind scores of other provider organizations that have divested their managed-care businesses, Novant said June 18 it was selling its 400,000-enrollee managed-care business to Blue Cross and Blue Shield of North Carolina. Blues officials said they intend to run Partners, a for-profit subsidiary of not-for-profit Novant, as a wholly owned subsidiary and maintain it as an independent business.

"Novant Health's primary mission is to provide healthcare services and provide patient care," said Jim Tobalski, Novant's spokesman. "In the future, we felt for Partners to continue to be successful that we would have to be linked up to an organization whose primary mission was to provide health plans to area residents." "Partners turned a $1.2 million profit on $623.4 million in premium revenue for 2000 and enjoyed a $3 million profit for its first quarter this year alone," said Stuart Veach, vice president of Partners.

With its HMO profits helping the delivery side of its business rather than hurting it, eight-hospital Novant last year reported overall net income of $4.9 million on revenue of $1.5 billion. The profitability of Novant's managed-care business stands in stark contrast to most of the other provider-owned plans in North Carolina, which have lost money in recent years. Novant's decision to sell Partners and its 116,000-enrollee third-party administrator business, ACS Benefit Services, was announced within weeks of a decision by Carolinas HealthCare System, its chief rival in the Charlotte, NC, market, to shut down its 29,000-enrollee Medicaid HMO, the Wellness Plan, by Sept. 30. Partners, meanwhile, was beginning to suffer from Novant's strategy of limiting its provider network to Novant hospitals in its two major markets, Charlotte and Winston-Salem, Tobalski said. In an environment where choice was becoming more highly valued among insurers, Partners was at a disadvantage because of its ties to Novant's hospitals.

Source: Barbara Kirchheimer, *Modern Healthcare*, June 25, 2001.

actual net income was $10,000. Though it is tempting to assume that the $10,000 increase in net income was due to changes in the number of enrollees and visits, often more than one factor is responsible for budget variances. The rest of this section presents an approach to systematically explain why a budget variance occurs.

As shown in Exhibit 11–7, it is common for health care organizations to separate their total budget variance (variance in net income) into the portion due to changes in revenue and the portion due to changes in expenses. The revenue variance is then broken down into the portion attributable to volume and the portion attributable to rate differences. The expense variance is subdivided into the portion due to volume and the part due to other factors. This model will now be used to explain the net income variance of $10,000 in Exhibit 11–6.

Revenue Variances

In Exhibit 11–6, both the number of enrollees covered and the revenues earned from them increased beyond what was budgeted. This resulted in a positive revenue

Exhibit 11–5 Typical Financial Performance Measures Used to Evaluate the Financial Performance of Responsibility Centers

	Cost Centers	Profit Centers	Investment Centers
Budget Variances	Volume Variances Cost Variances Acuity Variances	Volume Variances Cost Variances Acuity Variances Revenue Variances	Volume Variances Cost Variances Acuity Variances Revenue Variances
Liquidity Ratios		Current Ratio Quick Ratio Days Cash on Hand	Current Ratio Quick Ratio Days Cash on Hand
Activity Ratios		Asset Turnover Receivable Turnover Payables Turnover	Asset Turnover Receivable Turnover Payables Turnover
Capitalization Ratios		Debt to Equity Times Interest Earned Debt Service Coverage	Debt to Equity Times Interest Earned Debt Service Coverage
Profit & Profitability Ratios		Profit Operating Margin	Profit Operating Margin Return on Equity Return on Assets

Exhibit 11–6 Revenue and Expense Variance Information for an Ambulatory Care Clinic Serving HMO Enrollees

Givens:

		Budgeted	Actual	Variance	
A	Enrollees	25,000	26,000	1,000	
B	Visits	1,000	1,200	200	
C	Revenues	$100,000	$117,000	$17,000	Favorable
D	Expenses	$100,000	$107,000	$7,000	Unfavorable
E	Net Income	$0	$10,000	$10,000	Favorable

Exhibit 11–7 Common Variances Used by Health Care Organizations

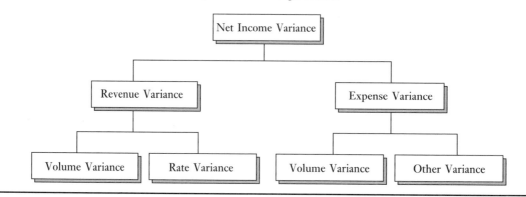

variance of $17,000. This is called a *favorable* variance because more income was received than was budgeted. Using just this information, it is tempting to conclude that the increase in revenues was due to the increase in employees covered. In fact, a variance analysis of the change in revenues shows that this is only partly the case.

Step 1. Develop the Flexible Budget Estimate for Revenues

In addition to the budgeted estimate and actual results, a variance analysis involves one more piece of information, called a flexible budget estimate. The **flexible budget estimate** adjusts for the actual volume being different from what was planned. The flexible budget estimate is what would have been budgeted had the actual volume been known ahead of time. Determining the flexible budget estimate involves two steps: calculating the budgeted rate and then using this number to determine how much would have been budgeted had the actual volume been known.

Flexible Budget: A budget which accomodates a range or multiple levels of activities.

Step 1A. Determine the Budgeted Revenue per Unit

To determine the budgeted revenue per unit, first determine what measure of volume will be used. In Exhibit 11–6, there are two measures of volume: enrollees and visits. Though in a fee-for-service or flat rate payment environment revenues might be expected to vary with the number of visits, in a capitated situation revenues fluctuate with the number of enrollees. Using enrollees as the measure of volume, the budgeted revenues are $4 per member per month (PMPM). This is determined by dividing budgeted revenues, $100,000, by the budgeted number of enrollees, 25,000 (see Exhibit 11–8, Step 1A).

Step 1B. Develop the Flexible Budget Estimate

The flexible budget estimate is the budgeted revenue PMPM multiplied by the actual volume ($4.00 PMPM × 26,000 = $104,000). This is the amount that would have been budgeted for revenues had it been known when the original budget was made that the actual volume would be 26,000 rather than 25,000 enrollees (see Exhibit 11–8, Step 1B).

A flexible budget estimates the revenues, expenses, or both over a range of volumes in order to forecast what the revenues would be at various levels. For example, by multiplying the $4.00 PMPM by a range of enrollees from 24,000 through 28,000, the clinic could develop a range of revenue estimates at selected levels (see Exhibit 11–8, rows D–F).

Both the range of volume estimates (in this case the number of enrollees) and the gap between each estimate are open to judgment. However, the range should include both the budgeted and actual volumes. Using this approach, the clinic just as easily could have estimated the results for a range of 24,500 to 27,500 using steps of 500. Either way, at 26,000 enrollees the budget estimate would have been $104,000.

Exhibit 11–8   Analysis of a Revenue Variance by Volume and Rate Variances

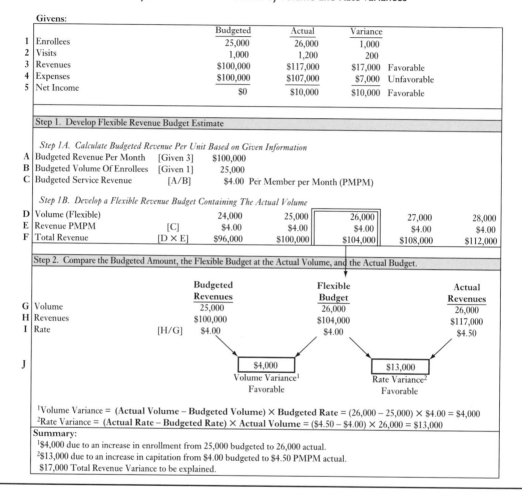

Givens:

		Budgeted	Actual	Variance	
1	Enrollees	25,000	26,000	1,000	
2	Visits	1,000	1,200	200	
3	Revenues	$100,000	$117,000	$17,000	Favorable
4	Expenses	$100,000	$107,000	$7,000	Unfavorable
5	Net Income	$0	$10,000	$10,000	Favorable

Step 1. Develop Flexible Revenue Budget Estimate

Step 1A. Calculate Budgeted Revenue Per Unit Based on Given Information

A	Budgeted Revenue Per Month	[Given 3]	$100,000
B	Budgeted Volume Of Enrollees	[Given 1]	25,000
C	Budgeted Service Revenue	[A/B]	$4.00 Per Member per Month (PMPM)

Step 1B. Develop a Flexible Revenue Budget Containing The Actual Volume

D	Volume (Flexible)		24,000	25,000	26,000	27,000	28,000
E	Revenue PMPM	[C]	$4.00	$4.00	$4.00	$4.00	$4.00
F	Total Revenue	[D × E]	$96,000	$100,000	$104,000	$108,000	$112,000

Step 2. Compare the Budgeted Amount, the Flexible Budget at the Actual Volume, and the Actual Budget.

			Budgeted Revenues	Flexible Budget	Actual Revenues
G	Volume		25,000	26,000	26,000
H	Revenues		$100,000	$104,000	$117,000
I	Rate	[H/G]	$4.00	$4.00	$4.50
J				$4,000 Volume Variance[1] Favorable	$13,000 Rate Variance[2] Favorable

[1]Volume Variance = **(Actual Volume – Budgeted Volume) × Budgeted Rate** = (26,000 – 25,000) × $4.00 = $4,000
[2]Rate Variance = **(Actual Rate – Budgeted Rate) × Actual Volume** = ($4.50 – $4.00) × 26,000 = $13,000

Summary:
[1]$4,000 due to an increase in enrollment from 25,000 budgeted to 26,000 actual.
[2]$13,000 due to an increase in capitation from $4.00 budgeted to $4.50 PMPM actual.
$17,000 Total Revenue Variance to be explained.

Step 2. Calculate the Revenue Variance Due to Changes in Volume and Rate

This step begins by laying out, side by side, the three revenue budget figures: budgeted amount, flexible budget, and actual revenues (see Exhibit 11–8, rows G–I).

All that remains is to compare these three figures. The difference between the original budget, $100,000, and the flexible budget, $104,000, shows how much of the revenue variance is due to volume: $4,000 (Exhibit 11–8, row J). The difference between the flexible budget, $104,000, and actual results, $117,000, is the amount of the revenue variance that is due to a change in rate: $13,000.

These differences can also be derived a different way. Looking at the volume variance, since the rate is held constant at $4.00 PMPM, the only difference between the original budget and the flexible budget is volume (26,000 rather than 25,000 enrollees). Thus, using the formula:

$$\textbf{Revenue Volume Variance = (Actual Volume - Budgeted Volume)} \times \textbf{Budgeted Rate}$$

the **revenue volume variance** is $4,000 [(26,000 – 25,000) × $4.00]. That is, since volume increased by 1,000 at $4.00 per member, $4,000 extra was earned.

The $13,000 rate variance can be analyzed similarly. Since the flexible budgeted revenue PMPM was $4.00 and the actual revenue is $4.50 PMPM ($117,000/26,000) there is a rate increase of $0.50 PMPM. Using the formula:

$$\textbf{Revenue Rate Variance = (Actual Rate - Budget Rate)} \times \textbf{Actual Volume}$$

the **revenue rate variance** is $13,000 [($4.50 – $4.00) × 26,000]. Thus, since the organization earned $0.50 more PMPM than was budgeted, and it served 26,000 enrollees, the variance due to a change in rate is $13,000.

The procedure to calculate revenue volume and rate variances is summarized in Exhibits 11–9a and b.

Expense Variances

This section explains why the ambulatory clinic was $7,000 over its budgeted expenses ($107,000 – $100,000). As shown in Exhibit 11–10, analyzing expense variances is quite similar to analyzing revenue variances.

Step 1. Explain the Amount of Variance Due to Fixed Costs

Though variable costs are directly affected by volume, fixed costs should not be. There are a number of reasons why fixed costs might have been incurred beyond what was budgeted. For example, there may be additional depreciation taken on the purchase of new equipment, unanticipated raises given, or new employees hired. (Consider that perhaps volume went beyond the relevant range into a higher "step" of

Revenue Volume Variance: The portion of total variance in revenues due to the actual volume being either higher or lower than the budgeted volume. It is the difference between the revenues forecast in the original budget and those in the flexible budget. It can be computed using the formula: (actual volume – budgeted volume) × budgeted rate.

Revenue Rate Variance: The amount of the total revenue variance that occurs because the actual average rate varies from the one originally budgeted. It is the difference between the revenues forecast in the flexible budget and those actually earned. It can be calculated using the formula: (actual rate – budgeted rate) × actual volume.

Exhibit 11–9a Derivation of the Revenue Volume and Rate Variances

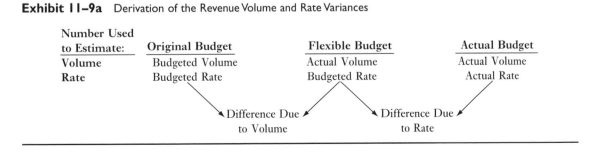

Number Used to Estimate:	Original Budget	Flexible Budget	Actual Budget
Volume	Budgeted Volume	Actual Volume	Actual Volume
Rate	Budgeted Rate	Budgeted Rate	Actual Rate

Difference Due to Volume   Difference Due to Rate

Exhibit 11–9b   Actual Numbers Used to Compute the Revenue Volume and Rate Variances

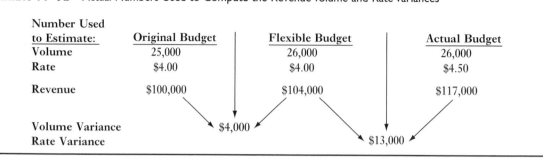

Number Used to Estimate:	Original Budget	Flexible Budget	Actual Budget
Volume	25,000	26,000	26,000
Rate	$4.00	$4.00	$4.50
Revenue	$100,000	$104,000	$117,000
Volume Variance		$4,000	
Rate Variance			$13,000

Exhibit 11–10   Breaking Down the Expense Variance into Fixed, Volume, and Cost Variances

Step 1. Explain the amount of variance due to non-variable expenses

		Budgeted	Actual	Variance	
A	Volume	1,000	1,200	200	
B	Non-Variable Expenses	$0	$5,000	$5,000	Unfavorable
C	Expenses	$100,000	$102,000	$2,000	Unfavorable
D	Total Expenses	$100,000	$107,000	$7,000	Unfavorable

Step 2. Develop Flexible Expense Budget Estimate

Step 2A. Calculate Budgeted Expense Per Unit Based on Information in Step 1.

E	Budgeted Total Variable Expenses	[C]	$100,000	
F	Budgeted Visits	[A]	1,000	
G	Budgeted Variable Expenses	[E/F]	$100.00 Per Visit	

Step 2B. Develop a Flexible Expense Budget Using Budgeted Expense Per Unit

H	Volume (Flexible)		1,000	1,100	1,200	1,300	1,400
I	Budgeted Variable Expenses per Visit [G]	[G]	$100	$100	$100	$100	$100
J	Total Variable Expenses [H × I]	[H × I]	$100,000	$110,000	$120,000	$130,000	$140,000

Step 3. Compare the Budgeted Expenses, the Flexible Budget at the Actual Volume, and Actual Expenses

			Budgeted Expenses	Flexible Budget	Actual Expenses
K	Volume	[A]	1,000	1,200	1,200
L	Total Variable Expenses	[C]	$100,000	$120,000	$102,000
M	Expense per Visit	[L/K]	$100.00	$100.00	$85.00

N $20,000   ($18,000)

Volume Variance[1]   Other Variance[2]

Unfavorable   Favorable

[1] Volume Variance = (Actual Volume – Budgeted Volume) × Budgeted Rate = (1,200 – 1,000) × $100.00 = $20,000
[2] Cost Variance = (Actual Cost – Budgeted Cost) × Actual Volume = ($85.00 – $100.00) × 1,200 = –$18,000

Summary:

Visits	1,200
Total Variance to be explained	$7,000
Non-Variable Variance	$5,000
Volume Variance	$20,000
Variance due to other factors	($18,000)
Total Unexplained Variance	$0

[1] $20,000 increase in expenses due to an increase in visits from the 1,000 which were budgeted to 1,200.
[2] $18,000 in other savings were gained due to a decrease in per visit cost from the $100.00 budgeted to $85.00 actual.

step-fixed costs.) This example assumes that fixed expenses increased because one contract nurse was hired for $5,000 per month.

Original expense variance (Exhibit 11–6, row D):	$7,000
Amount explained by fixed expenses (Exhibit 11–10, row B):	$5,000
Amount of expense variance still unexplained:	$2,000

This explains $5,000 of the $7,000 expense variance. The following steps explain the remaining $2,000 unfavorable expense variance – due to variable expenses.

Step 2. Develop a Flexible Expense Budget

This step involves developing a flexible budget in order to determine how much would have been budgeted had it been known at the time the budget was prepared that the actual number of visits would be 1,200 and not 1,000.

Step 2A. Determine the Budgeted Cost per Unit

Determining the budgeted cost per unit requires selecting the measure of volume. Whereas revenues vary with enrollees under capitation, expenses are more likely to vary with the number of visits. The budgeted cost per unit in the example then is calculated by dividing the $100,000 in budgeted expenses by the 1,000 budgeted visits (see Exhibit 11–10, Step 2A, rows E, F). Thus, the budgeted cost per visit is $100.00 (see Exhibit 11–10, Step 2A, row G).

Step 2B. Develop the Flexible Budget Estimate

The flexible expense budget estimate is the budgeted cost per unit multiplied by the actual volume ($100.00 × 1,200 = $120,000). This is the amount that would have been budgeted for expenses had it been known when the original budget was made that the actual volume would be 1,200 rather than 1,000 visits (see Exhibit 11–10, Step 2B, rows H–J).

Step 3. Calculate the Expense Variance Due to Changes in Volume and Other Factors

As in Step 2 of the revenue variance analysis presented earlier (Exhibit 11–8), this step begins by laying out, side by side, the three expense budget figures: budgeted, flexible, and actual expenses.

From Exhibit 11–10, Step 3, the difference between the original budget, $100,000, and the flexible budget, $120,000, is the amount of the variance due to volume, $20,000 (rows L, N). The difference between the flexible budget and the actual results ($120,000 – $102,000 = $18,000) is due to a change in costs per unit (also rows L, N). Note that this is a cost saving and is therefore considered *favorable*. Costs actually decreased from what was expected.

Expense Volume Variance: The portion of total variance in expenses due to the actual volume being either higher or lower than the budgeted volume. It is the difference between the expenses forecast in the original budget and those in the flexible budget. It can be computed using the formula: (actual volume - budgeted volume) × budgeted rate.

As with the revenue variances, expense variances can also be derived a different way. In regard to the volume variance, since the cost per unit is held constant ($100 per visit), the only difference between the original budget and the flexible budget is volume (1,200 rather than 1,000 visits). Thus, using the formula:

Expense Volume Variance = (Actual Volume − Budgeted Volume) × Budgeted Cost per Unit

the **expense volume variance** is $20,000 [(1,200 − 1,000) × $100.00]. This is because 200 more members than budgeted were seen at a $100 cost per visit. The expense volume variance is the portion of total variance in variable expenses that is due to the actual volume being either higher or lower than the budgeted volume. It is the difference between the expenses forecast in the original budget and those in the flexible budget. It can be computed using the following formula: (actual volume − budgeted volume) × budgeted cost per unit.

 Key Point In the formula for expense volume variance, the sign of the answer is crucial. A negative answer indicates a decrease in volume, but this is considered a *favorable variance* because it leads to a decrease in costs. A positive answer indicates an increase in volume, and this is considered an *unfavorable variance* because it leads to an increase in costs.

Expense Cost Variance: The amount of the variable expense variance that occurs because the actual cost per unit varies from that originally budgeted. It is the difference between the variable expenses forecast in the flexible budget and those actually incurred. It can be calculated by the formula: (actual cost per unit − budgeted cost per unit) × actual volume.

The $18,000 savings shown in the cost variance can be analyzed similarly. Since the flexible budgeted cost per visit was $100 and the actual cost per visit is $85 ($102,000/1,200), there is a decrease in the cost per visit of $15. Using the formula:

Expense Cost Variance = (Actual Cost per Unit − Budgeted Cost per Unit) × Actual Volume

the **expense cost variance** is −$18,000. Thus, since the organization spent $15 less per visit than had been budgeted, and it provided 1,200 visits, the variance due to a change in cost per visit is −$18,000 (−$15 × 1,200).

The procedure to calculate expense volume and cost variances is summarized in Exhibits 11–11a and 11–11b.

Though the amount of the cost variance was calculated, the reason for it is unclear. The cost variance could be due to a variety of factors, including changes in quality, case mix, intensity of services, efficiency, and wages. Although it is possible to decompose the cost variance into other variances, that methodology is beyond the scope of this text.

Summary of the Example

When considering both revenues and expenses, the total variance was $10,000. Of this, a change in volume resulted in increased revenues of $4,000 and increased costs of $20,000. On the other hand, the change in rate from $4.00 to $4.50 PMPM brought in an extra $13,000, and the change in cost per unit from $100 to $85 accounted for $18,000 in savings from what was budgeted. In addition, a step-fixed cost was incurred by hiring a contract nurse at $5,000 per month.

Exhibit 11-11a Derivation of the Expense Volume and Cost/Unit Variance

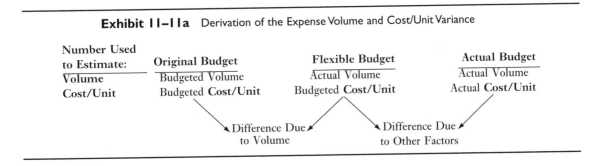

Number Used to Estimate:	Original Budget	Flexible Budget	Actual Budget
Volume	Budgeted Volume	Actual Volume	Actual Volume
Cost/Unit	Budgeted **Cost/Unit**	Budgeted **Cost/Unit**	Actual **Cost/Unit**

Difference Due to Volume   Difference Due to Other Factors

Exhibit 11-11b Actual Numbers Used to Compute the Expense Volume and Cost/Unit Variances

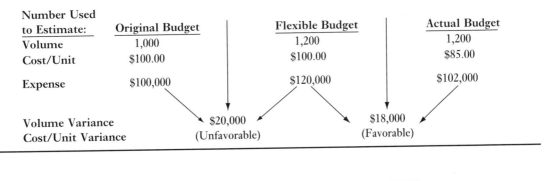

Number Used to Estimate:	Original Budget	Flexible Budget	Actual Budget
Volume	1,000	1,200	1,200
Cost/Unit	$100.00	$100.00	$85.00
Expense	$100,000	$120,000	$102,000
Volume Variance Cost/Unit Variance	$20,000 (Unfavorable)	$18,000 (Favorable)	

Total variance	$10,000	Favorable
Variance explained by a change in volume:		
Increase in enrollees from 25,000 to 26,000 (revenues)	$4,000	Favorable
Increase in visits from 1,000 to 1,200 (expenses)	$20,000	Unfavorable
Increase in rates from $4.00 to $4.50 PMPM	$13,000	Favorable
Decrease in cost per visit from $100 to $85 per visit	$(18,000)	Favorable
Increase in fixed costs by hiring a contract RN	$5,000	Unfavorable
Total variance explained	$ 10,000	Favorable

Key Point In the formula for expense cost variance, the sign of the answer is crucial. A negative answer indicates a decrease in variable cost per unit, but this is considered a *favorable variance* since it leads to decreased costs. A positive answer indicates an increase in variable cost per unit, but this is considered an *unfavorable variance* because it leads to increased costs.

Beyond Variances

Revenue Attainment: Earning the amount of revenue budgeted.

Budget variances are usually associated with the operating budget, which focuses on short-term **revenue attainment** (earning the amount of revenue budgeted) and **cost containment** (not spending more than budgeted). A more long-term focus is neces-

Cost Containment:
Not spending more
than is budgeted in the
expense budget.

**Revenue
Enhancement:** Finding
supplemental sources
of revenue.

Cost Avoidance:
Finding new ways to
run a business that
eliminate certain
classes of costs.

sary to effect major efficiencies in the organization. Measures must be implemented to promote **revenue enhancement** (finding new sources of revenue) and **cost avoidance** (finding new ways to operate that eliminate certain classes of costs) in the long term. For instance, just-in-time (JIT) inventory methods deliver supplies "automatically" to the organization as needed, and they avoid many of the traditional costs of ordering, storing, and keeping track of inventories that flow through health care organizations. If only a short-term focus were used, the initial costs might discourage an administrator from installing such a system; however, long-term measures might encourage such a decision.

Other Financial Performance Measures

Though budget variances are the most used financial measure, various ratios are increasingly being used as financial performance measures for profit and investment centers. Though the use of these indicators is basically the same for profit centers and investment centers as it is for the organization as a whole, some complications arise when using these measures to judge the financial performance of divisions within the organization. The most common are:

1. They may promote a lack of goal congruence; that is, they may encourage the organizational unit to make decisions that are in its own best interest, but not in the best interest of the organization as a whole.
2. They may introduce complicated measurement problems. For instance, when two organizational units share the same assets, it is difficult to partition the assets between the two units to calculate such measures as return on assets.
3. They may promote short-term thinking.

◀SUMMARY▶

A growing trend in the structure of health care providing organizations is decentralization, which presents some interesting problems in the measurement of financial performance of the organizational units. Decentralization is the degree of dispersion of responsibility within an organization.

The advantages of decentralization include: time, information relevance, quality, speed, talent, and motivation and allegiance. The disadvantages include loss of control, decreased goal congruence, increased need for coordination and formal communication, and lack of managerial talent.

A responsibility center is an organizational unit that has been formally designated with the responsibility to carry out one or more tasks and/or to achieve one or more outcomes. There are four major types of responsibility centers:

1. Service centers are responsible for ensuring that health care-related services are provided to a population in a manner that meets the volume and

quality requirements of the organization. They have no direct budgetary control.

2. Cost centers are responsible for providing services and controlling their costs. They are the primary level in the organization with direct budget control. The two types of cost centers in health care organizations are clinical cost centers and administrative cost centers. Clinical cost centers provide health care-related services to clients, patients, or enrollees. Administrative cost centers provide support to the clinical cost centers and the organization as a whole. Included in this category are general administration, the business office, information services, admitting, medical records, and housekeeping.

3. Profit centers are responsible for controlling costs and earning revenues. The three types of profit centers are traditional profit centers, capitated profit centers, and administrative profit centers.

4. Investment centers are responsible for attaining a return on investment.

The relationship between responsibility, accountability, and authority is straightforward. Ideally, managers should be given the authority to carry out their responsibilities. To the extent that this occurs, managers are held accountable for the performance of their responsibility centers. Responsibility refers to the duties and obligations of a responsibility center, authority is the power to carry out a given responsibility, and accountability means the sanctions, both positive and negative, attached to carrying out responsibilities.

Cost, profit, and investment centers, respectively, are held accountable for increasing levels of financial responsibility. (Service centers have no direct financial responsibilities.) Budget variances are the most universal measure of financial performance. A budget variance is the difference between what was budgeted and what actually occurred. It is common for health care organizations to separate their total budget variance (variance in net income) into revenue variances and expense variances. The revenue variance is broken down into volume and rate variances. The expense variance is separated into volume variance and other factors.

The revenue volume variance is the portion of total variance in revenues due to the actual volume being either higher or lower than the budgeted volume. It is the difference between the revenues forecast in the original budget and those in the flexible budget. It can be computed using the following formula: (actual volume − budgeted volume) × budgeted rate. The rate variance is the amount of the total revenue variance that occurs because the actual average rate received varies from that originally budgeted. It is the difference between the revenues forecast in the flexible budget and those actually earned. It can be calculated using the formula: (actual rate − budgeted rate) × actual volume.

The expense volume variance is the portion of total variance in variable expenses due to the actual volume being either higher or lower than the budgeted volume. It is the difference between the expenses forecast in the original budget and those in the flexible budget. It can be computed using the following formula: (actual volume − budgeted volume) × budgeted cost per unit.

The expense cost variance is the amount of the variable expense variance that occurs because the actual cost per visit varies from that originally budgeted. It is the difference between the variable expenses forecast in the flexible budget and those actually incurred. It can be calculated by the formula: (actual cost per unit – budgeted cost per unit) × actual volume. The cost variance could be due to a variety of factors including changes in quality, case mix, intensity of service, efficiency, and wages.

◀Key Terms▶

Accountability	Cost Centers	Revenue Attainment
Administrative Cost Centers	Cost Containment	Revenue Enhancement
Administrative Profit Centers	Decentralization	Revenue Rate Variance
Authority	Expense Cost Variance	Revenue Volume Variance
Budget Variance	Expense Volume Variance	Service Centers
Capitated Profit Centers	Profit Centers	Traditional Profit Centers
Clinical Cost Centers	Responsibility	
Cost Avoidance	Responsibility Center	

◀Key Equations▶

Expense Cost Variance: (Actual Cost per Unit – Budgeted Cost per Unit) × Actual Volume

Expense Volume Variance: (Actual Volume – Budgeted Volume) × Budgeted Cost per Unit

Revenue Rate Variance: (Actual Rate – Budgeted Rate) × Actual Volume

Revenue Volume Variance: (Actual Volume – Budgeted Volume) × Budgeted Rate

◀Questions and Problems▶

1. **Definitions.** Define the following terms:
   a. Accountability.
   b. Administrative Cost Centers.
   c. Administrative Profit Centers.
   d. Authority.
   e. Budget Variance.
   f. Capitated Profit Centers.
   g. Clinical Cost Centers.
   h. Cost Avoidance.

    i. Cost Centers.
    j. Cost Containment.
    k. Decentralization.
    l. Expense Cost Variance.
    m. Expense Volume Variance.
    n. Profit Centers.
    o. Responsibility.
    p. Responsibility Center.
    q. Revenue Attainment.
    r. Revenue Enhancement.
    s. Revenue Rate Variance.
    t. Revenue Volume Variance.
    u. Service Centers.
    v. Traditional Profit Centers.

2. **Advantages of decentralization.** List and discuss the advantages associated with decentralization.

3. **Disadvantages of decentralization.** List and discuss the disadvantages of decentralization.

4. **Types of responsibility centers.** Describe the four types of responsibility centers, including the characteristics of each.

5. **Responsibility centers.**
    a. What is the most common type of responsibility center?
    b. What is the most basic type of responsibility center?

6. **Identifying responsibility centers.** Identify each responsibility center below as either a service center, cost center (clinical or administrative), profit center (capitated or administrative), or investment center. Explain your choices:
    a. Radiology department that must control its own costs.
    b. Admitting department of a hospital.
    c. HMO.
    d. Stand-alone outpatient clinic that must earn a 10 percent ROI.
    e. Volunteer department with no budget.
    f. Development office.

7. **The relationship among accountability, responsibility, and authority.** What is the relationship of accountability, responsibility, and authority with respect to a responsibility center?

8. **Transfer prices.** What are transfer prices? Discuss their major disadvantages.

9. **Performance measures.** What is the most commonly used financial performance measure?

10. **Performance measures.** Name two financial measures used to judge the performance of investment centers that are not used to measure the financial performance of profit centers.

11. **Performance measures.** What are major disadvantages of using traditional performance measures?

12. **Variance analysis.** What does the term "variance analysis" mean when applied to financial performance of health care organizations?

13. **Budget variances.** What are the most common types of budget variances used in health care organizations?

14. **Cost variances.** What can account for cost variances?

15. **ROI for an investment center.** An outpatient clinic invests $2,300,000. The desired ROI is 12 percent. In the first year, revenues are $750,000 and expenses are $370,000. Does the clinic meet its ROI requirement that year?

16. **ROI for an investment center.** A new cardiac catheterization lab was constructed at Havea Heart Hospital. The investment for the lab was $450,000 in equipment costs and $50,000 in renovation costs. A desired return on investment is 12 percent. Once the lab was constructed, 5,000 patients were served in the first year and were charged $340 for each procedure. The annual fixed cost for the catheterization lab is $1 million and the variable cost is $129 per procedure. What is the catheterization lab's profit? Did this profit meet its desired ROI?

17. **Detailed variance analysis.** The following are planned and actual revenues for Cutting Edge Surgery Center. Since they are one of four surgery centers in the community, the administrator is very concerned with his rates in relation to those of his competitors.

	Planned	Actual
Surgical volume	1,200	1,400
Gift shop revenues	$12,000	$15,000
Surgery revenues	$500,500	$750,750
Parking revenues	$15,000	$17,000

a. Determine the total variance between the planned and actual budgets.

b. Determine the service-related revenues and calculate variance still unexplained.

c. Prepare a flexible budget estimate. Present side-by-side the budget, flexible budget estimate, and actual surgical revenue (and related volumes).

d. Determine what variance is due to change in volume and what variance is due to change in rates.

e. Determine the volume variance and rate variance based on per unit rates.

18. **Detailed variance analysis.** The administrator of Break-a-Leg Hospital is very aware of the need to keep his cost down, since he just negotiated a new capitated arrangement with a large insurance company. The following are selected planned and actual expenses for the previous month.

	Planned	Actual
Patient days	24,000	30,000
Pharmacy	$100,000	$140,000
Miscellaneous supplies	$56,000	$67,500
Fixed overhead costs	$708,000	$780,000

a. Determine the total variance associated with the planned and actual expenses.

b. Calculate the amount of unexplained variance and give a possible reason for the change in fixed expenses.

c. Prepare a flexible expense estimate for variable costs. Compare budget, flexible budget, and actual (show related volumes).

d. Determine what variance is due to change in volume and what variance is due to change in rates.

e. Determine the volume variance and rate variance based on per unit rates.

19. **Detailed variance analysis.** A dermatology clinic expects to contract with an HMO for an estimated 80,000 enrollees. The HMO expects 1 in 4 of its enrolled members to use the dermatology services per month. At the end of the year, the dermatology clinic's business manager looked at her monthly figures and saw that the number of enrolled members had increased by 5 percent over the budgeted amount, and that 1 in 3 of the total HMO members had used the dermatology services per month. Net monthly revenues of the dermatology clinic were budgeted at $260,000 but were actually $450,000. Monthly expenses for the clinic were budgeted at $200,000 but were actually $270,000.

a. Prepare a monthly revenue, expense, and net income variance budget for the clinic.

b. Are these variances favorable or unfavorable? Why?

Chapter Twelve

PROVIDER COST FINDING METHODS

LEARNING OBJECTIVES

After completing this chapter, you will be able to:

- ▶ Identify three methods for estimating costs.
- ▶ Calculate costs using the Step-down Method.
- ▶ Calculate costs using Activity-based Costing.
- ▶ Understand the major advantages and disadvantages of Activity-based Costing.

Chapter Outline

◀INTRODUCTION▶

Finding the costs to serve various populations (e.g. the elderly, Medicare patients, rehabilitation patients), to produce various goods and services, and to work with various payors (e.g. Medicaid, insurance companies) is an important activity for most health care providers. A *cost object* is anything for which costs are being estimated, such as a population, a test, a visit, a patient, or a patient day. This chapter discusses the three most commonly used approaches to find costs for various cost objects: 1) the Cost-to-Charge Ratio; 2) the Step-down Method; and 3) Activity-based Costing.

◀THE COST-TO-CHARGE RATIO▶

Historically, the cost to charge ratio, CCR, is one of the most common methods used by hospitals, dentists, and doctors to estimate costs. It is based upon an assumed relationship of costs to charges, usually determined by industry norms or special studies. CCR begins with charges (or reimbursement) and assumes that costs are a certain percentage of this amount. For example, a group planning a dental office might use the rule of thumb that all non-direct labor expenses amounted to 22 percent of charges.

The main advantage of this approach is simplicity. The disadvantages include: 1) to the extent that the ratio used is typical for the industry or segment of the industry, it may not apply well to any particular organization; 2) if the ratio were determined by a study, to the extent that volume or service mix deviates from the figures used in the study, the CCR may become inaccurate; 3) to the extent that the fixed/variable cost composition has changed, the ratio may provide an inaccurate measurement; and 4) to the extent that an overall ratio is used for all procedures, the CCR may underestimate or overestimate the cost of individual procedures.

While CCR is relatively simple to implement, more complex health care organizations usually use a Step-down or an Activity-Based Costing approach, either of which is commonly thought to be more accurate.

◀THE STEP-DOWN METHOD▶

The **Step-down Method** is a cost-finding method based on allocating those costs that are not directly paid for to those products or services that are. The example in Exhibit 12–1 shows three responsibility centers to which payment is *not* attached (utilities, administration, and laboratory) and three to which revenues *are* attached (walk-in services, pediatric services, and adolescent services). The goal of the step-down method is to allocate the costs of the support centers (utilities, administration, and laboratory) fairly among each of the three patient services. The full step-down allocation is shown in Exhibit 12–2.

There are four steps to allocate the costs of non-directly paid for costs to services for which payment is attached:

1. Determine an allocation base and compile basic statistics.
2. Convert basic statistics for the step-down.
3. Calculate allocation percentages.
4. Allocate costs from the support centers to each of the centers below it (thus, the "down" in "step-down").

Cost Object: Anything for which costs are being estimated, such as a population, a test, a visit, a patient, or a patient day.

Cost-to-charge Ratio (CCR): A method to estimate costs which assumes that costs are a certain percentage of charges (or reimbursements).

Step-down Method: A cost finding method based on allocating those costs that are not directly paid for to those products or services to which payment is attached. The method derives its name from the stair-step pattern that results from allocating costs.

These steps will now be followed to allocate utilities, administration, and laboratory costs, respectively.

Allocating Utilities

An **allocation base** is an item used to allocate costs, based upon its relationship to why the costs occurred. Some common allocation bases are listed in Exhibit 12–3. The better the cause-and-effect relationship between why the cost occurred and the allocation basis, the more accurate the cost allocation. Because of their causal relationship to costs, allocation bases are also called *cost drivers* (discussed in more detail below). A

Exhibit 12–1   Example of Costs for which Payment Is Not Directly Attached and Those to which Payment Is Directly Attached

	Direct Costs	
Utilities	$50,000	These costs, which are not paid for directly…
Administration	100,000	
Laboratory	175,000	
Walk-in Clinic Services	200,000	Must be folded into these services, to which payment is attached.
Pediatric Services	200,000	
Adolescent Clinic Services	300,000	
Total	$1,025,000	

Exhibit 12–2   The Step-down Method of Allocating Costs

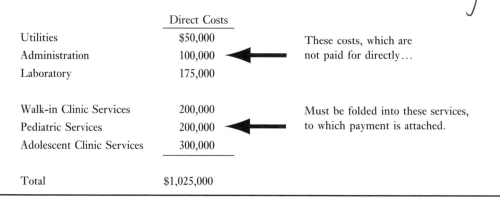

	Step 1: Compile Basic Statistics			Step 2: Compute Converted Statistics		
	A	B	C	D	E	F
	Sq. Feet	Direct Costs	Lab Tests	Sq. Feet	Direct Costs	Lab Tests
Utilities		$50,000				
Administration	1,000	$100,000		1,000		
Laboratory	2,000	$175,000		2,000	$175,000	
Walk-in services	2,000	$200,000	250	2,000	$200,000	250
Pediatric services	2,500	$200,000	450	2,500	$200,000	450
Adolescent services	2,500	$300,000	300	2,500	$300,000	300
Total	10,000	$1,025,000	1,000	10,000	$875,000	1,000

	Step 3: Compute Allocation %			Step 4: Allocate Costs[1]				
	G	H	I	J	K	L	M	N
	Utilities	Administration	Laboratory	Direct Costs	Utilities	Administration	Laboratory	Total
	[Sq. Feet]	[Direct Costs]	[Tests]					
Utilities				$50,000	($50,000)			
Administration	10%			$100,000	$5,000	($105,000)		
Laboratory	20%	20.0%		$175,000	$10,000	$21,000	($206,000)	
Walk-in services	20%	22.9%	25%	$200,000	$10,000	$24,000	$51,500	$285,500
Pediatric services	25%	22.9%	45%	$200,000	$12,500	$24,000	$92,700	$329,200
Adolescent services	25%	34.3%	30%	$300,000	$12,500	$36,000	$61,800	$410,300
Total	100%	100%	100%	$1,025,000	$0	$0	$0	$1,025,000

[1]Differences due to rounding.

Exhibit 12–3   Some Common Allocation Bases

Costs to Be Allocated	Allocation Basis
Billing Office	Number of Bills
General Administration	Direct Costs of Department
	Number of FTEs[1]
Laboratory[2]	Weighted Average Costs of Tests
	Number of Tests
Medical Records	Number of Records "Pulled"
Nursing[2]	Nursing Hours
	Acuity-weighted Hours
Purchasing	Number of Purchase Orders
Rent, Utilities, Cleaning	Square Feet

[1] Full-time Equivalent Employees.
[2] Laboratory and Nursing are frequently charged directly to patients, rather than being allocated.

common base to allocate utilities is square footage, on the assumption that actual utility usage is proportional to the size of the space a service occupies.

Exhibit 12–4 highlights those parts of Exhibit 12–2 relevant to allocating utilities. Since administration occupies 1,000 of the 10,000 square feet of the facility (see Exhibit 12–4, columns A and D), it is allocated 10 percent (column G) of the $50,000 direct cost of utilities, which is $5,000 (column K). Similarly, since the laboratory and

Exhibit 12–4   Steps in the Step-down Process Relevant to the Allocation of Utility Costs

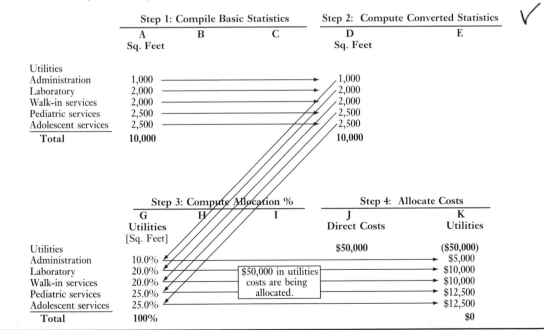

	Step 1: Compile Basic Statistics			Step 2: Compute Converted Statistics	
	A Sq. Feet	B	C	D Sq. Feet	E
Utilities					
Administration	1,000			1,000	
Laboratory	2,000			2,000	
Walk-in services	2,000			2,000	
Pediatric services	2,500			2,500	
Adolescent services	2,500			2,500	
Total	10,000			10,000	

	Step 3: Compute Allocation %			Step 4: Allocate Costs	
	G Utilities [Sq. Feet]	H	I	J Direct Costs	K Utilities
Utilities				$50,000	($50,000)
Administration	10.0%				$5,000
Laboratory	20.0%		$50,000 in utilities		$10,000
Walk-in services	20.0%		costs are being		$10,000
Pediatric services	25.0%		allocated.		$12,500
Adolescent services	25.0%				$12,500
Total	100%				$0

the walk-in services each occupy 2,000 of the 10,000 square feet (columns A and D), each is allocated 20 percent (column G), which is $10,000 (column K). Finally, since the pediatric and adolescent services each occupy 2,500 square feet (columns A and D), each is allocated 25 percent (column G), which is $12,500 (column K).

Allocating Administrative Costs

Exhibit 12–5 highlights those parts of Exhibit 12–2 relevant to allocating administrative costs. Note that instead of allocating just the $100,000 in direct administrative costs that were there at the beginning of the allocation (column J), $105,000 is allocated from Administration, $100,000 in direct administrative costs, and an additional $5,000 that has been allocated to Administration from Utilities.

The allocation base used to allocate administration is direct costs (see Exhibit 12–5, column E), based on the assumption that administrative costs are incurred by each of the other responsibility centers in the same proportion as are their direct costs. Another allocation base sometimes used to allocate administrative costs is the number of FTEs (full-time equivalent employees) in each responsibility center. This assumes that administrative costs are incurred in proportion to the number of employees working in each responsibility center.

Though the procedure here is similar to allocating utilities, there is one major difference. Note that in column B of Exhibit 12–5 there is $1,025,000 in direct costs, including $50,000 in utilities and $100,000 in administrative direct costs, while in col-

Exhibit 12–5   Steps in the Step-down Process Relevant to the Allocation of Administrative Costs

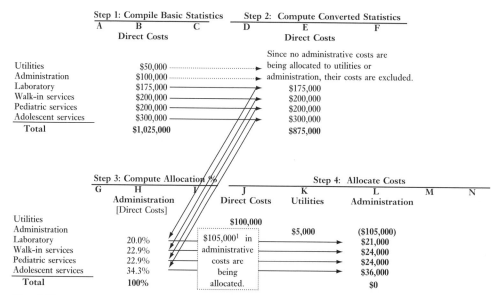

Note: Differences due to rounding.
[1]$100,000 Administrative Costs (Col. A) + $5,000 Allocated Utilities Costs to Administration (Exhibit 12–4, Col. K) = $105,000.

umn E there is only $875,000 in direct costs because utilities and administrative direct costs have been omitted. This is done for two reasons. 1) By convention, the step-down allocation method always proceeds downward from one responsibility center to those below it. Thus, no administrative costs are allocated (upward) to utilities. Therefore, the $50,000 in utilities cost is excluded (column E) when determining the proportional share of administration to be allocated on the basis of direct costs. 2) Since administration is fully allocated to the services below it, it cannot give any of its cost to itself. Therefore, in using direct costs as the basis to determine what percentage of the administrative costs being allocated go to the services below it, the $100,000 in administrative direct costs are omitted (column E).

Without the $150,000 of utilities and administration, there is $875,000 in direct costs over which to allocate administration. Laboratory has $175,000 in direct costs (column E), and thus it receives $175,000/$875,000 or 20 percent (column H) of the $105,000 in administration being allocated, which is $21,000 (column L). The walk-in services clinic has $200,000 of direct costs (column E), so it receives $200,000/$875,000 or 22.9 percent (column H) of the $105,000 in administrative costs being allocated, which is $24,000 (column L). The remaining administrative costs are allocated to the pediatric and adolescent services in a similar fashion (column L).

Allocating Laboratory

The only costs that have not yet been allocated are those of the laboratory. Note that in Exhibit 12–2, instead of the original $175,000 in direct laboratory costs, $206,000 is being allocated (column M). This is because in addition to its own direct costs, laboratory also includes $10,000 in costs allocated from utilities and $21,000 in costs allocated from administration.

Laboratory costs are allocated on the basis of lab tests under the assumption that the fair share of the laboratory costs due to each of the three services is in proportion to the number of tests each service ordered (see Exhibit 12–2, column C). Using lab tests as a basis, the walk-in services clinic is allocated 25 percent (column I) of the $206,000 (column M), which is $51,500 (column M). The pediatric services and the adolescent services clinics are allocated 45 percent and 30 percent, respectively (column I) of the $206,000 (column M), which are $92,700 and $61,800, respectively (column M).

Fully Allocated Cost

After all the costs of the services that are not directly paid for have been allocated to those services that are paid for, the totals are summed (see Exhibit 12–2, column N). Rather than the $200,000 it costs to deliver walk-in services when only direct costs are considered, the **fully allocated costs** are $285,500. Similarly, pediatric services changed from $200,000 to $329,200, and adolescent services changed from $300,000

Fully Allocated Cost: The cost of a cost object that includes both its direct costs and all other costs allocated to it.

to \$410,300 when allocated costs are included. Thus, the fully allocated cost reflects both the original direct costs as well as all allocated costs, but the total cost, \$1,025,000, remains the same as before.

Several final comments regarding the step-down allocation method:

1. In finding costs, the *order* in which the services are allocated makes a difference in the final costs. For example, if Administration were placed ahead of Utilities in the allocation order, the costs of Walk-in, Pediatric, and Adolescent Services would be different than in the example. There are two sometimes conflicting rules of thumb to help choose a reasonable order: a) rank-order the centers being allocated from highest dollar amount to lowest dollar amount (according to this rule, in the example, Laboratory and then Administration should have been listed ahead of Utilities); or b) list the centers, from highest to lowest, in an order that reflects the number of other centers they affect. It was for this reason that the centers were ordered as they were in the example, with Laboratory being last.

2. The *allocation basis* used to allocate costs makes a difference in the final costs. If the *number of FTEs* instead of *direct dollars* were the allocation basis for administration, and there were a low correlation between the two, then the costs of Walk-in, Pediatric, and Adolescent services would be different.

3. The number of centers to which costs are allocated makes a difference. For example, if there were four services instead of three, then the costs allocated to the original three services (Walk-in, Pediatric, and Adolescent) would be different (probably less).

4. Though the step-down method is the most widely used method because of its legacy from Medicare, there are several other related methods available to providers to calculate costs. These are the direct method, the double apportionment method, and the reciprocal method. Since they are used relatively infrequently, they are not discussed here.

5. The step-down method is useful for pricing and reimbursement-related decisions, but should not be used to control costs. There are other methods, including activity-based costing, that are better for this purpose.

Most inpatient facilities use the step-down method to report their Medicare costs. Though the Medicare Cost Report relies heavily on the step-down approach, in reality it combines the step-down and CCR methods, as alluded to in Perspective 12–1. As shown in Perspective 12–2, there is more to finding costs that just the cost allocation method, one key point being that the costs being reported are allowable.

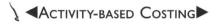

◄ACTIVITY-BASED COSTING►

Though the step-down method of cost allocation is widely used to find the cost of services for pricing and reimbursement purposes, a newer cost-finding

PERSPECTIVE 12–1

The Southwest Regional Consumers Union's Interest in the Use of the Medicare Cost Report

House Committee on Public Health
Recommendations relating to Hospital Charity Care
& Hospital System Sales, Conversions, Partnerships and Mergers
June 28, 2000

Consumers Union appreciates the opportunity to testify before the House Committee on Public Health regarding hospital charity care and the impact hospital system sales, conversions, partnerships and mergers have on the level of charity care in their communities. Consumers Union has been actively involved with the development, passage and implementation of the Texas charity care law since 1991. We currently serve on the Hospital Data Advisory Committee and monitor the annual levels of charity care provided by Texas hospitals.

Consumers Union also has actively pursued the preservation of charitable assets when nonprofit hospitals and other health care entities have changed their status due to a sale, conversion, partnership or merger, often referred to collectively as "conversions." Our expertise in this arena reaches beyond Texas, as our West Coast Regional Office has an active national project providing technical assistance to states and local communities experiencing conversions.

What do these numbers tell us? $544 million in charity care was delivered in Texas in 1998 (using the Medicare cost report method of calculation). It tells us that hospitals – nonprofit, for-profit DSH, and public – are contributing significantly towards helping the uninsured. But the numbers tell us more . . .

Too many of these hospitals hover around the 4% requirement, suggesting that, as a standard, it has become a ceiling rather than a floor. Of the 89 nonprofit hospitals required to meet the standard, 26 (13 of which reported as a system) were within two percentage points of the 4% standard. . . .

Is it enough? Probably not, since these nonprofit hospitals have a mission to serve people in their community regardless of the ability to pay. Charitable obligations go beyond simple tax deferment, the basis for the 4% of net patient revenue standard (based on the average tax benefit received by a nonprofit hospital). Also, considering the high numbers of uninsured Texans, we need help.

Recommendations relating to the charity care law.

1. Keep the charity care law in Texas. Consider raising the bar for charity and unreimbursed uncompensated sponsored care above 4% of net patient revenue, especially if the current calculation method is maintained (we oppose maintaining this method).
2. The Medicare Cost Report should be used to calculate the cost to charge ratio for hospital charity care. The Medicare Cost Report provides a more true reflection of costs of patient care than the current base using the hospital's audited financial statement. For example, the current standard in the law, using the hospital's audited financial statement, allows the inclusion of bad debt charges in calculating the cost to charge ratio. The Medicare cost report does not allow the inclusion of bad debt charges, but only the cost of providing the care that results in bad debt. In theory, bad debt charges above actual cost of providing care are not "expenses."

Standardization provided by the Medicare cost report is important in order to get a fair comparison of hospital charity care. For example: Hospital A provides luxury rooms, a specialty chef, a concierge, an office building for staff doctors, large new covered parking garage. Hospital B provides basic patient care without the frills. When using audited financial statements, all those Hospital A amenities are included in the base from which the hospital calculates its cost to charge ratio, while the base for Hospital B will not include such items. In the end this method will inflate Hospital A's charity care numbers without actually increasing the charity care delivered.

Source: Testimony by the Consumers Union on Its Website
June 28, 2000 (http://www.consumerism.org/health/charitysw700.htm).

PERSPECTIVE 12–2

Review of a Medicare Cost Report

This final report points out that Community Behavioral Services (CBS) claimed Medicare reimbursement totaling $4.5 million representing 31,951 services to 305 Medicare beneficiaries in Fiscal Year (FY) 1995. Our review of services provided to 43 of these beneficiaries disclosed that: 7,868 (71 percent) of the services were provided to 31 beneficiaries who, in the opinion of medical experts, did not meet the Medicare eligibility criteria for receiving partial hospitalization program (PHP) services; and 286 (3 percent) of the services provided to 6 beneficiaries were considered unallowable by medical review personnel because they were either not documented, the services were not reasonable and necessary, the services were not ordered, or the supporting documentation was not dated, not signed, or duplicated. We recommended that the fiscal intermediary (FI) recover the amount overpaid to CBS and place the four providers owned by CBS under focused medical review with special emphasis on beneficiary eligibility.

This final reports points out that CBS claimed costs totaling $2.3 million in FY 1994. Our review disclosed that the claimed costs included costs that were not allocable or reimbursable according to Medicare reimbursement requirements. The cost report included $1.4 million that was not related to patient care, not reasonable and necessary and costs that were not supported with sufficient documentation to determine whether the costs were incurred, reasonable and necessary, and related to patient care. The FI notified CBS of the unallowed costs and took recovery action. The Health Care Financing Administration took action to suspend payments to this provider until the overpayments are recovered. We recommended that the FI review subsequent cost reports for similar unallowable costs. The FI agreed with our recommendations.

Source: Department of Health and Human Services, Office of Inspector General – AUDIT, "Review of Partial Hospitalization Services and Audit of Medicare Cost Report for Community Behavioral Services, a Florida Community Mental Health Center" (A–04–96–02118 and A–04–96–02124).

Activity-based Costing: A method to estimate costs of a service or product by measuring the costs of the activities it takes to produce that service or product.

methodology, called **activity-based costing** (ABC), is receiving increased attention by health care providers (see Perspective 12–3). ABC is based on the paradigm that activities consume resources and products consume activities (see Exhibit 12–6). Therefore, if activities or processes are controlled, then costs will be controlled. Similarly, if the resources for an activity can be measured, a more accurate picture of the actual costs of services can be found, as compared to traditional cost allocation. Such information can be extremely useful, as shown in Perspective 12–4.

Traditional cost allocation is called a top-down approach because it begins with all costs and allocates them downward into various services for which payment will be received (see Exhibit 12–7a). ABC, on the other hand, is called a bottom-up approach because it finds the cost of each service at the lowest level, the point at which resources are used, and aggregates them upward into products (see Exhibit 12–7b).

For example, in Exhibit 12–8, the service "Normal Delivery" comprises three intermediate products (or processes): prenatal visit, labor and delivery, and postpartum care. Each of these intermediate products comprises a number of activities. For example, the prenatal visit includes urinalysis, complete blood count (CBC), vital signs, recent history, etc. Each of these activities might also include a portion of what are usually considered indirect costs, such as those associated with ordering supplies, medical records, or financial counseling.

PERSPECTIVE 12–3

An On-line Article Discusses Activity Based Costing in Healthcare

To achieve continuous improvement, management must be informed. In healthcare, as with other businesses, the key is understanding the interrelationships of activities and taking actions to minimize waste and eliminate non-value-added costs. Simply put, that's what activity-based costing and activity-based management are all about.

The ABC model

ABC provides a better and more detailed cost model by allocating costs to activities based on the resources they consume. The model . . . links processes and resources.

For example, the case management department may assign case managers to specific clinical departments of service lines. In the traditional cost accounting model the case manager cost is allocated to other departments based on some gross measure such as patient days. This "peanut butter" allocation method assumes that case management is a generic commodity that is the same for an OB patient as a frail elderly cardiac surgery patient. Not likely.

The ABC model would look at each patient population and examine the case management process for each. What are the activities involved? How much case management time is consumed by each activity? What other resources are consumed? From this, more detailed cost allocation a more accurate picture or cost emerges. **More importantly, the relationship between activities and resources is more clear, making cost reduction easier.** Adding appropriate quality, patient satisfaction, outcomes, and clinical performance measures makes any process improvement more intelligent and less likely to reduce the quality of care.

. . . In their quest to reduce costs and develop an advantaged marketplace position, healthcare providers are discovering ABC. It offers an approach and the type of information required to realize performance breakthroughs:

- It recognizes that cost and quality are the direct result of the activities providers undertake to deliver services to their patients.
- It is business-process and end-product focused, and invites cooperation, rather than competition, between functional departments.
- It is developed based on the process knowledge and insight of those directly involved in the delivery of the service. In the case of patient care, physicians, nurses, therapists, et al, participate and contribute to its development.

As a result, activity-based cost information is both intuitive and logical. In short, it makes sense to those charged with the responsibility for improving performance and provides them with transparent information on the cost ramifications of their decisions. Example applications include:

- Evaluating the cost implications of alternative clinical pathways
- Streamlining care delivery practices across the care continuum
- Decision-making regarding management levels and spans of control
- Enhancing staff utilization by time of day
- Resourcing consolidated departments/deployed functions

Source: Robert Luttman & Associates Online Articles, Activity Based Costing, pp. 1–4 (http://www.robertluttman.com/activity_based_costing.html#Feature).

Exhibit 12–6   Products Result from Activities and Processes, which Result from the Utilization of Resources

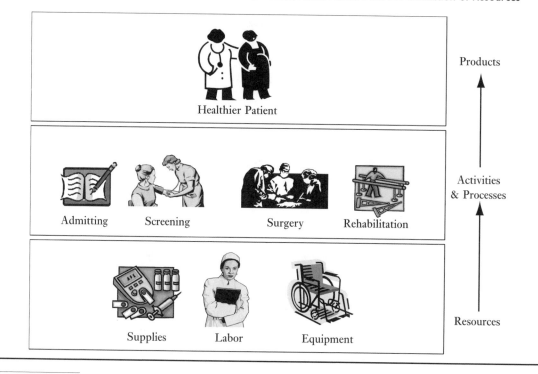

Products

Healthier Patient

Activities & Processes

Admitting   Screening   Surgery   Rehabilitation

Resources

Supplies   Labor   Equipment

Direct Costs: Costs which can be traced to a particular cost object.

Indirect Costs: Costs which cannot be traced to a particular cost object. Common indirect costs include billing, rent, utilities, information services, and overhead. Typically, these costs are allocated to cost objects according to an accepted formula (e.g. step-down method).

Cost Driver: That which causes a change in the cost of an activity.

Costing Terminology

Before continuing, it is important to understand three key terms: direct costs, indirect costs, and cost drivers. **Direct costs** are costs (e.g. nursing costs) that an organization can trace to a particular cost object (e.g. a patient). **Indirect costs** are costs that an organization is not able to directly trace to a particular cost object. For example, many health care organizations have great difficulty tracing to a particular patient or service such items as the cost of the billing clerk, rent, or information systems. Thus, a cost is direct or indirect not by its nature, but by the ability of the organization to trace it to a cost object.

An important difference between traditional cost allocation and ABC is how each handles indirect costs. Traditional cost allocation methods usually deal with indirect costs by allocating them to cost objects using relatively gross cause and effect relationships. ABC attempts to overcome this problem by more directly tracing costs to their cost objects and/or finding more precise cost drivers. **Cost drivers** are those things that cause a change in the cost of an activity.

For example, under traditional step-down costing, purchasing costs might be bundled with other administrative costs and allocated to a service based on the relative size of its budget. Under ABC it is more likely that the costs of purchasing would be allocated to that service more precisely on the basis of the number of purchase orders

PERSPECTIVE 12–4

Cost for Pricing at Blue Cross and Blue Shield of Florida

During the early 1990s, Blue Cross and Blue Shield of Florida, Inc. (BCBSF) faced an increasingly competitive and complex marketplace for its healthcare products and services, and its management structure and processes did not respond adequately to the market's different needs. To solve this problem, BCBSF identified specific objectives and strategies that divided the state into regions and market segments and sought to improve its management information tools and processes. . . .

BCBSF has a variety of products, customers, and delivery options that demand special services. Because the company has large work units and shared processes, managers need to be able to accurately identify the processes and administrative costs associated with the various products and customers. They do this through the CFP [Cost for Pricing] cost assignment process. . . .

Each activity in the company is undertaken for one of three general purposes: 1) to build or maintain a product, 2) to serve or sell to a customer, or 3) to perform general corporate duties. Furthermore, all costs incurred by the company must be recovered through the amounts that are charged to customers. Therefore, one policy decision made during the CFP design phase was to allocate all costs to products and customers.

Some of the company's activity costs relate directly to specific products and customers so are easy to allocate if the correct basis (that is, cost driver) data are provided. Other activities are conducted in support of broad categories of customers or products or even other cost centers. The allocations of these activity costs are more difficult to relate to specific products or customers and require that cost center managers identify who is supported and to what extent they consume the cost center resources. Finally, some activities are performed for the company as a whole or for the benefit of all customers and cannot be related to specific products or customers at all. These activity costs are allocated across all customers based on the total corporate activity.

A major advantage of cost for pricing is that it tracks and reports the costs associated with performing activities as they relate to particular products and customers in a timely, customized, and inexpensive manner. For example, the cost of providing customer service activities to a small group customer with a health maintenance organization (HMO) may be different from the cost of providing customer service activities to a larger, multi-state customer that has a preferred provider organization (PPO) product. This type of cost information is useful for pricing and profitability analysis. Also, management uses CFP information to identify and analyze cost variances and to benchmark and develop improvement programs. The model allows the company to manage and lower administrative expenses by providing more specific information about where these costs are incurred and their purpose. . . .

For example, the identification and costing of nonvalue-added administrative activities (processing unnecessary forms or performing redundant activities) can prompt management efforts to lower costs through the reduction and eventual elimination of such activities. The resources released could be used to improve the performance of value-added activities. Also, benchmarking may reveal high-cost activities that subsequent investigations show are the result of quality problems. For instance, low-quality explanations by associates to clients about their health insurance or the sale of inappropriate health insurance products to clients may lead to excessive written, telephone, and walk-in inquiries from subscribers. In addition to creating dissatisfied customers, these practices are likely to lead to higher salary costs from the increased staffing needed to address the extra customer service inquiries. . . .

Source: Kenneth L. Thurston, CPA, Dennis M. Deleman, and John B. MacArthur, *Management Accounting Quarterly*, Spring 2000, pp. 4–13.

Exhibit 12–7a　Comparison of Traditional and Activity-based Costing (Top Half)

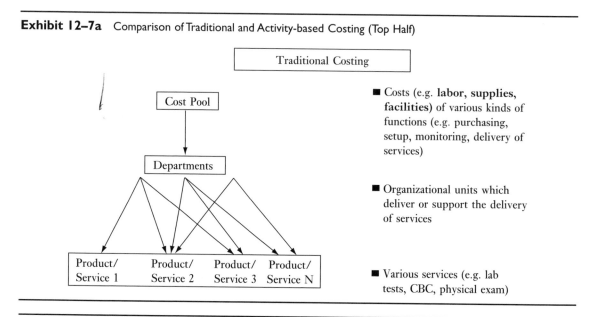

Traditional Costing

- Costs (e.g. **labor, supplies, facilities**) of various kinds of functions (e.g. purchasing, setup, monitoring, delivery of services)

- Organizational units which deliver or support the delivery of services

- Various services (e.g. lab tests, CBC, physical exam)

Exhibit 12–7b　Comparison of Traditional and Activity-based Costing (Lower Half)

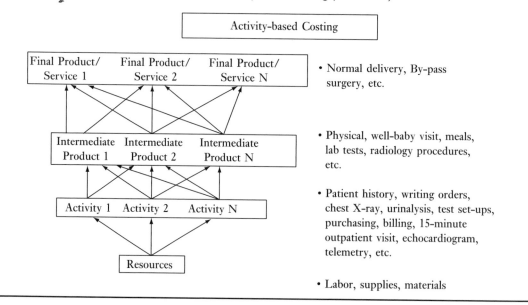

Activity-based Costing

- Normal delivery, By-pass surgery, etc.

- Physical, well-baby visit, meals, lab tests, radiology procedures, etc.

- Patient history, writing orders, chest X-ray, urinalysis, test set-ups, purchasing, billing, 15-minute outpatient visit, echocardiogram, telemetry, etc.

- Labor, supplies, materials

emanating from that service, or even more precisely by measuring the number of minutes spent processing purchase orders from that department.

An Example

Exhibit 12–9 compares the results of a more traditional cost allocation approach to that of an ABC approach. In this example, the organization is offering three outpatient

Exhibit 12–8 Examples of Intermediate Products and Activities for a Normal Delivery

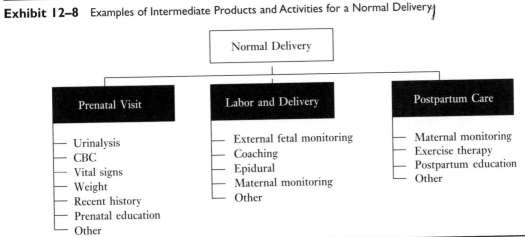

services: an initial visit, a routine regular visit, and an intensive visit. It is assumed that labor and materials can be directly traced to each type of visit, and, therefore, they do not vary between the two approaches. Thus, the main difference between the two approaches (as is often the case in practice) is the allocation of overhead. As explained below, the traditional approach uses a single cost driver, visits, and thus assigns the same overhead cost per visit, $17.50, to all three services (row 3, columns A, B, and C). The ABC approach, on the other hand, uses three cost drivers, and derives an overhead cost per visit of $28.88 for an initial visit, $13.65 for a regular visit, and $16.33 for an intensive visit (row 3, columns D, E, and F). Thus, relative to the traditional approach, the ABC approach estimates overhead cost to be $11.38 higher than the average $17.50 for an initial visit, and $3.85 and $1.17 lower for a regular and intensive visit, respectively (row 3, columns G, H, and I).

When spread across all 10,000 visits, these unit cost differences result in considerably different estimates of the total cost for each type of visit. Using the $17.50 estimate for overhead costs for each visit, the conventional method estimates the total costs of an initial, regular, and intensive visit to be, respectively: $130,000, $237,500, and $307,500 (row 8, columns A, B, and C). On the other hand, the ABC approach estimates the total cost of initial, regular, and intensive visits to be, respectively: $152,750, $218,250, and $304,000 (row 8, columns D, E, and F). Thus, the ABC approach estimates the initial visit cost $22,750 more than what was estimated using a conventional approach, and the regular and intensive visits cost $19,250 and $3,500 less, respectively, than the conventional approach's estimate (row 8, columns G, H, and I). Such differences can be highly significant when making decisions. In the case of the initial visits, the cost estimate differed by over 17 percent ($22,750/$130,000 = 0.175). Exhibit 12–10 illustrates more closely how the numbers in Exhibit 12–9 were derived.

In Exhibit 12–10, the total overhead cost is $175,000 (row 4, column D). Under the conventional method, it is assumed that all overhead costs are driven by visits. Thus, the $175,000 in overhead is divided by the 10,000 visits made during the year to calculate the average cost per visit for each type of visit, $17.50 (row 4, columns E, F, G, and H).

Exhibit 12-9 A Comparison of the Results of Using a Conventional versus an ABC Approach to Costing Three Services

	A	B	C		D	E	F
	Conventional Cost Method				**Activity-based Costing**		
	Visit Type				Visit Type		
Per Visit Costs	Initial	Regular	Intensive		Initial	Regular	Intensive
1 Direct Materials (etc.)	$2.50	$3.00	$10.00		$2.50	$3.00	$10.00
2 Direct Labor	$45.00	$27.00	$75.00		$45.00	$27.00	$75.00
3 Estimated Overhead	$17.50	$17.50	$17.50		$28.88	$13.65	$16.33
4 **Total Cost/Visit**	$65.00	$47.50	$102.50		$76.38	$43.65	$101.33
Total Visit Costs							
5 Direct Materials (etc.)	$5,000	$15,000	$30,000		$5,000	$15,000	$30,000
6 Direct Labor	$90,000	$135,000	$225,000		$90,000	$135,000	$225,000
7 Estimated Overhead	$35,000	$87,500	$52,500		$57,750	$68,250	$49,000
8 **Total Costs**	$130,000	$237,500	$307,500		$152,750	$218,250	$304,000

	G	H	I
	Difference in Cost Estimates		
	[ABC – Conventional]		
	Visit Type		
Per Visit Costs	Initial	Regular	Intensive
1 Direct Materials (etc.)	$0.00	$0.00	$0.00
2 Direct Labor	$0.00	$0.00	$0.00
3 Estimated Overhead	$11.38	($3.85)	($1.17)
4 **Total Cost/Visit**	$11.38	($3.85)	($1.17)
Total Visit Costs			
5 Direct Materials (etc.)	$0.00	$0.00	$0.00
6 Direct Labor	$0.00	$0.00	$0.00
7 Estimated Overhead	$22,750	($19,250)	($3,500)
8 **Total Costs**	$22,750	($19,250)	($3,500)

/ **Exhibit 12-10/** A Comparison of a Conventional and an ABC Approach to Costing Three Services

Basic Data and Calculation of Unit costs Using a Conventional Approach

	Total Cost by Visit Type				Calculation of Cost/Unit by Visit Type			
	Basic Data							
	A Initial [Given]	B Regular [Given]	C Intensive [Given]	D Total [A+B+C]	E Initial	F Regular	G Intensive	H Cost/Unit Formula:
1 Number of Visits	2,000	5,000	3,000	10,000				
2 Direct Materials (etc.)	$5,000	$15,000	$30,000	$50,000	$2.50	$3.000	$10.00	[Row 2/Row 1]
3 Direct Labor	$90,000	$135,000	$225,000	$450,000	$45.00	$27.00	$75.00	[Row 3 / Row 1]
4 Estimated Overhead [Total is a Given]				$175,000	$17.50	$17.50	$17.50	[D4/D1]
5 Cost/Visit: Conventional Method					$65.00	$47.50	$102.50	[Sum(Rows 2-4)]

1) Basic Data, Annual Projections of Overhead Costs by Activity; 2) Unit Cost Calculations for These Overhead Activities

Activity	I Cost [Given]	J Driver [Given]	K Units [Given]		L Unit Cost [I/K]	
6 Intake	$17,500	New Visits	2,500	New Visits	$7.00	Per New Visit
7 Medical Records	$17,500	Hours Spent	2,040	Hours	$8.58	Per Hour
8 Billing	$35,000	Hours Spent	4,080	Hours	$8.58	Per Hour
9 Other	$105,000	Visits	10,000	Visits	$10.50	Per Visit
10 Total	$175,000					

Additional Basic Data

Basic Data: Actual Annual Operating Results of Cost Drivers to Be Used in Assigning ABC Overhead Cost

| | | Visit Type | | |
	M Initial [Given]	N Regular [Given]	O Intensive [Given]	P Total [M+N+O]
11 New Visits	2,000	250	250	2,500
12 Medical Records	612	816	612	2,040
13 Billing	2,040	816	1,224	4,080
14 Other	2,000	5,000	3,000	10,000

(Continues)

Exhibit 12–10 *(Contd)*

Derivation of Unit Costs Using an ABC Approach

Calculation of Total and Per Visit Overhead Costs Using ABC

		Q	R	S	T	U
			Visit Type			
		Initial	Regular	Intensive	Total	Formula
15	New Visits	$14,000	$1,750	$1,750	$17,500	[L6 × Row 11]
16	Medical Records	$5,250	$7,000	$5,250	$17,500	[L7 × Row 12]
17	Billing	$17,500	$7,000	$10,500	$35,000	[L8 × Row 13]
18	Other	$21,000	$52,500	$31,500	$105,000	[L9 × Row 14]
19	Total	$57,750	$68,250	$49,000	$175,000	[Sum (Rows 15–18)]
20	Per Visit	*$28.88*	*$13.65*	*$16.33*	*$17.50*	[Row 19/Row 1]

Unit Cost Estimates ABC

		V	W	X	Y
	ABC		Visit Type		
		Initial	Regular	Intensive	Formula
21	Direct Materials	$2.50	$3.00	$10.00	[Row 2, Cols E,F,G]
22	Direct Labor	$45.00	$27.00	$75.00	[Row 3, Cols E,F,G]
23	*Overhead*	$28.88	$13.65	$16.33	[Row 20]]
24	Total using ABC	**$76.38**	**$43.65**	**$101.33**	[Sum(Rows 21–23)]

Comparison of Unit Costs: ABC v. Conventional

	Z	AA	AB	AC	AD
		Visit Type			
	Initial	Regular	Intensive		Formula
25 Total Conventional	$65.00	$47.50	$102.50		[Row 5, Cols E,F,G]
26 Amount ABC Estimate is More (Less) Than Conventional	$11.38	($3.85)	($1.17)		[Row 24 - Row 25]

Comparison of Total Costs: ABC v. Conventional

	AE	AF	AG	AH	AI
		Visit Type		Total	
	Initial	Regular	Intensive	[AE+AF+AG]	Formula
Acitivity Based Costing Method					
27 Number of Visits	2,000	5,000	3,000	10,000	[Row 1]
28 Direct Materials	$5,000	$15,000	$30,000	$50,000	[Row 2]
29 Direct Labor	$90,000	$135,000	$225,000	$450,000	[Row 3]
30 *Overhead*	$57,750	$68,250	$49,000	$175,000	[Row 27 × Row 23]
31 Total ABC	$152,750	$218,250	$304,000	$675,000	[Sum (Rows 28–30)]
Conventional Method					
32 Direct Materials	$5,000	$15,000	$30,000	$50,000	[Row 2]
33 Direct Labor	$90,000	$135,000	$225,000	$450,000	[Row 3]
34 *Overhead*	$35,000	$87,500	$52,500	$175,000	[Row 27 × Row 5, E,F,G]
35 Total Conventional	$130,000	$237,500	$307,500	$675,000	[Sum(Rows 32–34)]
36 Amount ABC Estimate is More (Less) Than Conventional	$22,750	($19,250)	($3,500)	$0	Row 31 - Row 35

Rather than assuming that overhead costs are driven solely by the number of visits, the ABC approach assumes multiple cost drivers. In this case, the ABC approach breaks down overhead costs into four categories and looks more closely at what may be driving the $175,000 overhead cost. The four categories are: the *intake process*, *medical records*, *billing*, and *other* (see rows 6–9). The *intake process* occurs when background information is gathered and an account is set up for each new patient. It is assumed that these costs occur each time a new patient visit occurs; thus, the cost driver is a new-patient visit (row 6, column J). Assuming that the total salaries and benefits of all the employees engaged in this process are $17,500 (row 6, column I) and there are 2,500 visits a year (row 6, column K), the intake process costs the organization $7.00 ($17,500/$2,500) for each new patient (row 6, column L). Since there were 2,000 new patients making initial visits, 250 new patients each making a regular visit (referrals), and 250 patients making an intensive visit (row 11, columns M, N, O, and P), it costs $14,000 for the intake process for these new patients ($7.00/patient × 2,000 new patients), and $1,750 each ($7.00/patient × 250 patients) for regular and intensive visits, respectively (row 15, columns Q, R, S, T, and U).

The second category, *medical records*, refers to the process of coding and charting the visit onto the medical records (row 7). Since it is assumed that these costs are driven by the time spent coding and charting, the cost driver is hours spent (row 7, column J). Since the salary and benefit costs associated with medical records are $17,500 and there are 2,040 hours devoted to this activity, the cost per hour is $8.58 (row 7, columns I, J, K, and L). The medical records staff estimates that it spent 30, 40, and 30 percent of its time with initial, regular, and intensive visit records, respectively. This equates to 612, 816, and 612 hours for each of the respective types of visits (row 12, columns M, N, O, and P). At $8.58 per hour, the initial visits medical record cost is $5,250 ($8.58/hour × 612 hours), while the regular and intensive visit medical record costs are $7,000 ($8.58/hour × 816 hours) and $5,250 ($8.58/hour × 612 hours), respectively (row 16, columns Q, R, S, T, and U).

The billing costs and other costs are derived in a similar manner to those just discussed. When this process is completed, the estimated total overhead cost of initial visits is $57,750, while those of regular and intensive visits are $68,250 and $49,000 respectively (row 19, columns Q, R, and S). Dividing these numbers by the number of visits in their respective categories (rows 1, 19, and 20) results in the per visit cost estimates of $28.88 ($57,750/2,000 visits) for initial visits, $13.65 ($68,250/5,000 visits) for regular visits, and $16.33 ($49,000/3,000 visits) for intensive visits. As can be seen, these numbers are quite different from the $17.50 overhead cost per visit estimated using the conventional approach.

The various parts are now in place to compare costs using a conventional approach and an ABC approach. Under the ABC approach, the per visit costs for an Initial, Regular, and Intensive visit, respectively, are $76.38, $43.65, and $101.33 (row 24, columns V, W, and X). Under the conventional method, they are $65.00, $47.50, and $102.50, respectively, for these same types of visits (row 25, columns Z, AA, and AB). Thus, on a comparative basis, the ABC approach estimates that the cost of an Initial visit is $11.38 higher than that of the cost calculated using the conventional approach, and the costs of a Regular and Intensive visit, respectively, are $3.85 and $1.17 lower (row 26, columns Z, AA, and AB).

The differences between the cost per visit estimates using ABC and a conventional approach are totally due to how the overhead is handled. The conventional approach used a single cost driver, total visits, to derive a $17.50 per visit overhead rate (row 4, columns E, F, and G). The ABC approach decomposed overhead into four separate categories of activities: intake, medical records, billing, and other. It then determined the unit cost of each type of activity based upon what was driving these costs: new visits for intake, hours worked for medical records and billing, and visits for all other overhead activities (rows 6–9, columns I, J, K, and L). Thus, the ABC approach more closely matched the actual usage of resources by each type of visit.

In today's environment, the importance of having the more accurate estimate from ABC cannot be overemphasized. For example, assume the practice was negotiating a contract for Initial visits with a managed care organization that offered to pay $75 per visit. If the provider thought its costs were $65.00, as derived by the conventional method, it might accept the offer. However, with the more accurate information of the cost being $76.38 per visit, the provider might very well reject the offer, or certainly negotiate a higher rate. If it could not negotiate a higher rate, and were it not for the ABC method, it might very well be satisfied under the conventional method, for it would assume it was making a profit on each visit. However, armed with the ABC cost estimate, it would be driven to look for cost reductions to reduce its unit cost from $76.38 to closer to or below the $75 being offered.

There are a number of other differences between the traditional step-down and ABC methods, but a discussion of these is beyond the scope of this text. However, in many cases these two methods are likely to yield vastly different estimates of cost. While the step-down method is relatively inexpensive to implement and may provide an adequate estimate in some cases, those using ABC feel it provides several advantages, including increased accuracy and insights on how to control processes and, thus, costs. In the future, the management of most health care facilities will be faced with weighing the relatively low costs of the step-down method against the added costs, greater precision, and cost-control of ABC. In an increasingly cost-driven health care system, it is likely that ABC will gain greater prominence.

◀SUMMARY▶

Because they are assuming more risk, providers must be able to measure their costs accurately. Providers generally use one of three approaches: the cost-to-charge ratio, the step-down method, or activity-based costing (ABC). The step-down method finds costs by allocating those costs that are not directly paid for into those products or services to which payment is attached. It is a top-down approach, because it begins with all costs and allocates them downward into various services for which payment will be received. As a result of methodological idiosyncrasies, those performing a step-down cost finding must pay considerable attention to the order of allocation, the allocation basis, and the number of cost centers. The step-down method is useful for pricing and reimbursement-related decisions, but should not be used to control costs.

Activity-based costing (ABC) not only finds costs, but also helps to control costs. ABC is a bottom–up approach, because it finds the cost of each service at the point at which resources are used and then aggregates them upward into products. ABC is based on the paradigm that activities consume resources and processes consume activities. Therefore, since the use of resources is what causes cost (by definition), if activities or processes are controlled, then costs will be controlled. Similarly, if the resource use of an activity can be measured, then a more accurate picture of the actual costs of services can be determined.

◀KEY TERMS▶

ACTIVITY-BASED COSTING	COST OBJECT	FULLY ALLOCATED COSTS
ALLOCATION BASE	COST-TO-CHARGE RATIO	INDIRECT COSTS
COST DRIVERS	DIRECT COSTS	STEP-DOWN METHOD

◀QUESTIONS AND PROBLEMS▶

1. **Definitions.** Define the following terms:
   a. Activity-based Costing.
   b. Allocation Base.
   c. Cost Driver.
   d. Cost Object.
   e. Cost-to-charge Ratio (CCR).
   f. Direct Costs.
   g. Fully Allocated Cost.
   h. Indirect Costs.
   i. Step-down Method.
2. **Cost-to-charge Ratio.** What is the basic concept of the cost-to-charge ratio method of estimating costs? Give an example.
3. **Cost-to-charge Ratio.** Discuss the four major concerns of using the cost-to-charge ratio method.
4. **Step-down Method.** Discuss how the step-down method of cost allocation derives its name.
5. **Cost Allocation and Cost Drivers.** What is the relationship between the concepts *cost allocation basis* as used in the step-down method and *cost driver* as used in ABC?

6. **Fully Allocated Costs.** What is the difference between a cost object's direct cost and its fully allocated cost? Give an example.

7. **Step-down Method.** Identify and discuss four points that must be considered when using the step-down method of cost allocation.

8. **ABC and Step-down Methods.** What are the advantages and disadvantages of ABC relative to the step-down method of cost allocation?

9. **Activity-based Costing.** In Exhibit 12–10, suppose that instead of 2,000, 5,000 and 3,000 visits for an initial, regular, and intensive visit, respectively, the number of visits was 3,000, 5,000 and 2,000. Assume that the intake, new visits, medical records, and billing costs do not change in number or distribution.
   a. Would there be a change in the overhead cost *per visit* of an initial visit using either the conventional or ABC methods?
   b. Would there be a change in the *total* overhead cost of initial visits using either the conventional or ABC methods?

10. **Activity-based Costing.** In Exhibit 12–10, suppose that instead of 2,000, 5,000 and 3,000 visits for an initial, regular, and intensive visit, respectively, the number of visits was 2,500, 6,000 and 1,500. Assume that the intake, new visits, medical records, and billing costs do not change in number or distribution.
   a. Would there be a change in the overhead cost *per visit* of an initial visit using either the conventional or ABC methods?
   b. Would there be a change in the *total* overhead cost of initial visits using either the conventional or ABC methods?

11. **Cost Allocation.** Use the information in Exhibit 12–11 to answer these questions.
   a. David Paul, the new administrator for the surgical clinic, was trying to figure out how to allocate his indirect expenses. His staff were complaining that the current method of taking a percentage of revenues was unfair. He decided to try to allocate utilities based on

Exhibit 12–11   Basic Statistics for Cost Allocation in Surgery Clinic A

	A Square Feet	B Direct Costs	C Lab Tests
Utilities		$200,000	
Administration	2,000	$500,000	
Laboratory	2,000	$625,000	
Day-op Suite	3,000	$1,400,000	4,000
Cystoscopy	1,500	$350,000	500
Endoscopy	1,500	$300,000	500
Total	10,000	$3,375,000	5,000

Exhibit 12–12 Basic Statistics for Cost Allocation in Surgery Clinic B

	Sq. Feet	Direct Costs	Lab Tests
Utilities		$100,000	
Administration	1,500	$400,000	
Laboratory	3,000	$725,000	
Day-op Suite	4,500	$1,200,000	4,000
Cystoscopy	2,500	$400,000	500
Endoscopy	3,000	$350,000	500
Total	14,500	$3,175,000	5,000

square footage for each department, to allocate administration based on direct costs, and to allocate laboratory based on tests. What would the results be?

b. Kathleen Aceti, the nurse manager of the cysto suite, was given approval to add more space to her current area by converting 500 square feet of administrative space into another cystoscopy bay. What will her new fully allocated expenses be? (Assume there are no new additional costs incurred by adding the 500 square feet.)

c. Mara Kelsey, the manager of the endoscopy suite, was concerned about adding more space to cystoscopy. She contends that if the two units were combined, fewer staff would be needed and direct costs could be reduced by $50,000 ($25,000 in each unit). She also feels that the Day-Op area is underutilized, and that 500 square feet could be used by a combined unit when excess capacity was needed. Assuming the 500 square feet were to be allocated equally between the endoscopy suite and cystoscopy, what would the total allocated costs for each of these two services be under this scenario?

12. **Cost Allocation.** Use the information in Exhibit 12–12 to answer these questions.

a. David Paul, the new administrator for the surgical clinic, was trying to figure out how to allocate his indirect expenses. He decided to try to allocate utilities based on square footage of each department, to allocate administration based on direct costs, and to allocate laboratory based on tests. How would indirect costs be distributed as a result?

b. Nick Zeeman, the Director of Labs, was given approval to add 250 square feet of space to the lab by expanding into the Day-Op Suite, which lost the space. What will his new fully allocated expenses be? (Assume there are no new additional costs incurred by adding the 250 square feet.)

c. Callie Zev, the Manager of the endoscopy suite, was concerned about adding more space to cystoscopy. She contends that if the two units were combined, fewer staff would be needed and direct costs could be reduced by $40,000 ($20,000 in each unit). She also feels that the Day-Op area is underutilized, and that 200 square feet could be used by a combined unit when excess capacity was needed. Assuming the 200 square feet were to be allocated equally between the endoscopy suite and cystoscopy, what would the total allocated costs for each of these two services be under this scenario?

13. **Traditional and Activity-based Costing.** Use the information in Exhibit 12–13 to answer these questions.
 a. What is the *per unit* cost of an initial, regular, and intensive visit using the conventional and ABC approaches?
 b. What is the *total cost* of initial, regular, and intensive visits using the conventional and ABC approaches?

14. **Traditional and Activity-based Costing.** Use the information in Exhibit 12–14 to answer these questions.
 a. What is the *per unit* cost of an initial, regular, and intensive visit using the conventional and ABC approaches?
 b. What is the total cost of initial, regular, and intensive visits using the conventional and ABC approaches?

Exhibit 12–13   Data for Clinic C

Basic Data and Calculation of Unit Costs Using a Conventional Approach

	Total Cost by Visit Type			
	Basic Data			
	A Initial [Given]	**B** Regular [Given]	**C** Intensive [Given]	**D** Total [A + B + C]
1 Number of Visits	5,000	10,000	5,000	20,000
2 Direct Materials (etc.)	$21,000	$14,000	$35,000	$70,000
3 Direct Labor	$80,000	$80,000	$240,000	$400,000
4 Estimated Overhead [Total is a Given]				$150,000
5 **Cost/Visit: Conventional Method**				

Additional Basic Data

Basic Data: Annual Projections of Overhead Costs by Activity

Activity	**I**	**J**	**K**
		Cost Driver Information	
	Cost [Given]	Driver [Given]	Units [Given]
6 Intake	$22,500	New Visits	2,500 New Visits
7 Medical Records	$22,500	Time Spent	2,040 Hours
8 Billing	$45,000	Time Spent	4,080 Hours
9 Other	$60,000	Visits	20,000 Visits
10 Total	$150,000		

Basic Data: Actual Annual Operating Results of Cost Drivers to be Used to Assign ABC Overhead Cost

	M	**N**	**O**	**P**
		Visit Type		
	Initial [Given]	Regular [Given]	Intensive [Given]	Total [M + N + O]
11 New Visits	1,500	750	250	2,500
12 Medical Records	204	612	1,224	2,040
13 Billing	2,040	816	1,224	4,080
14 Other	5,000	10,000	5,000	20,000

Exhibit 12–14 Data for Clinic D

Basic Data and Calculation of Unit Costs Using a Conventional Approach

| | Total Cost by Visit Type | | | |
| | Basic Data | | | |
	A Initial [Given]	B Regular [Given]	C Intensive [Given]	D Total [A+B+C]
1 Number of Visits	3,000	7,500	4,500	15,000
2 Direct Materials (etc.)	$5,000	$10,000	$35,000	$50,000
3 Direct Labor	$52,500	$70,000	$227,500	$350,000
4 Estimated Overhead [Total is a Given]				$125,000
5 Cost/Visit: Conventional Method				

Basic Data: Annual Projections of Overhead Costs by Activity

Activity	I Cost [Given]	J Driver [Given]	K Cost Driver Information Units [Given]
6 Intake	$25,000	New Visits	1,000 New Visits
7 Medical Records	$25,000	Time Spent	2,040 Hours
8 Billing	$37,500	Time Spent	4,080 Hours
9 Other	$37,500	Visits	15,000 Visits
10 Total	$125,000		

Basic Data: Actual Annual Operating Results of Cost Drivers to be Used to Assign ABC Overhead Cost

| | M Initial [Given] | N Regular [Given] | O Intensive [Given] | P Total [M+N+O] |
		Visit Type		
11 New Visits	800	100	100	1,000
12 Medical Records	612	816	612	2,040
13 Billing	2,040	816	1,224	4,080
14 Other	3,000	7,500	4,500	15,000

Additional Basic Data

Chapter Thirteen

PROVIDER PAYMENT SYSTEMS

LEARNING OBJECTIVES

After completing this chapter, you will be able to:

▶ Identify the history, theory, and characteristics of the major types of payment systems.
▶ Identify the tactics payors and providers use to reduce their financial risk.
▶ Determine the cost per member per month for specific procedures.
▶ Understand the new wave of innovations in health care payment systems.

Chapter Outline

(Continues)

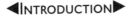

◀INTRODUCTION▶

This chapter provides an introduction to the development of the *health care payment system* in the United States and some of the basic methods used to determine health care payments. The evolution of the payment system will be emphasized in light of the ongoing public policy debate about the roles, responsibilities, and effects of the payment system on various stakeholders, including:

- Patients.
- Providers, including physicians, institutional providers, and ancillary providers (e.g. physical therapists, laboratories, hospices, and home care providers).
- Employers.
- Payors, including various levels of government agencies and managed care organizations.
- Regulators, including governmental and private agencies (e.g. the Joint Commission on Accreditation of Healthcare Organizations and the National Committee for Quality Assurance).

Simply put, this debate has been over "Who gets paid?," "How much?," "By whom?," "For what types of services?," and "With what consequence?"

All health care systems attempt to balance cost, quality, and access. Over the years, each of these three facets has received more or less emphasis in the US health care system as various stakeholders have asked and attempted to answer such questions as: "For the cost, are we getting sufficient quality and access?" (see Perspective 13–1) and "What would it cost to provide better quality care to the uninsured and underinsured?" While this debate continues, it largely focuses on the roles of governmental entities, payors and providers, not individual consumers (See Exhibit 13–1). Meanwhile, health care providers are on the front line every day, trying to balance their missions and their margins, walking a fine line between the art of healing, the science of medicine, and the business of health care.

In order to truly understand the current health care payment system, it is important to have insight into how it has evolved (see Exhibit 13–2).

Payor: An entity that is responsible for paying for the services of a health care provider. Typically, this is an insurance company or a government agency.

PERSPECTIVE 13–1

The World's Health Care: How Do We Rank?

The United States spends a great deal on health care but gains too little, says the World Health Organization.

    Health care in the United States is second to none. Right? Well, not according to the World Health Organization. A recent WHO survey ranked the United States 37th in overall health system performance – sandwiched between Costa Rica and Slovenia. This dismal showing occurred despite the fact that the United States spends more on healthcare – 13.7% of its gross domestic product – than any other of the 191 WHO nations.

Source: Susan Landers, AMNews staff, August 28, 2000.

Exhibit 13–1   Key Elements in the Debate Undergirding the Health Care Payment System in the United States

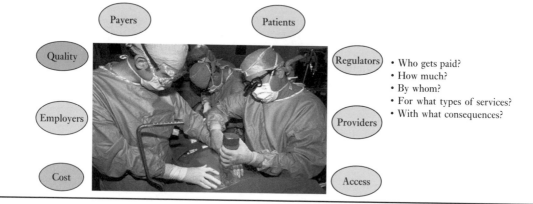

- Payers
- Patients
- Quality
- Regulators
- Employers
- Providers
- Cost
- Access

- Who gets paid?
- How much?
- By whom?
- For what types of services?
- With what consequences?

Prior to the late 1920s and early 1930s, health care was funded primarily by the patient. The growth of the country's population, however, brought additional costs in the form of more doctors and more health care facilities. The burden of paying for health care shifted to the employer and later to government. A summary of key events in this evolution follows, ending with some future trends.

◄HISTORICAL PERSPECTIVE ON PAYMENT SYSTEMS►

The "Early" Years (1929–1965)

Defining events	Industry trends
BC/BS established 1929	Advent of indemnity insurance
Kaiser established 1930s	Rapid growth of hospitals (inpatient focus)
Hill-Burton Hospital Construction Act 1946	Employers largely passive

Exhibit 13–2 Key Events in the Evolution of the Health Care Payment System in the United States

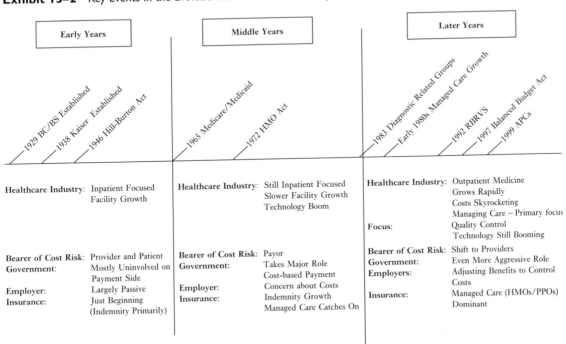

The payment system during this period was largely composed of a combination of **charge-based, fee-for-service**, and employer-based **indemnity insurance**. Typically, regardless of the extent of employer involvement in the payment for health services (whether the employer paid a portion, all, or none of the charges for the services), the provider was the price setter. Despite the massive amount of government funding created for facility development, there was relatively little federal or state government involvement as payors.

Charge-based: A method of payment which is based on the charge of the provider.

Blue Cross and Blue Shield Established

In 1929, Justin Ford Kimball, an official at Baylor University in Dallas, introduced a plan to guarantee schoolteachers 21 days of hospital care for $6 per year. Other groups of employees in the area soon joined the plan, known as the Baylor Plan, and the idea attracted national attention. By 1939, the Blue Cross symbol was officially adopted by a commission of the American Hospital Association (AHA) as the national emblem for plans like the Baylor Plan that met certain guidelines.

Blue Cross and Blue Shield (BC/BS) plans were attractive to both consumers and providers. They guaranteed that payment would be made for covered services (such as 21 days in the hospital). All covered individuals paid their **premium**

Fee-for-service: A method of reimbursement based on payment for services rendered, with a specific fee correlated to each specific service. An insurance company, the patient or a government program such as Medicare or Medicaid (discussed later) may make payment.

based on "**community rating**," and payment was made directly to the hospital. In terms common today, a **third party** (the payor, BC/BS in this case) would pay the **second party** (the provider, hospitals in this case) on behalf of the **first party** (the patient).

As a result of wage freezes (due primarily to the United State's involvement in the Second World War) labor forces resorted to bargaining for more benefits, including better health care coverage. It was at this time that private, for-profit, insurance companies began to be major competitors with BC/BS plans. It was during this period (the late 1930s) that the Kaiser Health Plan began. The Kaiser Engineering Company provided a health care benefit for its employees who were involved in the construction of the Grand Coulee Dam and the Los Angeles Aqueduct by providing physician services in a company-sponsored clinic and hospital services at local hospitals.

Along with a few other prepaid health care plans, the Kaiser Plan grew throughout the 1940s and 1950s, expanding beyond the realm of its own employees, and became the prototypical staff model *Health Maintenance Organization* (HMO). In the Kaiser Plan, physicians were salaried, patients received care in a controlled environment, and all services (except hospital services) were provided in a single facility. (HMOs are addressed in greater detail later in this chapter.)

With the population boom after the Second World War, and with the continued industrialization of the USA, a great need arose for the development of adequate health care facilities – in particular, hospital beds and support facilities. The *Hill-Burton Act* of 1946 provided government supported grants to build and upgrade hospitals.

Prior to 1946, the US hospital system had evolved with great disparities in facilities and accessibility. With about one-third of the country's counties without a hospital and many of the existing facilities of substandard quality, the intent of this legislation was to fund development in geographic areas that were without health care facilities. During the period between 1947 and 1975 (the end of Hill-Burton expenditures), almost 7,000 hospitals received assistance, with many rural areas gaining access to hospital care for the first time.

The "Middle" Years (1965–1983)

Defining events	Industry trends
Medicare/Medicaid established	Indemnity insurance growth
HMO Act	Managed care catching on
	Technology boom on the horizon
	Cost risk shifts to payor
	Employers concerned about costs

During the middle years, governments became heavily involved as payors through two new programs (Medicare and Medicaid), employers played a relatively passive role, and there was a trend toward trying to manage care and a movement away from the provider as a price-setter.

Because of the influence of the government as a payor, the late 1960s and 1970s represented a plateau in the evolution of payment systems. Medical costs, while still rising during this period, were relatively manageable. Employers, while concerned about cost, continued to pay for rich health care benefits. Technology was beginning to boom but had not yet advanced to the point where it materially affected the cost of providing or paying for services. Indemnity insurance dominated, and providers were generally satisfied with the payment systems employed during this time. For the most part, payment systems revolved around cost-based and charge-based methodologies, an overview of which can be found in Appendix H.

Increasing Concerns about Costs and Access

While the Hill-Burton Act improved access by catalyzing the construction of new hospitals, paying for the care provided at these new and improved facilities (and new technology associated with them) was becoming increasingly expensive. While being employed was one way to access health care coverage, there was a growing concern about the ability to pay for care by the unemployed, the under-insured (perhaps self-employed or employed by an employer not offering an insurance benefit, for example), the poor, the young, the elderly, and the disabled. Thus, much of the national debate focused on the issue of access to care.

Medicare and Medicaid

The government's role in the payment of health care, which to this point had been passive (on both a federal and a state-specific basis), changed dramatically in the mid-1960s with President Lyndon Johnson's administration. The formation of a "Medical Care" program (Medicare), established largely to help pay for care of those 65 years and older, and the creation of a companion "Medical Aid" program (Medicaid), designed to provide assistance to the medically indigent and those with certain categories of disabilities, marked the beginning of a new era in US health care (see Exhibit 13–3).

At its inception, Medicare paid hospitals based on the hospital's costs, using **Cost-based Reimbursement** paid on a retrospective basis. At the end of a period after care was provided (typically, at the end of a year), the hospital would submit a report, the *Medicare Cost Report*, detailing all of the costs associated with the provision of Medicare services throughout that period. The government, in turn, would scrutinize the costs being claimed and would allow or disallow costs on the basis of standards.

Also during this period, the HMO Act of 1972 was passed under the administration of Richard Nixon. This had a major impact on the management of care in later years by empowering the staff model HMO (discussed later) to become a common system practiced outside of the mainstream medical society. The Act allowed certain

The Third Party: Typically, the payor (insurance company/government agency) in a health care encounter.

Medicare: A nationwide, federally financed health insurance program for people age 65 and older. It also covers certain people under 65 who are disabled or have chronic kidney (end-stage renal) disease. Medicare Part A is the hospital insurance program; Part B covers physicians' services. Created by the 1965 amendment to the Social Security Act.

Medicaid: A federally mandated program, operated and partially funded by individual states (in conjunction with the federal government) to provide medical benefits to certain low-income people. The state, under broad federal guidelines, determines what benefits are covered, who is eligible, and how much providers will be paid.

Cost-based Reimbursement: Using the provider's cost of providing services (i.e. supplies, staff salaries, space costs, etc.) as the basis for reimbursement.

Exhibit 13–3   Medicare and Medicaid Entitlement Programs

	Medicare	Medicaid
Who Pays for Program?	Federal Tax on Income	Federal and State Tax on Income (Feds pay larger share based on State's per capita income)
Who Is Covered?	• People aged 65 and older • Some people with disabilities under age 65 • People with end-stage renal disease	• People with disabilities • The poor • Needy women and children
How Many Are Covered?	1980: 28.5 Million 1990: 34.2 Million 1999: 39.9 Million	1981: 20.2 Million 1990: 23.9 Million 1999: 42.2 Million
Percent of Americans Covered	14%	15%
Percent of Older Americans Covered (65+)	97%	–
Expenditures	1980: 36 Billion 1990: 108 Billion 1999: 212 Billion	1980: 24.7 Billion 1990: 71.2 Billion 1999: 159.2 Billion
Percent of Total Health Care Expenditures (1999)	17.6%	15.4%
Predicted Enrollment in 2010	46.6 Million (22% of total population)	46.7 Million (22.04% of total population)

Source: Webpage: http://www.hcfa.gov, August, 2000

Retrospective Payment: Method for reimbursing a provider after the service has been delivered.

Allowable Costs: Costs which are allowable under the principles of reimbursement under government (Medicaid, Medicare) and other payors.

Managed Care: Any of a number of arrangements designed to control health care costs through monitoring, prescribing, or proscribing the provision of health care to a patient or population.

competitive advantages for qualifying HMOs, but these generally languished and became more interested in cost containment.

The "Later" Years (1984 to the Present)

Defining events	Industry trends
Diagnosis Related Groups	Managed care is dominant theme
RBRVS	Government taking more aggressive role
Balanced Budget Act	Flat fee payment systems
APCs	Costs shift back to provider
	Technology booming
	Employers adjusting benefits to control costs
	Quality control becomes a major issue

Health care infrastructure and technology grew exponentially over the early and middle years of the modern health care era. Programs such as Medicare and Medicaid, which were originally designed to fill relatively small gaps in access, felt the brunt of this growth. Because of this, the government was experiencing unexpected difficulties trying to pay for the benefits it had created. Employers, as well, were growing increasingly concerned with the question of cost containment, as health care costs and employee health benefits began to eat into corporate profits. Other payors were also experiencing difficulties in matching the premiums they were receiving with the payments they were making to providers. This set the stage for a change of the locus of risk from the payor to the provider.

DRGs

It was at this point that the government changed its reimbursement methodology for Medicare from a cost-based payment system to a **Prospective Payment System,** commonly known as the **DRG (Diagnostic Related Groups)** system. Prospective payment shifts the risk from payor to provider. In this system, the provider is paid a predetermined flat amount for an inpatient admission. If the provider's costs are below that flat amount, the hospital retains the difference. However, they are at risk for the amount their costs exceed the payment they receive. Therefore, it becomes extremely important for the hospital to understand and control its costs, while maintaining appropriate levels of access and quality.

Under the DRG system, the government's payment to providers of inpatient services for Medicare recipients is based upon a *flat rate* (see below) for all services rendered in each of the over 500 diagnosis-based categories. Each DRG serves to group clinically similar services together in a way that accounts for predicted resource consumption. Each of these predetermined groupings is then assigned a DRG payment. DRGs are ultimately intended to account for case mix, or the acuity of services required in caring for the patient. For example, an inpatient stay involving neurosurgery and an intense recovery will be paid a much higher rate than will one involving a normal obstetric delivery.

DRG payments are based on an adjusted average payment rate. In essence, a relatively minor, commonly performed procedure is established as a baseline (1.000) against which all other procedures are weighted. These weights are then adjusted for geographic differences. For example, a relatively simple procedure/diagnosis, such a skin graft for injury, might be weighted slightly higher, at 1.709; a medical stay driven by asthma might be slightly lower, at 0.5873; and a heart transplant requiring extensive resources might be weighted at 19.0098 (see Exhibit 13–4). A hospital's payment is unaffected by the length of stay prior to discharge; it is expected that some patients will stay longer than others, and hospitals will offset the higher costs of a longer stay with the lower costs of a reduced stay. The government regularly updates both the DRG weights and the geographic adjustments.

These efforts by the government defined the third era of payment systems: "The Later Years" and the entry of many payors into the world of flat fee payment.

Prospective Payment System: A payment method that establishes rates, prices or budgets before services are rendered and costs are incurred. Providers retain or absorb at least a portion of the difference between established revenues and actual costs.

Predetermined Rates: A set fee paid to a provider for an inpatient episode of care.

Flat Fee: A predefined amount of money paid to a provider for a unit of service.

DRGs: A patient classification scheme used by Medicare that clusters patients into categories on the basis of patients' illnesses, diseases and medical problems. These classifications are then used to pay providers a set amount based on the diagnostic related group in which the patient has been classified.

Exhibit 13–4 Examples of Diagnostic Related Groups

DRG	DESCRIPTION	RELATIVE WEIGHT FY – 2001	Geographic Adjustment[1]	Average Payment per Weighted Unit	Total DRG Payment
439	Skin Graft for Injury	1.7090	0.97	$4,100	$6,797
97	Bronchitis and Asthma > 17 w/o Complications	0.5873	0.97	$4,100	$2,336
103	Heart Transplant	19.0098	0.97	$4,100	$75,602

[1] Geographic Adjustment varies by area.

Source: Webpage: http://www.hcfa.gov, August, 2000

Flat Fee Systems

Flat Fees for Hospitals

Flat fee systems in general pay a predefined amount for a unit of service. The fee may be established by the payor alone or as a result of negotiations between the payor and provider. As with cost-based systems, the units of service paid for vary widely and include the following:

- Per procedure.
- Per inpatient day.
- Per admission.
- Per discharge.
- Per diagnosis.

By paying a flat fee, the payor is limiting its liability. By accepting a flat fee, the provider is accepting the risk that it can offer the service for less than the payment. If a provider cannot offer a service for less than it is paid, it has several alternatives: 1) absorb the cost; 2) transfer the cost to another payor; 3) improve efficiency; and/or 4) drop the service.

Flat Fees for Physicians

RBRVS: A system of paying physicians based upon the relative value of the services rendered.

For professional (i.e. physician) services, the corresponding system is **RBRVS (Resource Based Relative Value System)**, which was developed by the government in 1992. This system assigns a relative value to every one of over 7,000 professional services (including pathology/laboratory and radiology), and establishes a flat fee for those services based on their relative weight compared to a standard **relative value unit** (RVU) of 1.000.

RVU: Relative Value Unit.

Flat Fees for Outpatient Care

APC: A flat fee payment system instituted by the government to control the payment for outpatient services provided to Medicare recipients.

APC, or the Ambulatory Payment Classification System, is a prospective payment system which was implemented in 1999 by the government in accordance with The Balanced Budget Act of 1997 (BBA 97). This legislation was enacted to reduce and stabilize the amount of reimbursement hospitals receive for *outpatient* care. The development of this system came in response to the exponential growth of the cost and the volume of outpatient medicine. With the stringent DRGs in place and improved technology that could not have been fully anticipated, an unexpected result was that hospitals converted many procedures from inpatient to outpatient (including free-standing ambulatory surgical centers). As seen in Exhibit 13–5, the amount of dollars spent for Medicare enrollees also saw a dramatic shift from inpatient to outpatient expenses. This rise in outpatient expenses drove the relatively speedy APC development and implementation.

Outpatient care previously reimbursed on a cost basis is now paid under the APC flat fee format, which has many similarities to the DRGs developed for inpatient care.

Exhibit 13–5   Percentage Increase in Medicare Expenditures (IP and OP), 1970–1998

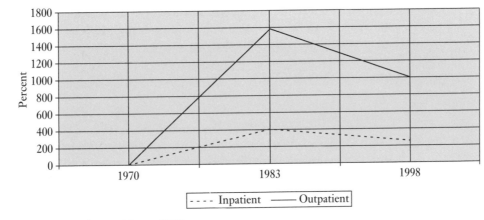

Source: http://www.hcfa.gov (accessed August, 2000).

The original intent was to cluster outpatient services into a manageable number of groupings. In the early stages of development, there were 290 total groups. Due to comments and feedback to the government from concerned providers about the lack of detail within these initial groupings, the total number of APCs is now over 900 (*Journal of AHIMA*, July/August 2000).

Services within these groups are clinically similar and require a comparable allocation of resources. They are categorized into the following groupings:

- Significant Procedures, Therapies, or Services.
- Medical Visits.
- Drugs and Biologicals.
- Medical Devices/Implants.
- Partial Hospitalization.
- Ancillary Tests and Procedures.

To gain acceptance by the provider community as a valid and equitable methodology, the new outpatient payment methodology needed a historical benchmark that would be viewed as a globally accepted standard among providers. It used actual 1996 outpatient cost data from a large group of hospitals as a baseline. The costs were grouped according to similar services (e.g. an outpatient MRI). A median was derived for each service grouping, and then a new "value" for each service grouping was established by determining a factor/percentage of the median average prospectively for the group in the future. For example, if among 250 hospitals nationally the government found a low cost of $500 for an outpatient MRI and a high cost of $1,000 and determined the median was $750, the prospective APC for that service might be 90 percent of the median, or $675.

As a safety measure, Medicare created an additional formula designed to guarantee slow growth in APC reimbursement levels. On a going-forward basis, it was determined that the APCs would be increased annually by a percentage that would be 1 percent less than the medical cost inflation factor specific to outpatient services. As an example, if the overall medical cost index for all services related to outpatient care was 4.5 percent, then the APCs would be adjusted by 3.5 percent.

The governmental department which oversees the Medicare payment systems (DRG and RBRVS, APCs and others) is known as the **Center for Medicare and Medicaid Services** (CMS). Until 2001, it was called the **Health Care Financing Administration** or HCFA.

Other Payors Follow Suit

Health care was so expensive that domestic employers complained they were spending a disproportionate amount on health care compared to their peer employers in other nations. Many US companies found it difficult to compete, when the cost of their products had to be artificially inflated in order to cover the monies spent on health care (see Exhibit 13–6). In 1995, General Motors noted that it was spending more on the health care benefits for its employees than it was for the steel for the production of its automobiles.

While some employers tried to organize in coalitions for leveraged buying power and economies of scale in health care purchasing, this movement never fully caught on nationally. The overall complaint against the fee-for-service medicine facing employers was that service providers have inherent incentives to perform more surgeries, hold patients in the hospital longer, and (arguably) even provide services that are not medically necessary.

Following the lead of the government and its cost containment efforts, its use of prospective payment on both the inpatient and outpatient sides, many commercial payors adopted the same methodologies. Again, the use of these methods limited the ability of the provider to a set dollar amount per inpatient stay or outpatient case. The

Exhibit 13–6   Health Care Expenditures as a Percentage of GNP, 1940–2000

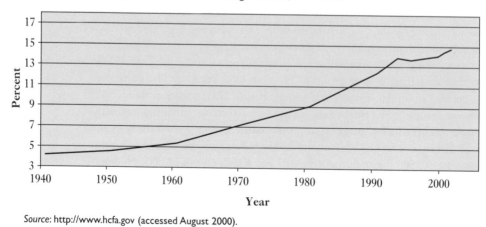

Source: http://www.hcfa.gov (accessed August 2000).

use of prospective payment also provided greater predictability of medical expenditures for payors.

Managed Care and Risk Sharing

During this period, the changing dynamic between payors and providers was driven by a desire to shift the financial risk from the payors (who traditionally held it) to the providers. The payment methodologies became increasingly creative and complex as payors and providers became focused on "managing care" and cost containment. This managed care concept created an entire industry devoted to controlling the expenditure of the health care dollar.

A number of managed care organizations were publicly traded and earnings pressures from Wall Street and/or demands from employers to keep fees "under control" drove many managed care organizations to walk a fine line between an overriding concern for patient/"member" care and the larger issues of profit and loss. America developed a "love/hate" relationship with managed care organizations. When President Clinton proposed a radical overhaul of the US health care system through a government-led "Managed Competition" system, there was a strong reaction to limit government involvement from a broad range of stakeholders in the health care system, including employers, employees, providers, and managed care companies. By the mid–1990s managed care, which had held considerable promise for controlling costs while maintaining quality, became fixed in the public's mind as a system which limited the quality of and access to care for the sake of financial gain (see Perspective 13–2).

Despite all the public outcry against restriction of provider choice/access, and for all the public distaste for some of the stringent medical management mechanisms that came into being, the fact is that in the early 1990s, medical costs plateaued in the USA for the first time in many years. By early in the next century, however, they began to rise again.

Overview of "Managed Care"

The predominance of managed care in the "later years" catalyzed the evolution of many payment schemes, a description of which follows.

The term **managed care** is often used as if it were referring to a specific type of care and payment arrangement. In fact, the term is used to describe a wide variety of options, with Health Maintenance Organizations (HMOs), Preferred Provider Organizations (PPOs), and Point of Service plans (POS) being the three dominant managed care models. They are arranged in Exhibit 13–7 according to the degree that they manage the care giving process and share risks between payors and providers, and are discussed in turn below.

Perhaps the easiest way to understand the structures and payment methodologies of managed care is to contrast them to typical fee-for-service models of care. As discussed previously, the fee-for-service arrangement is most commonly characterized

PERSPECTIVE 13–2

An Opinion of Managed Care

THE ISSUE: Some believe that the death knell is being sounded for managed healthcare.
OUR POSITION: The price pressures that gave us HMOs in the first place are still here.

Physicians who are hoping that managed care is dead, or at least losing its grip, need to think again.

All of the inflationary pressures that caused employers and the government to start herding people into HMOs in the first place are still there, from the high cost of medical technology to the severe cost shifting that occurs when large segments of the population have no insurance. And now, there are new pressures, such as the rising cost of drugs, and the effect that opening the door to litigation will have on HMOs.

Many employers are now seeing sharp hikes in their HMO rates. As the year ends, we've seen 20 percent increases locally. It won't take more than a year or two of that before the next wave of managed care – or some other form of medical rationing – takes place.

Rising medical costs have taken a huge cut of the nation's billfold. And make no mistake, the lower and middle classes have indirectly footed the bill for the lavish costs of healthcare in America. If not for managed care, where would we be right now? Through the 1980s, when traditional postwar indemnity health plans were still common, employers were seeing premium hikes of 15 percent to 25 percent a year. By 1990, $675 billion was spent on US healthcare, or 12.2 percent of gross domestic product. In 1993, the Congressional Budget Office forecast that the US would spend $1.6 trillion on healthcare by 2000 – 18.9 percent of projected GDP. At that rate of inflation, half the nation's gross domestic product would have gone to healthcare by 2050. But the tide was turned when employers started contracting with HMOs, and the HMOs started squeezing the system. The current forecast is that by next year, the US will spend $1.3 trillion. That's plenty, but not as much as was expected.

Make no mistake, managed care has been ruthless and too often greedy as all get-out. The HMOs for too long were able to insulate themselves from legal liability, for example, when they refused appropriate care and coldly rationed medical treatment. But greed hasn't been the exclusive domain of HMOs. A big part of what managed care has been about is trying to put price pressure on medicine. That's driven down some of the outrageous expenditures in the industry.

We still need a national healthcare policy. We still need to achieve coverage for every American so that the risks and costs can be spread more evenly among all of us. And we still need to be skeptical when medical specialists tell us that cost controls are not good for us.

Source: Sacramento Business Journal, December 17, 1999.

Exhibit 13–7 Managed Care Environments

PPO   POS   IPA HMO   Staff Model HMO

———————————————————————————————→

| Least Restrictive Provider Choice |
| More Expensive |
| Less Medical Management |
| Broader Provider Networkre |

| Most Restrictive Provider Choice |
| Less Expensive |
| More Medical Management |
| Smaller Provider Network |

by independent providers who are paid "reasonable charges" for providing "necessary" services to patients who make an unrestricted choice to go to them.

PPOs

The **PPO** is a network of independent providers approved in advance by the payor to provide a specific service or range of services at predetermined (usually discounted) rates. It is based upon some restriction of access and utilization in return for a discount.

HMOs

HMO is a term used to describe a specific type of company/insurer that offers medical care to a covered population. There are two general types of HMOs: the **group model HMO** (consisting of a loose affiliation of providers that act as an entity and contract to cover the health care needs of a covered population) and a **staff model HMO** (whereby the providers are actually employed by the HMO), where patients receive care in controlled/owned facilities (e.g. Kaiser Permanente plans).

POS

A **POS** arrangement is a hybrid between an HMO and a PPO. Though patients are encouraged to see **participating providers** in order to receive their most financially favorable benefit, at the *point-of-service* they may see a non-participating provider, though usually at some additional cost or reduced benefit.

Methods of Managed Care Payments

The following methods of payment are used in various ways by the entities described above to help manage care and share risk.

Steerage

Steerage is one of a variety of straightforward, market-driven techniques designed to increase or maintain market share. In order to increase volume (and thus reduce fixed costs per unit), providers give payors a discount in exchange for the payors agreeing to employ mechanisms that direct patients to the participating provider. An example of steerage is the "Center of Excellence" designation used by insurers. Typically, in this situation, a provider has distinguished itself as a high-quality provider of one or more services. This is most often accomplished by meeting or exceeding predetermined criteria established by a payor. Once a provider is chosen as a "Center of Excellence" by a payor, the payor agrees to *steer* those in need of the services covered to the provider. Providers also implement strict benefit differentials to ensure that their population utilizes participating providers who have joined the managed care organization's network. If a patient uses a participating provider, the copayments and benefits might be very favorable, whereas if a non-participating provider is used, there might be greatly reduced benefits, or even no benefits whatsoever. To help ensure that

Preferred Provider Organization (PPO): A network of independent providers preselected by the payor to provide a specific service or range of services at predetermined (usually discounted) rates to the payor's covered members.

Health Maintenance Organization (HMO): A legal corporation that offers health insurance and medical care. HMOs typically offer a range of health care services at a fixed price (see capitation).

Group Model HMO: An HMO which contracts with medical groups for services.

Staff Model HMO: An HMO which owns its clinics and employs its doctors.

Point of Service (POS): A hybrid between an HMO and a PPO in which patients are given the incentive to see providers participating in a defined network, but may see non-network providers, though usually at some additional cost.

Participating Provider: A provider who has contracted with the health plan to provide medical services to covered members at predetermined rates.

Steerage: The process of directing patients towards certain providers in exchange for discounts or other incentives.

Primary Care Provider (PCP): A physician (typically a Family Medicine, Internal Medicine, Pediatric and sometimes Obstetrics and Gynecology provider) who is the primary caregiver of a patient.

Gatekeepers: Providers (typically the PCP) who must preapprove care received by a patient, such as a visit to the specialist. Gatekeepers are utilized in most POS plans and HMO plans.

Members: People who are covered by a health care plan. Typically the member and/or the employer of the member pays a premium to the plan for the privilege of being covered.

Discounts: A reduction in the charge for services.

patients are "steered" in a certain direction, providers and insurers look to the beginning of the health care continuum: the patient's **primary care provider** (PCP).

Many providers, including hospitals, integrated networks, HMOs, and PPOs, purchase or affiliate with PCPs to make sure that the patient stays within their system. These providers are known as **gatekeepers**. The gatekeepers control both the level of care and who provides it. If the patient seeks care outside the network for anything other than an emergency, there is usually a penalty in the form of a hefty copayment or total denial of payment.

The **members**, then, have a very real financial incentive to stay within the network of participating providers, and, subsequently, the participating providers get the volume increases promised as a benefit of being in the managed care organization's network. In exchange for the added volume, the provider gives the payor a **discount**. Depending on the competition, discounts can range from 5 to 40 percent of normal charges. Though 40 percent seems like an enormous discount, many providers feel that if their variable costs are being met, then the additional volume is worth the discount. Steerage, discounts and allowances have only been partially successful in bringing down costs to employers.

Copayments and Deductibles

One of the simplest methods of risk sharing is through copayments and deductibles, where patients absorb some of the cost of service provision. With **copayments**, members covered by the plan are required to pay part of the cost of the service. For instance, if the fee for an office visit is $50, the patient may have to pay $10 and the insurance pays the remainder of the allowable reimbursement, up to the remaining $40. With **deductibles**, the person covered is responsible for paying a certain base amount before coverage begins. For instance, a patient may be required to pay for the first $250 of service before the third party pays any of the bill. Exhibit 13–8 shows an example of a health care plan that uses copayments and deductibles.

Two risk-reducing outcomes occur as a result of copayments and deductibles: 1) insurers do not have to pay the portion of the bill that the copayment and deductible amounts cover; and 2) copayments and deductibles are designed to encourage people to seek less care (especially in the common tiered copayment schedule, where a primary care visit may cost $10 while a specialty visit is $25 and an emergency room or urgent care copayment is $50). The copayments and deductibles are generally low enough to be affordable if care is really needed, but high enough to make people think twice before seeking unnecessary care and generally to make people consider whether they are seeking care in the most appropriate location.

Per Diem

Another method of payment is a **per diem** (or "per day") rate. Similar to case rates, a payor negotiates an amount that it will pay for one day of care, which includes all hospital charges associated with the inpatient day (nursing care, surgeries, medications, etc.). The day of care can be defined in several ways. Certainly a day in the

Intensive Care Unit (ICU) is more expensive than a day on a regular unit. Therefore, the per diem rate for the ICU might be $1,700 and for the regular unit might be $1,000. For a patient who spends seven days in the hospital, two in the ICU, and five on the regular unit, the payment would be:

2 Days @ $1,700	= $3,400
+ 5 Days @ $1,000	= $5,000
Total	$8,400

To reduce their financial risk under per diems, payors place limits on length of stay. They may even put limits within the length of stay. For example, in the seven-day stay, the insurer may say (based on its analysis of the situation compared to its national statistics) that a total of seven days is fine, but it may only allow one day in the ICU, not two. Typically, per diems favor the managed care organization, which has control over the number of days "allowed" as a benefit, even if it does not necessarily have the ability to discharge the patient.

Another way that insurers attempt to manage their risk is by encouraging outpatient treatment, only approving hospital admission for the sickest of patients. As the level of acuity rises, so do the expenses associated with care. This can be a very troubling aspect of per diems from the provider's perspective. They are concerned that though a rate will be negotiated on a wide variety of patient types, only the sickest and most complicated cases will end up at their hospital. Thus their costs will rise above the per diem.

Case Rates

Another form of managing care and sharing risk is to negotiate a rate that is all-inclusive of everything that the hospital provides during the entire inpatient stay.

Copayment: Requiring the patient to pay part of the health care bill. These payments are used to prevent overutilization of services.

Deductibles: When the patient covered is responsible for paying a certain base amount before coverage begins.

Per Diem: An amount a payor will pay for one day of care, which includes all hospital charges associated with the inpatient day (nursing care, surgeries, medications, etc.).

Exhibit 13–8 Example of Employee Benefits Using Copayments and Deductibles

Service	Plan Coverage		Employee Responsibility	
	Participating Provider	Non-participating Provider	Participating Provider	Non-participating Provider
MD Office Visit	100% after Copayment	70% after Copayment	$10 Copayment per Visit	$25 Copayment per Visit
Emergency Room Visit	100%	100%	Subject to Plan Approval	Subject to Plan Approval
Inpatient Stay	100% after Deductible	70% after Deductible	$200 Deductible per Stay/$1,000 Maximum per Year	$200 Deductible per Stay/$1,000 Maximum per Year
Prescription Drugs	100% after Copayment	70% after Deductible	$5 Copayment/ Prescription	$10 Copayment/ Prescription

Case Rates: A rate that covers everything that the hospital provides during the entire inpatient stay.

In this instance, the insurer and the provider agree to a fixed rate, which limits the liability of the payor and shifts some of the financial risk to the provider. This negotiated rate is known as a **case rate**. For example, a hospital might agree to accept $30,000 for a patient who needs a coronary artery bypass graft (CABG). Of particular concern to providers when considering case rates is the very complicated case, referred to as an *outlier*, or, informally, a *"train wreck,"* that ends up costing far more than the negotiated rate. The provider is taking a big risk if it is guaranteed only $30,000 for a given procedure, but unusual complications of the case cost hundreds of thousands of dollars.

The benefit to the provider, however, is that if the case is of lower severity or experiences a shorter length of stay than expected, then the provider may indeed receive a case rate well in excess of costs and sometimes even in excess of charges. While this is uncommon, providers often have a false sense of confidence that they can manage the care of the patients to such a level that they will "win" in the case-rate scenario. What they fail to realize, often, is that once the financial risk for the provision of health care services is handed from the payor to the provider, the payor may have no real incentive to assist in the medical management of the patient. In fact, every penny the managed care organization spends on administration by helping the hospital is really a penny of annual profit lost. It is easy to see why hospitals have become increasingly shy about contracting with this methodology unless they are *very* certain that they have the medical management protocol in place to allow them to benefit.

Stop-loss: A method providers use to limit the exposure that comes with the possibility that charges will go far beyond negotiated rates – a level of charges over which the provider is no longer totally liable.

One method providers use to limit the exposure that comes with the possibility that charges will go far beyond negotiated rates is to negotiate a level of charges over which the hospital is no longer totally liable, called a *stop-loss limit*. For example, in the case just described, a hospital and insurer might agree that $50,000 is the maximum amount for which the provider is totally liable (see Exhibit 13–9). If a patient's charges exceed $50,000, the insurer will pay the provider for charges over this amount. Many times insurers and providers share this risk by negotiating a discount – for example, 20 percent – off the excess charges. Continuing with the CABG example, if a patient incurs a total of $75,000 on a CABG case, this is a stop-loss case. The insurer pays the provider $30,000 (the negotiated case rate) plus 80 percent of the charges over the $50,000 stop-loss or $20,000 [80 percent × ($75,000 - $50,000)]. This stop-loss reduces the loss to the provider from $45,000 to $25,000. Risk is shared between the provider and the insurer.

Exhibit 13–9   Example of a Stop-loss Implementation

A	Total Charges		$75,000
B	Negotiated Case Rate Payment		30,000
C	Balance	[A – B]	45,000
D	Amount over Stop-loss ($50,000)	[A – $50,000]	25,000
E	Additional Payment from Insurer	[0.8 × D]	20,000
F	Total Insurance Payment	[B + E]	50,000
G	Remaining Balance (amount for which the provider is at risk)	[A – F]	$25,000

This stop-loss reduces the loss to the provider from $45,000 to $25,000. Risk is shared between the provider and the insurer. The patient could also be at risk for the balance, but the patient is not usually a part of the negotiation.

Capitation

In **capitation**, the basic premise is that a provider agrees in advance to cover the health care needs of a defined population for a set amount (often **per member per month** (PMPM) or per member per year (PMPY)), which is pre-paid to the provider. The gamble for the provider, of course, is that the cost of the medical expenditures provided to the HMO member will be less than the capitated payment amount pre-paid to the provider, in which case the provider is able to retain the difference. The philosophy is that this payment system will encourage prudent medical management and preventive care, which will prevent more expensive inpatient care in the future, for example.

Inherent in capitation, however, is that the very act of providing services in any form causes the provider to incur a cost that wouldn't have been incurred if the service had not been provided. In short, there is a perverse incentive in the short run to provide a minimum level of care or *not* to provide care at all: to withhold care, to settle for a less expensive but less effective course of treatment, or to create obstacles for the patients in being able to access care (only having appointments available weeks or months in advance, so as to discourage unnecessary utilization). In the instance of hospitals, patients have allegedly been discharged prematurely or, again, have not received a more expensive course of treatment when a cheaper "band-aid" approach would suffice. In short, while capitation was initially intended to force a new level of fiscal accountability on the providers – really forcing them to understand the costs of medical care and utilize only the most cost-effective treatments – it has become a controversial payment form because of the temptation it presents to focus more on the short-term financial aspects of medical care than on the care of the patient itself.

Premium Rate-setting Methodologies

The methodologies for deriving the premiums used by managed care companies for capitation (i.e. HMOs) are complicated, and accurate actuarial information is absolutely critical to pricing the coverage appropriately. There are two basic methodologies that payors use when developing premiums: community rating and **experience rating**. The obvious difference is that community rating evaluates the health risk of a population as a whole, whereas experience rating focuses on assessing the potential medical expenditures of individuals and then aggregates them into a group premium.

Managed care organizations attempt to know as much information as possible about the covered population in order to develop reliable predictions of how much health care will be utilized. For example, the cost to cover the hospital care required for colon and rectal cancer can be predicted if enough is known about the covered population. Information such as the number of men (particularly white males since incidence is higher among this group), 50 plus age group size (incidence increases over 50), general diet of the population (higher fat content causes higher incidence), and income level (income is a predictor of diet) can all provide valuable predictive input. Once a predicted number of potential cases is determined and a potential length of stay estimated, the potential cases are multiplied by the average length of stay, yielding the total number of expected hospital days. The insurer then seeks the lowest price it can find for this number of inpatient days. It often uses all the tools described in this

Capitation: A method of payment in which the provider is paid a fixed amount over a set period of time, usually a month or a year, for each person served no matter what the actual number or nature of services delivered.

Per Member per Month (PMPM): Generally used by HMOs and their medical providers as an indicator of revenue, expenses, or utilization of services per member per one-month period.

Experience Rating: The method of setting premium rates based on the actual health care costs of a group or groups.

chapter to obtain this rate, such as promising steerage and contracting via per diems and/or case rates.

For example, assume a payor covers 100,000 lives. After studying all the detailed demographic data (age, gender, etc.), it is determined that 19.1 individuals from this population could be diagnosed with colon or rectal cancer in a given year. The current treatment for this illness requires an average stay in the hospital of 6.5 days. Thus, the payor must be prepared to cover 124 days of hospital care (19.1 cases at 6.5 days/case). If the payor can negotiate a rate with providers of $1,000 per day, the total cost will be approximately $124,000 for the year. Taking this amount and dividing it by the number of covered lives (100,000) gives a figure of $1.24 per year or $0.103 per month that it must charge its members to cover this health care need. To cover its administrative costs and desired profit, the payor may add an additional 15 percent (ranges between15 and 25 percent) to the $0.103, creating a final figure of $0.12 PMPM (see Exhibit 13–10).

This methodology can be repeated for all covered health care needs to create the final monthly premium. All events resulting in health care costs such as the number of strokes, heart attacks, accidents, mental illnesses, and kidney failures must be accurately predicted and their costs analyzed to create a viable premium. The premium amount will obviously vary based on services covered and the size and demographics of the covered population. It is also very dependent on the provider climate.

When rating various groups, payors may also consider such things as the types of industry, applying conversion factors to account for potential differences in health care expenditures. For example, covering a group of 25 men who are in an accounting firm will probably result in fewer claims related to industrial accidents than covering a construction crew of 25 men. Likewise, groups with women in the 25–40 age group might be expected to have more pregnancy and subsequent well-child check-ups than

Exhibit 13–10   Premium Rate Setting Methodology

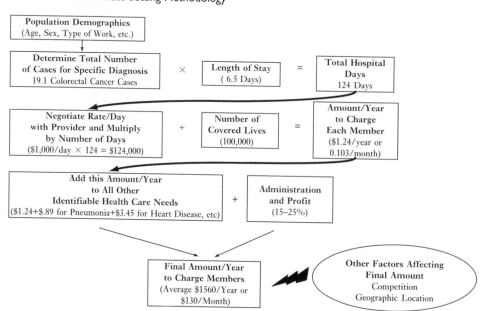

covering a group with older adults. Competition is also a factor which forces premiums to be lower. For example, a West Coast premium, where competition among HMOs for lives is fierce and competition between providers for patients is tight, might be under $100 PMPM, whereas a premium in an area where few HMO options are available for employees and benefit coverage levels are richer might exceed $130 PMPM.

Conversion Factor: Actuarial based formulas developed to adjust rates allowing for differences in population demographics.

Percent of Premium Capitation

To regain some of the control lost to insurers, in the early to mid–1990s a prominent trend was for providers to accept a *percentage of the managed care premium* to provide all of the care needed by that patient population. For example, if an insurer charges its members a monthly premium of $130, the provider may say, "If you pay me 80 percent of that premium [$104], I will provide everything your patient needs." While this saves both the provider and the payor from having to negotiate for every service the provider offers, it does, however, place the financial burden of supplying all the health care needs directly on the provider. This is similar to the case rates described earlier because it pays a fixed price for a service. In this instance, however, it is much more global, in that the provider is not simply accepting the risk for providing an entire episode of care, but rather is responsible for the financial risk associated with the patient's medical experience for a predetermined period for covered services (generally, one month increments for a year).

The advantage to the provider is that it has an ongoing cash flow from a pool of people who may or may not need health care. Again, this creates an incentive for the provider to prevent illness and reduce the odds that a patient will need to seek a more expensive form of care in the future. One of the disadvantages of these approaches is that often, by the time prevention occurs, the patient may have moved on to another provider, thus diminishing the reward to the initial provider for having provided preventive care. If a payor agrees to such an arrangement, it typically retains about 15–20 percent of the premium for administrative services such as billing, collections, utilization review, quality assurance, credentialing of providers, and, of course, profit.

To enter into an agreement such as a global percentage of premium contract, a provider must be able to control its costs and provide a full range of services at all levels of care. It must control through either ownership or affiliation anything a patient might need. Exhibit 13–11 lists several services that should be offered by a health care system to enable it to enter into this realm of risk-sharing.

The complexity and global nature of this type of arrangement was an important factor for a trend among providers in the 1990s: integration. Within a brief period, an entirely new set of acronyms sprang to life: PHOs (physician–hospital organizations), POs (physician organizations), Super PHOs (an aggregation of PHOs on a more regional basis), IDSs (integrated delivery systems), PSNs (provider sponsored networks), etc. Both "vertically integrated delivery systems," with health systems offering womb-to-tomb care, and "horizontally integrated delivery systems," with providers owning broad networks of primary and specialty care providers throughout a service region, were born. Providers became more organized and eager to provide a complete scope of services, partially in response to the need to be able to survive and compete in this changing environment.

Exhibit 13–11   Selected Services Offered by an Integrated Health Care System

Primary Care	Secondary Care	Tertiary Care	Quaternary Care	Ancillary Services
General Practitioners	Community Hospitals	Trauma Centers	Transplant Centers	Home Health
Nurse Practitioners	Birthing Centers	Intensive Care Units	Burn Centers	Nursing Homes
Physician Assistants	Emergency Services	Specialty Physicians	Emergent Air	Hospice Care
Urgent Care Centers	Ambulance Services		Transport	Dental Plans
				Prescription Plans
				Hotel Accomodations

Other Forms of Capitation

In the global percentage of premium capitation scenarios like the ones described above, a large hospital or health system is most often the holder of the risk (because hospitals and health systems typically are the only providers to have enough solvency to be able to cover the downside risk if the overall medical expenditures exceed the capitation revenues). However, often working beneath the surface of such global arrangements are smaller, more specialized versions of capitation. Global professional (physician) capitation, primary care or specialty care capitation, and ancillary capitation are some examples. In all these formats, the basic premise is the same: capitation is simply a prepayment for health care, with the provider being at risk for medical expenditures that exceed the amount prepaid based on anticipated expenditures. Physician capitation has some nuances, however, due to the many variations that exist.

In single-provider primary care capitation, the primary care gatekeeper physician (whether a family medicine, internal medicine, or pediatric physician) will receive a set amount for a fixed population and will have to provide all primary care services. Depending on how the contract is negotiated between the primary care provider and the payor, the capitated amount may also include all or some specialty services for the fixed population, which the primary care physician must subsequently pay. This payment may be on a fee-for-service or **subcapitated basis**, with the provider receiving either a fixed amount (e.g. $2 PMPM) or a variable amount (e.g. 4 percent of the professional capitation) to provide a subset of professional services, such as orthopedic services.

Subcapitation: Where the primary care physician pays a portion of the total capitated dollars received to another provider (i.e. specialist).

Often, multi-provider capitation agreements are structured on the same premise, except that a global amount will be allotted to the multi-provider group, and all professional (non-hospital, non-ancillary) care must be paid from that single pool. The individual providers within that group determine the most equitable way to divide the pool of dollars, which takes the payor out of the equation in terms of this subdivision of professional money but which often creates tensions and confusion among physicians who are trying to standardize the values of services. In this case, negotiations must occur between the primary care and specialty care physicians as a whole, in order to establish two smaller budgets within the professional capitation amount. Tensions can flare even more when the specialists themselves have to determine how to weight the value of the services they provide. Is glaucoma surgery more "valuable" than setting a broken bone? How much more difficult or simple is back surgery than urologic surgery?

One method that providers have employed to equitably divide the specialty portion of the professional capitation amount is through a **zero-based budget**, which is based on dividing the entire medical budget through a sliding scale of RVUs. The sliding scale is intended to equalize disparities between the ever-subjective assessment of how difficult one procedure is compared to another (particularly when attempting to compare two procedures or services which are dissimilar in nature, such as the back and urologic surgeries mentioned above). In such a scenario, monies are distributed retrospectively based on the number or "work units" that each physician has provided (with the RVUs simply taken from the RBRVS scale discussed earlier), so that each physician is rewarded commensurate with the number of RVUs provided.

A similar technique known as **contact capitation** creates a pool of funds for each specialty. These funds are then divided among the physicians in that specialty based on the number of "contacts" that the individual specialist receives during a specific period of time (e.g. a month, six months, or a year), with one "contact" being awarded during that time period for each specialty referral from a primary care physician. The specialty care physician is then responsible for that patient for the time period. Contact capitation, while interesting and effective in theory, has not been employed on a large-scale because of the effort required to monitor the comparative performance of the physicians within the group. Despite the administrative burden, zero-based budgets and contact capitation are indicative of the types of techniques being explored as providers seek more uniform and more equitable ways to be compensated for care (see Exhibit 13–12 for an example of a Global Capitation Model).

Zero-based Budget (Capitation): Dividing the entire amount of capitation (the "budget") among all the providers, essentially leaving nothing or "zero" left at the end of every accounting period.

Contact Capitation: A method of capitation whereby each specialty has its own capitation pool and use of services by a physician only affects that physician's compensation, not the whole specialty network's compensation.

Exhibit 13–12 Global Capitation Model

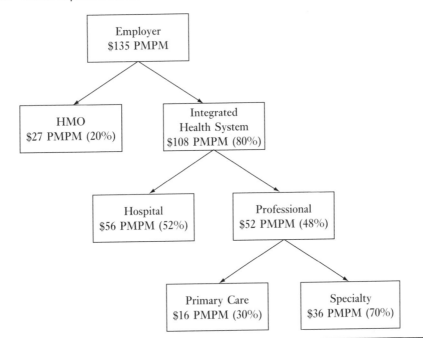

Despite its early success and popularity, capitation as a payment method has come under severe scrutiny by all parties and in the media in the past few years. While some had predicted it would become *the* managed care payment system, its use as the dominant method of payment for managed care in the future is uncertain. There is actually a shift of risk back towards the payors under way. Many of the current negotiations between payors and providers have returned to the methods of old such as "percentage discounts." Providers have seemed to reach their saturation point with risk and are turning away business associated with capitation type arrangements.

◀THE FUTURE IS NOW▶

In years to come, payment systems will continue to evolve in reaction to external forces, such as federal and state budgets and regulations, demands for various levels of access and quality, technology, the health status of the public, and costs.

Regulation

The struggle to balance cost, quality, and access will be an ongoing focus of our public policy debate. The questions noted at the beginning of this chapter will continue to be the focus of the ongoing evolution of payment systems in this country: "Who gets paid?," "How much?," "By whom?," "For what types of services?," and "With what effect?".

Demands and counter demands regarding the role of government as a regulator and payor can be anticipated in reaction to technological and pharmaceutical advances in reaction to changing disease complexities and consumer demand. Safety controls to monitor the efficacy and long-term outcomes of these new innovations will necessarily follow.

Medical Savings Accounts: A limited amount of money an employee can take as pre-taxed income to pay for medically related items such as physician visits, pharmaceuticals, eyewear, and dental visits. The pre-tax income is placed in an escrow account held by the employer. The employee must submit receipts for care received to get reimbursed.

Two current and evolving examples of regulatory measures that are being deliberated and implemented are HIPAA and the Patients' Bill of Rights.

HIPAA or the Health Insurance Portability and Accountability Act was introduced in 1996 to improve the portability and continuity of health insurance coverage, to combat waste, fraud, and abuse in the health insurance and delivery systems, to promote the use of **medical savings accounts**, to improve access to long-term care, and to simplify the administration of health insurance.

This legislation has evolved over time, with considerable national attention focusing on the *Administrative Simplification* element. These regulations involve major changes in how health care organizations handle all facets of information management, including reimbursement, coding, security, and patient records. They impact on every department of every entity that provides or pays for health care.

HIPAA is designed to ultimately lower the cost of administrative transactions by eliminating the time and expense of handling paper by standardizing software to accommodate all payors and plans, while protecting patients' confidential health care information.

As is often true, however, improvements are costly, and complying with the new HIPAA regulations has been predicted by some to cost more than ten times the amount spent on preparing for the year 2000 (see Perspective 13–3).

The Patients' Bill of Rights

Over the past decade, there has been a major public policy debate on a "Patients' Bill of Rights." Democrats and Republicans have quite different perspectives and have traditionally disagreed on the levels of controls that should be in place.

The primary substantive attributes of such a Bill of Rights include:

- An external appeals process to allow the patient to sue for damages that may have occurred due to treatment being withheld.

PERSPECTIVE 13–3

HIPAA Opinion

Praise HIPAA: Some providers embrace privacy regulations in hopes of securing long-term savings.

Jeremy Pierotti can envision a day when federal regulations will improve his health system's cash flow by some $68 million. Instead of subscribing to the notion that the Health Insurance Portability and Accountability Act of 1996 represents an expensive administrative nightmare, Pierotti views it as an opportunity. And he's not alone.

As the HIPAA program director of Allina Health System in Minneapolis, Pierotti undertook a rigorous analysis of one part of the regulation – the one that requires standardized electronic transactions – and found that it will cost much less to implement than it will reap in hard savings.

Pierotti is part of a growing chorus singing the praises of HIPAA rather than wailing about its potential to divert funds from other important areas and disrupt normal operations. Those have been some of the many criticisms of the law, which was passed at the behest of the industry but has since become the whipping boy of providers and payers alike.

HHS estimates that the industry will spend $3.8 billion complying with the controversial privacy regulations, but an analysis paid for by the American Hospital Association pegs the cost at $22.5 billion, which does not cover all of HIPAA's privacy provisions.

One privacy provision left out of HHS' estimate, the AHA says, is the "minimum necessary" rule, which limits the patient information hospitals and staff members can share with one another as well as with outside organizations such as insurers. Complying with that provision alone could cost hospitals as much as $19.8 billion over five years, according to the AHA analysis. . . .

The privacy regulation controls how and when physicians and administrative staff can share protected patient information, calls for formal agreements to ensure business partners use confidential data appropriately and requires patient consent prior to using information even for the most routine clinical and administrative purposes.

Both the AHA and the AMA, and groups such as the American Association of Health Plans, have problems with the privacy regulations, believing them to be administratively burdensome and a possible threat to clinical care. . . .

Snell and others argue that hospitals stand to benefit from aggressive implementation of the privacy regulations. By convincing patients that they're not just following the rules but placing a premium on protecting confidentiality, hospitals may be able to win over customers – and keep the ones they have.

Source: Jeff Tieman, *Modern Healthcare*, March 26, 2001.

- Mastectomy length-of-stay rights.
- Protection for the self-insured consumer.
- Emergency care and what constitutes an "in-network" versus an "out-of-network" provider.
- Access to specialists.
- Point-of-service plan descriptions.
- Direct access to obstetricians and gynecologists.
- Continuity of care.

The most contentious issue, however, is the patient's appeal process, which is fundamentally about a patient's right to sue his or her insurance company if a physician-recommended treatment regimen is either delayed or denied by the insurance company and ultimately causes harm to the patient.

Democrats have favored an appeals process that includes an external review by a third party that employs a broad definition of "medical necessity," and large damages are possible if the insurance company is found to be negligent.

Republicans have also favored an external review, but with a more limited definition of "medical necessity" and lower damages.

The potential awards by the courts have sparked the interest of very powerful groups to lobby on their respective sides. Insurers/payors favor more control and less damages, while lawyers have favored higher cap and less control by the insurers.

However, as a Patients' Bill of Rights evolves over time, it can be expected to have numerous and diverse impacts on health care costs. If patients are more aware of any right to sue insurance companies at any level, increased litigation could result. Awards against payors will be passed on to the employer/patient in the form of higher premiums. A concern is that employers may reduce benefit levels in an attempt to keep premiums reasonable, which could lead to more uninsured Americans and more costs being shifted to the government. Another concern is that physicians will be more defensive in their practices, ordering additional tests in an attempt to legally protect themselves.

The Continued Search for Quality in the New Millennium

There has been an ongoing effort to improve the quality of care and the data available to make cost/quality comparisons. The early days of health care relied mostly on "word of mouth" measurements of quality, which were limited to either cure or palliation. Today practically every health care issue has a quality component in some form.

Patients are concerned with safety, outcomes, and satisfaction, while many payors focus on the ability to differentiate which procedures and treatments provide the greatest value for the dollars spent. Providers want to please both patients and payors but are continually concerned about how to afford the quality that is being demanded of them under a payment system which favors cost containment. Information compilation and data mining are major industries, with organizations such as The National Practitioner Data Bank, JCAHO, and NCQA heavily involved.

As benchmarks have improved they have become much more complex. The focus has changed from such items as infant mortality, length of stay, readmission rates, and C-section rates to a new level of sophistication. Demographics and acuity of a patient population, even analyzing aspects of genetic differentiation, are now being considered when comparing providers. Episodes of care, including months and even years surrounding a disease process, rather than single events/procedures, are being analyzed and presented for consumption by providers, payors, and patients.

Health Care Enters the Digital Age: Technological Advancements Enable Efficiencies

Another area that shows great promise for the future can be found in the integration of technology into health care administration. While technology has enabled clinical solutions that were unimaginable even a few short years ago, less apparent is how technology is working "behind the scenes" to make health care more efficient and, in many ways, more cost-effective.

The Internet is one example of a technological improvement that has had great utility in health care already. From an administrative standpoint, for example, physician office personnel are now able to submit medical claims electronically by using EDI (electronic data interchange) technology, with software packages that have "rules matrices" built in, so that a provider cannot submit a "dirty" claim (one that has invalid medical coding or is lacking certain essential information for the claim to be processed). This has reduced the necessity to refile claims and enhanced cash flows by ensuring more timely payment. Claims filed through the Internet do not have to pass through the mail and then be sorted and processed manually, all of which are time consuming. As recently as the early 1990s, the average length of time between mailing and receiving payment could easily be a month. Electronic filing, processing, and payment transfer can reduce that time to a few days.

The Internet has also made it possible for providers to tackle administrative and clinical tasks like checking insurance eligibility information and claims status, implementing disease management programs, automatically reordering supplies (both medical and general office supplies through e-commerce transactions), and being connected with other providers (e.g. laboratory, radiology) via the Internet. With an entirely new realm of applications being developed with the Internet as a platform, the efficiencies and cost savings for providers and payors alike are likely to grow exponentially in the future.

Another fascinating use of technology which is likely to grow is the use of personal digital assistants (PDAs). With a simple handheld device, clinicians can have up-to-the-minute patient data, including an electronic copy of the patient medical record. Ready access to key information is or soon will be readily available, including patient medication history, drug formularies from different payors (stipulating which drugs are covered and not covered by the patient's benefit plan), drug interaction information, generic versus brand name drug information, and even electronic scripting capabilities (where prescriptions can be electronically transferred directly to a pharmacy). These capabilities can empower clinicians to make more informed decisions at the point of care, which ultimately can result in better clinical outcomes, higher patient and provider satisfaction, and perhaps a more efficient delivery of health care.

PDAs have also duplicated many of the other applications once available only via desktop computers, so now physicians can actually create and file electronic claims at the point of care from their PDA. As with the brief discussion of Internet-enabled technologies, this can reduce filing errors and enhance cash flow for the providers. While only a small percentage of practicing physicians utilize this technology as of 2002, all indications are that PDAs will become an integral part of the typical physician's day-to-day practice operations. Given the rapid progress in this field (the integration of medical record dictation capabilities into the same PDA, for example), the possibilities in the future seem unlimited.

Information Technology

The business of health care continues to evolve as providers, payors, and employers seek solutions to questions that have never previously been posed. While the introduction of new technology addresses some of these issues, it also raises new ones and often calls into question presumptions that were previously accepted as true. Nowhere is this clearer than in one of the growing fields in health care that offers astounding possibilities for the future: the area commonly known as "health care informatics" or "information technology" (see Perspective 13–4).

Where employers and providers once thought health care data was an inessential by-product of simple claims payment, today there is a strong, even urgent, need for information that is timely, informative, and in a usable format. Throughout the health care industry we see a constant need and desire to push the borders into areas that have never been explored before. The information services arena has evolved from an accounting-based, relatively basic means of analyzing charge and payment data to an integral part of modern health care delivery and payment.

Early efforts focused on how components of the delivery system (physicians, hospitals, etc.) performed and interacted financially with one another. Retrospective analysis of this sort depended on analyzing post-payment claims data, understanding where the health care dollar was spent, and comparing that to national and regional benchmarks of what the financial performance *should have been*, based on industry norms.

This was the next significant step beyond simply understanding cost structures and whether charges were appropriate for specific procedures and in the marketplace. Particularly with providers and payors involved in capitation arrangements, the need for this sort of intricate information was critical to their ability to implement successful medical management programs and, ultimately, to their financial success. An entire sector of information technology and health care informatics companies has grown to meet this need.

The level of complexity and sophistication of information available to providers, payors, and employers is evolving quickly. New forms and formats of information

PERSPECTIVE 13–4

Technology's Rip Van Winkles

First the dot-coms crashed. Then healthcare organizations learned they really would have to comply with sweeping new patient-privacy regulations. It wasn't too much longer before an Institute of Medicine report said the industry can and should use information technology to prevent patients from being harmed as a consequence of care.

Three events, all within the past year, may seem unrelated, but they're not: Each represents a challenge to employ information systems for more than registering patients and sending invoices. Often viewed as an industry that neglects or even abstains from such technology, healthcare finally may have little choice but to embrace computers and automation. And, for the first time, not doing so can mean running afoul of the law as well as putting patient safety at risk.

In a recent study, it is predicted that annual Healthcare Information Technology expenditures will gain momentum in 2002 and 2003, reaching $23 Billion by the end of 2003.

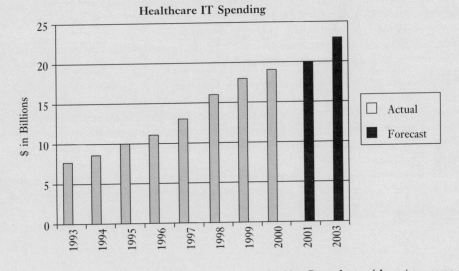

Healthcare IT Spending

Source: Jeff Tieman, *Modern Healthcare,* July 16, 2001. *Chart source:* Sheldon Dorenfest and Associates, same article.

are emerging to predict what *might* happen with the clinical and financial experiences of a population. In some of the new information technologies being developed and refined, the relationship between past and present medical data on a patient-specific level can even be used to prospectively assess the medical risk of a group population – information that was completely unavailable even two or three years ago.

While these companies in health care technology are reinventing the future of health care every day, it is important to stay vigilant in regard to patient confidentiality and security (see Perspective 13–5).

PERSPECTIVE 13–5

Innovations through Information

Integrated Healthcare Information Services, Inc. (IHCIS) in Waltham, Massachusetts is a prime example of how the healthcare informatics sector is creating an entirely new paradigm for our industry as we enter the new millenium. By expanding the information that is available, groups like IHCIS have reengineered information from being a rear window look at the road already traveled to being a tool that empowers payors, providers, and even employers to be proactive and informed as they work to create more cost-effective, higher quality patient care.

Today IHCIS is breaking new ground by having developed a new approach to health risk assessment, which is essentially using data and information to predict the medical expenditures and utilization of individuals and group populations. This information is absolutely invaluable because it enables:

- The establishment of health plan premiums that reflect the acuity and potential medical expenditures of a population more accurately than ever before;
- The identification of high-risk health plan enrollees (enabling both payors and providers to implement proactive medical management for the patient, which in turn results in the prevention of unnecessary health issues and expenditures); and
- The development of more accurate clinical and financial provider profiles that are more useful than anything that has ever been developed in the past.

The primary tool that IHCIS uses is a technology they developed called "Episode Risk Groups" or "ERGs™." Episode risk groups were developed based upon the leading episode grouping methodology in the industry – episode treatment groups or ETGs. In the same way that X-Ray technology paved the way for MRI technology, ERGs would never have been possible but for the efforts of other informatics groups that laid the foundation by looking at patient "episodes of care" as "events" defined by diagnoses and other work that has been done to categorize diagnoses into similar groupings.

IHCIS and similar informatics groups are pioneers on the frontier of a new era in health care. Information is power and may well be one of the most important pieces in finding a solution to the healthcare dilemma in our country.

Source: Matthew Ayotte, Strategic Planning, Duke University Medical Center, August 2001.

 ◀SUMMARY▶

Health care services have grown along with the growth in the American population. Different payment methodologies have been tried in order to find a reasonable balance among costs, quality, and access. Health care payment in the United States has remained a "living experiment", from the early days of private, cash-based exchange through the middle and later years where commercial and government payors were involved in a massive exercise of trial-and-error, testing different payment methodologies and structures of care delivery.

Systems include: charged-based payment, where providers receive payment based on actual charges and payors bear the risk; cost-based payment, where providers are paid based on the cost of providing services and payors still bear the risk; and finally flat fee systems, where the provider is paid a predetermined amount and the providers bears the risk.

There has also been a growth in the types of health care payors. Indemnity companies, governmental payors, and managed care have all played major roles in trying to balance cost, quality, and access. Discounts, steerage, per diems, case rates, community/experience rating, benchmarking, managed care, and capitation are all examples of these methods.

After nearly 100 years of experimentation, we have learned that balancing cost quality and access is an ongoing process and will be influenced in the future by the trends discussed in the first chapter of this text.

◄KEY TERMS►

ALLOWABLE COSTS	GATEKEEPER	PRICE SETTER
APCs	GROUP MODEL HMO	PRIMARY CARE PROVIDER (PCP)
CAPITATION	HEALTH CARE FINANCING	POINT-OF-SERVICE PLAN (POS)
CASE RATES	ADMINISTRATION (HCFA)	PROSPECTIVE PAYMENT SYSTEM
CHARGE-BASED	HEALTH MAINTENANCE	(PPS)
CMS	ORGANIZATION (HMO)	RETROSPECTIVE PAYMENT
COMMUNITY RATING	INDEMNITY INSURANCE	RBRVS (RESOURCE BASED RELATIVE
CONTACT CAPITATION	MANAGED CARE	VALUE SYSTEM)
CONVERSION FACTOR	MEDICAID	RVU
COPAYMENT	MEDICAL SAVINGS ACCOUNT	STAFF MODEL HMO
COST-BASED REIMBURSEMENT	MEDICARE	STEERAGE
COST SHIFTING	MEMBERS	STOP LOSS
DEDUCTIBLES	PARTICIPATING PROVIDER	SUBCAPITATION
EXPERIENCE RATING	PAYOR	THE FIRST PARTY
DIAGNOSIS RELATED GROUPS	PER DIEM	THE SECOND PARTY
(DRGs)	PREMIUM	THE THIRD PARTY
DISCOUNTS	PREDETERMINED RATES	USUAL, CUSTOMARY, AND
FEE-FOR-SERVICE	PER MEMBER PER MONTH (PMPM)	REASONABLE CHARGES
FINANCIAL REQUIREMENTS	PREFERRED PROVIDER ORGANIZATION	ZERO-BASED BUDGET (CAPITATION)
FLAT FEE	PREMIUM	

◄QUESTIONS AND PROBLEMS►

1. Define the "Key terms" found in this Chapter.
   a. Allowable Costs.
   b. APCs.
   c. Capitation.
   d. Case Rate.
   e. Charge-based.
   f. CMMS.
   g. Community Rating.
   h. Contact Capitation.
   i. Conversion Factor.
   j. Copayment.

k. Cost-based Reimbursement.

l. Cost Shifting.

m. Deductibles.

n. Experience Rating.

o. Diagnosis Related Groups (DRGs).

p. Discounts.

q. Fee-for-service.

r. Financial Requirements.

s. Flat Fee.

t. Gatekeeper.

u. Group Model HMO.

v. Health Care Financing Administration (HCFA).

w. Health Maintenance Organization (HMO).

x. Indemnity Insurance.

y. Managed Care.

z. Medicaid.

aa. Medical Savings Account.

bb. Medicare.

cc. Members.

dd. Participating Provider.

ee. Payor.

ff. Per Diem.

gg. Premium.

hh. Predetermined Rates.

ii. Per Member per Month (PMPM).

jj. Preferred Provider Organization (PPO).

kk. Premiums.

ll. Price Setter.

mm. Primary Care Provider (PCP).

nn. Point-of-service Plan (POS).

oo. Prospective Payment System (PPS).

pp. Retrospective Payment.

qq. RBRVS (Resource Based Relative Value System).

rr. RVU.

ss. Staff Model HMO.

tt. Steerage.

uu. Stop Loss.

vv. Subcapitation.

ww. The First Party.

xx. The Second Party.

yy. The Third Party.

zz. Usual, Customary, and Reasonable Charges.

aaa. Zero-based Budget (Capitation).

2. What were the major events and trends that defined the "Early," "Middle," and "Later" periods of the US health care system? In each period describe:

  a. The major events and trends.

  b. The price-setter.

  c. The risk bearer.

  d. The predominant method of payment and the unit to which payment is attached.

3. What was the driving force behind the development of Blue Cross/Blue Shield?

4. Name the units of service on which cost-based payers may pay providers.

5. What drove the development of Medicare? Who is covered under Medicare?

6. What drove the development of Medicaid? Who is covered under Medicaid?

7. Who pays for the Medicare and Medicaid programs?

8. How do copayments and deductibles reduce risk?

9. Why do providers desire "steerage"?

10. What do providers fear most under a case rate model?

11. What are some methods insurers use to limit their risk under per diem arrangements?

12. Who bears the risk under a flat rate system? Why?

13. What factors determine what a flat rate payment to a provider should be?

14. Why was the DRG system developed?

15. What are APCs? Why were they developed?

16. Why do HMOs use prevention and case management?

17. How do HMOs determine their premiums?

18. If an HMO covered 150,000 lives, expected 25 myocardial infarctions (MI) to occur each year within the covered lives, would expect a length of stay of 4.5 days for each MI, and had to pay an average of $950 per day for each day the MI patient was in the hospital, what would the PMPM cost to the HMO be? What would have to be charged to the patient/employer if the HMO had administrative costs equaling 10 percent of its costs and it wanted a profit margin of 7 percent?

19. Given the same scenario as in question 18, what if the HMO's shareholders demanded a 9 percent profit margin? What would the premium be in this case?

20. In question 19, what if the employer/patient refused to pay the new premium? What would the HMO offer to pay the hospital for an inpatient day?

21. What if, in question 20, the hospital refused to take the new rate, the employer refused to pay the new premium, and the employer decided to take its employees (10,000) to another HMO. Also, suppose these departing employees/members represented 6 percent of the MI total. What would the new PMPM premium be for the 140,000 remaining members.

22. Who bears the financial risk in a capitated payment system?

23. Name and describe four different types of capitation.

24. Why would a provider be willing to accept a global capitation payment?

◄QUESTIONS FROM APPENDIX H►

25. What are four factors to consider when developing charges in a charge-based system?

26. What charge method primarily uses the market price to establish a charge?
27. What charge method relies on the case mix, volume, and financial requirements of the institution?
28. What is the difference between determining charges on an average-cost basis and a weighted-cost basis?
29. What are the steps in determining weighted-average costs?
30. Describe the two margin-based approaches to developing charges.

Appendix H

Payment Systems

Cost-based Payment Systems

Reasonable and Allowable Costs

In establishing cost-based payment systems, the natural tension that exists between providers and payors revolves around five issues: reasonableness, case mix, service mix, staff mix, and efficiency.

Areas of Contention in Determining Allowable Costs

- **Reasonableness** issues are concerned with the cost of one provider versus others. In this regard, payors often set boundaries to establish what is usual, customary, and/or reasonable (UCR). For instance, a payor may only pay up to 85 percent of the cost of a procedure, based on an analysis of a profile of all providers who have submitted cost reports.
- **Case mix** issues revolve around patient eligibility. For instance, although a hospital incurs legitimate costs in treating a patient who has a deviated septum, a payor may decide to not pay for this surgery because the patient failed to receive all necessary preadmission certification. Similarly, if a health department treats a pregnant woman who resides outside its county, the county's prenatal care program may not pay for the treatment because the patient was outside the location eligibility guidelines.
- **Service mix** issues focus on the appropriateness of care. For instance, in treating stroke patients, the provider may feel that recreational therapy is an important part of treatment. Though it may be, the payor may not pay for this service because it does not consider it a necessary service within its guidelines.
- **Staff mix** issues pertain to the appropriateness of who provides service. In the mental health field, for example, although a payor may agree that a patient needs psychological services, it might not pay for care provided by a pastoral counselor who is not a licensed psychologist.
- **Efficiency** issues address questions of the appropriateness of the cost of service per unit rendered. A hospital with a low volume may have very high unit costs or a radiology center with old equipment may have to take several X-rays just to get one good one. In such instances, although the payor may agree to pay for some level of the service, it will not pay for what it feels are inefficiencies.

Under any of these five conditions, if the payor denies payment and the service has already been rendered, the provider has two choices: 1) absorb the cost; and/or 2) transfer the cost to another payor. This latter technique is called **cost-shifting** or **cross-subsidization**. Under this system "over"-reimbursement or reimbursement in excess of total costs is used for one service to cover the costs associated with "under"-reimbursement of another service where reimbursement is less than total costs. This technique has been one of the major reasons for a rise in the number of alternatives to cost-based systems.

Cost-shifting: Charging one group of patients more in order to make up for underpayment by others. Most commonly, charging some privately insured patients more in order to make up for underpayment by Medicaid or Medicare.

Unit-based Payment Systems

Two key issues that arise in cost-based payment systems are "What is the unit of service to which payments are attached?" and "What are reasonable and allowable costs?"

Unit of Service

There are a variety of units on which cost-based payors pay providers, including:

- Per procedure.
- Per inpatient day.
- Per admission.
- Per discharge.
- Per diagnosis.

Unfortunately for many providers, there is little consistency among third parties with respect to the unit of service on which payment is made. It is not unusual for a single provider to receive payments from Medicare on the basis of **Diagnosis Related Groups**, from private insurance companies on the basis of reasonable charges, and from **managed care** organizations in the form of capitation. Though it is relatively straightforward to have a cost-finding system that establishes the costs for any one of these payment schemes, it takes a very complicated information system to find costs along several of these bases at once.

Charge-based Systems

A charge-based system is based in large part on the assumption that a provider is entitled to a reasonable return for its efforts. It relies heavily on the market to ensure that profits are not excessive. While it would seem that charge-based payment systems are "reactionary" in nature from the payor perspective (since, after all, it is the providers who establish the charges on the front-end and seemingly dictate the level of payment), the dynamic is not that simple. Let us look first at the reasoning that underlies the establishment of provider charges.

In setting charges, a provider must consider a wide range of costs that must be covered. These fall into the same categories discussed in Chapter 5 (operations, opportunities, contingencies, and return on investment). Together, these comprise the organization's *financial requirements*.

Financial Requirements: For health care providers this is a combination of issues related to operations, opportunities, contingencies, and return on investment.

- **Operations.** This category includes covering all operating costs, now and into the future. That is, charges: must cover costs associated with supplies, equipment, labor, and working capital; have sufficient margin to ensure that staff remains current; and keep technology and facilities sufficiently up-to-date.
- **Opportunities.** Providers must build into their charges a reasonable markup so they can take advantage of opportunities to hold onto or expand existing markets, serve new markets, and/or exit existing markets.
- **Contingencies.** The changing health care environment presents not only various opportunities, but also various unforeseen events such as evolving payment systems,

labor shortages, and uncovered catastrophic events. Therefore, charges must build in a reasonable margin for such contingencies that siphon off the organization's capital.

● **Return on investment.** For for-profit providers, charges must also sufficiently compensate the organization and/or its owners for an investment.

Though all these methods have been employed, they all share a common concern from the point of view of payors: are they reasonable? Two ways of dealing with this problem have been: 1) to limit payments only to that part of charge considered reasonable; or 2) to employ another basis of payment altogether.

Historical/Market/Payor Method

The **historical/market/payor method** is extremely simple. Charges are established by a combination of: 1) what the organization has traditionally charged; 2) what similar organizations charge; and 3) what payors will pay. This approach to establishing charges is only loosely related to costs, but it is widely used, especially in ambulatory care settings.

Weighted-average Method

The **weighted-average method** sets charges as a function of the number and type of procedures an organization performs and the financial requirements of the organization. For instance, assume a small health care clinic expects 10,000 visits and anticipates having $1,000,000 in financial requirements next year (see Exhibit H–1). If visit type is ignored, the clinic could set its price by charging the same price for each visit, $100 ($1,000,000/10,000). However, charging each visit an average price of $100 overlooks questions of equity. Since each visit does not consume the same resources, some patients would pay more than their fair share while others would pay less.

An alternative to charging each visit the same amount is to take into account the type of visit and to weight these visits by the relative amount of resources they consume. This is accomplished through the following steps:

Step 1: **Categorize visits by resource consumption.** Exhibit H–1 assumes there are three types of visits: brief, routine, and complex. It further assumes that 60 percent (6,000) of the 10,000 visits are brief, 30 percent (3,000) routine, and 10 percent (1,000) complex.

Step 2: **Convert visits by category into weighted visit units by category.** Exhibit H–1 also assumes that routine visits consume twice the resources, and complex visits consume four times the resources of brief visits. Since the 3,000 routine visits consume twice the resources of brief visits, they count the same as if they were 6,000 brief visits (row H: 3,000 × 2). Similarly, since the complex visits consume four times the resources of a brief visit, the actual 1,000 complex visits count as if they were 4,000 brief visits (1,000 × 4). Thus, the actual 10,000 undifferentiated visits become 16,000 weighted visit units (6,000 brief + 6,000 routine + 4,000 complex visits, row H).

Step 3: **Determine charge per weighted visit unit and apply charges to categories.** Rather than spreading the $1,000,000 in financial requirements over 10,000 visits and charging $100, the $1,000,000 now can be spread over 16,000 weighted visit units and the charge reduced to

Exhibit H–1 Selected Services Offered by an Integrated Health Care System

	Given:						
A	*Number of Procedures*	[1]	10,000				
B	*Financial Requirements*	[2]	$ 1,000,000				
C	*Average Charge per Visit*	[B/A]	$ 100				
			Brief	**Routine**	**Complex**		**Total**
D	*Type of Visit*	[1]					
E	*% Distribution of Visit by Type*	[1]	60%	30%	10%		100%
F	*Relative Weight of Visit by Type*	[1]	1	2	4		
G	*Number of Visits*	[A × E]	6,000	3,000	1,000		10,000
H	*Number of Weighted Visits*	[F × G]	6,000	6,000	4,000		16,000
I	*Charge per Weighted Visit*	[3]	$ 62.50	$ 62.50	$ 62.50	$	62.50
J	*Total Charges*	[H × I]	$ 375,000	$ 375,000	$ 250,000	$	1,000,000
K	*Charges Using Average Charge*	[C × G]	$ 600,000	$ 300,000	$ 100,000	$	1,000,000
L	*Over or Under Charge Compared to Weighted Average Charge*	[J – K]	$ (225,000)	$ 75,000	$ 150,000	$	–

[1] Given.
[2] Includes all financial requirements of the organization, not just ongoing operating costs.
[3] The financial requirements ($1,000,000) in Row B/the total number of weighted visits (16,000) in Row H.

$62.50 ($1,000,000/16,000) per weighted visit unit. For instance, although there are 3,000 routine visits, they equal 6,000 weighted visits. At $62.50 each, they will raise $375,000 (row J).

Note in row L that there is a considerable difference between charging the average price ($100) to all visits, and charging by taking into account the amount of resources used. By weighting for resource consumption, those making a brief visit pay $225,000 less and those making routine and complex visits pay $75,000 and $150,000 more than they would under the undifferentiated system. Some would argue that this is more equitable. This is the logic Medicare used to establish the Resource Based Relative Value Scale (RBRVS) currently in use in ambulatory care reimbursement along with Ambulatory Payment Classifications (APCs).

Margin Approaches

There are two margin-based approaches to setting charges: cost-plus and coverage. The **cost-plus approach** starts with cost and adds a margin for profit. For instance, assume a freestanding radiology center desires to make a 10 percent profit over and above its cost. If it has determined that the cost of performing a certain radiological procedure is $125, then it adds a 10 percent surcharge of $12.50, creating a final charge of $137.50. The cost-plus approach is most often used with ancillary services such as radiology, pharmacy, and laboratory services.

Exhibit H–2   Illustration of the Coverage Approach to Setting Charges

A		Variable Cost per Unit:	$20						
	B	C	D		E	F	G	H	I
	Volume	Charge (1)	Total Charges		Financial Requirements	Direct Fixed Costs	Direct Variable Costs	Other Costs	Desired Profit
	[Given]	[D/B]	[E]	[F + G + H + I]					
	5,000	$48	$240,000		$ 240,000	$ 100,000	$ 100,000	$ 20,000	$ 20,000
	5,500	$45	$247,500		$ 250,000	$ 100,000	$ 110,000	$ 20,000	$ 20,000
	6,000	$43	$258,000		$ 260,000	$ 100,000	$ 120,000	$ 20,000	$ 20,000
	6,500	$42	$273,000		$ 270,000	$ 100,000	$ 130,000	$ 20,000	$ 20,000
	7,000	$40	$280,000		$ 280,000	$ 100,000	$ 140,000	$ 20,000	$ 20,000
	7,500	$39	$292,500		$ 290,000	$ 100,000	$ 150,000	$ 20,000	$ 20,000
	8,000	$38	$304,000		$ 300,000	$ 100,000	$ 160,000	$ 20,000	$ 20,000
	8,500	$36	$306,000		$ 310,000	$ 100,000	$ 170,000	$ 20,000	$ 20,000
	9,000	$36	$324,000		$ 320,000	$ 100,000	$ 180,000	$ 20,000	$ 20,000
	9,500	$35	$332,500		$ 330,000	$ 100,000	$ 190,000	$ 20,000	$ 20,000
	10,000	$34	$340,000		$ 340,000	$ 100,000	$ 200,000	$ 20,000	$ 20,000

The **coverage approach** essentially sets charges using a breakeven type of formula. Once the organization's cost structure, desired profit, and projected volume are known, charges can be set. Notice in Exhibit H–2 that the charge changes with volume. If the organization thought that 5,000 visits could be expected, it would establish a charge of $48 per visit, whereas if volume were forecast at 7,500 visits, it would establish a charge of $39 per visit.

GLOSSARY

Accountability: Sanctions, both positive and negative, attached to carrying out responsibilities.

Accrual Basis of Accounting: An accounting method which tracks the flow of resources and the revenues those resources helped to generate. It tracks revenues when earned and resources when used, regardless of the flow of cash in or out of the organization. This is the standard method in use today.

Accumulated Depreciation: The total amount of depreciation taken on an asset since it was put into use.

Activity-based Costing: a method of estimating costs of a service or product by estimating the costs of the activities it takes to produce that service or product.

Administrative Cost Centers: Cost centers that support clinical cost centers and the organization as a whole. They are often considered the *infrastructure* of the organization.

Administrative Profit Centers: Organizational units that do not provide health care-related services, but are responsible for their profit. There are two types: those that sell their services internally, and those whose primary responsibility is to bring revenues into the organization.

Aging Schedule: A table which shows the percentage of receivables being collected in each month.

Allocation base: a statistic (e.g. square feet, number of full-time employees) used to allocate costs, based on its assumed relationship to why the costs occurred.

Allowable Costs: Costs which are allowable under the principles of reimbursement of government (Medicaid, Medicare) and other payors.

Ambulatory Procedure Classifications (APCs): Enacted by the federal government in 2000, a prospective payment system for outpatient services, similar to DRGs, which reimburses a fixed amount for a bundled set of services.

Amortization: 1) The allocation of the acquisition cost of debt to the period which it benefits. 2) The gradual process of paying off debt through a series of equal periodic payments. Each payment covers a portion of the principal plus current interest. The periodic payments are equal over the lifetime of the loan, but the proportion going toward the principal gradually increases. The amount of a payment can be determined by using the formula to calculate the present value of an annuity.

Annuity Due: A series of equal annuity payments made or received at the beginning of each period.

Annuity: A series of equal payments made or received at regular time intervals.

APC: A flat fee payment system instituted by the government to control the payment for outpatient services provided to Medicare recipients.

Asset Mix: The amount of working capital an organization keeps on hand relative to its potential working capital obligations.

Assets: Resources that the organization owns, typically recorded at their original costs.

Authoritarian Approach: Budgeting and decision-making which are done by relatively few people concentrated in the highest level of the organizational structure. Opposite of the *participatory approach*.

Authority: Power to carry out a given responsibility.

Avoidable Fixed Cost: A fixed cost that is avoided if a particular alternative is chosen *Example:* full-time nursing costs saved if a service is closed.

Basic Accounting Equation: Assets = Liabilities + Net Assets.

Billing Float: Delay getting a bill to the patient or third-party payor (such as an insurance company). This includes the time to assemble the bill in-house, as well as the time to send the bill to the correct person or place.

Bond: A form of long-term financing whereby an issuer receives cash from a lender (an investor), and in return issues a promissory note (a "bond") agreeing to make principal and/or interest payments on specific dates.

Breakeven Analysis: A technique to analyze the relationship among revenues, costs, and volume. It is also called Cost–Volume–Profit or CVP analysis.

Breakeven Point: The point where total revenues equal total costs.

Budget Variance: The difference between what was planned (budgeted) and what was achieved (actual).

Cannibalization: When a new service decreases the revenues from other established services or product lines. These are considered cash outflows.

Capital Appreciation: Occurs whenever an investment is worth more when it is sold than when it was purchased.

Capital Budget: One of the four major types of budgets, it summarizes the anticipated purchases for the year. Typically, to be included, all items in this budget must have a minimum purchase price, such as $500.

Capital Investment Decision: Decisions involving major dollar investments that are expected to achieve long-term benefits for an organization.

Capital Investments: Large dollar, multiyear investments.

Capital Lease: A lease that lasts for an extended period of time, up to the life of the leased asset. This type of lease cannot be canceled without penalty, and at the end of the lease period, the lessee may have the option to purchase the asset. Also called a *financial lease*.

Capitated Profit Centers: Organizational units responsible for earning a profit by agreeing to take care of the health care needs of a population for a per-member fee (which is not directly tied to services). Examples include HMOs, PPOs, and various managed care organizations.

Capitation: 1) A system which pays providers a specific amount in advance to care for the health care needs of a population over a specific time period. Providers are usually paid on per member per month

(PMPM) basis. The provider then assumes the risk that the cost of caring for the population will not exceed the aggregate PMPM amount received. 2) A payment mechanism where the insurer prepays a health care provider an agreed-upon amount per member that covers a designated set of services over a defined time. Typically, these payments are made on a per member per month (PMPM) basis. If there are no terms to the contrary, in return for the capitated payments, the provider agrees to bear all the risk for the costs of services provided. If the provider's costs are below the capitation, the provider can keep the difference. If the provider's costs are more than the capitation, the provider is at risk for the difference. 3) A method of payment in which the provider is paid a fixed amount, over a set period of time, usually a month or a year for each person served no matter what the actual number or nature of services delivered.

Care Mapping: A process which specifies in advance the preferred treatment regimen for patients with particular diagnoses. This is also referred to as a **clinical pathway, clinical protocol,** or **practice guideline**.

Case Rate: A rate that covers everything that the hospital provides during the entire inpatient stay.

Cash Basis of Accounting: An accounting method which tracks when cash was received and when cash was expended, regardless of when services were provided or resources were used.

Cash Budget: One of the four major types of budgets, it displays all of the organization's projected cash inflows and outflows. The bottom line for this budget is the amount of cash available at the end of the period.

Charge-based: A method of payment which is based on the charge of the provider.

Charity Care Discounts: Discounts from Gross Patients Accounts Receivable given to those who cannot pay their bills.

Clinical Cost Centers: Cost centers that provide health care-related services to clients, patients, or enrollees.

CMS: The Center for Medicare and Medicaid Services. The acronym, CMS, is pronounced "sims."

Collateral: 1) A tangible asset which is pledged as a promise to repay a loan. If the loan is not paid, the lending institution as a legal recourse may seize the pledged asset. 2) An asset with clear value (such as land or buildings) which is pledged against a loan to reduce risk to the lender. If the loan is not paid off satisfactorily, the lender has a legal claim to seize the pledged asset.

Collection Float: The time between when a bill is paid and the time the payment is deposited.

Commitment Fee: A percentage of the unused portion of a credit line which is charged to the potential borrower.

Common Costs: Costs that benefit a number of services and whose costs are shared by all. Examples: rent, utilities, and billing. Also called **joint costs**.

Community Rating: A rating methodology required of indemnity and HMO insurers that guarantees that there will be equivalent amounts collected from members of a specific group without regard to demographics such as age, sex, size of covered group, and industry type.

Compensating Balance: A designated dollar amount on deposit with a bank which a borrower is required to maintain.

Compliance: The need to abide by governmental regulations, whether they be for the provision of care, billing, privacy, security, etc.

Compound Interest Method: A method which calculates interest on both the original principal and on all interest accumulated since the beginning of the investment time period.

Compounding: Converting a present value into its future value taking into account the time value of money. See Compound Interest Method. It is the opposite of discounting.

Contact Capitation: A method of capitation whereby each specialty has its own capitation pool and use of services by a physician only affects that physician's compensation, not the whole specialty network's compensation.

Contra-asset: An asset which, when increased, decreases the value of a related asset on the books. Two primary examples are Accumulated Depreciation, which is the contra-asset to Properties and Equipment, and the Allowance for Uncollectibles, which is the contra-asset to Accounts Receivable.

Contribution Margin per Unit: Revenue per unit minus variable cost per unit. If all other costs (fixed costs, overhead, etc.) remain the same, it is the amount of profit made on each additional unit produced.

Contribution Margin Rule: If the contribution margin per unit is positive and no other additional costs will be incurred, then it is in the best financial interest of the organization to continue to provide additional units of that service, even if the organization is not fully covering all of its other costs.

Contribution Margin: Revenue minus variable cost.

Controlling Activities: Activities which provide guidance and feedback to keep the organization within its budget once it has been approved and is being implemented.

Conversion Factor: Actuarial based formulas developed to adjust rates allowing for differences in population demographics.

Copayment: Requiring the patient to pay part of the health care bill. These payments are used to prevent overutilization of services.

Corporate Compliance: Mandated legislation and regulations bestowed upon health care institutions to ensure fairness, accuracy, honesty, and quality in the provision of and billing for health care services.

Corporate Compliance Officer: The individual (or department) responsible for knowing the corporate compliance rules and regulations, and for ensuring that the organization strictly abides by them.

Cost Avoidance: The ability of an organization to find new ways to operate that eliminate certain classes of costs.

Cost-based Reimbursement: Using the provider's cost of providing services (supplies, staff salaries, space costs, etc.) as the basis for reimbursement.

Cost of Capital: The rate of return required to undertake a project. The cost of capital accounts for both the time value of money and risk. Also called the *hurdle rate* or *discount rate*.

Cost Centers: Organizational units responsible for providing services and controlling their costs.

Cost Containment: Not spending more than is budgeted in the expense budget.

Cost Drivers: Those things that cause a change in the cost of an activity.

Cost Object: Anything for which the cost is being estimated, such as a population, a test, a visit, a patient, or a patient day.

Cost-shifting: Charging one group of patients more in order to make up for underpayment by others. Most commonly, charging some privately insured patients more in order to make up for underpayment by Medicaid or Medicare.

Current Assets: Assets which will be consumed (used up) within one year (or one time period).

Current Liabilities: Financial obligations due within one year (or one time period).

Decentralization: The dispersion of responsibility within a health care organization.

Deductibles: When the patient covered is responsible for paying a certain base amount before coverage begins.

Defensive Medicine: The tendency of health care practitioners to do more testing and to provide more care for patients than might otherwise be necessary, simply to protect themselves against potential litigation.

Depreciation: A measure of how much a tangible asset (such as plant or equipment) has been "used up" or consumed.

Diagnosis Related Groups (DRGs): A system to classify patients based upon their diagnoses. In the most pervasive system, which is used by Medicare, there are approximately 500 different diagnostic categories.

Direct costs: Costs (e.g. nursing costs) that an organization can trace to a particular cost object (e.g. a patient).

Disbursement Float: An organization's practice of delaying payment as long as possible to its creditors, without causing ill will.

Discount Rate: See *Cost of Capital*.

Discount: When the market rate is higher than the coupon rate, a bond is said to be selling at a discount from its par value. See also *Premium*.

Discounted Cash Flows: Cash flows that have been adjusted to account for the cost of capital.

Discounting: Converting future cash flows into their present value taking into account the time value of money. It is the opposite of compounding.

Discounts: A reduction in the charge for services.

Dividends: Represents the portion of profit that an organization distributes to equity investors.

DRGs: A patient classification scheme used by Medicare that clusters patients into categories on the basis of patients' illnesses, diseases and medical problems. These classifications are then used to pay providers a set amount based on the diagnosis related group in which the patient has been classified.

Effective Interest Rate: The approximate annual interest rate incurred by not taking advantage of a supplier's discount offer to pay bills early.

Expansion Decision: Capital investment decision designed to increase the operational capability of a health care organization.

Expense Budget: A subset of the operating budget, which is a forecast of the operating expenses that will be incurred during the current budget period.

Expense Cost Variance: The amount of the variable expense variance that occurs because the actual cost per visit varies from that originally budgeted. It is the difference between the variable expenses forecast in the flexible budget and those actually incurred. It can be calculated by the formula: (actual cost per unit − budgeted cost per unit) × actual volume.

Expense Volume Variance: The portion of total variance in variable expenses that is due to the actual volume being either higher or lower than the budgeted volume. It is the difference between the expenses forecast in the original budget and those in the flexible budget. It can be computed using the following formula: (actual volume − budgeted volume) × budgeted cost per unit.

Experience Rating: The method of setting premium rates based on the actual health care costs of a group of groups.

Factoring: Selling accounts receivable at a discount, usually to a financial institution. The latter then assumes the role of trying to collect upon the outstanding payment obligations.

Feasibility Study: A study which examines market and management factors that affect the issuer's ability to generate the necessary cash flows to meet principal and interest requirements.

Fee-for-service: A method of reimbursement based on payment for services rendered, with a specific fee correlated to each specific service. An insurance company, the patient, or a government program such as Medicare or Medicaid (discussed later) may make payment.

Financial Lease: See *capital lease*.

Financial Leverage: The degree to which an organization is financed by long-term debt.

Financial Requirements: For health care providers this is a combination of issues related to operations, opportunities, contingencies, and return on investment.

Financing Mix: How an organization chooses to finance its working capital needs.

First Party: Typically, the patient in a health care encounter.

Fixed Costs: Costs that stay the same in total over the relevant range, but change inversely on a per unit basis as activity changes.

Fixed Income Security: A bond which pays fixed amounts of interest at regular periodic intervals, usually semi-annually.

Fixed Labor Budget: A subset of the labor budget which forecasts the cost of salaried personnel.

Flat Fee: A predefined amount of money paid to a provider for a unit of service.

Flexible Budget: A budget which accommodates a range or multiple levels of activities.

Float: The time delay of the process of assembling a bill until depositing the payment in the bank and making subsequent payments to creditors.

Fully allocated cost: The cost of an item that includes both its direct costs and all other costs allocated to it.

Fund Balance: A term used until 1996 for owners' equity by not-for-profit health care organizations. It was replaced with the present term, *net assets*, for non-governmental, not-for-profit organizations.

Future Value (FV): What an amount invested today (or a series of payments made over time) will be worth at a given time in the future using the compound interest method, which accounts for the time value of money. See also *Present Value*.

Future Value Factor of an Annuity (FVFA): A factor that when multiplied by a stream of equal payments equals the future value of that stream. See also *Present Value Factor of an Annuity*.

Future Value Factor: The factor used to compound a present amount to its future worth. It is the reciprocal of the present value factor and is calculated using the formula $(1 + i)^n$.

Future Value of an Annuity Table: Table of factors which shows the future value of equal flows at the end of each period, given a particular interest rate.

Future Value of an Annuity: What an equal series of payments will be worth at some future date using compound interest. See also *Future Value Factor of an Annuity* and *Present Value of an Annuity*.

Future Value Table: Table of factors which shows the future value of a single investment at a given interest rate.

Gatekeepers: Providers (typically the PCP) who must preapprove care received by a patient, such as a visit to the specialist. Gatekeepers are utilized in most POS plans and HMO plans.

Global Payments: A system to pay providers whereby the fees for all providers (hospitals, physicians, home health care agencies) are included in a single negotiated amount. This is sometimes called "bundling" of services. In non-global payment systems, each provider is paid separately.

Goodwill: An amount paid above and beyond the book value of an asset when it is sold, in part to offset the seller from potential lost future earnings from the asset had it not been sold.

Gross Charges: The amount that an organization would bill its patients if they all paid full charges. See *Net Charges*.

Group Model HMO: An HMO which contracts with medical groups for services.

HCFA: The Health Care Financing Administration. The US government department that oversaw the provision of and payment for health care provided under its entitlement programs (Medicare, Medicaid) until 2001.

Health Insurance Portability and Accountability Act (HIPAA): A set of federal compliance regulations enacted in 1996 to ensure standardization of billing, privacy, and reporting as institutions enter a paperless age.

Health Maintenance Organization (HMO): A legal corporation that offers health insurance and medical care. HMOs typically offer a range of health care services at a fixed price. See *Capitation*.

Hedging: The art of offsetting high variable rate debt payments with returns from high-rate investments.

Horizontal Analysis: A method of analyzing financial statements which looks at the percentage change in a line item from one year to the next. It is computed by the formula (subsequent year − previous year)/previous year.

Hurdle Rate: See *Required Rate of Return*.

Incremental Cash Flows: Cash flows that occur solely as a result of a particular action such as undertaking a project.

Incremental costs: Additional costs incurred solely as a result of an action or activity or a particular set of actions or activities.

Incremental/Decremental Approach: A method of budgeting which starts with an existing budget to plan future budgets.

Indemnity Insurance: A plan which reimburses physicians for services performed, or beneficiaries for medical expenses incurred. Typically, the employer and/or patient pays a monthly premium to the plan for a predetermined set of healthcare benefits.

Indirect costs: Costs that an organization is not able to directly trace to a particular cost object. Common indirect costs include the cost of the billing clerk, rent, computer costs and many so-called overhead costs.

Interest: A payment to creditors, those who have loaned the organization funds or otherwise extended credit.

Internal Rate of Return Method: A method to evaluate the financial feasibility of an investment decision which compares the investment's rate of return to that return required by the organization.

Internal Rate of Return: That rate of return on an investment which makes the net present value equal to $0, after all cash flows have been discounted at the same rate. It is also the discount rate at which the discounted cash flows over the life of the project exactly equal the initial investment.

Joint costs: See *Common Costs*.

Labor Budget: A subset of the expense budget, this budget is composed of the fixed labor budget and the variable labor budget.

Lessee: An entity that negotiates the use of another's asset via a lease.

Lessor: An entity that owns an asset which is then leased out.

Letter of Credit: Offered through a bank, this can be used to enhance the creditworthiness of an institution, and, hence, a bond's rating.

Liabilities: The financial obligations of the organization (i.e. debts).

Line-item Budget: The least detailed budget, showing only revenues and expenses by category, such as labor or supplies.

Liquidity: A measure of how quickly an asset can be converted into cash.

Lockbox: A post office box located near a Federal Reserve Bank or branch, from which the bank will pick up and process checks quickly, but for a fee.

Managed Care: Any of a number of arrangements designed to control health care costs through monitoring, prescribing, or proscribing the provision of health care to a patient or population.

Market Value: What a bond would sell for in today's open market.

Medicaid: A federally mandated program, operated and partially funded by individual states (in conjunction with the federal government) to provide medical benefits to certain low-income people. The state, under broad federal guidelines, determines what benefits are covered, who is eligible, and how much providers will be paid.

Medical Savings Accounts: A limited amount of money an employee can take as pretaxed income to pay for medically related items such as physician visits, pharmaceuticals, eyewear, dental visits, etc. The pretax income is placed in an escrow account held by the employer. The employee must submit receipts for care received to get reimbursed.

Medicare: A nationwide, federally financed health insurance program for people age 65 and older. It also covers certain people under 65 who are disabled or have chronic kidney (end-stage renal) disease. Medicare Part A is the hospital insurance program; Part B covers physicians' services. Created by the 1965 amendment to the Social Security Act.

Members: People who are covered by a health care plan. Typically the member and/or the employer of the member pays a premium to the plan for the privilege of being covered.

Mission Statement: A statement which guides the organization by identifying the unique attributes of the organization, why it exists, and what it hopes to achieve. Some organizations divide these attributes between a vision and a mission statement.

Multi-year Budget: A budget which is forecast multiple years out, rather than just for the upcoming year.

Net Assets: In not-for-profit organizations, the difference between assets and liabilities (assets *minus* liabilities).

Net Charges: The amount that an organization bills its patients after accounting for discounts and allowances. See *gross charges*.

Net Income: Excess of revenues over expenses.

Net Present Value Method: A method to evaluate the financial feasibility of an investment decision based solely upon the resulting net present value. It uses a specific discount rate which may not be equal to the organization's required rate of return.

Net Present Value: The present value of future cash flows related to an investment net (less) the cost of the initial investment. It represents the difference between the initial amount paid for an investment, and the future cash inflows that the investment will bring in, after adjusting for the cost of capital.

Net Proceeds from a Bond Issuance: Gross proceeds less the underwriter's and others' issuance fees.

Non-avoidable Fixed Costs: A fixed cost that will remain even if a particular service is discontinued. Example: full-time nursing costs in an organization that will continue, even though one of several services is dropped.

Non-current Assets: The resources of the organization that will be used or consumed over periods longer than one year.

Non-current Liabilities: The financial obligations not due within one year.

Non-regular Cash Flows: Cash flows that occur spordically or on an irregular basis. A common non-regular cash flow is salvage value, receipt of funds following a one-time sale of an asset at the end of its useful life.

Notes to Financial Statements: Additional key information written out in detail which is not presented in the body of the financial statement.

Operating Budget: One of the four major types of budgets. It is comprised of the revenue budget and the expense budget. The bottom line for this budget is net income.

Operating Cash Flows: Cash flows that occur on a regular basis, oftentimes following implementation of a project. Also called **regular cash flows**.

Operating Income: Income derived from the organization's main line of business.

Operating Lease: A lease that lasts shorter than the useful life of the leased asset, typically one year or less. This type of leasing arrangement can be canceled at any time without penalty, but there is no option to purchase the asset once the lease has expired.

Opportunity Cost: Proceeds lost by forgoing other opportunities.

Ordinary Annuity: A series of equal annuity payments made or received at the end of each period.

Outstanding Bond Issue: A bond that trades in the marketplace.

Owner's Equity: In for-profit institutions, the difference between assets and liabilities (assets *minus* liabilities).

Par Value: The face value amount of a bond. It is the amount the bondholder is paid at maturity. It does not include any coupon payments.

Participating Provider: A provider who has contracted with the health plan to provide medical services to covered members at predetermined rates.

Participatory Approach: A method of budgeting in which the roles and responsibilities of putting together a budget are diffused throughout the organization, typically originating at the department level. There are guidelines to follow, and approval must be secured by top management. Opposite to the *authoritarian approach.*

Payback Method: A method to evaluate the feasibility of an investment by determining how long it would take until the initial investment is recovered, disregarding the time value of money.

Payor: An entity that is responsible for paying for the services of a health care provider. Typically, this is an insurance company or a government agency. Commonly referred to as third parties.

Per Diem: An amount a payor will pay for one day of care, which includes all hospital charges associated with the inpatient day (including nursing care, surgeries, medications, etc.).

Per Member Per Month (PMPM): Generally used by HMOs and their medical providers as an indicator of revenue, expenses, or utilization of services per member per one-month period.

Performance Budget: An extension of the program budget which also lays out performance objectives.

Perpetuity: An annuity for an infinite period of time. Also called a perpetual annuity.

Planning: The process of identifying goals, objectives, tasks, activities, and resources necessary to carry out the strategic plan of the organization over the next time period, typically one year.

Point of Service (POS): A hybrid between a HMO and a PPO in which patients are given the incentive to see providers participating in a defined network, but may see non-network providers, though usually at some additional cost.

Predetermined Rates: A set fee paid to a provider for an inpatient episode of care.

Preferred Provider Organization (PPO): A network of independent providers preselected by the payor to provide a specific service or range of services at predetermined (usually discounted) rates to the payor's covered members.

Premium: A monthly payment made by a person and/or an employer to an insurer that makes one eligible for a defined level of health care for a given period of time.

Premium: When the market rate is lower than the coupon rate, a bond is said to be selling at a premium. See also *discount*.

Present Value (PV): The value today of a payment (or series of payments) to be received in the future, taking into account the cost of capital.

Present Value Factor of an Annuity (PVFA): A factor that when multiplied by a stream of equal payments equals the present value of that stream.

Present Value Factor: The factor used to discount a future amount to its current worth. It is the reciprocal of the future value factor and is calculated using the formula $1/(1 + i)^n$.

Present Value of an Annuity Table: Table of factors which shows the worth today of equal flows at the end of each future period, given a particular interest rate.

Present Value of an Annuity: What a series of equal payments in the future is worth today taking into account the time value of money.

Present Value Table: Table of factors which shows what a single amount to be received in the future is worth today at a given interest rate.

Price Setter: The entity that controls the amount paid for a health care service.

Primary Care Provider (PCP): A physician (typically a Family Medicine, Internal Medicine, Pediatric and sometimes Ostetrics and Gynecology provider) that is the primary care giver of a patient.

Product Margin Decision Rule: If a service's product margin is positive, the organization will be better off financially if it continues with the service, *ceteris paribus*. Conversely, if a service's product margin is negative, the organization will be better off financially if it discontinues the service, *ceteris paribus*.

Product Margin: Total Contribution Margin – Avoidable Fixed Costs. It represents the amount which a service contributes to covering all other costs after it has covered those costs which are there solely because the service is offered (its total variable cost and avoidable fixed costs) and would not be there if the service were dropped.

Profit Centers: Organizational units responsible for controlling costs and earning revenues.

Program Budget: An extension of the line-item budget which shows revenues and expenses by program or service lines.

Prospective Payment System: The payment system used by Medicare to reimburse providers a predetermined amount. Several payment methods fall under the umbrella of PPS, including: DRGs (inpatient admissions); APCs (outpatient visits); RBRVS (professional services); and RUGs (skilled nursing home care). DRGs were the first category to fall under this type of predetermined payment arrangement.

Prospective Payment System: 1) The payment system used by Medicare to reimburse providers a set amount based upon the patient's DRG. This system is commonly referred to as the PPS or DRG payment system. 2) A payment method that establishes rates, prices, or budgets before services are rendered and costs are incurred. Providers retain or absorb at least a portion of the difference between established revenues and actual costs.

Ratio: An expression of the relationship between two numbers as a single number.

RBRVS: A system of paying physicians based upon the relative value of the services rendered.

Red Herring: A preliminary official statement offered to prospective buyers of a bond by the underwriters to help determine a fair market price for the bond.

Regular Cash Flows: See *Operating Cash Flows.*

Relative Value Units (RVUs): A standardized weighting applied to services which reflects the amount of resource consumption to provide that service. A service assigned 2 RVUs consumes twice the resources as does a service assigned 1 RVU.

Relevant Range: The range of activity over which *total fixed costs* and/or *per unit variable cost* do not vary.

Replacement Decision: Capital investment decision designed to replace older assets with newer ones.

Required Market Rate: The market interest rate on similar risk bonds.

Required Rate of Return: An organization's minimally acceptable internal rate of return on any investment to justify an initial investment. Also called **Cost of Capital** or **Hurdle Rate**.

Residual Value: See *Salvage Value.*

Responsibility Center: An organizational unit that has been formally given the responsibility to carry out one or more tasks and/or achieve one or more outcomes.

Responsibility: Duties and obligations of a responsibility center.

Retained Earnings: A second type of benefit to an investor. These are in the form of the portion of the profits the organization keeps in-house to use in growth and support of its mission.

Retrospective Payment: Method for reimbursing a provider after the the service has been delivered.

Revenue Attainment: Earning the amount of revenue budgeted.

Revenue Budget: A subset of the operating budget, which is a forecast of the operating revenues that will be earned during the current budget period.

Revenue Enhancement: Finding supplemental sources of revenue.

Revenue Rate Variance: The amount of the total revenue variance that occurs because the actual average rate charged varies from the one originally budgeted. It is the difference between the revenues forecast in the flexible budget and those actually earned. It can be calculated using the formula (actual rate – budgeted rate) × actual volume.

Revenue Volume Variance: The portion of total variance in revenues due to the actual volume being either higher or lower than the budgeted volume. It is the difference between the revenues forecast in the original budget and those in the flexible budget. It can be computed using the formula (actual volume – budgeted volume) × budgeted rate.

Risk Pools: A generally large population of individuals who are all simultaneously insured under the same arrangement, regardless of working status. Health care utilization – and therefore cost – is more stable for larger groups than it is for smaller groups, which makes larger groups' cost more predictable for insurers.

Rolling Budget: A multi-year budget which is updated more frequently than annually, such as semi-annually or quarterly.

RVU: Relative Value Unit.

Sale/Leaseback Arrangement: A type of capital lease whereby an institution sells an owned asset and then simultaneously leases it back from the purchaser. The selling institution retains rights to use the asset, but benefits from the immediate acquisition of cash from the sale.

Salvage Value: The amount of cash to be received when an asset is sold, usually at the end of its useful life. Also called **terminal value**.

Scrap Value: see *Salvage Value*.

Second Party: Typically, the provider (hospital/physician) in a health care encounter.

Service Centers: Organizational units that are primarily responsible for ensuring that health care-related services are provided to a population in a manner that meets the volume and quality requirements of the organization. They have no direct budgetary control.

Shareholders' Equity: Another name for Owners' Equity.

Short-term Plans: Specific plans which identify an organization's short-term goals and objectives in more detail, primarily in regard to marketing/production, control, and financing the organization.

Simple Interest Method: A method to calculate interest only on the original principal amount. The principal is the amount invested.

Sinking Fund: A fund into which monies are set aside each year to ensure that a bond can be liquidated at maturity.

Staff Model HMO: An HMO which owns its clinics and employs its doctors.

Static Budget: A budget which uses a single or fixed level of activity.

Statistics Budget: The first budget to be prepared. One of the four major types of budgets. It identifies the amount of services that will be provided, typically categorized by payor type.

Step Fixed Costs: Costs that increase in total over wide, discrete steps.

Step-down method: A cost finding method based on allocating those costs that are not directly paid for to those products or services to which payment is attached. The method derives its name from the stairstep pattern that results from allocating costs.

Stop Loss: A method providers use to limit the exposure that comes with the possibility that charges will go far beyond negotiated rates – a level of charges over which the provider is no longer totally liable.

Straight-line Depreciation: A method which depreciates an asset an equal amount each year until it reaches its salvage value at the end of its useful life.

Strategic Decision: Capital investment decision designed to increase a health care organization's strategic (long-term) position.

Strategic Planning: Identifying an organization's mission, goals, and strategy to best position itself for the future.

Subcapitation: Where the primary care physician pays a portion of the total capitated dollars received to another provider (i.e. specialist).

Sunk Costs: Costs incurred in the past. They should not be included in NPV-type analyses.

Target Costing: Controlling costs and/or decreasing profit margins in order to meet or beat a predetermined price or reimbursement rate.

Tax Shield: An investment which reduces the amount of income tax that has to be paid, often because interest and depreciation expenses are tax deductible.

Term Loan: A loan typically issued by a bank which has a maturity of one to ten years.

Terminal Value: See *Salvage Value*.

Third Party: Typically, the payor (insurance company/government agency) in a healthcare encounter.

Third Party Payors: Commonly referred to as third parties, these are organizations that pay on behalf of patients.

Time Value of Money: The concept that a dollar received today is worth more than a dollar received in the future.

Top-down Budgeting: See *Authoritarian Approach*.

Top-down/Bottom-up Approach: See *Participatory Approach*.

Traditional Profit Centers: Organizational units responsible for earning a profit by providing health care services. Revenues are earned on either a fee-for-service or flat fee basis. Examples include cardiology, women's and children's services, and oncology.

Trend Analysis: A type of horizontal analysis that looks at changes in line items compared to a base year. It is calculated: [(any subsequent year – base year)/base year] $\times$ 100.

Trustee: An agent for bondholders who ensures that the health care facility is making timely principal and interest payments to the bondholders and complies with legal covenants of the bond.

Variable Costs: Costs that stay the same per unit but change directly in total with a change in activity over the relevant range. Total Variable Cost = Variable Cost Per Unit $\times$ Number of Units of Activity.

Vertical Analysis: A method to analyze financial statements which answers the general question: what percentage of one line item is another line item? Also called common-size analysis because it converts every line item to a percentage, thus allowing comparisons among the financial statements of different organizations.

Working Capital Strategy: The amount of working capital that an organization determines it must keep available as a cushion to protect against unforeseen expenditures.

Yield to Maturity: The rate at which the market value of a bond is equal to the bond's present value of future coupon payments plus.

Zero-based Budget (Capitation): Dividing the entire amount of capitation (the "budget") among all the providers, essentially leaving nothing or "zero" left at the end of every accounting period.

Zero-based Budgeting (ZBB): An approach to budgeting that continually questions both the need for existing programs and their level of funding, as well as the need for new programs.

WEB LINKS OF INTEREST FOR HEALTH CARE FINANCIAL MANAGEMENT

◀By Source▶

1. Health Care Financial Alert Quarterly

URL: http://www.ushnet.com/programs/nl.htm
Steps: Click on the link to view the newsletter.
Other information: This is a quarterly publication of the US Health Network which provides up-to-date information concerning health care providers of all types. This eight-page newsletter is available without charge and is provided through the respective Network member in your area. Written by experienced health care professionals, Health Care Financial Alert will inform and alert the health care provider to reimbursement, strategic planning, accounting, tax, and management issues on a timely basis.

2. AHA Financial Solutions Press Releases

URL: http://www.aha.org/fsi/press.asp
Steps: Click on the "News and Press" link.
Other information: The American Hospital Association (AHA) is a not-for-profit association of health care provider organizations and individuals that are committed to the health improvement of their communities.

3. AHA HIPAA Standards

URL: http://www.aha.org/hipaa/hipaa_home.asp
Steps: Click on the link for the current topic of interest
Other information: The American Hospital Association (AHA) is a not-for-profit association of health care provider organizations and individuals that are committed to the health improvement of their communities.

4. HFMA On-line; Health Care Financial Management Links

URL: http://www.hfmaiowa.org/links/html

Steps: Click on the link of interest from the list.
Other information: HFMA is the USA's leading personal membership organization for health care financial management professionals.

5. National Association of Rural Health Clinics

URL: http://www.narhc.org/
Steps: Click on the HCFA RHC information link.
Other information: Legislative rules and regulations.

6. American Hospital Directory

URL: http://www.ahd.com/
Steps: Click to get free information or register for more detailed information.
Other information: The American Hospital Directory provides on-line data for over 6,000 hospitals. The database of information is built from Medicare claims data, cost reports, and other public use files obtained from the federal Centers for Medicare and Medicaid Services (CMS, formerly HCFA). The directory also includes AHA Annual Survey Data licensed from Health Forum, an American Hospital Association company.

7. US Department of Health and Human Services

URL: http://www.hhs.gov/
Steps: Search for a topic of interest.
Other information: Home page for this federal agency.

8. HCFA's Provider Reimbursement Review Board

URL: http://www.hcfa.gov/regs/prrb.htm
Steps: Click on the Board's decisions by year at the bottom of the page.

9. Health Care Finance On-line

URL: http://www.hcfinance.com/
Steps: Click on the story of interest.
Other information: Health care financial information for not-for-profit providers.

10. National Association of Health Underwriters

URL: http://www.nahu.org/
Steps: Click on the link "The Issues."
Other information: Provides numerous articles and information on governmental regulations, managed care, long-term care, health insurance, and privacy.

11. CMMS (HCFA) APC Information

URL: http://www.hcfa.gov/regs/hopps/default.htm
Steps: Click on any report to be downloaded (Adobe Acrobat format).
Other information: Provides links to other federal government sites.

12. Healthcare Finance Group (HFG)

URL: http://www.hfgusa.com/
Steps: Click on link to find out about available services.
Other information: Healthcare Finance Group Inc. (HFG) is a specialty finance company, investing exclusively in the health care industry.

13. North Carolina Healthcare Information and Communications Alliance (NCHICA)

URL: http://www.nchica.org/
Steps: Click on links of interest.
Other information: NCHICA is dedicated to improving health care through information technology and secure communications. It offers resources in HIPAA, privacy, EDI, etc.

14. Wall Street Journal

URL: http://public.wsj.com/home.html
Steps: Click on business news to find articles on health care finance.
Other information: Requires that the user become a subscriber to have on-line access to all the information provided in the daily newspaper.

◄By Type of Information►

1. Updated Hospital Bond Ratings Information

URL: http://www.standardandpoors.com/Forum/MarketAnalysis/Healthcare/index.html#FA
Steps: Click on featured articles and methodology and credit statistics and look for articles on non-profit median health care ratios.
Other information: Provides health care financial ratio information for non-profit hospitals.

2. Updated Information on Hospital Financial Data

URL: http://www.solucient.com/
Steps: Type in financial ratios in search menu to identify financial performance ratios of hospital and *100 Top Hospitals: Benchmarks for Success.*
Other information: Provides health care financial ratio information.

3. Selected Information on Hospital Financial Data from the State of California

URL: http://www.oshpd.cahwnet.gov/hid/infores/hospital/finance/annual_data/
Steps: Click on reports.
Other information: Provides detailed financial statement and utilization information for California acute-care hospitals.

4. Selected HMO Operating and Financial Data from Interstudy

URL: http://www.hmodata.com/

Steps: Click on sample reports and look for sample financial reports for selected HMOs.
Other information: Provides sample reports on HMO financial data and ratios.

5. Selected Information on Operating and Capital/Financial Leases

URL: http://www.fleethealthcare.com/content/page_render.asp?use_case=FHC2
Steps: Click on this site and it will provide further explanation of key terms used in leasing.
Other information: Useful site to understand the aspects of lease financing.

6. Selected Information on Tax-exempt Financing Process

URL: http://www.nchffa.com/financial_advisors.htm
Steps: Click on the site.
Other information: Provides information on structuring a particular bond issue and on hiring investment bankers and negotiating financing terms with investment bankers, rating agencies, and credit enhancers. The information is provided by the Financial Advisors from the National Council of Health Facilities Finance.

7. Selected Information on the Capital Budgeting Process and Hospital Balance Sheet

URL: http://www.gemedicalsystems.com/services/financial/education/hfs_khtrain_menu.html
Steps: Click on the site.
Other information: Provides information on financial statement analysis of hospitals and explanation of analyzing a capital budgeting decision using net present value. The source of this site is General Electric Healthcare Financial Services.

8. Selected Financial Statement Filings for US Securities and Exchange Commission (SEC) for Publicly Traded Health Care Companies

URL: http://www.sec.gov/edgar.shtml
Steps: Click on search for company filings and general purpose search, quick form lookups. Enter company name (for example, HCA-THE HEALTHCARE CO), and enter 10-k under form type, which will provide detailed financial statement information that is registered with the SEC.
Other information: Provides the annual financial reports submitted by publicly traded health care companies.

9. Selected Trend Data on Medicare Payments, Costs, Profit and Utilization Data

URL: http://www.medpac.gov/publications/
Steps: Click on publications, click on reports. Payment reports will be titled "Report to the Congress: Medicare Payment Policy (Date)", and be PDF files.
Other Information: Presents detailed analysis of changes in Medicare costs and utilization for acute care and post-acute care services. Also provides information on the effects of the Balanced Budget Act of 1997 on hospitals.

10. Key Financial, Inpatient, and Outpatient Services, Cost and Charge Measurements for a Specific Hospital

URL: http://www.ahd.com
Steps: Click on free services, and type the specific name of the hospital and its address.

11. Timely News Stories that Affect Hospitals Nationally from the American Hospital Association

URL: http://www.ahanews.com

12. Information on the Bond Rating Methodology for Moody Bond Rating Agency

URL: http://www.moodys.com/moodys/
Steps: Click on US public finance and then click on rating methodology and look for reports for non-profit hospitals.

13. Information on How to Compute Cash Flows and the Cost of Capital in Computing a Company's Stock Price

URL: http://www.valuepro.net
Steps: Click on Learn the Valuepro approach and look for free cash flow and cost of capital. Also in the initial page enter an investor-owned hospital management company's stock symbol (for example, HCA), and it will provide the company's projected stock price and weighted average cost of capital information.

14. Information on How to Find Information on Investor-owned Hospital Management Companies' Financial Measures and Weighted Cost of Capital Measures

URL: http://valuation.ibbotson.com
Steps: Click on "Learn about methodology," click on "View sample," click on "SIC code 8," to find sale growth rates, capital structure ratios, margins, return on equity, cost of capital, and beta values for large investor-owned hospital companies.

15. On-line Monthly Trade Journal Regarding Health Care Finance Topics in the Hospital Markets

URL: http://www.hcfinance.com
Steps: Click on web address.
Other information: Specific topics include rating changes, hospital performance and hospital acquisitions and mergers.

INDEX